C000279577

Mosby
Nurse's Pocket Dictionary

For Mosby:

Senior Commissioning Editor: Jacqueline Curthoys
Project Manager: Gail Murray
Senior Designer: Judith Wright

Mosby
Nurse's Pocket Dictionary

32ND EDITION

Edited by

Chris Brooker

BSc MSc RGN SCM RNT

Author of *Human Structure and Function*

Mosby

An affiliate of Elsevier Limited

EDINBURGH LONDON NEW YORK OXFORD PHILADELPHIA
ST LOUIS SYDNEY TORONTO 2002

MOSBY
An imprint of Elsevier Limited

Thirty-second edition 2002
   Reprinted 2002, 2003 (twice), 2004

ISBN 0 7234 3233 3

British Library Cataloguing in Publication Data
A catalogue record for this book is available from the British Library.

Library of Congress Cataloging in Publication Data
A catalog record for this book is available from the Library of Congress.

Note
Medical knowledge is constantly changing. As new information
becomes available, changes in treatment, procedures, equipment and
the use of drugs become necessary. The editor and the publishers have
taken care to ensure that the information given in this text is accurate
and up to date. However, readers are strongly advised to confirm that
the information, especially with regard to drug usage, complies with
the latest legislation and standards of practice.

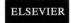

Printed in China
C/05

Contents

Preface

Health care and nursing practice continue to change at a rapid pace and nurses need access to information from many areas of nursing and other healthcare disciplines. This well established dictionary was due for revision and the opportunity has been taken to revise those entries most relevant to students undertaking the foundation and branch programmes, and registered nurses. Existing entries have been updated, those no longer relevant have been removed and many new entries have been added.

Several of the topics included for the first time in the 31st edition have been expanded, particularly research, legal terms, quality issues, information technology and those that reflect the changing culture of healthcare delivery.

The dictionary includes 90 clear and informative illustrations. The appendix material has been completely revised to ensure its continued relevance and usefulness to students and registered nurses. Blood glucose monitoring has been updated, and the useful addresses appendix now includes web addresses.

I hope that the 32nd edition will continue to be a valuable resource for students, registered nurses and others with an interest in health and health care, and that it will assist nurses in expanding their knowledge, fulfilling their professional development responsibilities and in the delivery of high-quality care.

Norfolk 2002   Chris Brooker

Acknowledgements

I would like to thank the staff at Harcourt Health Sciences for their support and enthusiasm. As always, my partner David was understanding about long hours spent working on this project and offered suggestions for the expansion of the information technology entries.

Comparative Temperatures

Celsius (°C)	Fahrenheit (°F)	Celsius (°C)	Fahrenheit (°F)
100 (boiling point)	212	38.5	101.3
95	203	38	100.4
90	194	37.5	99.5
85	185	37 (body temperature)	98.6
80	176	36.5	97.7
75	167	36	96.8
70	158	35.5	95.9
65	149	35	95
60	140	34	93.2
55	131	33	91.4
50	122	32	89.6
45	113	31	87.8
44	112.2	30	86
43	109.4	25	77
42	107.6	20	68
41	105.8	15	59
40	104	10	50
39.5	103.1	5	41
39	102.2	0 (freezing point)	32

To convert readings of the Fahrenheit scale into Celsius degrees subtract 32, multiply by 5, and divide by 9, for example:

$98 - 32 = 66 \times 5 = 330 \div 9 = 36.6$
Therefore $98°F = 36.6°C$

To convert readings of the Celsius scale into Fahrenheit degrees multiply by 9, divide by 5, and add 32, for example:

$36.6 \times 9 = 330 \div 5 = 66 + 32 = 98$
Therefore $36.6°C = 98°F$

The term 'Celsius' (from the name of the Swede who invented the scale in 1742) is now being internationally used instead of 'centigrade', which is the term employed in some countries to denote fractions of an angle.

A Guide to Pronunciation

The pronunciation guides in this dictionary are given for practical help. They appear in brackets after entries where the word is not in common use, and where the pronunciation is not easily deduced from the spelling. The stress mark ′ is given only where necessary. The basic vowel and consonant sounds are listed below.

Vowel sound	*Example*
ā as in bat	cataract *(kat′-a-rakt)*
a as in mate	flatus *(flā-tus)*
ah as in father	after *(ahf′-ter)*
ar as in far	carbon *(kar′-bon)*
ā-r as in air	aerosol *(ā′-ro-sol)*
aw as in fall	audiometer *(aw- dē-om′-et-er)*
e as in get	electric *(e-lek′-trik)*
ē as in been	ether *(ē-ther)*
ē-r as in ear	sclera *(sklē′-ra)*
i as in bit	nicotinic *(ni-kō-tin′-ik)*
ī as in bite	eye *(ī)*, hydro- *(hī-dro)*
o as in hop	optics *(op′-tiks)*
ō as in hope	isotopes *(ī-zo-tōps)*
oo as in soon	croup *(kroop)*
or as in for	orbit *(or′-bit)*
ow as in how	sound *(sownd)*
oy as in boy	boil *(boyl)*
u as in cup	tongue *(tung)*
ū as in mute	cubit *(kū-bit)*

Consonant sound	*Example*
f the sound of ph	as in phobia *(fō-bi-ah)*
j the sound of g	as in dermalgia *(der-mal′-ji-a)*
k the sound of c	as in catalyst *(ka′-ta-list)*
ks the sound of x	as in X-ray *(eks′-rā)*

kw the sound of qu   as in quintan *(kwin'-tan)*
s the sound of c   as in lucid *(loo'-sid)*
shon the sound of tion   as in ablution *(ab-loo'-shon)*
zhon the sound of sion   as in invasion *(in-vā'-zhon)*

A

AA, Alcoholics Anonymous.

abacterial, without bacteria.

abaissement, a depressing or lowering, displacement of the lens in ophthalmology.

A band, the dark bands of a sacromere, formed by overlapping of actin and myosin filaments.

abarticulation, 1. joint dislocation. **2.** freely movable or synovial joint. *See* DIARTHROSIS.

abdomen, body cavity between the thorax and pelvis. Contains many organs, including the lower oesophagus, stomach, intestines, liver, spleen, pancreas, other viscera, blood vessels, nerves and lymphatics. It is lined with a serous membrane called the peritoneum, which is reflected over many abdominal organs. The surface anatomy of the abdomen is divided into nine regions used to describe the location of organs or pain (Figure 1).

abdominal, pertaining to the abdomen. *A. aorta:* that portion of the aorta which runs through the abdominal cavity. *A. aortic aneurysm (AAA):* dilatation in part of the abdominal aorta. *See* ANEURYSM. *A. breathing:* respiratory effort mainly through contraction of the diaphragm and abdominal muscles. *A. reflex:* superficial reflex where the abdominal muscles contract when the overlying skin is stroked. *A. thrust: see* HEIMLICH MANOEUVRE.

abdominocentesis, aspiration of the peritoneal cavity. *See* PARACENTESIS.

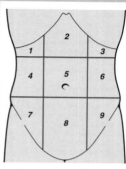

1 Regions of the abdomen

1. Right hypochondrium
2. Epigastrium
3. Left hypochondrium
4. Right lumbar
5. Umbilical
6. Left lumbar
7. Right iliac
8. Hypogastrium
9. Left iliac

abdominoperineal, *(ab-dōm-in-o-per-in-ē′-al)*, pertaining to abdomen and perineum. Rectal excision may be performed by utilizing both abdominal and perineal incisions.

abducens nerves, *(ab-dū′-senz)*, sixth pair of cranial nerves. They innervate the lateral rectus muscle which rotates the eyeball outwards.

abduct, to draw away from the midline. *See* ADDUCT.

abduction, act of moving a limb away from the midline of the body. *See* ADDUCTION.

abductor, a muscle which moves a limb away from the midline of the body, e.g. deltoid. *See* ADDUCTOR.

aberrant, an anatomical structure, e.g. nerve or blood vessel, which follows an unusual course.

aberration, 1. a deviation from normal. **2.** in optics, a defect in focus in a lens. **3.** in psychology, an unreasonable belief or thought.

ability, possessing the mental or physical powers to perform a specific act, such as those needed for the activities of daily living.

ablation, removal of a part or procedure that results in total loss of function. For example, the ablation of the endometrium using laser therapy.

ABO groups, *see* BLOOD GROUPS.

abort, to terminate a process before the full course is run, especially applied to pregnancy.

abortifacient, *(ab-or-te-fa-shent)*, an agent or drug which induces abortion.

abortion, expulsion of the products of conception from the uterus before the fetus is developed sufficiently to be capable of a separate existence (viable), i.e. 24 weeks' gestation. Some infants born before 24 weeks now survive because of advances in neonatal intensive care. An abortion may be spontaneous (often called a miscarriage) or therapeutic where a pregnancy is intentionally terminated. Abortion may be complete or incomplete; it may be threatened or inevitable, according to the dilatation of the cervix. It may be missed: where the fetus dies but is not immediately expelled, *see* CARNEOUS MOLE. Infection may complicate any type of abortion, but is more common in an illegally procured criminal abortion.

abortus, the aborted fetus, usually one weighing less than 500 g.

abortus fever, an undulant fever, also called brucellosis. Transmitted to humans from cows infected with *Brucella abortus.*

ABPI, abbreviation for **ankle–brachial pressure index**.

abrachia, *(ah-bra-kē-ah)*, without arms.

abrasion, a superficial injury to the skin or mucous membrane.

abreaction, a state of emotional release brought about by reliving painful experiences which have been previously repressed.

abruptio placentae, *(ab-rup-she-o-plas-en-te)*, *see* ACCIDENTAL HAEMORRHAGE.

abscess, a local collection of pus within a cavity, which results from inflammation. Surgical incision and drainage may be required before healing can occur.

absorption, 1. the take-up of a substance by another, e.g. the absorption of gases by liquids. **2.** the movement of substances across membranes or surfaces into body fluids or cells, e.g. water and nutrients into cells. **3.** transfer of energy to the tissues during exposure to ionizing radiation. *A. rate constant*: amount of drug absorbed in a given unit of time.

absorptive state, the fed state. Metabolic state occurring immediately after a meal and lasting for about 4 hours. Nutrients are absorbed and used for immediate energy, or in anabolic processes such as glycogenesis and lipogenesis. *See* POSTABSORPTIVE STATE.

abstinence, voluntarily refraining from taking a substance or performing an act from which the person has previously derived gratification, e.g. alcohol.

abulia, loss of or reduction in willpower and decision making ability.

abuse, 1. injury or assault as in the physical, psychological or sexual abuse, or neglect of vulnerable groups such as children or older adults. **2.** misuse of equipment, drugs and other substances, authority, power and position.

acanthoma, *(ak-an-thō-mah),* a tumour of the prickle-cell layer, the lowest stratum of the epidermis.

acanthosis, *(ak-an-thō'-sis),* thickening of the prickle-cell layer seen in conditions such as psoriasis. *A. nigricans:* hyperpigmented lesions seen in axillae, groin and perianal area.

acapnia, *(ā-kap'-ni-a),* a reduced level of carbon dioxide in the blood. May result from hyperventilation.

acardia, *(ā-kar'-di-ah),* congenital absence of the heart.

Acarus, a group of animal parasites belonging to the Arachnids. Includes many species of mites and ticks. *A. scabiei:* the parasite causing scabies *q.v.*

acatalepsy, *(ā-ka-ta-lep'-si),* uncertainty, lack of understanding.

acataphasia, *(ā-kat-a-fā'-zia),* difficulty in expressing ideas in logical sequence.

Access to Health Records Act (1990), allows access to both computerized and paper health records made since 1991. There are certain exceptions, e.g. where they may cause serious harm (mental or physical) to a person.

accessory nerves, eleventh pair of cranial nerves. They innervate the muscles of the pharynx, larynx, head, neck and shoulders.

accident/incident reporting, the legal and professional responsibility to report and record all accidents or incidents involving patients, visitors and staff. Each health care setting will have local policies, protocols and documentation to which staff must adhere.

accidental haemorrhage, bleeding from the uterus due to the premature separation of a normally situated placenta. May occur during the second half of pregnancy or after labour has commenced, but before the birth of the baby. The haemorrhage may be concealed, when bleeding is internal; or external, when bleeding occurs vaginally. *See* ANTEPARTUM HAEMORRHAGE.

accommodation, 1. in ophthalmology the power to adjust the eye to different distances. **2.** the physical and psychological processes by which we adjust to changes in our internal and external environment. **3.** in sociology the ability to reconcile conflicts between groups having differing beliefs or habits.

accouchement, *(ak-koosh-mon),* childbirth.

accountability, being responsible for actions and their results. The duty of care according to law. For nurses the professional and legal responsibility for the patient care they provide. *See* CODE OF PROFESSIONAL CONDUCT, MALPRACTICE, NEGLIGENCE.

accretion, accumulation of foreign matter in an organ, e.g. the formation of renal calculi.

ACE, angiotensin-converting enzyme *ACE* inhibitors: a group of drugs used to treat hypertension and heart failure, e.g. captopril.

acetabulum, *(a-se-tab'-ū-lum),* the cup-like socket in the hip or innominate bone into which the head of the femur fits.

acetaldehyde, *(as-et-al-de-hīd),* an intermediary product formed during the oxidation of ethyl alcohol by the liver enzyme alcohol dehydrogenase.

acetate, a salt of acetic acid.

acetic acid, the acid of vinegar. An organic acid.

acetoacetic acid, *(as-e-tō-a-sē'-tik),* a ketone formed when fatty acids are metabolized. It is converted to beta-hydroxybutyric acid and acetone, which can be used in small amounts as fuel molecules. In severe diabetes mellitus there is an excess which leads to elevation of blood levels and ketoacidosis, with severe disruption of pH, and fluid and electrolyte imbalance.

acetonaemia, *(as-ē-tō-nē-me-ah),* see KETONAEMIA.

acetone, an inflammable liquid with a characteristic 'pear drops' odour. A ketone present in small amounts in normal urine. Increased levels are found in the urine of poorly controlled diabetes mellitus and in starvation.

acetonuria, *(as'-ē-tō-nūr'-e-ah),* see KETOACIDURIA.

acetylcholine (ACh), *(as-ē-til-ko'-leen),* a neurotransmitter which allows the passage of nerve impulses across synapses in parasympathetic nerves and at the neuromuscular junction of skeletal muscle. Nerves using this neurotransmitter are described as cholinergic.

acetylcholinesterase, *(as-ē-til-ko'-leenest'-er-āz),* enzyme which inactivates acetylcholine after passage of the nerve impulse.

acetylcoenzyme A, *(as-ē-til-ko-en'-zīm),* an important metabolic molecule, involved in many vital cellular processes, e.g. glycolysis and Krebs' citric acid cycle. Also known as acetyl CoA.

acetylsalicyclic acid, *(as-ē'-til-sa-li-sil'-ik a-sid),* aspirin.

achalasia, *(ak-al-ā'-ze-ah),* failure of relaxation of a muscle sphincter. Applied particularly to the cardiac sphincter, often resulting in dilatation of the oesophagus. *See* CARDIOMYOTOMY, HELLER'S OPERATION.

achievement, attainment, accomplishment. *A. age:* testing the level of educational development compared with the norm for a person of that age. *A. quotient:* the number which expresses achievement age divided by actual age expressed as a multiple of 100. *A. test:* standardized tests used to determine attainment levels in a variety of skills.

Achilles tendon, the large tendon which attaches the calf muscles (gastrocnemius and soleus) to the calcaneus (bone of the heel).

achillorrhaphy, *(ak-il-or-af-e),* surgical repair of ruptured Achilles tendon.

achlorhydria, *(ā-klor-hī'-dre-ah),* absence of hydrochloric acid in the gastric juice; may occur in pernicious anaemia and gastric cancer.

acholia, *(ākō-li-a),* absence of bile.

acholuria, *(a-kol-ū'-ri-a),* the absence of bile pigment from the urine.

acholuric jaundice, *see* JAUNDICE.

achondroplasia, *(a-kon-drō-plā-zi-a),* an inherited condition characterized by arrested development of the long bones due to premature ossification of the episphyseal plates. It results in short stature due to long bones being abnormally short, but the skull and trunk are normal.

achromasia, *(a-krō-mā'-zi-a),* 1. absence of colour. 2. loss of staining reaction in a cell.

achromatopsia, *(a-krō-ma-top'-si-a),* colour blindness.

acid, substances having an excess of hydrogen ions over hydroxyl ions. They release hydrogen ions on dissociation in solution. Acids have a pH below 7 and turn blue litmus paper red. Acids combine with alkalis to form salts and water. *A. phosphatase*: an enzyme needing an acid medium found in the prostate gland, semen, kidney and serum. Levels rise in prostatic cancers with bone spread. *A. rebound*: hypersecretion of gastric acid after the buffering effects of an antacid have worn off.

acidaemia, (*as-id-e-me-ah*), the blood is abnormally acid, pH below 7.35.

acid–alcohol fast, in microbiology it describes organisms which, when stained, are resistant to decolorization by alcohol as well as acid.

acid–base balance, the balance between the acidic and basic components which determine the pH of body fluids. Normal pH of blood is 7.35–7.45.

acid-fast, a microbiological term for bacteria which retain stains after treatment with acid and counterstaining. *acid-fast bacilli (AFB)*: bacteria that can be identified by use of acid-fast staining techniques, e.g. *Mycobacterium tuberculosis*.

acidosis, (*as-id-ō'-sis*), a condition in which the acid–base balance of the body is lost. It may have a respiratory or metabolic cause. The alkali reserve is exhausted, hydrogen ion concentration increases and the blood pH falls.

Acinetobacter, a genus of Gram-negative bacteria. Causes a range of infections, such as meningitis, wound infections and pneumonia. It has developed drug resistance and is a particular hazard to very ill patients.

acinus (*pl.* acini), (*a-sē-nus, a-sē-nĕ*), a minute grape-like structure whose cells secrete; as in the breast. Also describes the sac-like structures of the terminal bronchioles; **alveolus,** *sing.* **alveoli,** *pl.*

acne, inflammation of the sebaceous glands of the skin. *A. vulgaris*: commonly seen during adolescence is characterized by comedones and papulopustular lesions, especially on the face and back.

acousma, (*a-kūs-ma*), the hearing of imaginary sounds.

acoustic, relating to sound or hearing. *A. impedance*: a disruption in sound wave transmission. *A. neuroma*: a tumour arising from the eighth cranial nerve (vestibulocochlear or auditory).

acquired, occurring after birth, not inherited.

acquired immune deficiency syndrome (AIDS), a complex syndrome caused by the human immunodeficiency virus (HIV). Cell-mediated immunity is compromised which leads to an increased susceptibility to opportunistic infections such as *Pneumocystis carinii* and unusual malignant diseases, e.g. Kaposi's sarcoma. Management involves the use of antiviral drugs, usually in combination to prevent resistance, and antimicrobial drugs to reduce the risk of opportunistic infection. The virus is spread by contact with blood and other body fluids. This may occur through sexual contact, drug users sharing equipment such as syringes, accidental exposure, such as through needlestick injuries, or by the transfusion of infected blood/blood products. Prophylactic treatment is offered following occupational exposure, and to pregnant women found to be HIV-positive to reduce the risk of transmission to the fetus. *See* ARC, HIV, KAPOSI'S SARCOMA, PNEUMOCYSTIS CARINII.

acrid, pungent, corrosive.

acrocentric, (*ak'-rō-sen-trik*), describing a chromosome in which the centrosome is positioned at one end.

acrocephaly, (ak'-rō-ke-fa-li), congenitally malformed cone-shaped head.

acrocyanosis, (ak-rō-sī-a-nō-sis), blueness of the extremities.

acromegaly, (ak-rō-meg-a-le), a condition caused by oversecretion of growth hormone by the pituitary gland after fusion of the epiphyses. It causes enlargement of the bones of the lower jaw, hands and feet and also the heart and liver. *See* GIGANTISM.

acromion, (ā-krō'-mi-on), the outward projection of the spine of the scapula. *See* SCAPULA.

acronyx, (ak'-rō-niks), an ingrowing of the nail.

acrophobia, (ak-rō-fō'-bi-a), morbid fear of being at a height.

acrosome, (ak-rō-sōm), structure which surrounds the nucleus of a spermatozoon. Carries enzymes required for passage through the cervical mucus and penetration of the oöcyte.

ACTH, abbreviation for **adrenocorticotrophic hormone,** *q.v.*

actin, (ak-tin), a contractile protein, one of the component filaments of a muscle myofibril.

actinism, (ak-tin-izm), chemical changes produced by radiant energy, e.g. light rays.

actinodermatitis, (ak-tin-ō-der-mat-ī'-tis), inflammation of the skin from ultraviolet or other rays.

Actinomyces, (ak-tin-ō-mī-seez), a genus of anaerobic, branching microorganisms. *A. israeli* is the causative organism of actinomycosis in humans.

actinomycosis, (ak-tin-ō-mī-kō-sis), disease due to infection with *A. israeli.* It commonly affects the face and neck, lungs or abdomen with the formation of pus, abscesses and sinuses and tissue destruction.

actinotherapy, treatment by ultraviolet and infrared radiations.

action potential, the change in electrical potential and charge which occurs across cell membranes when a nerve fibre conducts an impulse or a muscle fibre contracts.

activated partial thromboplastin time (APTT), a test of blood clotting factor function.

active, energetic, moving. *A. movements*: the normal movements of a limb or part of the body performed by the individual without outside assistance. *A. transport*: movement of substances across cell membranes that requires the expenditure of metabolic energy and use of carrier molecules. This process allows movement against concentration gradients, where no gradient exists, and of large complex molecules.

activities of daily living (ADLs), term used by occupational therapists to describe the activities required for self-care or home management. They include personal (PADLs), e.g. washing and dressing; domestic (DADLs), e.g. cooking and cleaning; and instrumental (IADLs), sometimes used synonymously with DADLs to describe a wider range of activities that include communication, shopping, etc.

activities of living (ALs), activities that meet the physical, psychological and social needs of an individual, e.g. breathing, working and playing etc. They form the basis of some commonly used behavioural models of nursing.

actomyosin, (ak-to-mī'-ō-sin), a protein complex formed by the combination of actin and myosin as muscle fibres contract.

acuity, (a-kū-it-i), sharpness and clearness. *Auditory acuity*: ability to hear clearly and distinctly. Tests include the use of tuning fork tests, whispered voice and audiometry. Hearing screening in neonates can be performed by otoacoustic emission (OAE) testing. *Visual acuity*: the extent of visual perception depends on clarity of retinal focus, integrity of nervous components and cerebral integration of the stimulus. Usually tested by Snellen's test types at 6 metres.

acupuncture, originally from China, it involves the insertion of fine needles into the skin. It is based upon a theory that the body contains various channels or meridians through which 'energy/life forces' flow.

acute, sudden, severe. *A. abdomen*: a surgical emergency resulting from disease or damage of abdominal viscera. *A. confusional state*: sudden confusion, loss of awareness and disorientation due to a physical or metabolic disturbance affecting brain function. *A. respiratory distress syndrome (ARDS)*: Diffuse lung injury usually seen in adults suffering from an extremely serious illness associated with multiple organ dysfunction syndrome. *A. yellow atrophy*: severe liver damage due to toxic agents such as viruses, poisons and pregnancy.

acyclic, (*ā-sīk-lik*), a process without a cycle, occurring randomly.

acystia, (*a-sis'-ti-a*), absence of bladder.

adactylia, (*ā-dak-til'-i-a*), absence of fingers or toes.

adaptation, 1. adjustment by structural or functional change in response to a stressor. **2.** a psychological adjustment to changed circumstances which preserves normal functioning. **3.** the process by which the eye adjusts to changes from light to dark and vice versa. *A. model*: a model of nursing which is based upon the person as an adaptive system. Nursing interventions, which are required when problems occur, aim to encourage a response that allows the person to cope by achieving an adapted state.

adaptive behaviour, beneficial or appropriate behaviour in response to a change.

addiction, physiological or psychological dependence on a substance, e.g. alcohol, heroin; or a practice.

Addison's disease, failure of adrenocortical hormone secretion due to disease affecting the adrenal glands, e.g. autoimmune failure, tuberculosis. It is characterized by wasting, weakness, bronze skin pigmentation, hypoglycaemia, gastrointestinal disturbances, fluid and electrolyte imbalance and hypotension.

adducent muscle of eye, (*a-dū-sent*), medial rectus muscle which turns the eyeball inwards.

adduct, to draw towards the midline. *See* ABDUCT.

adduction, the act of moving a limb towards the midline of the body. *See* ABDUCTION.

adductor, a muscle which draws towards the midline of the body, e.g. *a. muscles* of the thigh draw the legs together. *See* ABDUCTOR.

adenectomy, (*ad-en-ek'-to-mē*), excision of a gland.

adenine, (*ad-en-īn*), nitrogenous base derived from purine, with other bases, a sugar and one or more phosphate groups forms the nucleic acids DNA and RNA. *See* NUCLEIC ACIDS, DNA, RNA.

adenitis, inflammation of a gland.

adenocarcinoma, (*ad-en-ō-kar-sin-ō'-mah*), a malignant tumour arising in glandular epithelial tissue.

adenohypophysis, (*ad-en-ō'-hi-pof'-i-sis*), alternative name for anterior lobe of the pituitary gland.

adenoid, 1. glandular. **2.** an enlarged pharyngeal tonsil. *See* TONSIL.

adenoidectomy, operation to remove adenoids (enlarged pharyngeal tonsils).

adenoma, (ad-en-ō´-ma), normally a benign tumour arising in glandular epithelial tissue.

adenomyoma, (ad-en-ō-mī-ō-ma), a benign growth, especially in uterus, of glandular and muscle tissue.

adenopathy, (ad-en-ōp´-ath-ē), a disease or enlargement of a gland.

adenosine, (ad-en-ō-sīn), a nucleoside formed from adenine and ribose (a pentose sugar); with the addition of one, two or three phosphate groups it forms a. monophosphate (AMP), a. diphosphate (ADP) and a. triphosphate (ATP). These are nucleotides closely involved in cellular energetic processes. See CYCLIC ADENOSINE MONOPHOSPHATE (CAMP).

adenovirus, a virus of the Adenoviridae family. They cause conjunctivitis, gastrointestinal and respiratory infections.

ADH, abbreviation for **anti diuretic hormone.**

ADHD, abbreviation for **attention deficit hyperactivity disorder.**

adhesion, a sticking together of two parts or surfaces. Bands of fibrous tissue, usually resulting from inflammation. Abdominal adhesions may obstruct the intestine.

adiaphoresis, (a-dī-a-for-ē-sis), deficiency of perspiration.

adipocyte, a fat cell.

adipose, fatty. A. tissue: a connective tissue of fat cells in an areolar matrix.

adiposogenital dystrophy, see FRÖHLICH'S SYNDROME.

adipsia, without thirst.

aditus, (ad´-it-us), an entrance or portal.

adjustment, see ACCOMMODATION.

adjuvant, substance included in a prescription to aid the action of other drugs. A. therapy: a treatment (usually refers to cancer treatment) given in conjunction with another, usually after any obvious tumour has been removed, either by radiotherapy or surgery. The aim is to improve cure rate and prevent recurrence. See NEOADJUVANT THERAPY.

Adler's theory, the theory that people develop neuroses to compensate for some inferiority.

ADLs, abbreviation for **activities of daily living.**

adnexa, appendages. Usually applied to the uterine appendages.

adolescence, the period between puberty and adulthood.

ADP, abbreviation for **adenosine diphosphate.**

adrenal, (ad-rē´-nal), see SUPRARENAL GLAND. A. glands: endocrine glands, one on the upper pole of each kidney. Each gland has two parts: the medulla which secretes adrenaline (epinephrine) and noradrenaline (norepinephrine), and the cortex which secretes various corticosteroid hormones, e.g. cortisol.

adrenalectomy, (ad-rē-nal-ek´-to-mē), the removal of one or both adrenal glands.

adrenaline (epinephrine), (ad-ren´-a-lin), a catecholamine produced by the adrenal medulla which augments the effects of the sympathetic nervous system at times of physiological stress. Therapeutic uses include locally to constrict small blood vessels and systemically to treat anaphylaxis and during cardiac arrest.

adrenergic, (ad-ren-er-jik), applied to the sympathetic nerves that use noradrenaline (norepinephrine) as their neurotransmitter. A. drug: drugs which mimic the action of adrenaline (epinephrine). A. receptor: receptor sites in structures innervated by the sympathetic nerves are mainly of two basic types: alpha and beta. Both types, which react differently to neurotransmitters, are further subdivided into alpha 1, 2 and beta 1, 2.

adrenocortical steroids, the hormones secreted by the adrenal cortex. Also called **corticosteroids,** they belong to three groups: glucocorticoids, mineralocorticoids and sex hormones.

adrenocorticotrophic hormone (ACTH), (ad- rē-nō-kor-ti-kō-tro'- fik), a hormone secreted by the anterior pituitary gland which stimulates the release of certain corticosteroid hormones by the adrenal cortex.

adrenogenital syndrome, (ad-rē-nō-jen-i-tal sin'-drōm), also called **adrenal virilism.** In female infants there is pseudohermaphrodism present at birth and male children exhibit precocious penile development with small testes. Adult females become masculinized and males show feminization. These effects are due to overproduction of androgenic hormones caused by hyperplasia or adenoma of the adrenal cortex.

adrenolytic, (ad-rē-nō-li-tik), a drug antagonistic to adrenaline (epinephrine).

ADRs, abbreviation for **adverse drug reactions.**

adsorbent, substance causing adsorption.

adsorption, the property possessed by certain porous substances, e.g. charcoal, of taking up different substances.

adulteration, the fraudulent addition of unnecessary, impure or inferior substances to drugs or food.

advance directive, also called a living will. A written declaration made by a mentally competent person, which sets out his or her wishes with regard to life-prolonging medical interventions if the person is incapacitated by an irreversible disease or terminally ill, if this prevents the patient making his or her wishes known to health professionals at the time. It is legally binding if it is in the form of an advanced refusal and the maker is competent at the time.

advanced life support (ALS), resuscitation techniques used during cardiac arrest that follow on from basic life support. They include defibrillation and appropriate drugs, e.g. atropine, etc.

advancement, surgery where a tendon or muscle is divided and reinserted further forward. Usually applied to an operation to correct strabismus.

adventitia, (ad-ven-tish-ē-ah), the outer coat of a structure, e.g. a blood vessel.

adverse drug reactions (ADRs), any unwanted effects from a drug. They range from minor side-effects through to harmful or seriously unpleasant effects.

advocacy, the process by which a person supports or argues for the needs of another. Nurses may act as advocate for their patients or clients. There are variations, such as people being helped to develop self-advocacy skills.

Aëdes, (a-ē-deez), a genus of mosquito responsible for the transmission of diseases such as yellow fever.

aeration, charging with air or other gas.

aerobes, (ā-er-ōbs), microorganisms which will grow in the presence of oxygen. A strict or obligate aerobe must have oxygen to grow and survive. ANAEROBES, c.f.

aerobic, needing free oxygen or air to support life. A. exercise: physical activity which causes the lungs and heart to work harder in order to obtain and circulate the extra oxygen needed for contracting skeletal muscles.

aerocele, *(ā-ro-sēl),* collection of air within a diverticulum of the larynx, trachea or bronchus.

aerogen, *(ā-ro-jen),* any gas producing bacteria, e.g. *Clostridium welchii,* a cause of gas gangrene.

aerophagy, *(ā-ro-fa-ji),* excessive air swallowing.

aerosol, finely atomized droplets or solid particles suspended in a gas. Some aerosol sources, e.g. sneezing, are responsible for the spread of infection. *A. sprays:* used to deliver drugs by inhalation, especially those acting upon the respiratory tract. Aerosols containing antibacterial chemicals are used in the environment.

Aesculapius, *(ē-skū-lā-pē-us),* a Greek god, the founder of the art of healing.

aesthesia, *(es-thē′-zi-a),* feeling.

aetas, *(ā-tas),* Latin for age. Abbreviation *aet.*

aetiology, *(ē-tē-ol′-ō-ji),* the science of the causation of disease.

AFB, abbreviation for **acid-fast bacilli.**

afebrile, *(ā-feb′- rīl),* without fever.

affect, the outward appearance of mood, feelings or emotions. *See* COGNITIVE, CONATION.

affective disorders, in psychiatry disorders characterized by disturbances of mood, e.g. depression.

afferent, leading to the centre, applied to the lymphatic vessels and to sensory nerves, *c.f.* EFFERENT.

affinity, attraction. In chemistry the property of a substance which prefers to combine with some other particular substance. The attraction which binds antigen and antibody together.

afibrinogenaemia, *(a-fi-brin-ō-jen-ē′-mē-ah),* a deficiency of fibrinogen in the blood leading to serious impairment of normal coagulation mechanisms. May be associated with amniotic fluid embolus, sepsis and severe trauma, that cause disseminated intravascular coagulation (DIC).

AFP, abbreviation for **alpha-fetoprotein.**

afterbirth, the placenta, amnion, chorion and umbilical cord expelled from the uterus during the third stage of labour.

afterimage, a retinal impression persisting although the stimulus of light has ceased.

afterload, the resistance against which the left ventricle pumps its volume of blood during systole. *See* PRELOAD, STROKE VOLUME.

afterloading, in radiotherapy a technique where applicators are sited near the tumour prior to loading with the radioactive source.

afterpains, pain from uterine contractions occurring after childbirth. Associated with breast feeding, caused by the hormone oxytocin.

agammaglobulinaemia, *(ā-ga-ma-glo-bū-lin-ē′-mē-a),* absence or deficiency of gammaglobulin in plasma proteins, leading to inadequate response to infection.

agar, a polysaccharide from seaweed. In microbiology it is used as culture media for bacteria. Also used as a bulk-forming laxative.

ageing, the natural process of cellular changes and failures which result in the physical changes associated with old age. *See* SENESCENCE.

ageism, stereotyping people according to chronological age alone; overemphasizing negative aspects to the detriment of positive aspects.

Usually applied to older people, resulting in discrimination.

agenesis, (ā-je'-nē-sis), defective development of a structure.

agglutination, (a-gloo-tin-ā'-shon), the clumping together or aggregation of cells, e.g. red blood cells. It is due to the presence of specific antibodies known as agglutinins.

agglutinins, (a-gloo-tin-ins), antibodies which produce an agglutination reaction on contact with an antigen.

agglutinogen, (a-gloo-tin-ō-jen), an antigenic substance which stimulates antibodies (agglutinins) which cause agglutination.

aggregate, to group together.

aggression, a hostile attitude which may result from threats, frustration or fear.

agitation, chronic restlessness associated with dementia and depression.

aglutition, inability to swallow.

agnosia, (ag-nō-zi-a), a disturbance in recognizing sensory impression.

agonist, 1. a muscle (prime mover) which contracts and shortens. It is opposed by the action of another muscle. 2. a drug that causes a cell to act in exactly the same way as it would with its usual ligand (hormone/neuro-transmitter) i.e. the expected cell response occurs. See ANTAGONIST.

agoraphobia, (ag-or-ah-fō'-be-ah), neurotic fear of open spaces.

agranulocyte, (a-gran-ū-lō-sīt), leucocytes which have no granules in their cytoplasm, e.g. lymphocytes.

agranulocytosis, (a-gran-ū-lō-sī-tō'-sis), a decrease in the number of granulocytes (polymorphonuclear leucocytes). The causes include drugs and ionizing radiation. Leads to fever with mouth and throat ulceration and may be fatal.

agraphia, (ā-graf'-i-a), loss of the power to express words and ideas in writing, or inability to interpret the written word.

ague, (ā-gū). See MALARIA.

AHF/G, antihaemophilic globulin. See ANTIHAEMOPHILIC FACTOR/GLOBULIN.

AID, artificial insemination with semen from a donor (not husband/partner).

AIDS, see ACQUIRED IMMUNE DEFICIENCY SYNDROME.

AIDS-related complex, See ARC (AIDS-related complex).

AIH, artificial insemination with semen from husband/partner.

air, see ATMOSPHERE. *A. embolism*: caused by air entering the circulatory system. *A. hunger*: respiratory distress caused by lack of available oxygen especially in haemorrhage. *A. swallowing*: see AEROPHAGIA.

airway, 1. the passage that allows air to enter and leave the lungs. 2. a plastic/rubber/metal tube used to maintain a patent airway in an unconscious person. *A. obstruction*: a serious condition where a mechanical blockage prevents air entering the lungs.

akathisia, (ak-ath-iz-ē-ah), abnormal restlessness with agitation, the person is unable to stay still.

akinesis, (a-kin-ē-sis), loss of ability to make voluntary movements.

ala, (ā-la), a wing. *A. nasi*: the outer side of the external nostril.

alanine, (al-an-een), a nonessential amino acid.

alanine aminotransferase (ALT), (al-an-een), see AMINOTRANSFERASES.

Al-Anon, a self help group for the family and friends of people affected by alcohol misuse.

Alateen, self help group for the children (12–20 years) of people affected by alcohol misuse.

Albers-Schönberg's disease, (shon'-burg), osteopetrosis. Marble bone disease.

11

albinism, inherited condition characterized by a lack of melanin (pigment) in skin, hair and eyes. Affected individuals may have visual problems such as astigmatism.

Albright's syndrome, a condition characterized by abnormal bone growth, with cysts, areas of skin pigmentation and precocious puberty in females.

albumin, *(al-bū'-min),* a type of protein found in both animal and plant tissues. The most abundant plasma protein, it is concerned with the movement of water between the fluid compartments.

albuminuria, *(al-bū-min-ūr-ē-ah),* albumin in the urine. May be associated with renal disease, but has other causes. *Orthostatic a:* occurs only in the standing position. *See* PROTEINURIA.

alcohol, a group of organic compounds containing hydroxyl (OH) groups. *Ethyl a.* (ethanol): the intoxicating substance produced by the fermentation of sugars by yeasts.

Alcoholics anonymous (AA), self help group for people who have an alcohol related problem. Based upon group support in achieving and maintaining sobriety through abstinence.

alcoholism, a morbid state of dependence upon an excessive intake of alcohol. Poisoning resulting from alcoholic addiction may be acute or chronic.

aldehyde, *(al-dē-hīd),* a group of organic compounds formed by the oxidation of an alcohol, e.g. acetaldehyde is formed from ethyl alcohol. They all contain a carbonyl (-CHO) group.

aldosterone, *(al-dos'-ter-ōn),* a mineralocorticoid hormone produced by the adrenal cortex, which enhances the reabsorption of sodium accompanied by water and the excretion of potassium by the renal tubules. Its release is mainly controlled through the renin–angiotensin response.

aldosteronism, *(al-dos'-ter-ōn-izm),* an excess secretion of aldosterone resulting in electrolyte imbalance and hypertension. It may be due to adrenal disease or secondary to another condition, e.g. cardiac failure. *See* CONN'S SYNDROME.

Alexander technique, a 'psychophysical' health technique based upon individual differences in breathing, muscles and posture.

alexia, *(a-leks'-ē-a),* inability to understand the written or printed word, owing to a lesion of the brain.

algae, *(al-jē),* a group of simple water plants used in water purification. There is increasing interest in their medicinal and nutritional properties.

algesia, *(al-jē-si-a),* excessive sensibility to pain.

alginates, a seaweed derivative used in some wound dressings. They are absorbent, haemostatic and do not damage tissue when removed.

algorithm, *(al-gor-ith'-em),* a step-by-step plan, guide or protocol for the management of a particular situation or problem.

alienation, 1. insanity. 2. feeling strange or separate.

alignment, bringing into line.

alimentary, pertaining to the absorption of nourishment. *A. canal:* the whole digestive tract, extending from the mouth to the anus (Figure 2).

alimentation, *(al-im-en-tā'-shon),* nourishment. *See* ENTERAL, PARENTERAL.

alkalaemia, *(al-kah-lē-mē-ah),* abnormally alkaline blood with a pH above 7.45.

alkali, substances having an excess of hydroxyl ions over hydrogen ions.

2 Alimentary tract

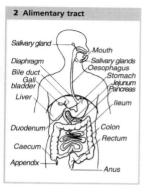

Salivary gland
Mouth
Diaphragm
Salivary glands
Bile duct
Oesophagus
Gall
Stomach
bladder
Jejunum
Liver
Pancreas
Ileum
Duodenum
Colon
Rectum
Caecum
Appendix
Anus

Also known as bases. Alkalis have a pH above 7 and turn red litmus paper blue. Alkalis combine with acids to form salts and water, they form a soap with fatty acids. *A. reserve*: the amount of alkali, normally bicarbonate (hydrogen carbonate), available in the blood for buffering acids and thus preventing changes in pH.

alkaline, containing an alkali, having a pH above 7. *A. phosphatase*: an enzyme produced by many tissues including bone, liver and kidneys. Levels in the blood may be elevated in certain bone and liver disorders.

alkalinity, proportion of alkali in a given substance.

alkaloid, *(al-kal-oid)*, organic compounds which have basic properties. A constituent of certain plants many of which are pharmacologically active, e.g. atropine, caffeine, morphine and quinine.

alkalosis, *(al-ka-lō'-sis)*, an abnormal increase in the pH of body fluids to above 7.45. It may be due to an increase in alkali reserve or loss of acids. Alkalosis may have a respiratory cause such as hyperventilation or a metabolic cause, e.g. vomiting gastric acid or excessive intake of alkali indigestion medicines.

alkapton, *(al-kap-ton)*, an abnormal metabolite of some amino acids, e.g. tyrosine, phenylalanine. Also known as **homogentisic acid.**

alkaptonuria, *(al-kap-ton-ūr'-ē-ah)*, the presence of alkapton in the urine due to a rare inherited disorder of amino acid metabolism where an enzyme is absent from the metabolic pathway. It is characterized by darkly stained urine.

alkylating agents, organic compounds containing alkyl groups. They are useful in anticancer chemotherapy, e.g. cyclophosphamide, busulfan, etc., as they damage DNA and interfere with cell division.

allantois, *(al-lan'-tō-is)*, a diverticulum formed as an outgrowth of the yolk sac of the developing embryo. It extends into the body stalk and is concerned with the formation of the umbilical cord and placenta.

allele, *(al-eel)*, originally used to denote inherited characteristics that are alternative and contrasting, such as normal colour vision contrasting with colour blindness. The basis of Mendelian inheritance of dominants and recessives. In modern usage allelomorph(s) is equivalent to alleles, namely the alternative forms of a gene at the same chromosomal location (locus). *See* MENDEL'S LAWS.

allelomorph, *see:* ALLELE.

allergen, *(al'-er-jen)*, any substance that stimulates an allergic state (hypersensitivity reaction). These substances, e.g. pollen, foods, drugs, house dust and animal hair/fur, are said to be allergenic.

allergic state, allergy. Hypersensitivity to a particular allergen, usually a protein. Examples include: asthma, eczema, hayfever and urticaria. Caused by the release of various chemical mediators, e.g. histamine, inflammation and an anaphylactic reaction. The results may be local, e.g. rashes and rhinitis or bronchospasm or, more unusually, systemic effects that result in anaphylaxis.

allograft, homograft. Graft with material obtained from a donor of dissimilar genotype, but of the same species.

allopathy, medical therapies which aim to produce a situation which counters the existing disorder or produces an environment which is unsuitable for that disease. It is the opposite to homoeopathy.

all-or-none law, the conduction of an action potential in excitable tissue, e.g. nerve or muscle fibres, obeys the rule that there are only two possible responses to a stimulus, either no response or a full response. There is no grading of response according to the strength or type of the stimulus.

alogia, poverty of thought. A negative symptom associated with mental illness such as schizophrenia. It is characterized by lack of spontaneous speech, etc.

alopecia, (al-ō-pē′-si-a), absence of hair, baldness.

alpha (α), first letter of the Greek alphabet. *A. antitrypsin*: a protein which normally opposes trypsin; low blood levels are associated with a genetic predisposition to emphysema and liver disease. *A. cells*: endocrine cells of the islets of Langerhans in the pancreas, they produce the hormone glucagon which raises blood glucose levels. *A. rays*: a type of ionizing radiation emitted as a radioactive isotope dis-

integrates. They consist of rapidly moving particles with a positive charge. It has very limited penetrating ability and is rarely used for therapeutic purposes. *A. receptor*: a type of receptor found in tissues innervated by sympathetic nerves. *See* ADRENERGIC RECEPTOR. *A. redistribution phase*: the point following an intravenous injection when blood concentrations of the drug will start to fall below the peak levels achieved. *A. state*: relaxed wakefulness without stimulation or concentration. *A. wave (rhythm)*: brain wave patterns seen when the individual is in the alpha state. They are slow, synchronous waves which typically have a frequency between 8–13 Hz and a low amplitude.

alpha (α)-adrenoceptor agonists, a group of drugs that stimulate alpha-adrenoceptors, e.g. adrenaline (epinephrine), which produces vasoconstriction and a rise in blood pressure.

alpha (α)-adrenoceptor antagonists, also known as alpha-blockers. A group of drugs that prevent stimulation of the alpha-adrenoceptors, e.g. doxazosin. They are vasodilators and are used as long-acting anti-hypertensive drugs.

alpha-fetoprotein (AFP), a protein produced by the human fetus. It is detectable in maternal blood and amniotic fluid. Elevated levels may indicate certain fetal abnormalities arising in the neural tube, e.g. spina bifida. Also a tumour marker for testicular and hepatocellular cancer.

ALS, abbreviation for **advanced life support.**

ALs, abbreviation for **activities of living.**

ALT, abbreviation for **alanine aminotransferase,** *see* AMINOTRANSFERASES.

alternating pressure pad/mattress, a device used to reduce the risk of pressure ulcer development. It aims to reduce the time a particular part of the body is subjected to pressure.

alternative therapies, *see* COMPLEMENTARY THERAPIES.

altitude sickness, *see* MOUNTAIN SICKNESS.

altruism, being unselfish, having concern for others.

aluminium (Al), a white metal. *A. salts:* used as antacids, e.g. aluminium hydroxide.

alveolar, pertaining to an alveolus. *A. air:* gases present within an alveolus. *A. capillary membrane:* the membrane between the alveoli and capillaries across which the respiratory gases diffuse. *A. ventilation rate:* the volume of inspired air reaching the alveoli in one minute available for gaseous exchange. Alveolar ventilation = (tidal volume – dead space) × respiratory rate. *See* DEAD SPACE, TIDAL VOLUME.

alveoli (*sing.* **alveolus**), *(al-vē'-ō-lī)* 1. tooth sockets. 2. secreting units of the breast. 3. minute air sacs in the lung. The site of gaseous exchange between alveolar air and pulmonary capillary blood (Figure 3). *See* EXTERNAL RESPIRATION.

alveolitis, *(al-vē-ō-lī-tis),* inflammation of the alveoli. *Extrinsic allergic a.:* caused by inhalation of an antigenic substance, e.g. mouldy hay spores in farmer's lung.

Alzheimer's disease, previously called senile dementia, it is a degenerative condition affecting the brain. Characterized by memory loss, confusion, restlessness, speech problems, agnosia, depression and personality changes. It is primarily a problem associated with older adults but may occur earlier.

amalgam, an alloy of mercury and other metals. *Dental a.* is of silver, tin and mercury. Used for filling teeth.

amasesis, unable to chew food for any reason.

amastia, *(à-mas-ti-a),* absence of breasts.

amaurosis, *(am-aw-rō'-sis),* blindness due to disease of the optic nerve or brain and systemic disease, e.g. uraemia, rather than problems within the eye.

amaurotic family idiocy, *see* TAY–SACHS DISEASE.

ambidextrous, equally skilful with each hand.

amblyopia, *(am-blī-ō-pē-ah),* indistinct vision in an eye which has no obvious defect.

amblyoscope, instrument used in orthoptics for the correction of squint.

ambulant, able to walk.

ambulatory, relating to walking, moving about. *A. surgery (day case surgery):* patients have minor surgery on the day of adminission and where no problems exist they are discharged home on the same day.

amelia, congenital absence of a limb or limbs.

amelioration, *(a-mēl-i-or-ā'-shon),* general improvement in the condition of the patient.

3 Alveoli

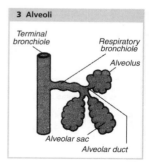

Terminal
bronchiole

Respiratory
bronchiole

Alveolus

Alveolar sac

Alveolar duct

amelogenesis, the development of dental enamel. *A. imperfecta*: inherited condition characterized by brown discoloration of the teeth due to a defect in enamel development.

amenorrhoea, *(a-men-o-re′-a),* absence of menstruation. In *primary a.,* menstruation has never been established. *Secondary a.* occurs after menstruation has commenced. There is amenorrhoea in pregnancy, and it may occur in certain endocrine disorders, anorexia nervosa, anaemia etc.

amentia, *(a-men′-she-a),* old term which describes absence of intellect with accompanying learning disability.

ametria, absence of uterus.

ametropia, *(a-mē-trŏ′-pi-a),* defective vision due to an error in refraction.

amines, group of organic compounds containing an amine (NH$_2$) group. They include many important biochemical molecules, e.g. histamine.

amino acids, nitrogenous organic acids from which all proteins are formed. They contain an amine (NH$_2$) group and a carboxyl (COOH) group. There are twenty common amino acids of which eight are considered essential or indispensable in adults as they are not synthesized by the body in sufficient quantities: isoleucine, leucine, lysine, methionine, phenylalanine, threonine tryptophan and valine; during childhood, histidine is considered to be essential and arginine is also considered to be essential because it is only synthesized in small amounts. They must be obtained from the dietary intake of high quality protein. The remaining can be synthesized by the body from essential amino acids: alanine, arginine, asparagine, aspartate, cysteine, glutamate, glutamine, glycine, proline, serine and tyrosine (Figure 4).

---

4 Amino acids

Indispensable/essential amino acids (not synthesized by the body in sufficient quantities)

Isoleucine	Phenylalanine
Leucine	Threonine
Lysine	Tryptophan
Methionine	Valine

Additional indispensable/essential amino acid during infancy and childhood
Histidine

Dispensable/non-essential amino acids (synthesized from indispensable amino acids)

Alanine	Glutamine
Arginine (semi-essential)	Glycine
Asparagine	Proline
Aspartate (aspartic acid)	Serine
Cysteine	Tyrosine
Glutamate (glutamic acid)	

aminoaciduria, *(am-īn-ō-as-id-ūr'-ē-ah),* amino acids in the urine, an abnormality associated with inborn errors of metabolism.

aminoglycosides, group of bactericidal antibiotics, e.g. gentamicin, streptomycin, etc. They have toxic side-effects on kidney function and hearing.

aminopeptidases, intestinal enzymes involved in protein digestion.

aminotransferases, transaminases. A group of enzymes which facilitate the movement of NH_2 groups from one amino acid to another, e.g. *alanine a.* (ALT), *aspartate a.* (AST). They are released from certain damaged cells and when measured in the blood are useful in diagnosis of liver and heart disease. *See* CARDIAC ENZYMES, LIVER FUNCTION TESTS.

amitosis, *(a-mit-ō'-sis),* simple cell division by fission.

ammonia, a pungent smelling gas produced during the breakdown of nitrogenous matter. It consists of hydrogen and nitrogen.

amnesia, loss of memory. Many types exist which include anterograde, retrograde and hysterical.

amniocentesis, *(am-nē-ō-sen-tē-sis),* aspiration of amniotic fluid from the uterus for the diagnosis of fetal abnormalities such as those due to chromosomal defects, e.g. Down's syndrome. It is usually performed around the sixteenth week of gestation, but can be done earlier (Figure 5).

amniography, *(am-nē-og-raf-ē),* radiographic demonstration of amniotic sac by injection of radiopaque medium.

amnion, the inner fetal membrane; contains the fetus and amniotic fluid.

amnioscopy, *(am-nē-os-ko'-pē),* endoscopic examination using an amnio-

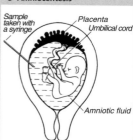

5 Amniocentesis

Sample taken with a syringe

Placenta

Umbilical cord

Amniotic fluid

scope which allows visualization of the amniotic sac and fetus. Uses either an abdominal or cervical approach.

amniotic fluid, *(am-nē-ot-ik),* the fluid surrounding the fetus within the amniotic sac. Also known as **liquor amnii.** *See* EMBOLISM.

amniotomy, *(am-nē-ot-ō-mē),* procedure to artificially rupture the fetal membranes (ARM), usually performed for the induction of labour.

amoeba, *(am-ē-bah),* a microscopic unicellular protozoon. Some species are pathogenic to humans, e.g. *Entamoeba histolytica.*

amoebiasis, *(am-ē-bī-a-sis),* infection with pathogenic amoeba such as *Entamoeba histolytica.* It may cause gastrointestinal symptoms, jaundice and weight loss.

amoebicide, substance lethal to amoeba, e.g. metronidazole.

amorph, a gene which does not express any trait. Inactive gene.

amorphous, formless.

AMP, abbreviation for **adenosine monophosphate.**

ampere (A), a measurement of electrical current. One of the base units in the International System of Units (SI).

17

amphiarthrosis, *(am-fē-ar-thrō'-sis),* a slightly movable joint, e.g. joints between the vertebrae. Cartilaginous joint.

amphipathic, *(am-fē-path'-ik),* a molecule with parts that have very different characteristics, e.g. a polar end and a non-polar end.

amphoric sounds, an abnormal sound in the chest, heard when a pneumothorax or other abnormal cavity is present.

amphoteric, a molecule capable of acting either as acid or base.

ampoule, a sealed phial containing some drug or solution sterilized ready for use.

ampulla, any flask-shaped dilatation. *A. of Vater.* see VATER'S AMPULLA.

amputation, the removal of an appending part, e.g. limb, breast.

amu, abbreviation for **atomic mass unit**.

amygdala, *(am-ig-dal-ah),* mass of grey matter situated in the caudate nucleus of the brain. It is part of the limbic system.

amylase, digestive enzyme present in saliva and pancreatic juice, it converts starch to maltose. *Serum a.:* test which measures amount of amylase in the serum, elevated in pancreatitis.

amyloidosis, amyloid disease. Deposits of a waxy glycoprotein called amyloid occur within various organs, e.g. heart, kidneys and liver. It may be primary or secondary when it is associated with malignant disease, chronic infection and inflammation.

amyotrophic, *(ā-mī-ō-trō'-fik),* pertaining to muscular atrophy. *A. Lateral sclerosis:* a degenerative motor neurone disease.

anabolic compound, a chemical involved in the synthesis of complex molecules from simple substances,

e.g. anabolic steroids; nandralone, etc.

anabolism, a metabolic process which involves the synthesis of other more complex substances. Requires the use of energy. *See* METABOLISM.

anacrotism, *(an-a',-krot-izm),* a small additional wave or notch found in the ascending limb of the tracing of the pulse curve.

anadipsia, excessive thirst, seen in certain psychotic conditions.

anaemia, diminished oxygen carrying capacity of the blood, due to a reduction in the number of red cells or the amount of haemoglobin, or both. The cause may be loss of blood, a deficiency of certain substances, e.g. iron, a failure of the bone marrow, or excessive breakdown of red cells. *See* APLASTIC ANAEMIA, BLOOD COUNT, HAEMOLYTIC, MACROCYTIC MEGALOBLASTIC ANAEMIA, MICROCYTIC.

anaerobe, *(an-ā'-er-ōb),* a microorganism that can live and multiply in the absence of free oxygen, e.g. *Clostridium tetani.* Microorganisms may be obligatory or facultative anaerobes.

anaerobic, *(an-ā'-er-ō'-bik),* **1.** absence of oxygen. **2.** able to survive without oxygen. *A. exercise.* Vigorous physical activity where oxygen supply to skeletal muscle tissue is inadequate; fuel molecules are broken down anaerobically with the formation of lactic acid.

anaesthesia, *(an-es-thē-zē-ah),* absence of sensation; loss of feeling. *Epidural a.:* anaesthesia of lower half of the body by injecting drugs into the epidural space. *General a.:* one that produces unconsciousness. *Inhalation a.:* the administration of anaesthetic agents via a mask (face or laryngeal) or a tube (endotracheal or tracheostomy) to produce general anaesthesia. *Intravenous a.:* drugs administered intravenously to produce general anaesthesia. *Local a.*: regional anaesthesia produced in certain areas of the body without alteration in consciousness. *Nerve block a.*: local anaesthesia produced by injecting drugs into a sensory nerve. *Rectal a.*: administration of anaesthetic drugs via the rectum. *Refrigeration a.*: anaesthesia produced by intense cold. *Spinal a.*: anaesthesia produced in the lower part of the body by injecting drugs into the subarachnoid space.

anaesthetic, 1. an agent which produces insensibility. **2.** *adj.* insensible to touch.

anaesthetist, a physician specially trained to administer anaesthetics.

anal, pertaining to the anus. *A. canal*: last part of gastrointestinal tract. *A. character*: in psychology a personality type characterized by orderliness, perfection, stubbornness, cleanliness and meanness. *A. phase.* the second stage of psychosexual development characterized by the child's sensual interest in the anal area and all matters connected with defecation. *A. reflex*: contraction of external anal sphincter when the perianal area is stroked.

analgesia, *(an-al-jē'-zīēa)*, diminished sensibility to pain. A symptom in certain nervous diseases. Patient-controlled analgesia (PCA) allows patients to self-administer a preset dose of a pain-relieving drug. Safety precautions prevent overdose.

analgesic, relieving pain; remedy for pain, e.g. morphine, paracetamol.

analogous, *(an-al-o-gus)*, similar in function but not in origin.

analogue, 1. a tissue or organ which performs similar functions as another structure but has different physical features or origin. **2.** a substance which has a similar structure to

another but differs in respect of one constituent.

analysis, in chemistry, the breaking down of a substance into its constituent parts. In psychiatric medicine, psychoanalysis. *A. of variance (ANOVA)*: a statistical method of comparing sample means. Used to compare more than two means.

analyst, the person who analyses.

anaphase, the third stage of nuclear division occurring during mitosis and meiosis.

anaphoresis, *(a-na-for-ē'-sis)*, diminished activity of the sweat glands.

anaphylactic, *(an-ah-fil-ak'-tik)*, pertaining to anaphylaxis. *A. shock*: *see* ANAPHYLAXIS.

anaphylaxis, *(an-ah-fil-aks-is)*, life-threatening situation resulting from an extreme hypersensitivity reaction to a previously encountered allergen, e.g. foreign protein in bee stings, penicillin, etc. It is characterized by laryngeal oedema, bronchospasm, severe dysponea and vasodilation leading to hypovolaemia and shock. Life-saving measures include: administration of adrenaline (epinephrine), provision of an airway, e.g. by tracheostomy and antihistamines such as chlorphenamine (chlorpheniramine).

anaplasia, *(an-a-plā'-zi-a)*, the reversion of a special tissue or cells to a less differentiated type.

anarthria, loss of ability to pronounce words though difficulties with the motor movements needed for speech.

anasarca, *(an-ah-sar-kah)*, extensive oedema associated with renal disease.

anastomosis, *(an'-as-to-mō'-sis)*, in anatomy the intercommunication of the terminal branches of two or more blood vessels. In surgery the establishment of some artificial connection, as, for instance, between two parts of the intestine.

anatomical, pertaining to anatomy. *A. dead space: see* DEAD SPACE. *A. position:* used as a reference point when describing the position of body parts. The person stands erect, faces forward, with arms at the side with palms uppermost.

anatomy, the science of body structure. Types of anatomy include: applied, comparative, gross, microscopic and surface.

anconeus, *(an-kō´-nē-us),* a small extensor muscle of the forearm.

Ancylostoma, (an-sil-os-tō-mah), hookworm. A genus of nematode worm. *A. duodenale* is parasitic in the human duodenum and jejunum.

ancylostomiasis, *(an-sil-os-'tō-mī´-a-sis),* infestation with the hookworm which can cause malnutrition and severe anaemia. Common in tropical and subtropical areas.

androgen, a group of steroid hormones, e.g. testosterone, which produce the male secondary sexual characteristics. They are secreted by the testes, the adrenal and to a lesser extent, the ovary.

android pelvis, shaped like a male pelvis. The narrow forepelvis, shallow posterior segment and straight lateral walls make child-bearing difficult.

androsterone, *(an-dros-ter-ōn),* a breakdown product of testosterone.

anencephalous, *(an-en-kef-a-lus),* having no brain; not compatible with life.

anergic, 1. inactivity **2.** a decreased immunological response to an antigen.

aneuploidy, *(an-ū-ploid´-ē),* a genetic abnormality where the chromosome number is not a multiple of the haploid number (23). Examples are: **1.** trisomy, where there are 47 chromosomes, e.g. Down's syndrome.

2. monosomy, where there are 45 chromosomes, e.g. Turner's syndrome. POLYPLOIDY, *c.f.*

aneurysm, *(an´-ūr-izm),* a permanent, abnormal dilatation of an artery which may be congenital or more usually due to degenerative arterial disease. It may be fusiform, sacculated or dissecting (Figure 6). *Arteriovenous a.:* a communication between an artery and a vein, usually the result of injury. *Berry a.:* congenital condition of the cerebral blood vessels, may rupture causing subarachnoid haemorrhage.

angiectasis, *(an-ji-ek´-ta-sis),* dilatation of blood vessel.

angiitis, *(an-ji-ī-tis),* inflammation of blood vessels.

angina, suffocating feeling, pain or constriction felt in the throat. *A. pectoris:* a condition characterized by sudden chest pain which may radiate to the arms; due to insufficient oxygenated blood reaching the myocardium, the coronary arteries being narrowed by disease or spasm. It is induced by physical effort, stress and cold. Usually subsides with rest. Management includes: lifestyle changes, e.g smoking cessation; low-dose aspirin;

6 Types of aneurysm: fusiform, sacculated and dissecting

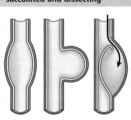

nitrates; beta-adrenoceptor antagonists, e.g. atenolol; calcium antagonists, e.g. nifedipine and surgical treatment. *See* ANGIOPLASTY. *Ludwig's a:* streptococcal cellulitis affecting the floor of the mouth. *Vincent's a:* bacterial infection of the gums with necrosis and spread to associated structures which may include the throat.

angiocardiogram, *(an-jĕ-ō-kar-dĕ-ō'-gram),* a radiograph showing the heart and great vessels.

angiocardiography, *(an-jĕ-ō-kar-dĕ-og'-raf-ē),* radiographic technique which demonstrates the structure and functioning of the chambers of the heart and great vessels, after the injection of a radiopaque contrast medium.

angiogenesis, formation of new blood vessels, such as during wound healing. Also occurs in malignant disease.

angiogram, radiograph showing blood vessels.

angiography, radiographic technique to show the internal structure of blood vessels after a radiopaque contrast medium has been injected.

angioma, a tumour composed of blood vessels, often called a **naevus.**

angio-oedema, angioneurotic oedema. Acute painless swelling of face, lips, eye lids, larynx, hands and feet. Occurs as a result of allergy or infection.

angioplasty, plastic surgery of blood vessels. *Balloon a.:* procedure to reopen a blood vessel by means of a catheter with inflatable balloon. When the technique is used on the coronary arteries it is called percutaneous transluminal coronary angioplasty (PTCA).

angiosarcoma, a sarcoma composed of vascular tissue.

angiospasm, a spasm of blood vessel causing constriction.

angiotensin, *(an-ji-ō-ten-sin),* a polypeptide formed by the action of renin on a precursor plasma protein.

It causes vasoconstriction and increased aldosterone secretion by the adrenal cortex. *A.-converting enzyme: see* ACE.

Angleman syndrome, an inherited condition that arises from a mutation of the maternal chromosome 15. It is characterized by severe learning disability and poor muscle tone with ataxia. *See* PRADER-WILLI SYNDROME.

anhedonia, inability to feel normal pleasure from events that would normally cause this response.

anhidrosis, *(an-hī-drō'-sis),* deficiency of perspiration.

anhidrotics, drugs which reduce the amount of perspiration.

anhydrous, *(an-hī'-drus),* without water.

anima, 1. in Jungian psychology, the personality, inner self or soul, rather than the public persona. **2.** the female part of the male personality.

animal pole, that part of the ovum which contains the nucleus and most of the cytoplasm.

animus, 1. the male part of the female personality. **2.** deeply hidden feelings of hostility which may be revealed under stress.

anion, *(an'-ī-on),* an ion with a negative charge. During electrolysis it is attracted to the positive electrode (anode). *A. gap:* the difference between the amount of anions and cations in the blood. *See* CATION.

aniridia, *(a-ni-ri-di-a),* absence or defect of iris.

anisocoria, *(an-is-ō-ko'-ri-a),* inequality of the pupils.

anisocytosis, *(an-is-ō-sī-tō'-sis),* inequality of size of the red blood cells.

anisomelia, *(an-is-ō-me'-li-a),* unequal limbs which should be a pair.

anisometropia, *(an-is-ō-me-trō-pi-a),* refraction of the two eyes is different.

ankle, joint between the tibia, fibula and talus.

ankle-brachial pressure index (ABPI) test used as part of leg ulcer assessment to confirm the diagnosis and inform decisions regarding the use of compression therapy. The systolic blood pressure at the ankle is divided by the brachial systolic blood pressure to give the ABPI.

ankyloblepharon, *(an-ki-lō-blef´-a-ron),* adhesion of the edges of the eyelids.

ankyloglossia, *(an-kil-ō-glos´-ē-ah),* inability to protrude the tongue fully, 'tongue tie'.

ankylosing spondylitis, *(an-kil-ōz-ing-spon-dil-ī-tis),* joint disease of unknown aetiology. Loss of joint space leads eventually to fusion with loss of movement. Commonly affects the sacroiliac joints and those of the spine.

ankylosis, *(an-ki-lō-sis),* **1.** fixation and immobility of joint due to disease, injury or disuse. **2.** surgical fixation of a joint, also called an arthrodesis.

annular, ring-shaped.

anode, electrode with positive charge.

anodyne, a pain-relieving drug.

anogenital, pertaining to the anal and the genital region.

anomalous, irregular. Out of the ordinary.

anomia, *(a-nō-mi-a),* inability to name objects and recall names.

anomie, sociological term applied in situations where the norms guiding behaviour are absent. The situation of 'normlessness' caused by weak social controls and moral obligations leads to disturbances in social behaviour. Also called **anomy.**

anonychia, *(ā-nō-ni´-ki-a),* without nail formation.

anoperineal, relating to anus and perineum.

Anopheles, *(an-of-el-eez),* genus of mosquito which transmits the malaria parasite to humans.

anophthalmos, congenital absence of a true eyeball.

anorchism, congenital absence of one or both testes.

anorectal, relating to the anus and rectum.

anorexia, loss of appetite. *A. nervosa:* a serious psychological condition characterized by refusal to eat, self-induced vomiting, use of laxatives and exercise. May be associated with a distorted body image, fear of obesity and an obsession with thinness. Can progress to severe emaciation and life-threatening metabolic consequences. *See* BULIMIA NERVOSA.

anosmia, loss of sense of smell.

anosognosia, inability to accept or recognize a physical defect such as paralysis of one side of the body.

anovular, without ovulation. Especially a menstrual cycle where ovulation has not occurred.

anovulation, cessation of ovulation.

anoxaemia, *(an-ok-sē´-mi-a),* insufficient oxygen in the blood.

anoxia, absence of oxygen in the tissues is the strict definition, but is more often used to describe the lack of tissue oxygen available for metabolic processes. *See* HYPOXIA.

antacid, a substance used to neutralize an acid, e.g. magnesium trisilicate.

antagonist, 1. a muscle which opposes or reverses the action of an agonist (prime mover) muscle. **2.** a drug or substance that opposes the action of another substance. *See* AGONIST.

ante mortem, before death.

antecubital, front of the elbow.

anteflexion, bending forward, such as the position of the uterus.

antenatal, before birth, the time from conception to birth. *A. care*: regular care and monitoring given to women during pregnancy.

antepartum, before parturition. In obstetrics usually applied to events occuring in the last trimester of pregnancy. *A. haemorrhage*: bleeding from the genital tract (for any reason) occurring after 24 weeks of pregnancy and before labour. There are many causes which include: abruptio placentae, placenta praevia and cervical lesions.

anterior, in front of. Ventral. *A. chamber of eye*: space between the cornea in front and the iris and lens behind, contains aqueous humour. *A. fontanelle*: see FONTA-NELLE. *A. poliomyelitis*: see POLI-OMYELITIS.

anterograde, proceeding forwards.

anteroinferior, lying in front and below.

anterointerior, lying to the front and internally.

anterolateral, in front and to the side.

anteromedian, lying in front and near the midline.

anteroposterior, from front to back.

anterosuperior, in front and above.

anteversion, tilted forward, such as the position of the uterus.

anthelmintic, *(an-thel-min-tik)*, drug used to treat worm infections e.g. mebendazole.

anthracosis, *(an-thra-kō-sis)*, a lung disease of coal miners. See PNEUMO-CONIOSIS.

anthrax, an infectious disease caused by *Bacillus anthracis*, it affects domestic animals who pass the spores in their faeces. It causes a skin lesion (malignant pustule), pyrexia, toxaemia and lung complications. Certain occupations are high-risk: farmers, veterinary sur-geons, butchers and those working with hides and wool.

anthropoid, manlike. *A. pelvis*. has narrowed transverse inlet which is long anteroposteriorly.

anthropology, the science and study of mankind.

anthropometry, *(an-thro-po-met-rē)*, the comparative measurement of different features of the body, e.g. weight, height, skin-fold thickness and areas, etc.

antiarrhythmic, *(an-tē-ā-rith-mik)*, drug used to correct an abnormal cardiac rhythm.

antibacterial, substance which des-troys or inhibits the growth of bacteria. Used to combat bacterial infections.

antibiotic, a substance obtained from microorganisms which is effective in the treatment of bacterial diseases. Generally used to describe all anti-bacterial drugs.

antibodies, immunoglobulins. Specific protein substances, usually circulat-ing in the blood, which destroy or inactivate the corresponding antigen.

anticholinergic, *(an-tē-kō-li-ner-jik)*, term applied to drugs inhibiting the action of acetylcholine. See MUS-CARINIC.

anticholinesterase, enzyme that destroys cholinesterase, enabling acetylcholine to accumulate at the nerve endings, thus allowing the resumption of normal muscle con-traction.

anticipatory adaptation, efforts made to adapt to a potentially diffi-cult or distressing event prior to dealing with the situation. *A. grief*: bereavement process which com-mences prior to the inevitable death of a loved one.

anticoagulant, *(an-tē-kō-ag-ū-lant)*, substance that prevents or delays blood clotting.

anticodon, in genetics, the triplet of bases in tRNA (transfer ribonucleic acid) which is involved in the translation stage of protein synthesis. *See* CODON.

anticonvulsant, *See* ANTIEPILEPTIC DRUGS.

anti-D, antibody formed when rhesus negative (Rh–ve) individuals are exposed to rhesus positive (Rh+ve) blood, e.g. transfusion, pregnancy, *A. (Rh$_o$) immunoglobulin*: used to prevent the production of rhesus antibodies in Rh-ve women during pregnancy, after delivery or termination of pregnancy, or spontaneous miscarriage.

antidepressant, substances or techniques used to reduce depression. Antidepressant drugs are of three main types: monoamine oxidase inhibitors; selective serotonin reuptake inhibitors and tricyclic antidepressants.

antidiuretic hormone (ADH), *(an-tē-dī-ū-re-tik)*, a hormone made in the hypothalamic nuclei and stored in the posterior lobe of the pituitary gland, from where it is released. Its antidiuretic action is achieved through increasing the permeability of the renal tubules to water. It also causes vasoconstriction which increases blood pressure, hence the alternative name vasopressin.

antidote, a drug or agent which opposes the effects of a poison.

antiembolic, against embolism. *A. hose*: elastic stockings which exert a linear trend graduated compression on the superficial veins of the leg. They improve venous return and help to prevent the venous stasis which predisposes to the development of the thromboembolic complications of surgery and immobility. Also known as thromboembolic deterrents (TEDs).

antiemetic, drug used to control nausea and vomiting.

antiepileptic, also known as anticonvulsant. Used to prevent seizures, e.g. valproate, or to control seizures, e.g. diazepam.

antifungal, any agent that destroys fungi, e.g. nystatin.

antigen, *(an'-ti-jen)*, a substance, usually a protein (e.g. a bacterium), capable of stimulating antibody production. The specific antibody inactivates the antigen in various ways, but all involve the formation of an antibody–antigen complex.

antigenicity, *(an-tē-jen-is'-it-ē)*, the ability or power to stimulate antibody production, as in a vaccine.

antihaemophilic factor/globulin (AHF/G), *(an-tē-bē-mō-fil-ik)*, blood clotting factor VIII prescribed to prevent or control bleeding in individuals with haemophilia A.

antihistamine, drug used to counteract the effects of histamine release in allergic conditions.

antihypertensive, a drug or technique that reduces an abnormally high blood pressure.

anti-inflammatory, a drug which suppresses or reduces the inflammatory process.

antilymphocyte immunoglobulin, an immunosuppressive preparation occasionally used to prevent rejection of organ transplants.

antimalarials, drugs used in the prophylaxis and treatment of malaria.

antimetabolites, chemicals which prevent cell division. They are similar to essential metabolites and are able to interfere with their use by cells. Used in malignant conditions.

antimicrobial, substance which destroys or inhibits the growth of microorganisms.

antimitotic, *(an-tē-mī-to-tik)*, a substance which prevents mitosis.

antimycotic, *(an-tē-mī-ko-tik),* see ANTI-FUNGAL.

antineoplastic, a substance used to kill or prevent the growth of malignant cells.

antinuclear antibody (ANA), an autoantibody detected in conditions such as rheumatoid arthritis. It specifically attacks the cell nucleus.

antioestrogen, *(an-tē-ē-strō-jen),* a substance which inhibits oestrogen production. See: SELECTIVE (O)ESTRO-GEN RECEPTOR MODULATORS.

antioxidant, a chemical which inhibits oxidation. Added to foods containing fats to prevent deterioration. Certain vitamins (A, C and E), eaten in a balanced diet, act as antioxidants, as do some minerals, e.g. zinc.

antiparkinson(ism) drugs, drugs used in the treatment of parkinsonism, e.g. L-dopa, bromocriptine and benzatropine.

antiperistalsis, *(an-tē-pe-ri-stal'-sis),* reverse peristalsis, i.e. from below upward, See PERISTALSIS.

antiperistaltic, a substance which inhibits or reduces peristalsis.

antiprotozoal, substance used to treat diseases caused by protozoa. See MALARIA.

antipruritic, *(an-tē-proor-it'-ik),* substance relieving itching.

antipsychotic, drug used to treat psychotic illness. See NEUROLEPTICS.

antipyretic, a drug which reduces the high temperatures of feverish conditions.

antisepsis, prevention of sepsis (infection) by destruction of microorganisms or inhibition of their growth and multiplication.

antiseptic, a substance opposing sepsis by inhibiting the growth and multiplication of microorganisms.

antiserum, serum, prepared from the blood of animals, which contains antibodies for a specific disease. Previously used to provide passive immunity. Now replaced by the use of human immunoglobulins.

antisocial, against society. *A. behaviour:* behaviour which is contrary to the accepted standards or social norms. *A. personality disorder:* one where the individual repeatedly demonstrates a disregard for social norms, rules, the law and the needs or wishes of others. These individuals are aggressive, indifferent to the effects of their actions and show no remorse. Psychopathic personality.

antispasmodic, agent preventing spasm, usually of smooth muscle.

antistatic, measures which prevent a build-up of static electricity.

antithrombin III, a substance normally present in the blood which limits coagulation to areas where it is needed.

antithyroid drugs, substances which restrict the secretion of thyroid hormones.

antitoxin, a specific antibody produced in the blood in response to a toxin or poison. The antibody is capable of neutralizing that particular toxin.

antitussive, *(an-tē-tus-iv),* drugs which relieve a cough.

antivenin (antivenom), antiserum used as an antidote to snake or insect venom.

antiviral, substance used to destroy viruses, e.g. aciclovir, zidovudine, ritonavir, etc.

antrectomy, excision of an antrum, e.g. maxillary antrum or pyloric antrum.

antrostomy, incision to drain an antrum.

antrum, a cavity, usually in bone. Also used to describe the lower part of the stomach, the pyloric antrum. *Mastoid a.:* air filled space in mastoid part of temporal bone which communicates with the middle ear. *A. of Highmore*: the maxillary air sinus.

anuria, cessation of urine production or a reduction in volume to a level insufficient for normal waste excretion. Also called **suppression.**

anus, the opening of the anal canal. *Imperforate a.*: congenital anomaly where an infant does not have a patent anal opening or the anus does not communicate with the bowel above. It exists in varying degrees of severity and requires surgical correction.

anxiety, a normal reaction to stress or threat. Clinical anxiety is said to be present if the threat is minimal or non-existent. Anxiety may be persistent (anxiety state) or it may occur in discrete attacks (panic attacks).

anxiolytics, *(ang-zi-ō-li-tiks),* drugs which reduce anxiety, e.g. benzodiazepines. *See* TRANQUILLIZERS.

aorta, *(ā-or′-ta),* the large artery arising from the left ventricle of the heart. It supplies oxygenated blood to all parts of the body.

aortic, relating to the aorta. *A. bodies*: chemoreceptors situated in the aortic arch which monitor blood pH and oxygen levels. *A. regurgitation*: ineffective closing of aortic valve which allows blood to regurgitate back into the heart. *A. stenosis*: narrowing of the aortic valve which reduces the blood flow into the aorta. *A. valve*: a three cusp semilunar valve between left ventricle and aorta, which normally prevents back flow of blood.

aortitis, inflammation of the aorta.

apathy, listlessness. Lack of feeling and activity.

apatites, inorganic calcium salts (phosphate, carbonate and hydroxide) which are deposited in bone tissue to provide its extreme hardness.

APEL, abbreviation for **accreditation (assessment) of prior experiential learning.**

aperient, drug used to stimulate defecation. *See* LAXATIVE.

aperistalsis, cessation of peristalsis.

apex, top or extreme point. *A. beat*: contraction of the left ventricle felt, seen or heard against chest wall. Usually located in the mid-clavicular line at the level of the fifth intercostal space. *A. of the heart*: narrow end of the heart, inclined to the left. *A. of the lung*: top of conical lung, level with clavicle.

Apgar score, system for assessing physical condition of infants immediately after birth. A maximum of two points is awarded for five criteria (heart rate, respiratory effort, muscle tone, reflex irritability and colour), giving a possible score of ten for infants in good condition (Figure 7).

aphagia, *(a-fā′-ji-a),* inability to swallow.

aphakia, *(a-fă-ki-a),* absence of lens of eye.

aphasia, *(a-fā-zi-ā),* inability to use language. Types include: nominal, expressive and receptive.

apheresis, *(a-fer-ē′-sis),* separation of blood into its components following temporary removal. Selected components are removed prior to reinfusion.

aphonia, loss of voice.

aphrodisiac, an agent which stimulates sexual excitement.

aphthae, *(af′-thē),* small white ulcers in the mouth.

aphthous stomatitis, *(af-thus stō-ma-fi′-tis),* inflammation of the mucosa of the mouth with painful ulceration.

apical, *(ā′-pi-kal),* pertaining to the apex. *A. abscess*: of tooth root. *A. pulse*: heart rate recorded over the apex of the heart.

7 Apgar score

Signs/Criteria	Score		
	0	1	2
Heart rate	absent	slow, below 100/min	over 100/min
Respiratory effort	absent	slow, weak irregular	good chest movements or crying.
Muscle tone	limp	poor tone, some movement	active resistance, strong movement
Reflex irritability (response to stimulation such as sole flicks)	none	slight withdrawal	vigorous movement, cries
Colour (designed for Caucasian newborns)	pale or blue	extremities blue	completely normal colour

apicectomy, *(ā-pi-sek-to-mi),* excision of the root of a tooth.

APL, abbreviation for **accreditation (assessment) of prior learning**.

aplasia, *(ā-plā'-si-a),* non-development of an organ or tissue.

aplastic anaemia, *(ā-plas-tik),* anaemia caused by the failure of the bone marrow to produce blood cells. Causes include: idiopathic, radiation, drugs, infection and malignancy.

apneustic centre, *(ap-nū-stik),* a respiratory centre in the pons which ensures a smooth respiratory rhythm. *See* PNEUMOTAXIC CENTRE.

apnoea, *(ap-ne'-a),* cessation of spontaneous breathing. *See* SLEEP APNOEA.

apocrine glands, specialized sweat glands found in the axillae and genital regions. After puberty their secretions are responsible for body odour.

apolipoprotein, *(ap-ō-li'-pō-prō-teen),* the protein part of a lipoprotein.

aponeurosis, *(ap-o-nūr-ð'-sis),* a flat sheet of white fibrous tissue which forms attachments for muscles, e.g. abdominal muscles, and binds muscles together. *See* TENDON.

apophysis, a bony protuberance or outgrowth.

apoplexy, *(ap-ō-pleks-ē)* obsolete term for a stroke or cerebrovascular accident.

apoprotein, a protein before it binds to the prosthetic group required for its biological activity.

apoptosis, programmed cell death. For example, immune cells (many lymphocytes) that would react against body tissues are destroyed in the thymus gland during maturation of immune cells.

appendicectomy, *(ap-pen-di-sek'-to-mē),* surgical removal of the vermiform appendix.

appendicitis, inflammation of the appendix vermiformis.

27

appendix vermiformis, a worm-like offshoot from the caecum, ending blindly, and 2.5–12.5 cm long.

apperception, 1. perception or recognition of sensory stimuli. **2**. in psychology the modification of perception by past experiences.

appetite, pleasant anticipation of taking food or fluids; it can be fickle in illness; maintaining oral hygiene and hydration and offering small attractive portions will be helpful. *A. suppressant*: drugs sometimes used in the management of severe obesity, e.g. dexfenfluramine. Dependence and misuse are particular problems.

appliance, an implement or device which performs a specific role.

application, in computing, the programs that allow the computer to perform a specific function, e.g. word processing.

applicator, an instrument for applying local remedies, e.g. radium.

apposition, the lying together or the fitting together of two structures.

appositional growth, increase in size by the production of new cells around the outside, as in the increase in bone girth.

appraisal, process of making a valuation, such as during performance appraisal or review.

approved name, the non-proprietary (generic) name for a drug, e.g. carbimazole. *See* RECOMMENDED INTERNATIONAL NON-PROPRIETARY NAME.

apraxia, inability to perform purposeful movements.

aptitude, a natural ability, skill or talent.

apyrexia, without fever.

aqueduct, certain canals of the body, such as the *a. of Sylvius* which leads from the third to the fourth ventricle of the brain.

aqueous humour, watery fluid which fills the anterior and posterior chambers of the eye.

arachidonic acid, *(a-ra′-kid-on-ik)*, a polyunsaturated fatty acid used by the body for the synthesis of important regulatory lipids: prostaglandins and thromboxanes. It is synthesized from linoleic acid in the body, but may be considered to be an essential fatty acid when linoleic acid is deficient.

arachnodactyly, *(a-rak′-no-dak-til-ē)*, an inherited disease characterized by abnormally long and slender bones of the extremities; Marfan's syndrome.

arachnoid, *(a-rak′-noyd)*, resembling a web. *A. membrane*: the middle meninges between the pia and dura mater, covers the brain and spinal cord.

arborization, branching of processes of nerve cells.

arboviruses, arthropod-borne viruses causing diseases such as yellow fever.

ARC (AIDS-related complex), also linked to infection with HIV but there is less damage to the immune system than seen in AIDS. May progress to full AIDS.

arcus, an arch or ring. *A. senilis*: an opaque circle round the edge of the cornea, occurring in the aged.

ARDS, abbreviation for **acute respiratory distress syndrome.**

arenavirus, a family of RNA viruses which include the Lassa fever virus.

areola, *(ā-re′-ō-la)*, the pigmented skin around the nipple of the breast.

areolar tissue, a loose woven connective tissue with a semi-solid matrix containing cells and fibres.

arginine, *(a-jin-ēn)*, an amino acid. *See* AMINO ACIDS.

Argyll Robertson pupil, pupil of the eye which is small, reacting to accommodation but not to light. Seen in diseases of the nervous system, e.g. neurosyphilis.

Arnold–Chiari syndrome, congenital anomaly affecting the central nervous system. There is herniation of parts of the brain through the foramen magnum.

aromatherapy, a therapy which utilizes fragrances derived from essential oils. These may be combined with a base oil, inhaled or massaged into the skin.

arrectores pilorum, involuntary muscles attached to the hair follicles. They contract to cause erection of the hair and 'goose-flesh'.

arrest, to stop. *Cardiac a.*: a cessation of effective cardiac contraction and output, due to ventricular fibrillation or asystole, or electromechanical dissociation.

arrhenoblastoma, *(a-rā-nō-blas-tō-ma)*, a neoplasm of the ovary associated with masculinization. Also called androblastoma.

arrhythmia, *(a-rith'-mi-a)*, without rhythm. Usually used to describe a disturbance of heart rhythm. *Sinus a.*: an increase in heart rate with inspiration and a decrease with expiration.

arsenic, a poisonous metallic element present in preparations which include pesticides and herbicides. Small amounts may be present in fruit, vegetables and other foods.

arterial, pertaining to an artery. *A. blood gases*: amount of oxygen and carbon dioxide dissolved in arterial blood, and the pH. *A. blood pressure*: the pressure exerted by the blood on the arterial walls. *A. ulcer*: leg ulcer with an arterial aetiology. Usually on the foot, near the ankle or between the toes. The skin is discoloured, shiny and hairless. Ulcers are small, deep and produce some exudate.

arteriectomy, *(ar-tēr-ē-ek-to-mi)*, excision of part of an artery.

arteriography, a radiographic technique to demonstrate arteries following an injection of radiopaque contrast medium.

arterioles, small arteries with muscular walls which control arterial blood flow to the capillary network. Their ability to constrict and dilate controls peripheral resistance and influences blood pressure.

arteriopathy, disease of the arteries.

arterioplasty, surgery to reform an artery.

arteriorrhaphy, *(ar-tēr-ē-or'-raf-ē)*, suture of an artery.

arteriosclerosis, *(ar-tēr-ē-ō-skler-ō'-sis)*, a degenerative disorder of arteries characterized by hardening of the walls, narrowing of the lumen and loss of elasticity which results in decreased blood flow. Commonly affects the cerebral vessels and those of the lower extremities. *See* ATHEROMA, ATHEROSCLEROSIS.

arteriotomy, incising an artery.

arteriovenous, pertaining to an artery and a vein. *A. aneurysm*: *see* ANEURYSM. *A. shunt*: a communication between an artery and a vein which may be natural, or formed artificially when regular vascular access is required, e.g. for haemodialysis.

arteritis, *(ar-ter-i'-tis)*, inflammation of the arteries.

artery, a vessel carrying blood from the heart.

arthralgia, *(ar-thral'-ji-a)*, joint pain.

arthrectomy, surgical excision of a joint.

arthritis, inflammation of a joint. There are many causes and treatment varies with the cause. *See* JUVENILE CHRONIC ARTHRITIS, OSTEOARTHRITIS, RHEUMATOID ARTHRITIS, SEPTIC ARTHRITIS, STILL'S DISEASE.

arthrocentesis, (ar-thrō-sen-tē′-sis), removal of fluid from within a joint for diagnostic purposes.

arthroclasia, (ar-thrō-klā-si-a), an operation for breaking up an ankylosed joint to produce free movement.

arthrodesis, (ar-thrō-dē′-sis), fixation of a joint by surgery.

arthrodia, a gliding joint.

arthrodynia, (ar-thrō-din′-i-a), pain in the joints.

arthrography, radiographic technique to demonstrate the joint cavity following injection of radiopaque medium.

arthropathy, a joint disease.

arthroplasty, a surgical procedure to form an artificial joint. Commonly performed on the hip and knee joints where plastic, carbon fibre, metal or biological materials are used to refashion or replace diseased or damaged joint structures.

arthropod, a member of the Arthropoda which includes insects, spiders, ticks, mites and crabs.

arthroscopy, endoscopic joint examination using an arthroscope to view the inside of a synovial joint.

arthrotomy, incision into a joint.

Arthus reaction, a localized hypersensitivity (type III) reaction involving immune complexes. It occurs at the site of antigen injection.

articular, pertaining to a joint or joint structures, e.g. articular cartilage.

articulation, 1. a joint between two or more bones. **2.** the enunciation of words.

artifact, an extraneous entity or product produced by artificial means.

artificial insemination, artificial introduction of semen into the vagina. *See* AID, AIH.

artificial pneumothorax, *see* PNEUMOTHORAX.

artificial respiration, a method of life support where spontaneous breathing has ceased or is failing to maintain the blood gases within the normal range. It may be carried out by mouth to mouth/nose respiration or by use of ventilation therapy.

art therapy, the use of a wide range of artwork activities in the restoration of mental health.

arytenoid, (ar-ē-tē-noyd), the two funnel-shaped cartilages of the larynx.

asbestos, a fibrous mineral which is incombustible and a non-conductor of heat. The development of lung cancers and other serious diseases is linked to exposure to the substance. Previously used in fireproofing. *See* MESOTHELIOMA.

asbestosis, chronic lung diseases caused by the inhalation of asbestos dust. Seen in asbestos miners and workers in the building and demolition industries. In the UK asbestosis is a prescribed industrial disease.

ascariasis, (as-kar-ī-a′-sis), infestation of the bowel by nematodes (roundworms) of the genus *Ascaris*. They pass through and may affect the lungs during the larval stage.

ascaricide, (as-kar-ri-sīd), lethal to roundworms, e.g. levamisole.

Ascaris, (as′-kar-is), a genus of parasitic roundworm. *A. lumbricoides*: long roundworm.

Aschoff nodules, (ash-off), the focal necrotic lesions found in the tissues of the heart in rheumatic fever.

ASCII, in computing an acronym for **American Standard Code for Information Interchange.** A format where each text character is represented by a number. Referred to as 'askey'.

ascites, (as-sī′-tēz), excess fluid collection in the peritoneal cavity.

ascorbic acid, vitamin C. A water-soluble vitamin needed in the body for collagen formation and wound healing. Present in fresh fruit and vegetables, especially blackcurrants, potatoes and citrus fruit. *See* NUTRITION APPENDIX.

asepsis, (*ā-sep'-sis*), the state of being free from living pathogenic microorganisms.

aseptic, relating to asepsis. *A. technique*: procedures which exclude pathogenic microorganisms from an environment such as non-touch technique and the use of sterilized equipment.

asexual, (*ā-sek-shūal*), having no sex. A method of reproduction in which there is no gamete formation.

asparagine, (*as-par-aj-ēn*), an amino acid.

aspartame, artificial sweetener. It should be avoided by people with phenylketonuria as it is metabolized to phenylalanine.

aspartate, aspartic acid, an amino acid.

aspartate aminotransferase (AST), (*as-par-tait am-in-ō-tranz-fer-āz*), *see* AMINOTRANSFERASE.

Asperger's syndrome, a syndrome classified as part of the autistic disorders. Associated with various problems with social interaction, communication, expressing emotion and clumsiness.

aspergillosis, (*as-per-gil-ō-sis*), infection caused by a fungal species of the genus *Aspergillus*. May affect the skin, lungs, eyes and ears.

Aspergillus, (*as-per-gil-us*), a genus of fungi; some species are pathogenic to humans.

aspermia, 1. inability to produce or ejaculate semen. **2.** lack of spermatozoa in semen.

asphyxia, (*as-fix-ē-ah*), suffocation. A lack of oxygen and a build up of carbon dioxide in the blood. Causes include: drowning, electrocution, smoke inhalation, blocked airway and poisoning.

aspiration, 1. taking a breath in, inspiration. **2.** procedure to withdraw fluid, by suction or siphonage, from a body cavity. **3.** the entry of fluids or solids into the airway.

aspirator, the apparatus used for aspiration.

assault, threat of unlawful contact.

assay, quantitative test to determine the amount of a specific substance present or its potency, e.g. hormones, drugs.

assertiveness, the ability to express views and achieve needs and recognition in a confident, positive and emphatic manner whilst respecting the views and rights of others. *A. training*: techniques directed at helping individuals to achieve assertiveness and confidence in coping with interpersonal difficulties.

assessment, 1. an appraisal or judgement made about a particular situation or circumstances. A stage of the nursing process involving the collection of information and data relating to patients and their healthcare needs. **2.** a test or measurement of competence.

assimilation, 1. the utilization of digested food molecules by the cells and tissues. **2.** in psychology the process by which new experiences are consolidated into the consciousness.

assisted fertility/conception, techniques which aim to assist infertile couples achieve conception and a successful pregnancy, e.g. in vitro fertilization.

associate nurse, one who assists the primary nurse by effecting an agreed care plan or by acting in their absence. *See* PRIMARY NURSE.

association, coordination. *A. areas of the cortex*: areas of the motor and sensory cortex which integrate impulses. *A. fibres*: fibres which allow communication between individual gyri and between lobes of the same cerebral hemisphere. *A. of ideas*: a link between ideas, where the generation of one idea will trigger a previously connected idea.

AST, abbreviation for **aspartate aminotransferase.** See AMINOTRANSFERASE.

astereognosis, *(a-stēr-ē-og-nō'-sis)*, loss of power to recognize the shape of objects by touch.

asthenia, *(as-the-ne-ah)*, **1.** failure of strength; debility. **2.** in psychiatry a personality which lacks force or drive.

asthenopia, *(as-then-o-pe-ah)*, weakness of sight.

asthma, reversible airflow obstruction characterized by dyspnoea, cough and expiratory wheeze due to bronchospasm. Various types exist which may be precipitated by: extrinsic allergens such as dust or pollen, infection, exercise, poor air quality, cold air and intense emotions. See SEVERE ACUTE ASTHMA (STATUS ASTHMATICUS).

astigmatism, *(as-tig'-ma-tizm)*, a refractive problem caused by defects in the curvature of the lens, it is difficult to focus horizontal and vertical lines at the same time without blurring.

astringent, a substance applied to produce local constriction of blood vessels. Used on heavily exudating wounds.

astrocyte, a neuroglial cell. Supporting star-shaped cells of the central nervous system, they form part of the blood–brain barrier.

astrocytoma, *(as-tro-sī-tō-ma)*, a type of malignant tumour arising in the neuroglia (astrocytes) of the central nervous system.

astrophobia, a phobia involving a fear of stars.

asymmetry, lack of symmetry.

asymptomatic, without any symptoms.

asynclitism, *(a-sin-klit-izm)*, engagement in the pelvis of a diameter of the fetal head other than the biparietal. It may occur with a contracted pelvis.

asynergy, a situation where organs or structures whose functions are normally coordinated stop working together.

asystole, *(a-sis-to-le)*, one form of cardiac arrest where the heart ceases to contract; no PQRST complexes are seen on ECG. See CARDIAC ARREST, ELECTROMECHANICAL DISSOCIATION, VENTRICULAR FIBRILLATION.

atavism, *(at-av-izm)*, the recurrence of some hereditary trait which has missed one or more generations.

ataxia, ataxy, literally, disorder; applied to any defective control of muscles and consequent irregularity of movements. See also LOCOMOTOR ATAXIA and FRIEDREICH'S ATAXIA.

atelectasis, *(at-el-ek-ta-sis)*, **1.** imperfect lung expansion in the newborn. **2.** collapse of lung tissue with consequent reduction in gaseous exchange.

atherogenic, *(a-the-rō-jen-ik)*, applied to factors which may cause atheroma.

atheroma, plaques of fatty (lipid) material deposited in the walls of arteries.

atherosclerosis, *(a-the-rō-skle-rō-sis)*, coexisting atheroma and arteriosclerosis, extremely common degenerative arterial disease. It is characterized by the deposition of atheromatous plaques with damage, calcification and hardening of the walls of large and medium sized arteries (Figure 8). These changes lead to narrowing of the vessel

8 Atherosclerosis

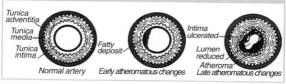

Tunica adventitia
Tunica media
Tunica intima
Fatty deposit

Normal artery

Early atheromatous changes

Intima ulcerated
Lumen reduced
Atheroma

Late atheromatous changes

lumen and reduced blood flow. A major cause of coronary heart disease; angina pectoris and myocardial infarction.

athetoid, relating to athetosis.

athetosis, *(ath-e-tō'-sis)*, a condition marked by continous and purposeless movements, especially of the hands and feet.

athlete's foot, *see* TINEA PEDIS.

atlas, first cervical vertebra.

atmosphere, 1. the air surrounding the earth, consisting of nitrogen (78%), oxygen (20%), carbon dioxide (0.04%) and inert gases with variable amounts of water vapour. **2.** a unit of gas pressure which is equal to average atmospheric pressure at sea level—101.3 kPa (760 mm Hg). Atmospheric pressure decreases with altitude and increases with depth, e.g. deep mines or under the sea.

atom, the smallest part of an element that exhibits the characteristics of that element and is capable of existing individually, or in combination with one or more atoms of the same or another element.

atomic, pertaining to atoms. *A. mass unit (amu) or Dalton*: a relative unit of weight used for measuring atoms and subatomic particles. The weight of a neutron and a proton have each been designated as being 1 amu. *A. number*: the number of protons (which always equal the number

of electrons) in an atom of a particular element. *A. weight or mass*: also known as *relative atomic mass*. The relative average mass of an atom based on the mass of an atom of carbon-12.

atomizer, nebulizer.

atonic, weak. Lacking tone, e.g. a flaccid muscle.

atony, wanting in muscular tone or vigour; weakness.

atopy, a familial condition where some individuals have an increased allergic response to certain allergens. There is a tendency to eczema, allergic rhinitis (hayfever) and asthma.

ATP, abbreviation for **adenosine triphosphate.**

atresia, absence of a natural passage. Closure of a duct.

atria, *(sing.* **atrium***)*, *(ā-tri-a)*, two thin-walled upper receiving chambers of the heart.

atrial, pertaining to the atria. *A. fibrillation*: cardiac arrhythmia caused by the independent contraction of the muscle bundles in the atrial walls. There is no coordinated atrial contraction and the ventricular contractions are stimulated irregularly. *A. flutter*: an arrhythmia where the atria contract in a rapid but regular manner, usually between 250 and 300/min. Only one in two or three impulses reach the ventricles. *A. natriuretic peptides*: peptides

33

produced by the cardiac atria. They help to control blood pressure by inhibiting the release of vasopressin and aldosterone when the blood pressure rises. *A. septal defect (ASD)*: congential heart defect in which there is an opening between the atria.

atrioventricular (A-V), *(a-trē-ō-ven-trik'-ū-lar)*, pertaining to the heart chambers; atria and ventricles. *A-V block*: a defect in the conduction of impulses between the atria and ventricles. Results in varying degrees of heart block. *A-V bundle/bundle of His*: part of the cardiac conduction system. Specialized non-contractile muscle cells in the ventricular septum which conduct impulses from the A-V node to the ventricles. *A-V node*: part of the cardiac conduction system. Specialized cells, situated at the bottom of the right atrium, which conduct the impulse from the sinoatrial node to the A-V bundle. *A-V valves*: the valves between the atria and ventricles; bicuspid and tricuspid.

atrophy, *(at'-ro-fi)*, wasting of an organ or structure from disuse, disease or injury. Atrophy also occurs as part of normal ageing.

atropine, principal alkaloid of belladonna. *See* MUSCARINIC.

attachment, 1. state of being joined. **2.** in psychology the dependent relationship which one person forms with another, originating from the unique bonding between infant and parent figure.

attention, ability to select some stimuli for closer inspection while discarding others deemed less important.

attention deficit hyperactivity disorder (ADHD), behavioural disorder of children. It is characterized by poor attention/concentration, increased motor activity and impulsive behaviour. Also known as attention deficit syndrome.

attenuation, in microbiology the process by which vaccines are prepared which retain the antigenicity of the microorganism without its pathogenicity.

attitude, 1. position or posture of body. **2.** an opinion or perspective. A way of thinking.

atypical, not typical, e.g. *A. pneumonia* which does not follow the usual pattern.

audiology, science dealing with hearing ability and the non-medical management of hearing defects.

audiometry, measurement of hearing ability. Using an audiometer the results obtained are plotted as an audiogram to show how the ear responds to sounds of a different pitch.

audit, the investigative methods used to measure outcomes and review performance. *A. commission*: promotes 'best practice' in terms of economy, effectiveness and efficiency within the NHS. *A. trail*: a way of working and record keeping that allows the process to be transparent and clear. *Nursing a.*: an investigation into outcomes and standards of nursing care. It may be concurrent or retrospective.

auditory, pertaining to the sense of audition (hearing). *A. canal*: the canal leading from the outside to the tympanic membrane. *A. nerve*: vestibulocochlear. The eighth cranial nerve which innervates the cochlea (audition) and the vestibular apparatus (balance).

aura, a sensation; auditory, optic, olfactory etc. which may precede an epileptic seizure or migraine.

aural, pertaining to the ear.

auricle, 1. the pinna of the external ear. **2.** an appendage to the atrium. *See* HEART.

auricular, pertaining to the ear.

auriscope, *See* OTOSCOPE.

auscultation, listening to sounds of the body for the purpose of diagnosis. Usually a tube is employed, e.g. a stethoscope.

Australia antigen, term previously used to describe hepatitis B surface antigen (HBs Ag).

autism, a spectrum of disorders usually first recognized in childhood. It is characterized by poor social skills, communication difficulties, poor language development, fantasy, isolation and withdrawal frequently continuing into adult life. *See* ASPERGER'S SYNDROME.

autistic, pertaining to autism.

autoantibodies, immunoglobulins which destroy part of the body, e.g. red blood cells in autoimmune haemolytic anaemia.

autoclave, an apparatus for sterilizing by steam under pressure.

autoeroticism, *(awt-ō-er-ot'-is-izm),* sexual self-gratification through masturbation, fantasy etc.

autogenics, a complementary therapy which combines relaxation and self-hypnosis.

autogenous, *(aw-to'j-en-us),* self-produced.

autograft, a graft using tissue transplanted from one site to another in the same person, e.g. skin graft.

autohypnosis, self-induced hypnotism.

autoimmune, the production of immunoglobulins (autoantibodies) or cell mediated immunity against some body component. *A. diseases:* group of diseases where body cell antigens stimulate an immunological reaction within the body. They include: Hashimoto's thyroiditis,

rheumatoid arthritis, haemolytic anaemia and Addison's disease.

autoinfection, infection caused by a microorganism already present on or in the body.

autointoxication, poisoning by toxins produced by the body, e.g. products of metabolism.

autologous blood transfusion (ABT), a transfusion of a person's own blood that had been withdrawn previously and stored until required.

autolysis, a process of tissue digestion by enzymes produced in the body. It may occur as a physiological process, e.g. the uterus during the puerperium or as a pathological process.

automatism, *(awt-ōm-at-izm),* a condition in which actions are performed without consciousness or regulated purpose; sometimes follows an epileptic seizure.

autonomic nervous system, the part of the nervous system which controls involuntary functions such as heart rate, glandular secretion and smooth muscle. *See* SYMPATHETIC, PARASYMPATHETIC.

autonomy, ability to act independently and without supervision or control.

autoplasty, *see* AUTOGRAFT.

autopsy, a post-mortem examination.

autoregulation, the homeostatic mechanisms by which certain organs control their immediate environment, e.g. renal blood flow is regulated by mechanisms initiated by the kidney.

autorhythmic, describes cells such as those in the sinoatrial node, capable of producing an action potential without innervation.

autosome, one of forty-four (twenty-two pairs) non-sex chromosomes. With the two sex chromosomes (one pair) they form the full complement of forty-six (twenty-three pairs) found in somatic cells. Autosomal inheritance occurs through the expression or not of genes situated on an autosome.

autosuggestion, self-suggestion with the uncritical acceptance of the ideas originating within the person's own mind.

autotransfusion, infusion, after suitable treatment, of blood collected from a sterile site during haemorrhage from the body.

avascular, (*ā-vas-kū-la*), bloodless, e.g. heart valves, cornea. *A. necrosis*: tissue death caused when it is deprived of blood, as in the femoral head following some types of femoral neck fractures.

aversion, an intense dislike. *A. therapy*: a treatment using deconditioning. May be effective in some forms of addiction.

avian, pertaining to birds. *A. tubercle* or *Mycobacterium avium intracellulare*: an atypical mycobacterium that can infect humans.

avidin, substance in raw egg white which inhibits the absorption of biotin.

avirulent, not virulent.

avitaminosis, (*ā-vi-ta-mi-nō'-sis*), lacking in vitamins. Usually the particular vitamin deficiency is specified, e.g. *a.A.*

Avogadro's number, (*av-ō-gad-rōz*), *See* MOLE.

avoidance, the use of a defence mechanism to avoid feelings, thoughts or situations that the person finds difficult.

avulsion, a tearing apart.

axilla, the armpit.

axillary, pertaining to the axilla. Applied to the artery, vein and nerve.

axis, 1. a straight line through the centre of a body. **2.** the second cervical vertebra.

axon, (*aks-on*), the long process of a nerve cell conducting impulses away from the cell body.

axonplasm, the cytoplasm in an axon.

axonotmesis, (*ak-son-ō-tmē- sis*), damage causing the break-up of nerve fibres but leaving the supporting tissue intact.

azoospermia, (*ā'-zo-ō-sper'-mi-a*), absence of viable sperms in the semen causing male sterility.

azotaemia, (*az-ō-tē-mi-a*), abnormal amounts of nitrogenous compounds such as urea in the blood.

azygous, (*ā-zī'-gus*), not paired but single, e.g. a. vein.

B

Babinski's reflex, extensor plantar reflex. Extension instead of flexion of the great toe on stroking the sole of the foot. The sign is normal in infants and abnormal after about 2 years.

bacillary, pertaining to bacilli. *B. dysentery*: serious gut infection caused by bacteria of the *Shigella* genus. *See* SHIGELLA.

Bacille-Calmette-Guérin, *See* BCG.

Bacillus, a genus of Gram-positive microorganisms belonging to the family Bacillaceae. *B. anthracis*: bacterium causing anthrax. *B. cereus*: produces exotoxins which cause food poisoning.

bacillus, a general term applied to any rod-shaped bacterium.

back-up, in computing, data storage by copying from the hard disk to floppy disk or tape. Back-ups should form part of a regular and frequent routine and be kept safely in case the original data is lost.

bacteraemia, *(bak-ter-ē-mi-a),* bacteria in the blood.

bacteria, *(sing.* **bacterium),** microscopic unicellular organisms widely distributed in a variety of different environments. May be pathogenic (disease producing) in humans, other animals and plants or non-pathogenic; some serve useful functions, e.g. production of an environment which is hostile to pathogens such as lactobacilli in the adult vaginal flora. Non-pathogens may become pathogenic if they move from their normal site, a common example being a urinary infection caused by organisms normally found in the gut flora. Bacteria generally multiply by simple binary fission when environmental conditions are suitable. Some types have developed various physical and biochemical adaptations which allow them to exploit environments and survive hostile conditions, e.g. flagella, waxy outer capsules, spore formation and enzymes which destroy antibacterial drugs. Bacteria are classified and identified by criteria which include: shape and outer coat staining characteristics with Gram stain (positive or negative). The main forms (Figure 9) are: **1.** cocci, round in shape; some are paired – diplococci; some form chains – streptococci; and others bunches – staphylococci. Some important pathogenic cocci include: *Staphylococcus aureus, Streptococcus pyogenes* and *Neisseria meningitidis*. **2.** bacilli, rod-shaped. Important pathogenic bacilli include: *Escherichia coli, Haemophilus influenzae, Clostridium tetani* and *Mycobacterium tuberculosis* (acid-fast bacilli). **3.** spiral forms – spirilla, curved vibrios and spirochaetes which are corkscrew-shaped. This group includes *Vibrio cholerae, Treponema pallidum* and *Leptospira icterohaemorrhagiae*.

bacterial, pertaining to bacteria.

bactericidal, *(bak-teer-ē-sī'-dal),* capable of destroying bacteria.

bacteriologist, one who specializes in the study of bacteria.

9 Bacterial shapes

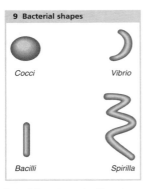

Cocci   Vibrio

Bacilli   Spirilla

bacteriology, the study of bacteria.

bacteriolysin, a specific antibody developed in the blood to destroy bacteria.

bacteriolytic, capable of dissolving bacteria.

bacteriophage, *(bak-teer-ē-ō-fāj)*, viruses which are parasitic on bacteria; they are specific to a particular bacterial strain and may be used to identify certain bacteria. *See* PHAGE TYPING.

bacteriostatic, *(bak-teer-ē-ō-stat´-ik)*, capable of preventing bacterial growth or multiplication.

bacteriuria, presence of bacteria in the urine, but for the purposes of diagnosing an asymptomatic urinary infection there must be at least 10^5 colony-forming organisms per ml of freshly voided urine.

Bainbridge reflex, increased venous return to the heart causes a reflex increase in heart rate. It operates through stretch receptors in the right atrium and sympathetic nerves.

Baker's cysts, cysts associated with the knee joint, they are formed when synovial fluid escapes from a bursa.

balance of probabilities, the standard of proof needed in civil legal proceedings.

balanitis, *(bal-an-ī-tis)*, inflammation of the glans penis.

Balkan beam/frame, frame fitted over a bed for the attachment of slings or to support the weights and pulleys required for traction.

balloon angioplasty, *see* ANGIOPLASTY.

ballottement, technique used to palpate a floating object or organ. Used in pregnancy, the uterus is pressed and the fetus can be felt as it floats back to its original position. May be elicited abdominally and vaginally.

bandage, an appliance made from a variety of materials, used to give support, immobilize, apply pressure or secure a dressing.

Bandl's ring, *see* RETRACTION RING.

Bankart's operation, operation to repair the glenoid cavity after repeated dislocation of the shoulder joint.

Banti's syndrome, characterized by anaemia, gastrointestinal bleeding, leucopenia, splenomegaly, hepatic portal hypertension and liver cirrhosis.

barbiturates, *(bar-bit-ūr-āts)*, sedative/hypnotic drugs derived from barbituric acid, use limited to general anaesthesia and epilepsy due to addiction problems.

barbotage, *(bar-bo-tahzh)*, a technique to ensure dilution and mixing of the drug with cerebrospinal fluid by repeated partial injection and withdrawal during the administration of a spinal anaesthetic.

barium sulphate, salt which is insoluble in water and opaque to X-rays. Used as a contrast agent for gastrointestinal radiographic examination, e.g. *B. enema, B. meal* and *swallow.*

Barlow's disease, infantile scurvy.

Barlow's sign, used as one of the tests for the diagnosis of developmental dysplasia of the hip (congenital dislocation) in the newborn. See ORTOLANI'S TEST, DEVELOPMENTAL DYSPLASIA OF THE HIP.

baroreceptors, specialized nerve endings able to monitor pressure changes, they are situated in the aortic arch, carotid sinus, cardiac atria, venae cavae and the internal ear.

barotrauma, (bar-ō-traw-mah), trauma caused by environmental pressure changes, e.g. the damage to the tympanic membrane following an explosion.

Barr body, in normal females a small condensation of sex chromatin present in the nucleus of non-dividing cells; an inactive X chromosome.

barrier nursing, precautions used to contain an existing infection: isolation, handwashing, protective clothing and proper disposal of excreta/body fluids, etc. See ISOLATION.

bartholinitis, inflammation of Bartholin's glands.

Bartholin's glands (greater vestibular glands), (bah-to-lins), two small glands situated either side of the vagina whose ducts open into the vestibule. They produce lubricating mucus which increases during sexual stimulation to facilitate coitus. See SKENE'S GLANDS

basal cell carcinoma, (bā-sal sel kahsin-ō-ma), a malignant epithelial tumour. See RODENT ULCER.

basal ganglia, (bā-sal gan-gli-a), see BASAL NUCLEI.

basal metabolism, the energy consumed at complete rest for the essential physiological functions, e.g. respiration. Basal metabolic rate (BMR) is the rate at which energy is used at rest. BMR is calculated indirectly by measuring the amount of oxygen used over a given time and is expressed as kJ or kcal per square metre body surface area per hour (kJ or kcal/m^2 per h). Adult males need about 40 kcal/m^2 per h and females 37 kcal/m^2 per h.

basal nuclei, isolated masses of grey matter deep within the white matter of the cerebral hemispheres. Part of the extrapyramidal motor pathways are important in modifying voluntary movements and initiating slow and prolonged motor activities. Their proper functioning depends upon the release of the neurotransmitter dopamine. Sometimes called **ganglia,** which more properly describes structures in the peripheral nervous system.

base, (bās), **1.** the bottom. **2.** the main constituent of a mixture. **3.** alkali substance which reacts with an acid to form a salt and water. See ALKALI.

basement membrane, a very thin tissue layer which separates epithelium from underlying structures.

BASIC, in computing an acronym for **Beginner's All-purpose Symbolic Instruction Code.** A computer language used for writing programs.

basic life support (BLS), a term describing the maintenance of a clear airway and cardiopulmonary resuscitation.

basilar, pertaining to the base. B. artery: formed by the unification of the two vertebral arteries. B. membrane: forms part of the cochlea.

basilic, superficial veins of the forearm. They are often used for taking blood samples and for intravenous infusions and injections.

basophil, (ba-so-fil), a polymorphonuclear leucocyte with an affinity for basic dyes, it is the least abundant leucocyte. Its cytoplasm contains granules of histamine and heparin. Basophils bind to antibodies prior to releasing chemicals involved in inflammation and anaphylaxis. *See* MAST CELLS.

basophilia, *(ba-so-fil-ē-ah),* **1.** an increase in basophil numbers. **2.** abnormal basophilic staining seen in red blood cells in conditions such as lead poisoning.

Batchelor plaster, type of double abduction plaster, with the legs in full abduction and medial rotation.

bath, 1. vessel used for bathing. **2.** immersion of the body or part of the body in water for various purposes: cleansing, analgesic and sedative effects. **3.** medicated baths: antiseptic as infection prophylaxis prior to invasive techniques, wax baths for the hands to relieve pain and joint stiffness in arthritis.

battered baby syndrome, *see* NON-ACCIDENTAL INJURY.

battledore placenta, a placenta in which the umbilical cord is inserted into the edge instead of the centre.

battery, an unlawful touching.

Bazin's disease, erythema induratum, a recurrent tuberculous infection of the skin. Reddish or purple nodules, which may ulcerate, appear on the legs.

BBVs, abbreviation for **blood-borne viruses,** such as hepatitis B and C, and HIV, that are transmitted in blood and body fluids.

BCG, abbreviation for **Bacille of Calmette-Guérin,** live attenuated strain of *Mycobacterium bovis* used to produce a vaccine against tuberculosis.

BEAM, abbreviation for **brain electrical activity mapping,** a technique used during electroencephalography.

bearing down, popular term for the expulsive contractions during the second stage of labour.

beat, applied to the beating of the heart and pulsation of blood within arteries. *See* APEX BEAT

Beck depression inventory, self-administered inventory for measuring depression.

Beck's triad, signs of cardiac tamponade: decrease in arterial pressure, increase in venous pressure and reduction in heart sounds.

becquerel (Bq), *(bek-er-el),* derived SI unit of radioactivity, equals radioactive disintegration per second. Replaces the curie.

bed, 1. device used for support during sleep and rest. Some have specialized uses such as pressure relief. **2.** in anatomy, a supportive structure such as the nail bed. **3.** capillary bed, the term applied to the network of small blood vessels within an organ or structure, which connect arteries and veins.

bedbug, a blood-sucking insect, *Cimex lectularius.* Lives in furniture and bedding.

bedpan, device used by bedbound patients for the reception of urine and faeces.

bed sore, obsolete term. *See* PRESSURE ULCER.

bedwetting, *see* ENURESIS.

behaviour, conduct; or response to stimuli. *B.* modification: forms of therapy which seek to change undesirable or maladaptive behaviour patterns. Also called *b.* therapy.

behaviour change, health education approach that encourages people to make lifestyle changes, e.g. dietary.

behaviourism, a set of psychological theories associated with the use of conditioning to change behaviour.

bejel, a form of non-venereal syphilis found in the Middle East, Asia, sub-Saharan Africa and Australia.

beliefs, a set of ideas and thoughts which individuals use to construct their views and behaviour. They are formed by culture, family, life experiences and many other factors.

belle indifference, *(bel),* a lack of concern or emotion in an obviously distressing situation. A feature of hysteria.

Bell's paralysis, paralysis of the facial nerve (VIIth cranial).

Bence Jones protein, an abnormal protein produced by myeloma cells, excreted in the urine in some cases of malignant myeloma. *See* MULTIPLE MYELOMA, MYELOMATOSIS.

benchmarking, a quality assurance process. Involves the identification of best practice in similar areas. Benchmark scores are identified, against which individual units can compare their practice.

bends, decompression sickness. *See* CAISSON DISEASE.

beneficence, doing good. An ethical ideal which also involves preventing harm and promoting good. *Cf.* NON-MALEFICENCE.

benign, non-malignant, innocent. *B. hyperplasia of the prostate,* common cause of prostatic enlargement, leading to urethral obstruction in older men.

Bennett's fracture, fracture of the base of the first metacarpal due to a blow on the base of the thumb.

benzene, a toxic hydrocarbon derived from coal tar. Exposure can lead to anaemia and leukaemia.

benzodiazepines, a large group of anxiolytic drugs widely used to reduce anxiety, e.g. diazepam. Dependence and withdrawal symptoms may occur following prolonged use. They are subject to considerable misuse.

benzyl benzoate, *(ben-zō-āt),* liquid preparation used in the treatment of scabies.

bereavement, the response to the death of a loved one, but could also be applied to some other considerable loss.

beriberi, a disease due to deficiency of vitamin B_1 (thiamine) characterized by polyneuropathy, muscle wasting, oedema, dyspnoea and eventual heart failure. *See* KORSAKOFF'S PSYCHOSIS, WERNICKE'S ENCEPHALOPATHY.

beryllosis, *(ber-il-ē-ō'-sis),* industrial lung disease due to the inhalation of beryllium which causes interstitial fibrosis.

bestiality, 1. animal-like or brutal behaviour. **2.** sexual relations between a human and an animal.

beta (β), second letter of Greek alphabet. *B. blocker. See* BETA (β)-ADRENOCEPTOR ANTAGONISTS. *B. cells:* endocrine cells of the islets of Langerhans in the pancreas, they produce the hormone insulin which lowers blood glucose levels. *B. lactamase:* enzyme produced by some bacteria, e.g. *Staphylococcus aureus,* that allows them to inactivate B. lactam antibiotics. *B. oxidation:* a process by which fatty acids are converted to acetyl CoA prior to the production of energy (ATP). *B. phase:* the period which follows the alpha redistribution phase of drug administration, it is characterized by a slow decline in drug blood levels during its metabolism and excretion. *B. rays:* a type of ionizing radiation emitted as a radioactive isotope disintegrates. They consist of electrons which penetrate tissue to a greater depth than alpha rays. *B. receptors: see* ADRENERGIC RECEPTORS. *B. state:* alert wakefulness associated with thinking and concentration. *B. stimulators. See* BETA (β)-ADRENOCEPTOR AGONISTS. *B. wave (rhythm):* brain wave pattern seen when the individual is in the beta state. The waves are more irregular than alpha waves and have a frequency between 14 and 25 Hz.

beta (β)-adrenoceptor agonists, drugs that stimulate beta-adrenoceptors (adrenergic), e.g. dobutamide and terbutaline. Also known as beta-stimulators.

beta (β)-adrenoceptor antagonists, drugs that prevent stimulation of beta-adrenoceptors (adrenergic) in the myocardium and other sites, e.g. atenolol, etc. Also known as beta-blockers.

beta (β)-lactam antibiotics, antibiotics such as penicillins, cephalosporins and others used less commonly, such as the carbapenems. They all contain a beta-lactam ring in their structure which many bacteria can destroy to stop the antibiotic working.

Betz cells, pyramidal cells. Neurones in the motor cortex which control voluntary muscle contraction.

bibliographical databases, details of papers, etc., but abstracts and full article sometimes available electronically via CD-ROM or the internet, e.g. CINAHL, Medline.

bicarbonate, hydrogen carbonate. Salt of carbonic acid. *Serum b.*: an important buffer system in the blood. *See* ALKALI RESERVE.

bicephalus, (*bī-kef-al-us*), having two heads.

biceps, the two-headed muscle anterior to the humerus.

biconcave, hollow or concave on both sides, usually of a lens.

biconvex, bulging or convex on both sides, usually of a lens.

bicornuate, having two horns. *B. uterus*: a developmental abnormality where the uterus has two horns or has two compartments.

bicuspid, having two cusps or points. *B. teeth*: the premolars. *B. value* or *mitral*: the left atrioventricular valve.

bifid, cleft, two parts.

bifocal, with a double focus. *B. spectacles* can be used for near and distant vision.

bifurcate, forked.

bigeminal, (*bī-je-mi-nal*), occurring in two pairs.

bilateral, two-sided. Pertaining to both sides.

bile, green/yellow viscous alkaline fluid produced by the liver as a result of red blood cell breakdown. Between 500 and 1000 ml of bile is produced daily; it consists of water, bile acids, bile salts, mucin, lecithin, bile pigments, cholesterol, enzymes, electrolytes and molecules for excretion such as drug metabolites. Bile drains into the intestine where it helps to provide an alkaline environment, emulsifies fat globules prior to their digestion, facilitates the absorption of fat-soluble vitamins, stimulates peristalsis and deodorizes faeces. *B. acids*. organic acids; cholic and chenodeoxycholic found in bile. *B. ducts*: hepatic, cystic and common bile ducts which convey bile from the liver, via the gallbladder, to the duodenum (Figure 10). *B. pigments*: bilirubin (red) and biliverdin (green) derived from the haem molecule during red cell breakdown. *B. salts*: conjugated bile acids (joined with glycine and taurine) form the sodium salts – sodium glycocholate and sodium taurocholate.

Bilharzia, (*bil-harts-ē-ah*), *see* SCHISTOSOMA, SCHISTOSOMIASIS.

biliary, pertaining to bile, gallbladder and ducts *B. atresia*: congenital narrowing or absence of bile duct or other biliary structure. Requires surgical treatment, including liver transplant in some cases. *B. calculus*: Stone which form in the gallbladder and may move to the ducts. *B. colic.*

---

10 Bile ducts

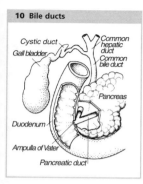

severe pain caused by the movement of a gallstone within the biliary tract.

bilious, connected with bile. Term often used to denote nausea.

bilirubin, *(bil-ē-rū'-bin), see* BILE PIGMENTS.

bilirubinuria, *(bil-ē-rū'-bin-ur'-ē-a),* presence of bilirubin in the urine.

biliuria, *(bil-ē-ūr'-ē-a),* presence of bile in the urine. Choluria.

biliverdin, *(bil-ē-ver'-din), see* BILE PIGMENTS.

Billroth's gastrectomy, 1. a partial gastrectomy where the remaining part of the stomach is joined to the duodenum. **2.** part of the stomach and duodenum are removed, the gastric remnant being joined to the jejunum.

bimanual, with the use of both hands.

binary, having two parts. *B. fission:* division of a cell into two equal daughter cells. *B. system:* the base 2 system of numbers where digits are either 0 or 1. For example 1, 2, 3, 4, 5, 6, 7 become 1, 10, 11, 100, 101, 110, 111. Used in digital computer processes. *B. digit: see* BIT, BYTE.

binaural, pertaining to both ears.

binge – purge syndrome, *see* BULIMIA.

binocular, relating to both eyes.

binovular, produced by two ova. *B. twins.* develop from two separate ova fertilized at the same time. The twins are no more alike than siblings born at separate times and may be different sexes.

bioassay, quantitative estimation of biologically active substances such as hormones.

bioavailability, the proportion of substance, e.g. nutrient or drug, that enters the circulation in an active form.

biochemistry, the chemistry of living organisms and organic molecules.

biofeedback, a conditioning process by which an individual may gain control over an autonomic function, e.g. blood pressure, following the provision of sufficient positive stimuli when optimal levels are reached.

biofilm, the collection of microorganisms and their protein products adhering to a surface, such as an indwelling urinary catheter.

bioflavenoid, general term for the coloured substances found in many fruits and vegetables, e.g. grapes, citrus fruits, broccoli and tomatoes. Also present in red wine and tea, they may be protective against cancer and heart disease and some have antibacterial properties.

biohazard, a hazard to health posed by biological material, e.g. body fluids contact, needstick injuries.

biological, 1. pertaining to biology. **2.** any substance prepared from a living organism or its products. *B. half-life:* the time taken for the body to excrete or inactivate half the amount of an administered substance. *See* HALF-LIFE. *B. response modifier (BRM):* cancer therapies based on manipulation of the immune processes. Substances, such as interferons, are used to stimulate the person's immune cells to destroy the cancer cells.

biology, the science of life and living organisms.

biopsy, 1. tissue removed from the living body for examination. **2.** the removal of tissue from the living body for examination.

biorhythms, the cyclical pattern of biological functions unique to each individual, such as variations in body temperature, sleep–wake cycles and menstrual cycle.

BIOS, in computing an acronym for **Basic Input/Output Systems**. Describes programs which are permanently embedded in a chip (ROM) and are used by operating systems to perform basic input/output tasks.

biosocial, pertaining to biological and social components of life.

biotin, a vitamin of the B complex. *See* NUTRITION APPENDIX.

Biot's respiration, (bē'-ō), abnormal breathing pattern characterized by irregular pauses in respiration.

bipolar, having two poles. *B. affective disorder.* a major affective condition with both depression and mania. *B. nerve cell:* nerve cell with both afferent and efferent processes. *B. version: see* VERSION.

birth, act of being born. *B. mark:* congenital naevus. *B. paralysis.* paralysis caused by birth injury. *See* ERB'S PALSY. *B. rate:* the number of births as a proportion of a population. Expressed as numbers of live births per 1000 of population in one year. It can be applied to women aged 15–44 years to calculate a fertility rate.

bisexual, 1. being of both sexes, hermaphrodite. **2.** being sexually attracted to both male and female.

bismuth, a grey metal used as a mild astringent and in preparations for the treatment of peptic ulcers.

bistoury, (bis-too-re), a surgical knife.

bit, acronym for binary digit. In computing the smallest unit of data storage. It represents 1 or 0 and can be viewed in simple terms as an on/off switch. *See* BINARY, BYTE.

Bitot's spots, (bī-tōz), shiny spots on the conjunctiva associated with vitamin A deficiency.

bivalent, 1. pair of synapsed homologous chromosomes. Also called divalent. **2.** in chemistry any substance with a valence of two.

bivalve, having two valves or blades. A plaster cast divided into two.

bivariate statistics, descriptive statistics that compare the relationship between two variables.

blackwater fever, a form of malaria characterized by haemolysis of red blood cells. There is high fever, haemoglobinuria which causes dark urine, jaundice and renal failure.

bladder, a hollow organ for the reception of fluid. *atonic b.:* urinary bladder with no tone – the detrusor muscle has lost its contractility, resulting in incomplete voiding or an inability to void at all. *Urinary b.:* receives and acts as temporary storage for urine from the kidneys. *See also* GALLBLADDER.

Blalock–Taussig procedure, formation of a shunt – the subclavian artery is anastomosed to the pulmonary artery. Performed in cases of congenital pulmonary stenosis. *See* FALLOT'S TETRALOGY.

blast cell, an immature cell.

blastocyst, (blas-tō-sist), early embryonic stage that follows the morula. Consists of trophoblast cells around a fluid filled cavity and an inner cell mass.

blastoderm, layer of cells forming the blastocyst. It eventually gives rise to the primary germ layers, ectoderm, mesoderm, endoderm, from which the embryo will develop.

blastoma, a tumour which originates from primitive embryonic tissue of an organ.

Blastomyces, (blas-tō-mī-sēz), a genus of pathogenic fungi, *B. dermatitidis.*

blastomycosis, (blas-tō-mī-kō'sis), the granulomatous condition caused by the fungus *B. dermatitidis.* It affects the lungs, lymph nodes, skin, viscera and bones.

blastula, see BLASTOCYST.

bleb, large blister.

bleeding time, the duration of bleeding following puncture of the skin as of the ear lobe.

blennorrhoea, (blen-o-rē-ab), **1.** purulent conjunctivitis. **2.** excess discharge of mucus.

blepharadenitis, (blef-ar-ad-en-ī'-tis), inflammation of the Meibomian glands.

blepharitis, inflammation of the eyelids.

blepharoptosis, (blef-ar-op-tō'-sis), see PTOSIS.

blepharospasm, spasm of the muscle around the eye.

blind loop syndrome, associated with situations leading to intestinal stasis, e.g. gastrointestinal surgery or small bowel abnormalities. Excessive proliferation of bacteria occurs, causing diarrhoea and malabsorption of nutrients. Also called stagnant loop syndrome.

blind spot, point where the optic nerve fibres leave the retina; without rods or cones it is insensitive to light.

blindness, lack of sight or visual impairment. Causes worldwide include: macular degeneration, retinopathy, glaucoma, cataracts, infections such as trachoma, trauma, vitamin A deficiency and tumours. *Colour b.*: an inability to distinguish certain colours. *Cortical b.*: blindness due to a lesion of the visual centre in the brain. *Night b.* or *nyctalopia*: vision subnormal at night, may be due to a deficiency of vitamin A in the diet. *Snow b.*: dimness of vision with pain and lacrimation due to the glare of sunlight upon snow. *Word b.*: inability to recognize familiar written words owing to a lesion of the brain.

blister, a collection of serum between the layers of the skin. A bleb, a vesicle.

blood, the red alkaline (pH 7.35–7.45 in health) fluid connective tissue which circulates within the vascular system; the normal adult volume is approximately 5–6 litres dependent on body size. Blood transports nutrients, water and oxygen to the cells and removes the waste products of metabolism. It distributes heat and carries various substances – hormones, drugs and antibodies – to areas where they are needed. It is divided into two parts, a fluid called plasma and a cellular component. Plasma is yellow and consists of water, proteins which include albumin, globulin and fibrinogen and electrolytes (inorganic ions) such as sodium, chloride and potassium. Blood cells form approximately 45% of the volume and are of several types: **1.** red cells or erythrocytes which contain the pigment haemoglobin; they are concerned with the transport of oxygen, some carbon dioxide and buffering pH changes. **2.** white cells or leucocytes, of which there are five main types: polymorphonuclear cells (granulocytes) of three varieties (neutrophils, basophils and eosinophils), monocytes and lymphocytes large and small. White cells provide protection against infection by their ability to destroy microorganisms by phagocytosis and the production of specific antibodies. Certain white cells are able to differentiate between 'self and non-self', a process known as cell-mediated immunity. The white cell will attempt to destroy foreign tissue or material entering the body; during transplant surgery drugs are given to suppress this function and prevent rejection of the donor tissue. **3.** platelets or thrombocytes are cell fragments involved in the clotting process. *See* BLOOD CLOTTING, BLOOD COUNT and BLOOD GROUPS.

blood–brain barrier (BBB), a protective barrier which helps the brain maintain a stable internal chemical environment. A special structural arrangement of capillary endothelial cells and astrocytes ensures that the capillary wall is relatively impermeable. It allows the entry of nutrients but generally prevents the passage of harmful substances. There are, however, exceptions – alcohol and certain drugs. In babies and young children the barrier is less effective and allows the passage of harmful substances, e.g. bile pigment and lead.

blood casts, casts containing blood cells which form in the renal tubules. They appear in the urine in some renal diseases.

blood clotting, involves a very complex system of chemical reactions which use enzyme cascades to initiate clotting. When tissue is damaged or platelets break down, enzyme complexes known as thromboplastins are released. These, in the presence of calcium ions, convert inactive prothrombin to the active enzyme thrombin. The plasma pro-

tein fibrinogen reacts with thrombin to become insoluble fibrin which forms a network of strands in which blood cells are trapped to form a clot. There are several other factors active in the process, e.g. anti-haemophilic globulin (factor VIII).

blood count, microscopic examination of a venous blood sample to determine the types, condition and numbers of cells present. A typical count for a healthy adult would be: red cells: $4.5–6.5 \times 10^{12}$ litre; white cells: $4.0–11.0 \times 10^9$ litre. If the number of the different white cells is determined it is called a differential white cell count; this is expressed in percentages: neutrophils 60–70%, basophils 0–1%, eosinophils 1–4%, lymphocytes 25–35%, monocytes 4–8%, and immature cells 4%. Platelets or thrombocytes $150–400 \times 10^9$ litre. *See* HAEMOGLOBIN, COLOUR INDEX, MCV, MCH, MCHC.

blood culture, incubation of a blood sample to allow the growth of any bacteria, which can then be examined and identified using a microscope. *See* BACTERAEMIA, SEPTICAEMIA.

blood groups, blood groups are genetically determined by the presence or not of certain antigens (agglutinogens) upon the red blood cell surface. In 1900 Landsteiner discovered that human blood can be classified into four groups – A, B, AB and O, according to the presence of A and B antigens. Group A = A antigen, group B = B antigen, group AB = A and B antigens and group O = none. In addition the plasma contains antibodies (agglutinins) which are specific to the antigens not carried by the person; group A = anti B, group B = anti A, group AB = none and group O = anti A and anti B. It is this antibody which agglutinates (clumps) donor red cells if an incompatible transfusion occurs. For most transfusion purposes group A can have A and O blood, group B can have B and O blood, group AB can have blood of any group and group O may only have O blood (Figure 11). The rhesus factor (Rh) with further antigens (agglutinogens), coded for by genes designated CDE/cde, was identified by Landsteiner and Wiener in 1940. For general purposes only the D antigen is of significance and is present in around 85% of the Caucasian population, who are said to be rhesus positive (Rh+ve). Those individuals without the D antigen are termed rhesus negative (Rh−ve). In contrast to the ABO system there are no pre-formed antibodies to the D antigen; anti-D only appears following exposure of rhesus negative individuals to rhesus positive blood such as might occur in pregnancy with a rhesus positive fetus or where rhesus positive blood is transfused. Other blood group systems include:

11 Blood group compatibility				
		Recipient		

	Group	A	B	O	AB
Donor	A	+	−	−	+
	B	−	+	−	+
	AB	−	−	−	+
	O	+	+	+	+

+ = compatible
− = non-compatible

MNS, Kell, Duffy and Lewis, but these are not part of routine testing.

blood-letting, bleeding, phlebotomy, venesection. The withdrawal of blood from a vein for therapeutic purposes.

blood plasma, fluid part of blood, forms around 55% of the total volume.

blood pressure, pressure exerted by the blood on the arterial walls as the heart pumps blood into the aorta. The pressure is produced when flow meets resistance: blood pressure = peripheral resistance × cardiac output. Factors contributing to blood pressure include: peripheral resistance, cardiac output, blood volume, venous return, blood viscosity and the elasticity of arterial walls. There are two readings: the systolic which represents the highest pressure in the left ventricle during systole; and the diastolic which is the lowest pressure as the ventricles fill during diastole. It is generally recorded indirectly in the brachial artery using a stethoscope and sphygmomanometer and recorded in millimetres of mercury pressure (mmHg). A typical blood pressure for a young adult would be 120/70 mmHg. Arterial blood pressure may also be recorded directly by the use of an arterial pressure transducer. See HYPERTENSION, HYPOTENSION, KOROTKOFF'S SOUNDS.

blood serum, see SERUM.

blood sugar, the amount of sugar (glucose) in the blood. A normal fasting level would be 3.9–5.8 millimoles/litre (mmol/l); this is elevated after meals and in diabetes mellitus. See HYPERGLYCAEMIA, HYPOGLYCAEMIA.

blood transfusion, the replacement of blood volume, cells or any component with blood collected from healthy (voluntary in UK) donors. It is stored in sterile bags at 4°C for a maximum of 35 days (whole blood), but many blood components have a much shorter shelf-life. Whole blood is anticoagulated prior to storage. Before transfusion the donor red cells are crossmatched against the patient's serum to ensure compatibility and prevent mismatched transfusions. *See* BLOOD GROUPS. Most is used from blood banks but occasionally a transfusion of fresh blood is required.

blood urea, the amount of urea in the blood. It is normally 2.5–6.5 millimoles/litre (mmol/l), it is raised where renal function is impaired and lower than normal in serious liver disease. *See* UREA.

BLS, abbreviation for **basic life support**.

blue baby, an infant born with a congenital heart abnormality causing cyanosis, such as Fallot's tetralogy.

BNF, abbreviation for **British National Formulary**.

Bodecker index, the ratio between the number of tooth surfaces (five to a tooth) which are carious and the total number of surfaces of the teeth which could be affected.

body, 1. the whole person. **2.** the trunk. **3.** the main part of an organ such as the body of the uterus.

body image, the mental image that an individual has of his or her body. May be seriously affected by trauma, certain surgical procedures such as mastectomy and affective disorders.

body language, non-verbal communication by means of facial expression, eye contact, gestures, clothes, touch and body posture.

body mass index (BMI), a measurement derived from weight and height: weight in kg divided by height in m². Used with other criteria to determine whether a person is within a healthy weight range and as part of a nutritional assessment.

body surface area, calculated from a special nomogram using the child's weight and height. Can be used to calculate drug dosage in children.

Boeck's disease, *(berks)*, *see* SARCOIDOSIS.

Bohr effect, the right shift of the oxygen dissociation curve as the pH of the blood falls (becomes more acid as hydrogen ion concentration increases) and the affinity of haemoglobin for oxygen decreases. This effect ensures that haemoglobin releases oxygen more easily in metabolically active tissue.

boil, furuncle. A staphylococcal infection of the skin, causing inflammation round a hair follicle.

Bolam test, the test laid down in the case of Bolam *v.* Friern HMC on the standard of care expected of a professional in cases of alleged negligence.

bolus, a large mass such as food prior to swallowing. *B. dose*; large dose of a drug given at the start of treatment to raise the concentration in the blood rapidly to therapeutic levels.

bonding, the special attachment which forms between a baby and its parents, especially the mother.

bone, hard connective tissue formed from an organic matrix which is mineralized with calcium salts, *see* APATITES. It has great tensile strength and is able to withstand considerable compressive forces. There are two types: hard, dense compact bone (Figure 12), and spongy cancellous bone. Bone is a dynamic tissue which is continually remodelled by cells that produce new bone (osteoclasts) and cells that absorb bone (osteoclasts). *B. graft*: a portion of

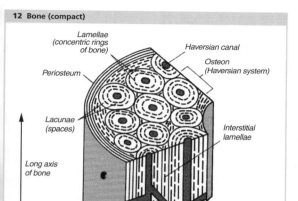

12 Bone (compact)

Lamellae (concentric rings of bone)

Haversian canal

Osteon (Haversian system)

Periosteum

Lacunae (spaces)

Interstitial lamellae

Long axis of bone

Nutrient foramina

Volkmann's canals

Haversian canal

bone is transplanted to repair a defect.

bone marrow, substance which fills the medullary cavity and spaces in cancellous bone. It is of two types: red marrow which is the site of haemopoiesis and yellow fatty marrow which replaces red marrow in certain bones in adults. *See* HAEMOPOIESIS. *B. m. transplant*: transplantation of marrow containing stem cells from healthy matched donors to treat a variety of conditions, including leukaemia.

boot, in computing the start-up routine that a PC follows whilst it runs some checks and loads the operating system when it is first switched on.

borborygmus, borborygmi, *(bor-bor-ig-mī),* audible bowel sounds, rumbling of flatus and fluid.

Bordetella, *(bor-de-tel-ah),* a genus of Gram-negative bacteria. *B. pertussis* causes whooping cough.

Bornholm disease, epidemic diaphragmatic pleurodynia (myalgia).

Borrelia, a genus of spiral (spirochaete) bacteria. *B. burgdorferi*: causes Lyme disease, a tick-borne relapsing fever.

botulism, *(bot-ū-lizm),* food poisoning caused by the bacterium *Clostridium botulinum.*

bougie, *(boo'-jē),* a slender solid instrument which is flexible and yielding, used for dilating contracted passages.

bovine, pertaining to an ox or cow. *B. spongiform encephalopathy (BSE):* an infective, fatal neurological disease of cattle which may have similarities with Creutzfeldt–Jakob disease in humans. *B. tuberculosis:* a form of tuberculosis passed to humans via milk from infected cows. It affects the bones and lymph nodes.

bowel, the intestine or gut. *Small b.:* is 5–6 m in length and has three parts: duodenum, jejunum and ileum. It is concerned with digestion of food and absorption of nutrients. *Large b.:* is 1.5 m in length and runs from the ileocaecal valve to the anus. It consists of the caecum, vermiform appendix, colon, rectum and anal canal. The large bowel stores food residues, eliminates waste as faeces and absorbs water, vitamins and some drugs. *B. sounds:* the sounds heard, on auscultation, as fluid and gas are moved through the bowel. Different sounds may be characteristic of certain disorders such as bowel obstruction.

bowleg, genu varum.

Bowman's capsule, the cup-like end of the renal tubule which encloses the glomerulus (tuft of capillaries).

Boyle's law, at a given temperature the pressure of a gas varies inversely to its volume.

brace, 1. an orthodontic device used in the realignment of teeth. **2.** in orthopaedics any device used to support a body part in its correct position.

brachial, (brā'-ki-al), pertaining to the arm. *B. artery:* main artery of the upper arm, used in recording arterial blood pressure. *B. plexus:* found in the neck and axilla is formed from spinal nerves C5–C8 and T1. It supplies the shoulder, arm, forearm and hand. *B. plexus paraylsis:* see ERB'S PALSY.

brachium, (brā'-ki-um), the arm.

brachytherapy, (brak-ē-ther-ap-ē), radiotherapy delivered from a small radioactive source(s) which is implanted in or adjacent to the tumour. Used to treat cancers of the cervix, tongue, oesophagus, etc.

Braden scale, pressure ulcer risk scale based on the Norton scale used in the United States.

Bradford frame, a special device for immobilizing the spine and/or pelvis in a variety of conditions.

bradycardia, (brad-ē-kar-de-ah), abnormally slow heart rate, usually below 60/min in an adult.

bradykinesia, slowness of voluntary movement such as in parkinsonism.

bradykinin, (brad-ē-kī-nin), an inflammatory peptide mediator, it causes vasodilatation, increased vessel permeability, smooth muscle contraction and induces pain.

braille, a printing method which produces a pattern of raised dots representing the letters of the alphabet. Visually impaired individuals are able to read by feeling the dots.

brain, the part of the central nervous system contained within the cranium (Figures 13 and 14). It consists of the cerebral hemispheres, cerebellum, and brainstem consisting of the pons varolii, midbrain and medulla oblongata.

brain death, a state characterized by complete lack of brain stem activity due to irreversible damage. It can be ascertained by testing certain reflexes, e.g. gag reflex. Diagnosis is confirmed when there is no evidence of brain stem or cerebral activity according to strict criteria.

brain scan, diagnostic imaging techniques which utilize various technologies: radionuclides, computed

50

13 Lateral view of the brain

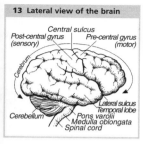

Central sulcus
Post-central gyrus (sensory)
Pre-central gyrus (motor)
Cerebrum
Lateral sulcus
Temporal lobe
Cerebellum
Pons varolii
Medulla oblongata
Spinal cord

14 The brain from above

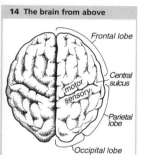

Frontal lobe
Central sulcus
motor
sensory
Parietal lobe
Occipital lobe

axial tomography, magnetic resonance and position emission.

branchial, *(brain'-ki-al),* pertaining to gills. Fissures and clefts that occur on each side of the neck of the human embryo and which are involved in the development of the mouth, nose and ears. Abnormal development may lead to cyst formation.

Braun's splint, a combined splint and extension apparatus for the lower limb.

Braxton Hicks, painless uterine contractions occurring during pregnancy.

breast, 1. the anterior surface of the thorax. **2.** mammary gland. Milk secreting glands. *B. awareness:* a self-care technique where women are encouraged to notice and report breast changes (skin changes, pain, lumps, nipple changes and discharge) in an effort to detect cancers at an early and treatable stage. *B. feeding:* suckling, feeding a baby milk from the breast. It has considerable advantages including nutritional balance and bonding.

breath, air taken into and expelled from the lungs. *B. holding:* a behaviour disorder of infants and children. *B. sounds:* the sounds heard by auscultation of the chest during respiration. *B. tests:* non-invasive tests for gastrointestinal disorders, e.g. malabsorption and the presence of *Helicobacter pylori.*

breathing, the alternate inspiration (inhalation) and expiration (exhalation) of air to and from the lungs.

breech, the buttocks. *B. presentation:* presentation of buttocks of the fetus.

bregma, *see* FONTANELLE.

Bright's disease, outdated term for glomerulonephritis.

British National Formulary **(BNF),** a twice-yearly publication detailing current prescription drugs. Published jointly by the Royal Pharmaceutical Society of Great Britain and the British Medical Association.

British Pharmacopoeia **(BP),** *(far-mah-ko-pe'-ah),* the official drugs reference available in the UK.

British sign language, a form of signing used widely in the UK.

broad ligaments, folds of peritoneum which enclose and support the uterus, uterine tubes, ovaries, blood vessels and lymphatics.

Broadbent's sign, retraction of the lower left part of the chest wall when the pericardium is adherent.

Broca's area, the motor speech area normally on the left side of the brain in right handed people.

Brodie's abscess, chronic abscess of bone. The tibia is most commonly affected.

bromidrosis, *(bro-mī-drŏ'-sis),* offensive sweating, most common in the feet.

bronchial, pertaining to a bronchus. *B. tree.* the network of bronchi and small bronchial tubes within the lung.

bronchiectasis, *(bron'-ke-ek'-tas-is),* a disease where the bronchi and bronchioles become dilated and filled with copious amounts of offensive purulent sputum.

bronchiole, one of the small airways which eventually terminate in an alveolus.

bronchiolitis, *(bron-ke-ō-lī'-tis),* inflammation of the bronchioles. Usually caused by a virus e.g. respiratory syncytial virus (RSV), it can cause serious respiratory problems in small children.

bronchitis, inflammation of the bronchial mucosa. *Acute b.:* often follows a respiratory tract infection or other illness such as measles. *Chronic b.:* caused by smoking and atmospheric pollutants, it belongs to the larger group of chronic obstructive pulmonary disease. It is characterized by excess mucus production and reduced ciliary clearance which will eventually lead to serious impairment of gaseous exchange in the lungs and heart failure.

bronchocele, *(bron'-kō-sēl),* a diverticulum of a bronchus.

bronchoconstrictor, any agent that constricts the bronchi.

bronchodilator, an agent that causes the smooth muscle of the bronchi to relax and the air passages to dilate e.g. salbutamol.

bronchogenic, originating from bronchus.

bronchomycosis, *(bron-kō-mī-kō'-sis)* fungal infection affecting the lung and bronchi.

bronchopleural fistula, an abnormal communication between a bronchus and the pleural cavity.

bronchopneumonia, acute inflammation of bronchioles and lung tissue it affects scattered areas in the lungs Often seen at the extremes of age or secondary to an existing condition or debilitated state.

bronchopulmonary, pertaining to the respiratory tract; bronchi and lungs *B. dysplasia:* chronic respiratory condition, seen in preterm babies born with immature lungs who have had long-term treatment with high-concentration oxygen and positive pressure ventilation.

bronchoscope, an endoscopic instrument used to view the bronchi, take specimens or remove foreign bodies

bronchoscopy, *(bron-kos-kŏ-pē),* endoscopic examination of the bronchi Commonly utilizes a flexible fiberoptic scope but rigid metal instruments may still be used in some situations.

bronchospasm, sudden, but temporary, constriction of the bronchial smooth muscle resulting in narrowing of the airways. There is dyspnoea, cough and wheezing such as in asthma.

bronchospirometry, *(bron-ko-spi-rom'-et-rē),* the measurement of the capacity of a lung or one of its lobes.

bronchus, *(pl.* **bronchi),** one of the two large air passages formed by the bifurcation of the trachea. Each bronchus enters a lung at its hilum where it further subdivides to supply individual lobes and segments.

Broselow paediatric resuscitation system, a US-designed system for use during paediatric resuscitation. A special tape measure with colour segments is placed alongside the child. This allows the medical team to read off the correct size equipment and drug doses for a child of that length. The colour coding is used on the equipment packaging.

brow, forehead. *B. presentation*: very unfavourable, but unusual presentation in labour. The large mentovertical diameter presents, which makes vaginal delivery practically impossible.

brown fat, a special type of adipose tissue, seen mainly in newborn infants, which is easily metabolized to release energy.

Browne, Denis, splints, splints designed to correct congenital talipes equinovarus.

Brown-Séquard's syndrome, syndrome seen after damage to the lateral part of the spinal cord. It is characterized by ipsilateral motor paralysis and postural problems with contralateral loss of temperature sense and anaesthesia.

Brucella, (broo-sel-a), a genus of bacteria causing brucellosis. *B. abortus* a bovine form causes abortion in cattle and undulant fever in humans. *B. melitensis* a goat form causes Malta fever in humans. Both organisms are transmitted via infected milk.

brucellosis, (broo-sel-ō-sis), infection with an organism of the *Brucella* group.

Brudzinski's sign, seen in meningeal irritation, when the hips and knees flex when the head is raised from the bed.

bruit, (broo-ē′), an abnormal sound heard during the auscultation of a structure or organ, e.g. blood vessel.

Brunner's glands, compound glands of the duodenum which secrete alkaline mucus.

Brushfield's spots, white or yellow spots seen on the iris in Down's syndrome.

bruxism, (brooks-izm), clenching of the teeth, especially during sleep.

Bryants' 'gallows' traction, fixed skin traction applied to the lower limbs; the legs are suspended vertically from a beam so that the buttocks are clear of the bed. May be used for fractures of the femur in children (usually under 12 months of age). It has been largely replaced by loop traction.

bubo, inflammatory swelling of lymph nodes, particularly of groin.

bubonic plague, a type of plague characterized by the formation of buboes. *See* PLAGUE, PNEUMONIC PLAGUE.

buccal, (buk-kal), pertaining to the mouth.

buccinator, (buk′-sin-ā-tor), the muscle of the cheek; one of the muscles of mastication.

Budd–Chiari syndrome, a serious liver condition, with hepatic portal hypertension caused by hepatic venous obstruction.

Buerger's disease, (ber-gerz), thromboangiitis obliterans. Rare disease of blood vessels resulting in reduction of blood supply to extremities.

buffer, substances which limit pH change by their ability to accept hydrogen ions or donate hydrogen as appropriate. In the body they prevent swings in pH which would inhibit cell function. The important buffer systems in the body include: hydrogen carbonate (bicarbonate) system, hydrogen phosphates and proteins such as haemoglobin.

bug, in computing an error within a program or system which causes it to crash or not run properly.

bulbar, pertaining to the medulla oblongata. *B. palsy*: neurological degenerative condition resulting in paralysis of tongue, difficulty in swallowing and speech problems.

bulbourethral glands, *(bul-bo-ūr-ē'-thral),* Cowper's gland. Two mucus secreting glands which open into the male urethra.

bulimia, morbid hunger. *B. nervosa:* a serious psychological condition characterized by binge-eating, self-induced vomiting and the use of laxatives. *See* ANOREXIA.

bullae, large blisters.

bundle of His, *See* ATRIOVENTRICULAR BUNDLE.

bunion, hallux valgus. Inflammation of the bursa associated with metatarsophalangeal joint of the great toe. *See* KELLER'S OPERATION.

burden of proof, the duty of a party to litigation to establish the facts, or, in criminal cases, the duty of the prosecution to establish the facts.

Burkitt's lymphoma, a non-Hodgkin's lymphoma, principally affecting children in tropical Africa, but it does occur elsewhere. It mainly affects the jaw and abdomen and is often seen in people previously infected with the Epstein–Barr (EB) virus.

burnout, a state of chronic stress characterized by ineffective coping strategies, extreme tiredness, apathy and lack of motivation seen in healthcare professionals and others with emotionally demanding work roles.

burns, burns may be partial or full-thickness, according to the depth of skin and other structures destroyed the latter requiring skin grafts Causes include: **1.** chemical; **2.** physical agents such as fire; **3.** electrical **4.** radiation. Prognosis depends on the percentage of body area burnt age and general condition. Priorities of treatment include fluid replacement and prevention of shock, pain relief, emotional support, preventing infection and later maintaining nutritional needs, and minimizing scarring and impaired function. *See* LUND AND BROWDER'S CHART, WALLACE'S RULE OF NINE.

burr hole, a hole drilled in the skull to relieve raised intracranial pressure or gain access to the brain.

bursa, a small sac lined with synovial membrane secreting synovial fluid Interposed between joint structures and muscles they act to reduce friction.

bursitis, inflammation of a bursa.

bypass, surgery that diverts flow, usually to overcome an occlusion such as in an artery: coronary, femoral and aorta. *Cardiopulmonary b.:* device which bypasses the heart and lungs to oxygenate blood during open heart surgery.

byssinosis, *(bi-sin-ō-sis),* a type of pneumoconiosis caused by inhalation of cotton dust.

byte, a unit of computer data storage capacity. It contains eight bits Larger units include the the kilobyte (kb), containing 1024 bytes, and the megabyte (Mb) which has 1 048 576 bytes. *See* BINARY, BIT.

C

C, 1. Celsius. **2.** Centigrade. **3.** Calorie. **4.** a complex but powerful computer language.

Ca-125, a substance that can be detected in the blood and can act as a tumour marker for cancer of the ovary.

cachexia, (ka-chek-si-a), extreme emaciation and debility, seen in serious illnesses such as cancer.

cadaver, a corpse.

cadmium (Cd), poisonous metallic element; industrial exposure may cause lung and renal problems.

caecal, (sē-kal), pertaining to the caecum.

caecosigmoidostomy, (sē'-kō-sig-moyd-os-to-mi), operation for establishing direct communication between the caecum and sigmoid colon.

caecostomy, (sē-kos'-to-mi), operation to provide an opening into the caecum through the abdominal wall.

caecum, (sē-kum), a blind pouch forming the first part of the large bowel, separated from the small bowel by the ileocaecal valve. See BOWEL, APPENDIX VERMIFORMIS.

caesarean section, (se-zār-ē-an), delivery of the fetus through an incision in the abdominal and uterine walls.

caesium (Cs), (sē-si-um), the radioactive isotope (^{137}Cs) of this element is used in radiotherapy to treat malignant disease.

café-au-lait spots, flattened pale brown spots on the skin, seen in neurofibromatosis and as part of the ageing process.

caffeine, alkaloid found in tea, coffee and cola drinks; a stimulant and diuretic.

caisson disease, decompression sickness or 'the bends'. Affects those working under heavier atmospheric pressure than normal, e.g. divers and those, such as air crew, who ascend rapidly to a lower atmospheric pressure. The sudden decompression causes nitrogen bubbles to form in the blood with variable, but sometimes fatal, consequences.

calamine, zinc carbonate used as an astringent.

calcaneus, the os calcis or heel bone.

calcareous, (kal-ka-re-us), containing compounds of calcium.

calciferol, (kal-sif-er-ol), See CHOLECALCIFEROL, ERGOCALCIFEROL and NUTRITION APPENDIX.

calcification, (kal-si-fi-kā-shon), deposition of calcium salts in bone. May occur abnormally in other tissue, e.g. blood vessels.

calcitonin, (kal-si-tō-nin), thyrocalcitonin. Thyroid hormone, concerned with calcium and phosphorus homeostasis.

calcitriol, 1,25-dehydroxycholecalciferol, the active form of vitamin D. Involved in calcium homeostasis.

calcium (Ca), metallic element required by the body; for neuromuscular action, for blood clotting and as a constituent of bone and teeth. *C. channel blocker:* a drug which inhibits

55

the flow of calcium in smooth muscle, used to treat angina and hypertension, e.g. nifedipine. Also known as calcium antagonists. *C. salts*: used as antacids and replacement in rickets and tetany.

calculus, concretion or stone found in various organs: gallbladder, kidney, ureter, bladder and salivary gland.

Caldwell–Luc operation, radical operation previously used to drain the maxillary sinus.

calibrate, to graduate an instrument for measuring by a given standard.

caliper, in orthopaedics, **1.** a supportive metal device worn on the leg to facilitate mobility. **2.** two-prong device inserted into bone, used to fix bones or apply traction in the treatment of fractures.

calipers, an instrument for measuring thickness or distances, e.g. skin fold thickness.

callosity, a thickened horny layer of epidermis formed on palmar and plantar surfaces subject to much friction.

callus, 1. *see* CALLOSITY. **2.** new bony deposit around a fracture site during healing.

calor, heat.

caloric, pertaining to heat. *C. test*: a test of vestibular function. When water at a certain temperature is poured into the ear nystagmus occurs if the ear is normal, but no reaction is seen where vestibular disease exists.

calorie, unit of heat. One large Calorie (C) or kilocalorie (kcal) is that amount of heat required to raise the temperature of 1 kilogram (kg) of water through 1° Celsius. The energy of food and metabolic needs are sometimes measured in large Calories/kilocalories, e.g. 1 gram (g) of fat releases 9 Calories/kcal. *See* NUTRITION APPENDIX. The small calorie (c) is

that amount of heat required to raise the temperature of 1 gram (g) of water through 1° Celsius; 1000 calories = 1 Calorie/kilocalorie. Calories/kilocalories have been replaced by an SI derived unit, for heat, energy and work, the joule (J) or kilojoule (kJ). Approximately 4.2 kilojoules = 1 kilocalorie/large Calorie = 1000 small calories.

calorific, producing heat. *C. value*: energy content of food.

calvaria, upper part of the skull, the cranial vault.

Calve's disease, osteochondrosis affecting the femur or vertebrae.

calyx, *(ka-liks)*, a cup-shaped organ or cavity such as the recesses of the renal pelvis.

cAMP, abbreviation for **cyclic adenosine monophosphate**.

Campylobacter, *(kam-pil-ō-bak-ter)*, a genus of Gram-negative bacteria of the family Spirillaceae. *C. jejuni*: a common cause of food poisoning in humans.

canal, in anatomy a narrow tube, e.g. auditory canal.

canaliculus, *(kan-al'-ik-ū-lus)*, a small canal or groove, e.g. passage leading from the eyelid to the lacrimal sac or one of the minute canals of the haversian systems in bone.

cancellous, *(kan-sel-us)*, has a lattice-like structure with many spaces. Forms the light spongy bone found in the extremities of long bones, irregular and flat bones. *See* BONE.

cancer, lay term used to describe the various forms of malignant disease. *C. units*: in the UK. Units in District General Hospitals that support the work of the Regional Cancer Centres by managing patients with common cancers, e.g. lung, colorectal, etc.

cancroid, *(kan'-kroyd)*, like a cancer.

cancrum oris, gangrenous stomatitis of the cheek as a result of dental sepsis.

andela (cd), SI base unit for luminous intensity.

andida, a genus of fungi (yeast). *C. albicans* causes candidiasis or thrush.

andidiasis, *(kan-did-i-as-is),* the disease caused by *Candida*. It affects various sites: mouth, gastrointestinal tract, lungs, skin and urogenital tract, especially in patients who are debilitated or immunosuppressed and following long-term or extensive use of antimicrobial agents and other drugs, e.g. oral contraceptives. The presence of oesophageal or pulmonary candidiasis is an AIDS-defining condition. *See* MONILIA, THRUSH.

anicola fever, disease in humans caused by *Leptospira canicola*, an organism carried by pigs and dogs.

anine teeth, the four eye-teeth, next to the incisors.

annabinoids, antiemetic drugs derived from cannabis, e.g. nabilone.

annabis indica, marijuana, pot, hash etc.; a psychoactive drug which is usually smoked, it produces hallucinations and euphoria. In the UK its supply, possession or cultivation are criminal offences under the provisions of the Misuse of Drugs Act 1971. There is considerable interest in the possibility of medicinal uses, e.g. relief of the effects of multiple sclerosis, and trials are currently underway.

annula, a hollow tube of plastic or metal for the introduction of fluids or their withdrawal from the body. *See* TROCAR.

annulation, insertion of a cannula, such as into a vein.

anthus, the angle of the eyelids, outer or inner.

apacitation, structural changes in a spermatozoon which allow the release of enzymes required for oöcyte penetration.

CAPD, *see* CONTINUOUS AMBULATORY PERITONEAL DIALYSIS.

capillaries, network of tiny blood vessels which connect arteries to veins (Figure 15). As their walls are only one cell thick, this facilitates the exchange of molecules between blood and cells.

capitate, like a head. One of the carpal or wrist bones.

capitation funding, a way of allocating money and other resources based on the number of people in a geographical area. This may be weighted to take account of age profile or the relative economic and social conditions, e.g. areas of social deprivation would attract extra funds.

capsaicin, substance found in sweet peppers. Acts to block pain impulse transmission. Applied topically to alleviate the pain following shingles.

capsule, 1. ligaments surrounding a movable joint. **2.** outer coat of some organs, e.g. liver. **3.** soluble container, e.g. gelatin.

capsulotomy, an incision of the capsule of the lens of the eye.

caput, term meaning head or superior part. *C. medusae*: a dilated knot of veins around the umbilicus, associated with hepatic portal hypertension. *C. succedaneum*: serous swelling on an infant's head caused by pressure during labour.

carbamino compound, *(kar-ba-min-o),* compound formed by carbon dioxide and plasma proteins.

carbaminohaemoglobin, *(kar-ba-min-o hē-mo-glo'-bin),* compound formed by haemoglobin and carbon dioxide. Some carbon dioxide is transported in this form.

carbohydrate, organic compounds consisting of carbon, oxygen and hydrogen. They include the sugars

15 Capillaries

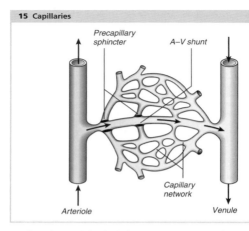

Precapillary sphincter

A–V shunt

Capillary network

Arteriole

Venule

and starches used by the body to produce energy. *See* MONOSACCHA-RIDE, DISACCHARIDE, POLYSACCHARIDE.

carbolic acid, phenol. A powerful anti-septic derived from coal tar. Highly poisonous.

carbon (C), non-metallic element; occurs in many forms, e.g. diamond and charcoal. A component of all organic compounds. *C. dioxide*: gaseous product of cellular metab-olism, combustion and fermenta-tion. Excreted via the lungs, it stimulates breathing by its action on the respiratory centres in the brain. *C. d. snow*: formed by compressing the gas at low temperature. Used to treat some superficial skin condi-tions. *C. monoxide*: poisonous gas present in the exhaust from internal combustion engines, coal gas and from the incomplete combustion of natural gas, wood and coal.

Poisoning, e.g. from car exhaust, characterized by dizziness, hypoxi cardiac arrhythmias, flushed ski convulsions and coma.

carbonate, a salt of carbonic acid.

carbonic anhydrase, *(kar-bon-ik an-h dräz),* enzyme which catalyses th reversible conversion of carbo dioxide and water to carbonic aci It facilitates the transfer of carbo dioxide from tissues to blood an from blood to alveolar air for excr tion.

carboxyhaemoglobin, *(kar-bok-si-h mo-glo-bin),* a stable compoun formed by carbon monoxide an haemoglobin. In this form haem globin is unable to transport oxyge and hypoxia occurs as in carbo monoxide poisoning.

carbuncle, *(kar-bun-kl),* severe sup purative inflammation of the ski and subcutaneous tissues caused by staphylococcal infection. Commonly affects the back of the neck.

carcinoembryonic antigen (CEA), *(kar-sin-ō-em-brē-o-nik),* a fetal antigen, but normally present in small amounts in adult blood. Elevated levels are indicative of certain malignancies, e.g. colorectal, or of liver cirrhosis.

carcinogen, *(kar-sin-ō-jen),* an agent that causes or predisposes to cancer, e.g. certain chemicals, viruses.

carcinogenic, pertaining to an agent causing or predisposing to cancer.

carcinoid syndrome, a clinical syndrome which occurs following the development and spread of carcinoid tumour which secretes 5-hydroxytryptamine (5-HT; also called serotonin). It is characterized by flushing, bronchospasm and diarrhoea.

carcinoma, *(kar-si-nō-ma),* malignant tumour arising from epithelial tissue. *C.-in-situ:* previously known as preinvasive cancer. It is a very early cancer that is asymptomatic and that has not invaded the basement membrane.

carcinomatosis, *(kar-sin-ō-ma-tō-sis),* disseminated malignant disease.

cardia, 1. the heart. **2.** the aperture between the oesophagus and the stomach.

cardiac, pertaining to the heart. *C. arrest:* cessation of an effective output from the heart; asystole, electromechanical dissociation, pulseless ventricular tachycardia or ventricular fibrillation. *C. arrhythmias:* any abnormal heart rhythm. *C. catherization:* introduction of a radiopaque catheter into the heart via a large artery or vein. Used to measure: pressures, cardiac output, oxygen concentration, and for angiography. *C. cycle:* events occurring during one heart beat; lasts for 0.8 s if the rate is

approximately 70/min. *See* SYSTOLE and DIASTOLE. *C. enzymes:* chemicals such as asparate aminotransferase normally present in myocardial and other cells. They are released into the blood after cell damage and the presence of elevated levels can be useful in the diagnosis of myocardial infarction. *See* AMINOTRANS-FERASES, TRANSAMINASES. *C. failure:* inability of either side of the heart to pump blood effectively. May occur in isolation or both sides may fail together, can be acute or (more commonly) chronic. Common causes include: ischaemia as in coronary heart disease, cardiomyopathies, valve defects and chronic respiratory disease. *See* COR PULMONALE, CON-GESTIVE CARDIAC FAILURE. *C. massage (external):* compression of the heart between the sternum and spine by pressure applied to the chest; used during cardiac arrest to provide an adequate circulation. *C. murmur:* abnormal heart sound heart on auscultation as blood passes through a defective heart valve or septal defect and during valve functioning. *C. output:* the amount of blood pumped by the ventricles in one minute (stroke volume × heart rate). *C. pacing:* see PACEMAKER. *C. tamponade:* compression of the heart caused by a collection of blood or other fluid within the pericardial sac. *C. transplant:* replacement of a diseased heart with a well matched donor organ. Combined heart/lung transplants are often performed.

cardinal, chief or principal. *C. ligaments:* the transverse cervical ligaments which run from the cervix to the side walls of the pelvis.

cardiogenic, of cardiac origin. *C. shock:* shock produced by an insufficient cardiac output such as following a severe myocardial infarction.

cardiogram, the tracing obtained by the use of the cardiograph.

cardiograph, instrument used to record various features of heart action, e.g. force, movements.

cardiology, the study of the heart and circulatory disorders.

cardiomegaly, *(kar-dē-ō-meg-a-lē),* enlarged heart.

cardiomyopathy, *(kar-dē-ō-mī-op'-ath-ē),* acute or chronic disease of the myocardium. It may be inherited, secondary to infections such as pneumonia and serious generalized disorders, or of unknown aetiology.

cardiomyotomy, *(kar-dē-ō-mī-ot'-ō-mi),* surgical relief of muscular spasm at the lower end of the oesophagus. *See* HELLER'S OPERATION.

cardiopathy, disease of the heart.

cardiopulmonary, *(kar-dē-ō-pul'-mon-ar-ē),* pertaining to heart and lungs. *C. bypass:* used to facilitate open heart surgery by isolating the heart and lungs. *See* BYPASS. *C. resuscitation (CPR):* life support procedures; artificial respiration and cardiac massage. Used during cardiac arrest to maintain the circulation of oxygenated blood to vital organs.

cardiospasm, spasm affecting the gastro-oesophageal (cardiac) sphincter. *See* ACHALASIA.

cardiothoracic, *(kar-dē-ō-thor-as-ik),* pertaining to the heart and thorax.

cardiotocography (CTG), *(kar-dē-ō-to-ko-gra-fē),* monitoring during labour to detect fetal hypoxia; fetal heart rate, movements and uterine contractions are recorded simultaneously.

cardiovascular, pertaining to the heart and circulatory system.

cardioversion, the use of direct current electricity to convert an arrhythmia, such as atrial fibrillation, to sinus rhythm.

carditis, inflammation of the heart. *See* PERICARDITIS, MYOCARDITIS, ENDOCARDITIS.

care pathway, integrated plan or pathway agreed locally by the multidisciplinary team for specific patient/client groups. The pathway is based on available evidence and guidelines.

care plan, the individualized plan of nursing interventions for a specific patient/client. It is based on data obtained from a variety of sources and should define care needs, set goals, describe appropriate nursing activities and state the desired outcomes. *See* NURSING PROCESS.

carer, a person taking responsibility for caring for another person (child, sick, disabled or older person). Describes unpaid family, friends and neighbours.

caries, dental decay, or inflammatory bone decay.

carina, a keel-shaped structure, especially the base of the trachea where it is joined by the bronchi.

carneous, *(kar-ne-us),* flesh-like. *C. mole:* missed abortion. The fetus dies but is not expelled, it becomes surrounded by blood clot.

carotenes, yellow or orange pigments found in deep yellow and dark green leafy vegetables. One is a provitamin converted to vitamin A in the body.

carotid, *(kar-ot-id),* the main arteries on each side of the neck. *C. body:* situated at the bifurcation of the carotid arteries it contains chemoreceptor tissue which monitors oxygen levels and pH in the blood. *C. sinus:* situated at the bifurcation of the carotid arteries it contains baroreceptor tissue. *See* BARORECEPTORS.

carpal, pertaining to the wrist. *C. tunnel syndrome:* numbness and tingling in the hand caused by compression of the median nerve at the wrist.

carpometacarpal, *(kar-pō-met-ah-kar'-pal),* relating to a carpus and metacarpus.

carpopedal spasm, *(kar-pō-pē-dal),* cramp and spasm in the hands and feet, due to a reduction of serum calcium levels. *See* CHVOSTEK'S SIGN, TETANY, TROUSSEAU'S SIGN.

carpus, the wrist. The eight bones of the wrist: scaphoid, lunate, triquetral, pisiform, trapezium, trapezoid, capitate and hamate.

carrier, 1. an individual who carries a pathogenic microorganism. He or she may be a source of infection whilst remaining asymptomatic or the carrier state may follow the disease. **2.** an individual who is heterozygous for a recessive gene. He or she does not exhibit the trait/disease, but may pass the gene to any children, e.g. cystic fibrosis gene. *See* HETEROZYGOUS.

cartilage, a dense and tough connective tissue of three types: yellow elastic, hyaline and white fibrous.

cascara sagrada, *(kas-kar'a sa-gra'-da),* a bark with laxative properties. Used to treat constipation.

case, *c. conference:* a meeting where the various professionals involved with the care and management of a specific person meet to discuss progress and coordinate their actions. *C. control study:* retrospective study which compares outcomes for a group with a particular condition with those of a control group without that condition. *C. study:* research study that examines data from one or a small number of cases.

caseation, *(kā-sē-ā'-shon),* necrosis characterized by tissue conversion to cheese-like material, associated with tuberculosis.

casein, *(ka-sēn),* protein formed by the action of rennin on caseinogen in milk.

caseinogen, *(ka-zin-ō-jen),* principal protein of milk, precursor of casein.

cast, 1. a rigid bandage containing material such as plaster of Paris. **2.** material which takes the shape of the cavity from which it was expelled, e.g. renal casts formed from epithelial debris and exudate are found in the urine in certain kidney diseases. **3.** the turning of an eye in strabismus.

castration, removal of testes or ovaries.

CAT, *see* COMPUTED AXIAL TOMOGRAPHY.

catabolic, pertaining to catabolism. *C. state:* produced when protein turnover in the body increases during severe illness or injury, such as trauma or sepsis. Dietary intake of protein is insufficient and the person is said to be in negative nitrogen balance.

catabolism, *(kat-ab-ol-izm),* metabolic processes in which complex molecules are broken down to release energy. *See* METABOLISM.

catalase, an enzyme, found in most cells, responsible for the decomposition of hydrogen peroxide to oxygen and water.

catalyst, a substance such as an enzyme which influences the rate of a chemical reaction without itself being permanently altered.

catalytic, something which causes another event to occur, such as a type of therapy which may encourage a person to act. *See* CATALYST.

cataplexy, *(kat-ah-pleks-ē),* muscular rigidity produced by fear or shock.

cataract, opacity or clouding of the lens of the eye; a common cause of impaired vision, it may be congenital or acquired. Treatment is by removal/destruction of the lens and replacement of focusing ability with an intraocular lens implant, contact lens or glasses.

catarrh, (kat-ahr), inflammation of the mucous membranes, usually applied to the upper respiratory tract.

catatonia, a state characterized by immobility or impulsive motor activity. Seen in schizophrenia.

catatonic, a form of schizophrenia.

catchment area, the geographical area served by a particular organization, e.g. health centre, health authority or school.

catecholamines, (ka-te-kol-ā-mēnz), substances such as dopamine, adrenaline (epinephrine) and noradrenaline (norepinephrine) produced in the body. They are physiologically important as neurotransmitters and for their effects upon blood sugar, heart rate and blood pressure which they increase. Abnormally high amounts are produced by certain adrenal and other tumours and can be detected in the urine. See 4-HYDROXY, 3-METHOXY-MANDELIC ACID, PHAEOCHROMOCY-TOMA.

categorical data, data that can be put in categories, e.g. hair colour.

catgut, material prepared from sheep's intestine and used for absorbable ligatures.

catharsis, (kath-ar-sis), **1.** in psychology the purging of emotion through experiencing it deeply. **2.** purging or cleansing.

catheter, hollow tube inserted into a vessel or body cavity for many purposes including the introduction or drainage of fluids; its introduction is known as catheterization. The many types include: Cardiac c.: see CARDIAC. Central venous c.: used for measuring central venous pressure, parenteral feeding and drug administration. Nasal c.: used to administer oxygen.

Swan–Ganz c.: used to monitor various haemodynamic criteria such as pulmonary wedge pressures. Urinary c.: used to drain urine from the bladder.

cathode, electrode with a negative charge.

cation, (kat-i-on), an ion which has a positive electrical charge, e.g. sodium (Na^+), attracted to the negative pole or cathode of a battery. See ANION.

CATS, abbreviation for Credit Accumulation and Transfer System.

cat scratch fever, minor condition which follows a cat scratch or bite. There is local inflammation and later lymph node swelling.

cauda equina, (kaw-da ek-wi-na), the bundle of lumbar, sacral and coccygeal nerves at the lower end of the spinal cord. Resembles a horse's tail.

caudal analgesia, anaesthetic administered into the epidural space by an approach through the caudal canal in the sacrum.

caul, fetal membranes about the face and head of some infants at birth.

causalgia, (kaw-sal-ji-a), severe pain persisting after an injury to a cutaneous nerve, e.g. following herpes zoster (shingles).

caustic, a substance, usually a strong alkali or acid, which destroys cells and causes chemical burns, e.g. silver nitrate used to remove excess granulation tissue.

cautery, an agent or device, e.g. electricity, chemicals or extremes of temperature, which destroys cells and tissues. May be used to destroy diseased tissue or to arrest haemorrhage during surgery.

cavernous, relating to or resembling a cavity. C. haemangioma: a benign tumour consisting of thin-walled blood vessels. *C. respiration*: a hollow sound, heard on auscultation, indicates a cavity in the lung. *C. sinus*: one of the venous sinuses enclosed in dura mater, drains venous blood from the brain. *C. sinus thrombosis*: usually follows an infection near the nose or eye.

cavitation, process whereby cavities are formed.

cavity, 1. an enclosed area within the body, e.g. cranial, thoracic, abdominal, peritoneal and pelvic. **2.** lay term for hole caused by dental caries.

CCU, abbreviation for **coronary care unit.**

CD, abbreviation for **controlled drug.**

CD-ROM, in computing an acronym for **Compact Disk Read-Only Memory.** Used as a storage and dis-

tribution device for data and programs which a PC can read.

cell, the basic structural unit of any living organism (Figure 16a). Consists of a mass of protoplasm, known as cytoplasm, contained within a plasma membrane. Inside the cytoplasm is a nucleus (usually) and various subcellular structures known as organelles, e.g. mitochondria, endoplasmic reticulum and ribosomes. Cells divide by mitosis (somatic cells) or meiosis (gametes). *C. cycle*: the sequence of events from the formation of a new cell through the replication stages to its own division (Figure 16b). *See* MITOSIS, MEIOSIS.

cell-mediated immunity, part of the immune response involving the

---

16a A cell

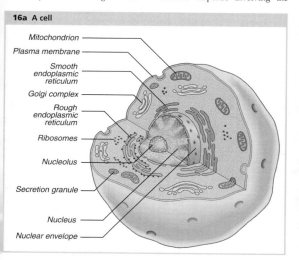

Mitochondrion

Plasma membrane

Smooth endoplasmic reticulum

Golgi complex

Rough endoplasmic reticulum

Ribosomes

Nucleolus

Secretion granule

Nucleus

Nuclear envelope

16b The cell cycle

G_1 (gap1)	variable-length period between mitosis and synthetic phase
S (synthetic)	period of DNA replication and growth
G_2 (gap2)	preparation for complete separation, growth and maturation
M (mitotic)	phase when mitosis and cytokinesis occur
G_0 (quiescent)	resting phase, but some cells rejoin the cell cycle when extra cells are required, e.g. liver cells following surgical resection

action of specific T lymphocytes which destroy abnormal/foreign cells and release of regulatory chemicals.

cellulitis, *(sel-lū-lī-tis),* diffuse inflammation of the skin and connective tissue.

cellulose, a polysaccharide found in plant cell walls. It is not digested by humans and provides the nonstarch polysaccharide (NSP dietary fibre) required to increase the faecal mass, stimulate peristalsis and reduce bowel transit time.

Celsius, derived SI unit for temperature.

cementum, connective tissue that helps to support and secure teeth in their sockets.

censor, Freudian term for the barrier preventing repressed memories, ideas and impulses from easily coming into consciousness.

centesis, puncture of a body cavity, e.g. amniocentesis, thoracocentesis.

centigrade, having 100 divisions or degrees. A thermometric scale in which water freezes at 0°C and boils at 100°C. Usually known as Celsius in science and medicine.

centimetre (cm), metric unit of length, 100th part of a metre.

central limit theorem, in research. Sampling distribution becomes more normal as more samples are taken.

central nervous system (CNS), general term for the brain and spinal cord.

central tendency statistic, averages. The tendency for observations to centre around a specific value rather than across the whole range. *See* MEAN, MEDIAN, MODE.

central venous pressure (CVP), monitoring technique whereby the pressure in the large veins (superior vena cava) or the right atrium is measured via a catheter attached to a manometer (Figure 17). Readings obtained are used to assess circulatory function, blood volume and fluid replacement requirements.

centrifugal, efferent. Having a tendency to move out from the centre, such as nerve impulses leaving the CNS.

centrifuge, a device which separates substances of different densities by high speed rotation.

centriole, cell organelle involved with spindle formation during cell division.

centripetal, afferent. Having a tendency to move to the centre, such as the rash of chickenpox.

centromere, *(sen-trō-meer)*, a structure which joins the double chromosome (two chromatids) and eventually attaches to the equatorial region of the spindle during cell division.

centrosome, *(sen-trō-sōm)*, an area within the cell situated near the nucleus, it contains the centrioles.

cephalhaematoma, *(kef-al-hē-ma-tō-ma)*, a subperiosteal haemorrhage on the head of an infant, usually due to pressure during a long labour. It is gradually absorbed.

cephalic, *(kef-al-ik)*, pertaining to the head. *C. presentation*: where the fetal

---

17 Central venous pressure

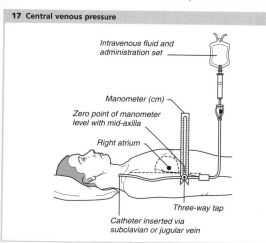

Intravenous fluid and administration set

Manometer (cm)

Zero point of manometer level with mid-axilla

Right atrium

Three-way tap

Catheter inserted via subclavian or jugular vein

head is the presenting part at the cervix. *C. version*: an obstetric manoeuvre which seeks to convert a breech or transverse lie to a cephalic presentation.

cephalocele, *(kef'-al-ō-sēl),* hernia of the brain.

cephalometry, *(kef-al-om-e-tri),* measurement of the head.

cephalopelvic, pertaining to the size of the fetal head and the maternal pelvis. *C. disproportion*: a situation where the fetal head is too large or the maternal pelvis is too small to facilitate a vaginal delivery, requires caesarean section.

cephalosporins, *(kef-al-ō-spor-in),* a large group of broad-spectrum beta-lactam antibiotic drugs related to the penicillins.

cerclage, *(ser-klahjh),* **1**. a technique where fractured bone ends are bound together with wire. **2**. a procedure where a circular suture is inserted into an incompetent cervix. *See* SHIRODKAR SUTURE.

cerebellar, pertaining to the cerebellum.

cerebellum, *(ser-ē-bel'-lum),* outgrowth from the hindbrain occupying the posterior cranial fossa. Concerned with motor coordination, posture and balance.

cerebral, *(ser-ē-bral),* pertaining to the cerebrum. *C. cortex*: outer layer of grey matter. *C. embolus*: an embolus, usually of blood clot (rarely fat or air) which becomes lodged in the cerebral circulation. It may arise from clots forming in the left side of the heart. *C. haemorrhage*: bleeding into the brain from a ruptured blood vessel, with tissue destruction. *C. hemisphere*: one of the two halves of the cerebrum. *C. lateralization*: most functional areas are duplicated in both hemispheres but some, such as speech, appear on the dominant side only. There are functional differences between the hemispheres with lateralization of functions. *C. oedema*: swelling of brain tissue due to fluid accumulation. Causes include: trauma, tumour and infection. *C. palsy*: an abnormality of motor control caused by prenatal defect, hypoxia or birth injury. There are varying degrees of spasticity or flaccidity affecting mobility and problems with speech, hearing and vision. *See* ATHETOSIS. *C. thrombosis*: thrombus formation in the cerebral vessels; associated with arterial disease. *See* CEREBROVASCULAR ACCIDENT.

cerebration, *(ser'-ē-brā-shon),* activity of the brain.

cerebrospinal, *(ser-ē-brō-spī'-nal),* pertaining to the brain and spinal cord. *C. fluid*: clear fluid produced in the ventricles of the brain by the specialized capillaries of the choroid plexus; it circulates in the subarachnoid space surrounding the brain and spinal cord providing protection and nourishment.

cerebrovascular accident (CVA), a general term referring to any defects in the cerebral circulation such as those caused by cerebral embolism, thrombosis or haemorrhage. Clinical presentation depends upon cause, severity and site and may include headache, hemiparesis, hemiplegia, coma, aphasia and visual problems. *See* APOPLEXY, STROKE, TRANSIENT ISCHAEMIC ATTACK.

cerebrum, *(ser-ē-brum),* the largest part of the brain, divided into two hemispheres. Mass of nerve fibres covered by a thin layer of nerve cells – the cerebral cortex. Contains major motor and sensory areas and controls the higher functions of the brain. *See* BRAIN.

ceruloplasmin, *(se-rū-lō-plaz-min),* a plasma protein concerned with copper transport.

cerumen, *(se-rū'-men),* ear wax. Sticky yellow-brown substance secreted by ceruminous glands (modified sweat glands) sited in the external auditory canal.

cervical, *(ser-vī'-kal),* pertaining to the neck or cervix of the uterus. C. *cap*: *see* DIAPHRAGM. C. *collar*: a semi-rigid neck appliance worn to maintain position and give support. C. *intraepithelial neoplasia (CIN)*: staging of cellular changes which occur in the cervix prior to the development of carcinoma-in-situ and invasive cancer; abnormal cells are detected by a smear test and colposcopy, treatment is with lasers or cone biopsy. *See* COLPOSCOPY. C. *nerves*: first eight pairs of spinal nerves. C. *rib*: a bony outgrowth from a cervical vertebra, may cause various symptoms, e.g. pressure on nerves. C. *smear*: *see* PAPANICOLAOU SMEAR. C. *spondylosis*: degenerative changes in the cervical joints and intervertebral discs which result in nerve root compression. C. *vertebrae*: first seven vertebrae of the spinal column.

cervicectomy, *(ser-vi-sek'-to-mi),* excision of the cervix uteri.

cervicitis, *(ser'-vi-sī-tis),* inflammation of the cervix of the uterus.

cervix, *(ser'-viks),* a neck. C. *uteri*: the neck of the uterus. The lowest third of the uterus, about 2.5 cm in length. It is traversed by a canal which opens into the vagina.

cestode, tapeworm. *See* TAENIA.

chaining, a technique used to teach skills in sequence to individuals with learning disabilities. *Forward c.*: where the skill is learnt in the sequence that it normally occurs with each step linking to the next. *Backward c.*: where the skill is learnt by working backwards from the final step.

chalazion, *(kal-ā-zi-on),* Meibomian cyst. A small retention cyst in the eyelid, due to blocking of a Meibomian follicle.

challenging behaviour, behaviour which by nature of its character, frequency or severity may seriously threaten the safety of the individual or other people, or behaviour which hinders the integration of the individual into the community by preventing his or her access to various facilities, e.g. mainstream education.

chalone, a polypeptide hormone-like substance that inhibits rather than stimulates.

chancre, *(shan'-ker),* syphilitic ulcer of the first stage; occurs at the site of infection. Contagious.

chancroid, *(shan-kroyd'),* see SOFT SORE.

character, in computing a numeral, letter or any other mark which can be displayed on the computer screen or printed.

charcoal, highly absorbent activated charcoal is used in the treatment of poisoning and certain wound dressings, reducing odour and exudate.

Charcot's joint, *(shar-kō),* painless destructive joint changes associated with tabes dorsalis or syringomyelia.

Charles' law, at a constant pressure the volume of a specific mass of gas is directly proportional to the temperature. Also known as **Gay-Lussac's law.**

chart, 1. a patient's record which includes: nursing actions, observations, treatments, drugs and investigations. 2. to record data in patient records.

CHD, abbreviation for **coronary heart disease.**

cheilitis, *(kī-li-tis),* inflammation of the lip.

cheiloplasty, *(kī'-lo-plas-ti),* plastic operation on the lips.

cheilorrhaphy, *(kī-lo-ra-fi),* operation to repair a cleft lip or lacerated lip.

cheiloschisis, *(kī-lō-skī-sis),* cleft lip (hare lip).

cheilosis, *(kī-lō-sis),* condition affecting the lips and angles of the mouth which can be caused by vitamin B deficiency.

cheiropompholyx, *(kī-rō-pom'-fo-liks),* a disease characterized by the appearance of small vesicles on the hands.

chelating agents, *(ke-la-ting),* substances which combine with certain metals to form complexes which can be eliminated safely from the body. Used as treatment for poisoning or overload, e.g. desferrioxamine for iron.

chelation, process by which an organic substance combines with a metal to form a ring structure.

chemical name, the name which indicates the chemical structure of a drug. This is in addition to approved (generic) and proprietary names.

chemoprophylaxis, use of drugs to prevent infection, e.g. antibiotics for certain surgical procedures and after contact with meningitis.

chemoreceptor, *(ke-mo-re-sep-tor),* sensory nerve endings or cells able to respond to chemical stimuli, e.g. oxygen levels in the blood, taste and smell. *C. trigger zone (CTZ):* brain area involved in the vomiting reflex. It responds to chemical stimuli, e.g. cytotoxic drugs and endogenous toxins.

chemosis, *(kē-mō'-sis),* oedema of the conjunctiva.

chemotaxis, *(ke-mo-tak-sis),* the attraction or repulsion of living cells for chemical substances, e.g. white blood cells are attracted to an infected area by bacterial chemicals.

chemotherapy, *(ke-mo-the-ra-pi),* use of chemical agents for cure or palliation of disease. Covers both antimicrobial and cytotoxic drugs, but usually the term is applied only to cytotoxic drugs used in malignant disease.

chenodeoxycholic acid, *(ken-ō-dē-oks-ē-ko-lik),* a bile acid. Used to disperse certain types of gallstones.

chest, the thorax. *C. cavity:* the thoracic cavity contains the heart, lungs and great vessels. *C. drain:* tube inserted into the chest to drain air, fluid or blood. *Flail c.:* unstable ribcage, usually resulting from multiple fractures, it is characterized by paradoxical breathing.

Cheyne–Stokes breathing, abnormal breathing pattern in which breathing waxes and wanes. It is characterized by periods where depth of breathing increases followed by decreasing depth and cessation of breathing (apnoea).

CHI, abbreviation for **Commission for Health Improvement**.

chi-square statistic, analyses the relationship between expected frequency and the actual frequency of data obtained. A test of statistical significance used to assess the probability of results occurring by chance.

chiasm, *(kī-azm),* **1.** a crossing such as the optic nerves. **2.** crossover points between chromatids during meiosis.

chiasma, *(pl.* chiasmata*),* *(ki-az-mah),* *see* CHIASM. *C. opticum:* see OPTIC CHIASMA.

chickenpox, varicella, a viral disease primarily of young children. There is mild pyrexia and a skin rash which develops through various stages to pustule formation and possible scarring. Incubation period 12–21 days. *See* HERPES. SHINGLES.

chilblain, pernio. Inflammation with swelling, burning and itching which affects toes, fingers and ears in cold weather.

68

child abuse, the physical, emotional or sexual maltreatment of children by their parents, other adults and sometimes by other children. Also includes neglect. *See* ABUSE, NON-ACCIDENTAL INJURY.

Child protection officer/co-ordinator, a suitably qualified and experienced individual (with a nursing, health visiting or social work background) employed by social services to oversee/co-ordinate the interagency child protection activities in an area. In addition, many NHS trusts employ designated nurses with a child protection role.

childbirth, giving birth to a child.

Children Act 1989, an Act of Parliament (became law in 1991) which clearly defines the rights of children, their protection, welfare and care.

chip, in computing an integrated circuit where electronic components are formed from a single silicon wafer. Their functions vary from control of simple tasks to extremely complex procedures.

chiropodist, *(ki-rop′-ō-dist),* podiatrist.

chiropractic, *(kī-ro-prak-tik),* manipulation of the spine and other structures to relieve pressure on nerve roots. Treatment given by a chiropractor.

Chlamydia, *(klam-id-ia),* microorganisms of the genus *Chlamydia*. They are intracellular parasites and have features common to both bacteria and viruses. *C. psittaci*: infects birds and causes psittacosis in humans. *C. trachomatis* causes trachoma. It commonly infects the genitourinary tracts of both sexes, leading to non-specific urethritis, epididymitis, prostatitis in men and salpingitis and pelvic inflammatory disease (PID) with infertility in women. Infants infected during birth can develop serious eye infections and pneumonia. *See* LYMPHOGRANULOMA VENEREUM, OPHTHALMIA NEONATORUM.

chloasma, *(klō-az′-ma),* pigmentation of the skin. *C. gravidarum*: brown pigmentation occurring during pregnancy. Also associated with the use of oral contraceptives.

chlorhexidine, *(klor-heks-i-dēn),* bactericidal solution used for hand hygiene and as a surgical scrub.

chlorhydria, *(klor-hī-drē-ah),* high levels of hydrochloric acid in gastric juice.

chloride, salt of hydrochloric acid. A major extracellular anion. *C. shift*: movement of chloride ions into the red blood cell, to restore electrical balance, as hydrogen carbonate ions move out into the blood as part of carbon dioxide transport.

chloropsia, *(klor-op-sē-ah),* a defect of colour vision where all objects appear to be green.

choana, *(kō-an-ah),* funnel-shaped cavity or opening.

chocolate cyst, a cyst, usually ovarian, containing degenerated blood. *See* ENDOMETRIOSIS.

cholagogue, *(kōl-a-gog),* drug which increases the flow of bile.

cholangiogram, *(kō-lan-jē-ō-gram),* X-ray showing the bilary system.

cholangiography, radiographic examination of the biliary ducts following the administration of radiopaque contrast medium by various methods, e.g. oral, intravenously, directly at operation, via a T tube, endoscopically or by the percutaneous transhepatic route.

cholangiopancreatography, *(kō-lan-jē-ō-pan-krē-at-og′-raf-ē),* radiographic examination of the biliary and pancreatic ducts following the endoscopic retrograde administration of radiopaque contrast medium.

cholangitis, *(kō-lan-jī-tis),* inflammation of the bile ducts.

cholecalciferol, *(ko-le-kal-sif′-er-ol),* vitamin D₃ produced by the action of sunlight on 7-dehydrocholesterol in the skin or obtained from diet. The active form, 1, 25-dihydroxycholecalciferol, results from biochemical processes which occur in the liver and kidneys. Required for calcium absorption by intestinal cells.

cholecystectomy, *(ko′-lĕ-sis-tek′-to-mi),* removal of the gallbladder.

cholecystenterostomy, *(ko′-lĕ-sist-enter-os′-to-mi),* operation to establish an anastomosis between the gallbladder and small intestine.

cholecystitis, *(ko′-lĕ-sis-tī′-tis),* inflammation of the gallbladder.

cholecystoduodenostomy, *(ko′-lĕ-sis-tō-dū-ō-dĕ-nost′-o-mi),* operation to establish an anastomosis between the gallbladder and the duodenum.

cholecystogastrostomy, *(ko′-lĕ-sis-tō-gas-tros′-to-mi),* operation to establish an anastomosis between the gallbladder and the stomach.

cholecystogram, *(ko′-lĕ-sis-tō-gram),* an X-ray of the gallbladder.

cholecystography, *(ko-lĕ-sis-tog-ra-fi),* radiographic examination of the gallbladder following the oral or intravenous administration of radiopaque contrast medium.

cholecystojejunostomy, *(ko′-lĕ-sis-to-jej-oon-os′-to-mi),* operation to establish an anastomosis between the gallbladder and the jejunum.

cholecystokinin (CCK), *(ko′-lĕ-sis-to-kī-nin),* hormone produced by the duodenal mucosa, it stimulates gallbladder contraction and relaxation of the sphincter of Oddi with release of bile into the duodenum and pancreatic enzyme secretion. *See* PANCREOZYMIN.

cholecystolithiasis, *(ko′-lĕ-sis-to-li-thī′-a-sis),* stones in the gallbladder.

cholecystostomy, *(ko′-lĕ-sis-tos′-to-mi),* operation for making the gallbladder open to the exterior.

cholecystotomy, *(ko′-lĕ-sis-tot-o-mi),* an incision into the gallbladder.

choledochoduodenostomy, *(ko-lĕ-do-kō-dū-ō-dĕ-nos′-to-mi),* operation to establish an anastomosis between the common bile duct and the duodenum.

choledocholithotomy, *(kol-ē-dok-ō-li-thot′-o-mi),* incision of the common bile duct for the removal of gallstone.

choledochotomy, *(ko′-lĕ-do-kot′-o-mi),* incision of the common bile duct.

cholelithiasis, *(ko-lē-li-thī′-a-sis),* stones in the gallbladder or bile ducts.

cholera, acute enteritis caused by the bacterium *Vibrio cholerae.* Endemic and epidemic in Asia and Africa where it is associated with faecal contamination of water and poor hygiene conditions. It is characterized by severe diarrhoea (rice-water stools) with agonizing cramp and vomiting which lead to dehydration, electrolyte imbalance and severe collapse. Mortality rates are high where patients do not have access to adequate fluid replacement.

cholestasis, *(ko-le-stā-sis),* an obstruction to the free flow of bile.

cholesteatoma, *(kol-es-tē-a-tō′-ma),* collection of abnormally sited squamous epithelium in the middle ear.

cholesterol, a sterol found in many animal tissues. It is important as a constituent of cell membranes and as the precursor of many biological molecules, such as steroid hormones, bile salts and vitamin D. High levels in the blood have, however, been linked with an increased incidence of arterial disease and gallstones.

cholic acid, a bile acid.

choline, *(kō-lēn),* an organic base which is a constituent of some important substances, e.g. phospho-glycerides, acetylcholine. It is used in fat metabolism and in the formation of plasma (cell) membrane.

cholinergic, *(ko-lin-er'-jik),* pertaining to nerves that use acetylcholine as a neurotransmitter. *C. drugs:* prevent the breakdown of acetylcholine. *C. receptors:* receptor sites on structures innervated by parasympathetic and voluntary motor nerves. The receptors are termed muscarinic or nicotinic according to how they respond to acetylcholine. *See* ACETYLCHOLINE.

cholinesterase, *(ko-lin-es-te-rāz),* an enzyme which breaks down and inactivates the neurotransmitter acetylcholine.

choluria, *(ko-lū'-ri-a),* bile in the urine.

chondral, *(kon-dral),* pertaining to cartilage.

chondralgia, *(kon-dral'-ji-a),* pain in a cartilage.

chondritis, *(kon-drī-tis),* inflammation of cartilage.

chondroblast, *(kon-drō-blahst),* the immature blast cell forming cartilage.

chondrocyte, *(kon-drō-sīt),* a cartilage cell.

chondroma, *(kon-drō'-ma),* a benign tumour of cartilage cells.

chondromalacia, softening of cartilage.

chondrosarcoma, *(kon-drō-sar-kō'-ma),* a malignant growth arising in cartilage.

chorda tympani, a branch of the facial nerve, supplying part of the tongue. It may be damaged during middle ear surgery.

chordae tendineae, *(kor-dē ten-di-ni-ē),* thin tendinous bands which stabilize the bicuspid and tricuspid valves by securing them to the papillary muscle of the heart.

chordee, *(kor-dē),* **1.** congenital structural defect of the penis. **2.** painful penile erection associated with urethritis.

chorditis, *(kor-dī'-tis),* inflammation of vocal cords or spermatic cord.

chordotomy, *(kor-do-to-mi),* division of the anterolateral tracts of the spinal cord.

chorea, *(ko-rē-a),* involuntary muscular twitching with uncoordinated movements. May follow rheumatic fever in children – *Sydenham's c.* – or in adults it may be due to degeneration in the nervous system as in *Huntington's* disease, an inherited disorder.

choreiform, resembling the uncoordinated jerky movements of chorea.

choriocarcinoma, also called **chorioepithelioma.** A malignant tumour of chorionic cells which may develop following abortion or evacuation of a hydatidiform mole or, rarely, following a normal pregnancy. Metastatic spread, e.g. to lung or brain, is common but treatment with cytotoxic drugs offers a very high cure rate. *See* HYDATIDIFORM MOLE.

chorion, *(ko-rē-on),* formed from the trophoblast it develops into the placenta and the outer membrane surrounding the fetus.

chorionic, *(kor-rē-on-ik),* pertaining to the chorion. *C. epithelioma: see* CHORIOCARCINOMA. *C. gonadotrophin:* (hCG) hormone secreted by the trophoblast layer and later the chorion, it maintains the corpus luteum. Its presence in blood or urine forms the basis of pregnancy testing. Elevated levels are associated with choriocarcinoma (chorioepithelioma), also a tumour marker for testicular cancer. *C. villi:* vascular processes developing from the chorion through which substances diffuse between fetal and maternal blood. They invade the uterine lining (decidua), eventually becoming placental tissue. *C. villus sampling (CVS)*: a screening test for genetic disorders, performed in early pregnancy (around 11 weeks) on samples obtained via the cervix.

choroid, *(ko'-royd)*, the posterior five-sixths of the middle coat of the eye. It is vascular and pigmented, lies between the sclera and retina, and absorbs light.

choroid plexus, specialized capillaries which produces cerebrospinal fluid, situated within the ventricles of the brain.

choroiditis, *(ko'-royd-ī'-tis)*, inflammation of the choroid.

choroidocyclitis, *(ko'-roy-dō-si-klī-tis)*, inflammation of the choroid and ciliary body.

Christmas disease, an inherited defect of blood coagulation where factor IX is deficient. Also called **haemophilia B.**

chromaffin cell, *(krō-maf-in)*, those cells which take up and stain with chromium salts. They are found in the adrenal medulla and the sympathetic nerves.

chromatid, one of the strands resulting from chromosome duplication during nuclear division.

chromatin, nuclear material which forms chromosomes, it has a DNA and protein component.

chromatography, *(krō-mat-og-raf-ē)*, analytical technique. Various methods of separating different gaseous or dissolved substances which include: *gel filtration c., gas c.* and *ion exchange c.*

chromatosis, pigmentation of the skin, e.g. as in Addison's disease.

chromophobe, *(krō-mo-fob)*, cell that resists staining. *C. adenoma*: anterior pituitary tumour affecting chromophobic cells.

chromosomes, genetic material present in the nucleus; when the cell divides they appear as microscopic threads. They consist of connected strands of DNA molecules known as genes. Humans have 23 pairs of chromosomes per cell: 22 pairs of autosomes and 1 pair of sex chromosomes (males XY and females XX) (Figure 18). The gametes have half the normal number (haploid) so that the fusion of oocyte and sperm results in an individual with 46 chromosomes. Genetic material is also present in other organelles, e.g. mitochondria, where it codes for metabolic processes and can be responsible for some inherited conditions, e.g. optic nerve atrophy.

chronic, a condition from which complete cure is not obtained. It develops slowly and tends to worsen. It may be subject to acute exacerbations *C. fatigue syndrome*: *see* MYALGIC ENCEPHALOMYELITIS. *C. obstructive pulmonary disease (COPD)*: a group of respiratory diseases where airway resistance is increased with impaired airflow, e.g. chronic bronchitis and emphysema. It is characterized by dyspnoea, expiratory problems, wheeze, cough and poor gaseous exchange.

chronic wounds, wounds such as leg-ulcers and pressure ulcers. Often have delayed healing and more complex aetiology than acute wounds.

chronological age, an individual's age expressed as the time from birth, e.g. weeks, months or years.

Chvostek's sign, *(shfos-teks)*, spasm of the facial muscles when the facial nerve is tapped. Present in tetany.

chyle, *(kīl)*, creamy (fat containing) fluid formed from chylomicrons within the lymphatic lacteals of the intestinal villi.

18 Normal chromosomes (male)

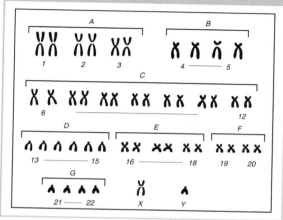

chylomicrons, *(kī-lo-mī-kronz),* tiny particles formed from triacylglycerols (triglycerides), cholesterol and lipoproteins within the intestinal cells after fat absorption. They enter the lymphatic lacteals to form chyle.

chyluria, *(kī-lū'-ri-a),* passing of chyle in the urine.

chyme, *(chīm),* food which has been partially digested in the stomach.

chymotrypsinogen, *(kī-mo-trip-sin'-ō-jen),* an inactive proteolytic enzyme secreted by the pancreas; it is activated by trypsin.

cicatrix, *(sik'-a-triks),* the scar of a healed wound or ulcer.

cilia, *(sil'-ē-a),* **1.** eyelashes. **2.** microscopic processes of certain cells, e.g. those lining the respiratory tract. *See* CILIATED EPITHELIUM.

ciliary body, *(sil'-ē-a-ri),* part of the eye which joins the iris to the anterior choroid, it contains the ciliary muscles that control accommodation and processes which secrete aqueous humor.

ciliated epithelium, *(sil'-ē-ā-ted),* epithelium with microscopic hair-like projections on its surface which move in one direction only. Found lining the respiratory tract and uterine tubes.

Cimex lectularius, *(sē-meks-lek-tū-lā-rē-us),* the common bed bug.

CINAHL, abbreviation for **Cumulative Index to Nursing and Allied Health Literature.**

cineradiography, radiographic technique where moving images are portrayed on a television monitor. Used in gastrointestinal studies, during cardiac catheterization and for urinary studies such as cystourethrography.

73

circadian rhythm, *(ser-kā-dē-an),* the periodic rhythm of biological functions over a 24 hour period, e.g. hormone levels, sleep patterns.

circinate, *(ser-kin-āt),* ring-shaped.

circle of Willis, circular intercommunication of arteries supplying the brain (Figure 19).

circulation, movement of an object or fluid around a circular route, e.g. circulation of blood. *See* HEART. *Coronary c.:* the blood supply to heart muscle via coronary arteries. *Extracorporeal c.:* diversion of blood outside the body as with cardiopulmonary bypass. *Hepatic portal c.:* venous blood from the digestive tract, spleen and pancreas, which is rich in nutrients and hormones passes through the liver, via the hepatic portal vein, prior to its return to the systemic circulation. *Lymph c.:* the collection and transport of lymph, in lymphatic vessels, back to the venous system. *Pulmonary c.:* deoxy-

genated blood leaves the right ventricle via the pulmonary artery which branches to each lung. The artery branches again within the lung eventually to form capillary networks around the alveoli. Gaseous exchange occurs – oxygen into the blood and carbon dioxide into the alveoli and oxygenated blood returns to the left atrium via the pulmonary veins. *Systemic (general) c.:* oxygenated blood returned to the left atrium passes into the left ventricle and is pumped out to the body via the aorta. It moves through smaller arteries to the capillary networks where nutrients, oxygen and waste diffuse between the blood and cells. The blood with high levels of waste returns via veins, eventually forming the venae cavae which empty into the right atrium.

circumcision, surgical removal of the male prepuce (foreskin) or the female clitoris and labia.

---

19 Circle of Willis

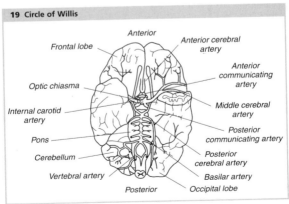

- Anterior
- Frontal lobe
- Anterior cerebral artery
- Anterior communicating artery
- Optic chiasma
- Middle cerebral artery
- Internal carotid artery
- Posterior communicating artery
- Pons
- Posterior cerebral artery
- Cerebellum
- Basilar artery
- Vertebral artery
- Posterior
- Occipital lobe

circumduction, circular movement where a limb traces a cone in space.

circumflex, having a winding path, such as a vessel or nerve.

circumoral, around the mouth. *C. pallor:* a pale area around the mouth in marked contrast to the rest of the face.

circumvallate, surrounded by a wall.

cirrhosis, *(sir-rō'-sis),* **1.** hardening in an organ. **2.** chronic diffuse damage to an organ. Usually applied to the degenerative changes which occur in liver. The fibrosis and structural damage leads to loss of liver cells and obstruction to the hepatic portal circulation. Causes include: alcohol misuse, viral hepatitis, drugs and metabolic disorders.

cisterna, *(sis-ter'-na),* a reservoir holding body fluids. *C. chyli:* a dilation at the start of the thoracic duct which receives lymph. *C. magna:* subarachnoid space between the medulla and cerebellum, contains cerebrospinal fluid.

cisternal puncture, *(sis-ter'-nal),* a puncture made through the neck into the cisterna magna to obtain a sample of cerebrospinal fluid.

citrate, *(sit-rāt),* formed from citric acid and a base. Used to prevent the in vitro coagulation of blood.

citric acid, organic acid found in citrus and soft fruit. *C. acid cycle: see* KREBS' CYCLE, TRICARBOXYLIC ACID CYCLE.

citrulline, *(sit-rul-een),* an intermediate of the urea cycle in the liver.

civil law, law relating to non-criminal. matters. *C. action:* proceedings brought in the civil courts. *C. wrong:* act or omission which can be pursued in the civil courts by the person who has suffered the wrong.

CJD, abbreviation for **Creutzfeldt–Jakob disease.**

claim form, the start of a civil action. Previously called a writ.

Clark's rule, a formula for calculating paediatric drug doses—

$$\frac{\text{weight of child (kg)}}{\text{average adult weight (70 kg)}} \times \text{adult dose}$$

clasp-knife reflex, the reflex observed in a spastic limb which at first resists passive movement and then suddenly gives way, very much like the closing of a clasp-knife.

class, a sociological term describing the socioeconomic variation between groups that accounts for differences in the level of affluence and influence. *See* SOCIAL CLASS.

claudication, limping. *Intermittent c.:* limping with severe pain on walking which disappears with rest; due to insufficient blood supply to the limb.

claustrophobia, irrational fear of a confined space, such as a room. Opposite of agoraphobia.

clavicle, collar bone. Articulates with the scapula and sternum.

clavus, *(klā-vus),* a corn.

claw foot, pes cavus. The foot is shaped like a claw and has a very pronounced arch.

claw hand, claw-shaped deformity due to flexor spasm followed by contracture of the muscles flexing the fingers; often due to ulnar nerve damage.

clean-catch specimen, method of obtaining a specimen of urine with as little bacterial contamination as possible without using invasive means.

clearance, the ability of the kidney to clear the blood of a particular substance. *Renal c.:* measurement of glomerular filtration rate and kidney function by calculating the volume of blood cleared of a substance, e.g. creatinine, in a given time, usually one minute.

cleavage, 1. process occurring in the ovum where it divides by mitosis following fertilization. *C. lines*: a pattern of lines occurring in the dermis. *C. furrow*: indentation which forms around a dividing cell just prior to cytokinesis.

cleft, narrow fissure. *C. lip*: congenital defect where the top lip fails to fuse in the midline during development. Frequently associated with cleft palate. *C. palate*: congenital defect where the palate fails to fuse in the midline during development (Figure 20). The cleft may vary, but when complete extends through both soft and hard palates into the nasal cavity. Cleft lip/palate are treated surgically.

cleidocranial dysostosis, *(klī-dō-krā-nē-al dï-sos-tō-sis)*, rare hereditary condition characterized by a failure of ossification in the cranial bones and a partial or total absence of clavicles.

client, a person who uses professional services such as those provided by a nurse. *C.-centred therapy*: a type of

20 A cleft palate

Hard palate

Soft palate

Uvula

Line of cleavage

psychotherapy where the therapist acts in a non-directive, reflective and supportive manner.

Clifton Assessment Procedure for the Elderly, a series of tests used to measure cognitive function and behaviour.

climacteric, *(klī-mak-ter-ik)*, in the female, describes the period of time during which ovarian activity declines and eventually ceases. It generally occurs between the mid-40s and mid-50s. The cessation of menstruation is a distinct event during the climacteric. *See* MENOPAUSE.

clinical, 1. pertaining to a clinic, or observation and treatment of patients. *C. equipment*: used in the treatment or nursing of patients. *C. nurse specialist*: a nurse with advanced knowledge, skills and qualifications in a particular field of nursing. *C. thermometer*: see THERMOMETER.

clinical audit, part of quality assurance. A critical analysis of the quality of clinical care and treatment. It includes diagnostic procedures, treatment, resource use and outputs, including quality of life for the individual.

clinical governance, describes the framework introduced into the NHS within which all organizations are accountable for their services, and are required to have in place an active programme of continuous quality improvement within an overall/coherent framework of cost-effective service delivery.

clinical supervision, aimed at the delivery of high-quality healthcare, the process of clinical supervision assists practitioners to develop skills, knowledge and professional values throughout their careers, and implies a requirement to reflect and measure risk. Enables individuals to develop a deeper understanding of what it is to be an accountable practitioner.

clitoris, small erectile organ situated in the anterior part of the labia minora. Homologous to the penis. It contains abundent nervous tissue, is very sensitive and is involved in the female sexual response.

cloaca, (klo-ō-ka), aperture through which both urine and faeces are discharged, or in diseased bone, the opening in newly formed bone which discharges pus.

clone, cells or organisms of identical genetic makeup produced, by successive mitotic divisions, from a single common cell.

clonic, characteristic of clonus. Muscle contraction and relaxation seen in some types of epilepsy.

clonus, spasmodic, rapid contraction and relaxation of muscle.

Clostridium, (klos-trid-ē-um), a genus of spore-forming anaerobic bacteria which include: *C. tetani* (tetanus), *C. botulinum* (botulism), *C. difficile* (pseudomembranous colitis) and *C. perfringens* (gas gangrene).

clot, 1. jelly-like mass of fibrin and blood cells. **2.** to coagulate.

clotting, the process by which blood clots or coagulates. *C. factor*: one of twelve factors required for blood clotting, e.g. calcium ions, prothrombin. *C. time*: the time taken for a clot to form when bleeding occurs. *See* BLOOD CLOTTING.

clubbing, enlargement of the terminal phalanges of the fingers and sometimes the toes. Associated with chronic cardiovascular and respiratory conditions.

clubfoot, *see* TALIPES.

clumping, packing together of cells (usually red blood cells), due to loss of membrane charge resulting from reaction with antibody. *See* AGGLUTININS.

Clutton's joints, swelling of the knee joints found in congenital syphilis.

CMV, abbreviation for **cytomegalovirus** and **controlled mandatory ventilation**.

CNS, abbreviation for **central nervous system** and **clinical nurse specialist**.

coagulant, any substance which causes blood clotting.

coagulase, (kō-ag-ū-lāz), a bacterial enzyme, present in some staphylococci, which clots plasma. *C. test*: a test for identifying pathogenic staphylococci based on their ability to produce coagulase.

coagulation, clotting. *See* BLOOD CLOTTING, CLOTTING.

coalesce, (kō-a-les), to converge or come together as may occur with a skin rash.

coarctation, (kō-ark-tā'-shon), contraction or compression of a vessel wall. *C. of the aorta*: a congenital narrowing of the aorta in the region of the ductus arteriosus (fetal structure).

cobalamin, a constituent of the molecules having vitamin B_{12} activity. Needed for normal red cell production and neurological function.

cobalt (Co), essential trace element utilized as a constituent of vitamin B_{12}. Required for healthy red blood cell formation and neurological function. A radioisotope (^{60}Co) is used to treat some malignant conditions.

cocaine, a powerful local anaesthetic. Controlled drug under the Misuse of Drugs Act (1971) and Misuse of Drugs Regulations (1985). It is addictive and subject to considerable criminal misuse. *Crack c.*: a highly potent and addictive form.

coccidiodomycosis, (kok-sid-ē-oid-ō-mī-kō'-sis), infection caused by the spores of the fungus *Coccidioides immitis*. Seen in the southern United States and south America.

coccus, *(kok'-us),* any spheroidal-shaped microorganism. *See* BACTERIA.

coccydynia, *(kok-si-din'-ē-a),* pain in the coccyx.

coccygeal, pertaining to the coccyx. *C. nerves*: last pair of spinal nerves.

coccygenus, a muscle forming part of the pelvic floor.

coccyx, *(kok'-siks),* last part of the spinal column formed from four or five fused vestigial tail bones.

cochlea, *(kok'-lē-a),* spiral fluid-filled tube (like a snail's shell) within the inner ear. It contains the auditory receptors of the organ of Corti which connect with fibres of the cochlear branch of the VIIIth cranial nerve.

code of practice, guidelines about how a healthcare professional should fulfil their role, duties, obligations and responsibilities, such as those produced by the statutory bodies set up to regulate the registration and work of healthcare professionals.

codon, in genetics the triplet of complementary bases in messenger RNA (mRNA) involved in the transcription stage of protein synthesis.

coeliac, *(sēl-ē-ak),* related to the abdominal cavity. *C. disease*: a bowel condition caused by a sensitivity to gluten, seen in infants after weaning but may occur in adults. Characterized by malabsorption, poor growth, weight loss, anaemia and bulky, offensive fatty stools. *See* GLUTEN-SENSITIVE ENTEROPATHY.

coenzyme, an organic non-protein substance which activates an enzyme. Many vitamins perform this role, e.g. B vitamins needed for the biochemical processes which liberate energy from nutrients.

cofactor, a coenzyme or a substance which functions with another.

coffee ground vomit, vomit which contains partly digested blood.

cognition, part of the mental process—thinking, awareness, knowing, judgement, memory and reasoning. *See* AFFECT, CONATION.

cognitive, involved with thought processes. *C. behavioural therapy*: a therapy where the patient learns to modify thought processes as a way of dealing with unwanted feelings and maladaptive behaviour. *C. development*: the development of intellect: thinking and reasoning skills during a person's lifespan.

cogwheel rigidity, a rigidity seen in certain neurological conditions. When a muscle is passively stretched it resists with jerky movements.

cohabitation, when a couple live together without marriage.

cohort, a group of people who have some common characteristic, e.g. age. *C. study*: research that investigates a population that shares a common feature.

cohorting, infection control measure where people in hospital with the same infection are located together.

coitus, *(ko-it'-us),* sexual intercourse. *C. interruptus*: unreliable contraceptive method where the penis is withdrawn from the vagina prior to ejaculation.

colectomy, *(ko-lek'-to-mē),* excision of the colon (part or all).

colic, severe abdominal pain due to muscular spasm in a hollow organ, often due to obstruction. *Biliary c.*: due to the presence of a gallstone in the cystic or common bile duct. *Intestinal c.*: due to gut irritation, as in food poisoning. *Renal c.*: due to a stone obstructing the ureter. *Uterine c.*: see DYSMENORRHOEA.

coliform, resembling enterobacteria such as *Escherichia coli*.

colitis, *(ko-lī-tis),* inflammation of the colon. It may be acute or chronic, and may be accompanied by ulcerative lesions. *See* ULCERATIVE COLITIS.

collagen, (kol'-a-jen), a protein constituent of fibrous tissue. *C. diseases*: a group of autoimmune diseases in which there is inflammation of the small blood vessels, e.g. systemic lupus erythematosus, polyarteritis nodosa, dermatomyositis, rheumatoid arthritis.

collapse, 1. severe sudden prostration. **2.** collapse of the walls of a hollow structure such as a lung.

collar bone, clavicle.

collateral, accessory or secondary. *C. circulation*: blood flowing in accessory vessels, generally when primary vessels are blocked.

Colles' fracture, (kol-es), fracture of the radius just above the wrist with displacement of the hand backwards and upwards, giving the characteristic dinner fork deformity.

collodion, inflammable liquid that forms a clear, flexible film when applied to skin.

colloid, a glue-like non-crystalline substance; diffusible but not soluble in water; unable to pass through animal membranes. Therapeutic uses include: **1.** various metals in their colloidal state, e.g. gold; **2.** colloid solutions given intravenously to increase extracellular volume.

coloboma, (kol-ob-ō'-ma), a fissure or gap in the eyeball or in one of its component parts, particularly the uvea.

colon, (kō'-lon), the part of the large intestine between the caecum and the rectum (Figure 21). *See* BOWEL.

colonic, pertaining to the colon.

colonization, the establishment of microorganisms in a specific environment, such as a body site, with minimal or no response. There is no disease, but colonization leads to a reservoir of microorganisms that may cause infection.

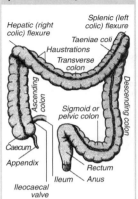

21 Large intestine (showing parts of the colon)

Hepatic (right colic) flexure
Splenic (left colic) flexure
Taeniae coli
Haustrations
Transverse colon
Ascending colon
Descending colon
Sigmoid or pelvic colon
Caecum
Appendix
Rectum
Ileum
Anus
Ileocaecal valve

colonoscopy, (ko-lon-os'-ko-pi), an endoscopic examination of the colon, using a fibreoptic colonoscope.

colony, a mass of bacteria growing in culture medium. *C.-stimulating factor (CSF)*: growth factors that stimulate blood stem cells to produce a particular cell line, e.g. granulocyte-CSF stimulates neutrophils.

coloproctitis, (ko-lō-prok-tī'-tis), inflammation of the colon and rectum.

colorectal, pertaining to the colon and rectum.

colostomy, operation to make an artificial opening so that the colon opens on to the anterior abdominal wall.

colostrum, (kol-os-trum), fluid secreted from the breasts during the first three days after delivery. It contains maternal antibodies, more protein, minerals and vitamins, but less lactose and fat than 'true' milk.

colotomy, *(kol-ot'-o-mi),* an incision into the colon.

colour blindness, various conditions where there is an inability to distinguish certain colours. *See* ACHROMATOPSIA, DALTONISM.

colour index, an index used to express the relative amount of haemoglobin contained in the red blood cells.

colpectomy, excision of the vagina.

colpitis, *(kol-pī'-tis),* inflammation of the vagina.

colpocele, prolapse of either the bladder or rectum so that it presses on the vaginal wall.

colpohysterectomy, *(kol-pō-his-ter-ek'-to-mi),* removal of the uterus through the vagina. A vaginal hysterectomy.

colpoperineorrhaphy, *(kol'-pō-per-i-nē-ōr'-a-fi),* operation for repairing a torn vagina and deficient perineum.

colporrhaphy, *(kol-por-a-fi),* an operation to repair a vaginal prolapse or tear. *Anterior c.:* repair of anterior vaginal wall and treatment for a cystocele. *Posterior c.:* repair of posterior vaginal wall and treatment for a retocele.

colposcopy, an examination of the cervix and vagina. A colposcope (low-powered microscope) is used to detect abnormal cells and give local laser treatment. *See* CERVICAL INTRAEPITHELIAL NEOPLASIA (CIN).

colpotomy, incision of the vagina.

coma, a state of altered consciousness where the individual is insensible and does not respond to painful stimuli. Causes include: trauma, drugs and alcohol, brain pathology and metabolic disorders. *See* GLASGOW COMA SCALE.

comatose, in a state of coma.

comedones, accumulations of sebaceous secretions in the hair follicles, commonly called blackheads (open) or whiteheads (closed).

commensal, a microorganism adapted to grow on the skin and mucous surfaces of the host, forming part of the normal flora. They cause no harm in the correct site and may have beneficial effects. May be pathogenic in other locations.

comminuted fracture, *see* FRACTURE.

Commission for Health Improvement, a body with powers to inspect and support the implementation of clinical governance in Health Authorities and NHS Trusts.

commissure, a connecting structure, such as a bundle of nerves connecting different sides of the brain or spinal cord. **2.** the point at which two structures meet, such as the corner of the lips, eyelids or labia.

Committee on the Safety of Medicines (CSM), the body that monitors drug safety and advises the UK Licensing Authority about quality, efficacy and safety of medicines. *See* YELLOW CARD REPORTING.

common law, that part of law that is derived from decisions made by judges, case law.

communicable disease, a microbial disease which is transmitted directly or indirectly from one person or animal to another.

community, a social group of people living in a particular geographical area and/or a group sharing common values and interests. *C. Health Council (CHC):* a body comprising lay members of the community who monitor local health services and represent the views of local consumers to the relevant health authority. Replacement by patient forums, patient advocacy liaison services in NHS and primary care trusts, and relevant local government authority is planned for 2002 depending on the necessary legislation. *C. nurse*: any nurse who provides professional services in a community setting, such as the patient's home or health centre. *C. psychiatric nurse*: a specialist mental health nurse who provides support, supervision and therapy for patients living in the community. *C. mental handicap nurse*: a specialist nurse who provides support, therapy and other services for individuals with learning disabilities and their families within the community.

compact tissue, the hard, external portion of a bone. *See* BONE.

comparative study, study comparing two populations.

compartment, an enclosed space. *C. syndrome*: compromised circulation and tissue function in a closed space, usually a muscle compartment, leading to muscle necrosis. *Fluid c.*: either the intracellular or extracellular compartments which contain body fluids.

compatibility, able to be mixed together without adverse result such as blood crossmatched prior to transfusion, tissue for transplant or two different drugs. *See* BLOOD GROUPS, BLOOD TRANSFUSION.

compensation, 1. the counterbalancing of a structural or functional defect, e.g. cardiac compensation, where the heart enlarges by hypertrophy to maintain an adequate cardiac output when disease is present. **2.** a mental defence mechanism, employed to cover up a weakness, by exaggerating a more socially acceptable quality.

competence, the state of being competent. Being properly qualified, knowledgeable, capable and skilful in a particular area such as a nursing action.

complement, a group of proteins present in the plasma, which, when

activated, enhance the immune response, inflammation and bacterial lysis. *C. fixation test*: serological test where the fixation of complement is used to detect the presence of specific antigen–antibody complexes.

complemental, complementary. *C. air*: additional air drawn into the lungs on deep inspiration.

complementary, an addition, making complete. *C. feeding*: extra feeds given to an infant where breast milk supplies are inadequate. Now generally accepted to impede the establishment of lactation. *C. Medicine*: a range of holistic therapies which include: acupuncture, reflexology, aromatherapy and homoeopathy.

complex, a series of emotionally charged ideas, repressed because they conflict with ideas acceptable to the person. *See* ELECTRA COMPLEX, OEDIPUS COMPLEX.

compliance, 1. the extent to which the lungs and thorax can stretch and distend. Healthy lungs need only a very small inflating pressure to move a tidal volume of around 500 ml. **2.** the degree to which a patient will follow a treatment regimen, drug course or lifestyle modification prescribed by a healthcare professional.

complicated fracture, *see* FRACTURE.

complication of disease, an accident or second disease occurring in the course of some other disease and more or less dependent upon it.

compos mentis, of sound mind. Being mentally competent.

compound, a chemical substance formed by the combination of two or more elements and having new properties. *C. fracture*: *see* FRACTURE.

comprehension, the understanding of ideas and the relationship between them.

compress, a folded pad of gauze or other material used to stop bleeding or apply pressure, medication, heat, cold or moisture.

compression, the state of being compressed *C. bandage*: used in the management of venous leg ulcers to increase venous return and reduce venous hypertension. Compression stockings are used to prevent venous leg ulcers, or to reduce the risk of deep vein thrombosis postoperatively or during immobility.

compromise, mental defence mechanism whereby a conflict is avoided by disguising the repressed wish to make it acceptable in consciousness.

compulsion, an urge to carry out an act recognized to be irrational. Resisting the urge leads to increasing tension which is only relieved by carrying out the act. *See* NEUROSIS.

computed axial tomography (CAT), *See* COMPUTED TOMOGRAPHY.

computed tomography (CT), computer-constructed imaging technique of a thin horizontal slice through the body, derived from X-ray absorption data collected during a circular scanning motion.

conation, part of the mental process – the will, desire and volition. *See* AFFECT, COGNITION.

concave, with outline curved like interior of a circle.

concavity, a depression.

conceive, 1. become pregnant. 2. to understand or appreciate something.

concentric, with a common centre.

conception, 1. the penetration of an oocyte by a spermatozoon. 2. an abstract idea or mental image, or its formation.

concha, *(kong-kah),* shell-like structure. *C. auris*: external ear, surrounds external auditory canal. *Nasal c.*: one of three bones (turbinate) protruding into the nasal cavity.

concrete operations, according to Piaget, a stage in cognitive development occuring between 7 and 12 years where thinking becomes more rational, but is based on concrete rather than abstract ideas.

concretion, *see* CALCULUS.

concurrent, events occurring or acting together. *C. audit*: a type of nursing audit where care in progress is assessed and evaluated.

concussion, a violent jarring or shaking, e.g. from a blow. The term is usually applied to the brain. It interferes with brain function and may cause: altered consciousness headache, dizziness, vomiting and visual problems.

condensation, 1. transformation of a gas to a liquid, or a liquid to a solid 2. becoming denser or thicker. 3. in psychology the combining of two or more concepts to form a single symbol, as in dreams.

conditioned reflex, a reflex in which response occurs, not to the sensory stimulus which caused it originally but to another stimulus which the subject has learned to associate with the original stimulus. It may be acquired by training and repetition.

conditioning, a process by which individuals learn to modify their behaviour in response to stimuli. *Classical c.*: a process by which a neutral stimulus, which was used with the original stimulus, will eventually produce the required response when used alone. *Operant c.*: a process by which the desired response to stimulus is rewarded. The desired behaviour, thus associated with reward, is more likely to be repeated.

condom, a thin sheath worn over the penis which prevents conception and reduces the spread of sexually transmitted infections (STIs). *Female c.*: polyurethane tube that fits into the vagina to provide contraception and protection against STIs.

conduction, 1. passage of heat, sound or light waves through a suitable medium. **2.** transmission of electrical impulses within the body, such as a nerve impulse.

conductor, a substance which allows the passage of electricity, heat, sound and light.

condyle, a round projection at the ends of some bones.

condyloma, *(kon-de-lo-ma),* warts. *C. acuminata*: caused by a virus are seen around the genital area and anus. *C. lata*: is a syphilitic lesion found in moist areas such as genitalia, anus, mouth and axilla.

cone biopsy, cone-shaped excision of the uterine cervix. Used to treat certain CIN stages.

cones, types of photoreceptors within the retina responsible for high definition colour vision in bright light. *See* RODS.

confabulation, the narration of fictitious events, seen in confusional states where the person fabricates information to compensate for loss of recent memory.

confidence interval, in statistics, a level, e.g. 95%, that indicates the level of confidence that the test result, e.g. sample mean, will fall within a specified range.

confidentiality, a legal and professional requirement to protect all confidences concerning patients and clients obtained in the course of professional practice, and make disclosures only with consent, where required by a court order, or by law, or where [they] can justify disclosure in the wider public interest.

confinement, 1. labour and childbirth. **2.** keeping someone within a designated area.

conflict, a mental struggle caused by the presence of two antagonistic or contradictory desires, goals or ideas. May be suppressed with the development of neuroses.

confounding variable, outside factor, apart from the variables already taken into account, that distorts the results of research.

confusion, inability to think clearly. It may be associated with clouding of consciousness, loss of decision making and disorientation.

confusional state, may be acute, such as with anaemia or infection. Chronic states have a slow onset, e.g. hypothyroidism.

congenital, existing at birth, e.g. developmental dysplasia of the hip (DDH) (previously known as congenital dislocation of the hip), congenital heart disease.

congestion, hyperaemia. Accumulation of blood in a part of the body. May be active, which involves dilatation of arterioles and capillaries, or passive, which is due to venous stasis.

congestive cardiac failure, cardiac failure characterized by venous congestion in organs and vessels which results in both systemic and pulmonary oedema and poor tissue oxygenation.

conization, *See* CONE BIOPSY.

conjugate, the diameters of the pelvis: true, diagonal and external conjugates, important in obstetrics.

conjugation, 1. joining of one substance to another to form a different chemical. Important body process, usually occurring in the liver, which allows toxic substances to be excreted safely. **2.** a method by which bacteria use sex pilli to transfer genetic material during sexual reproduction. Allows genes for drug resistance to pass between bacterial strains.

conjunctiva, transparent vascular membrane which lines the eyelids and is reflected over the anterior surface of the eyeball.

conjunctivitis, inflammation of the conjunctiva.

connective tissue, diverse group of tissues situated throughout the body which include: areolar, adipose, reticular, fibrous, elastic, cartilage, bone and blood/blood-forming tissue. They are characterized by a matrix containing cells and fibres.

Conn's syndrome, a primary oversecretion of aldosterone from the adrenal cortex. *See* ALDOSTERONISM.

consanguinity, blood relationship.

conscious, 1. being awake, alert and aware. **2.** mental processes of which the individual has full awareness.

consent, the voluntary agreement given by a patient or an authorized person, for an action, diagnostic procedure, treatment or surgical intervention. *Informed c.*: that agreement given only after a full discussion of the relevant facts, e.g. possible surgical complications or side effects from medication.

conservative, aiming at preservation or repair, e.g. conservative treatment of a tooth.

consolidation, becoming solid, as with a lung in lobar phenumonia.

constipation, infrequent or incomplete bowel action leading to hard faeces filling the rectum; caused by lack of non-starch polysaccharides (NSP), fluids and exercise or by ignoring or being unable to respond to the urge to defecate, medication, systemic illness, depression and anorectal conditions that cause pain on defecation.

constrict, contract or draw together.

contact, one who has been exposed to an infectious disease. *C. dermatitis*: a skin reaction caused by exposure to an irritant or antigen. *C. lens*: glass or plastic corrective lens worn on the anterior surface of the eyeball.

contagious, a highly infectious disease, transmitted easily by direct or indirect contact.

containment isolation, separation of patient with, or suspected of having, a communicable disease to prevent the spread of infection to others.

contaminate, to infect with pathogens, pollute or soil objects, food or water.

continence, 1. ability to control the voiding of urine and defecation until appropriate. **2.** voluntary restraint.

continuing care, nursing and other care required by a person with a chronic condition.

continuing professional development (CPD), also known as continuing education (CE), regular updating and advancement of skill and knowledge. Necessary for a registered nurses, midwives and health visitors as part of their professional accountability for practice. *See* APPENDIX 1: CODE OF PROFESSIONAL CONDUCT.

continuous, extended, uninterrupted. *C. ambulatory peritoneal dialysis (CAPD)*: a type of dialysis carried out each day by patients, with renal failure, at home. *C. positive airway pressure (CPAP)*: a respiratory therapy, using the administration of gases at positive pressure via a respirator to increase functional lung capacity by preventing alveolar collapse at the end of expiration.

contraception, preventing conception.

contraceptive, a device, appliance or drug which prevents conception

Oral c.: drugs, either combined oestrogens and progestogens or progestogen only, which prevent conception by inhibition of ovulation, prevention of endometrial proliferation, reduction of uterine tube motility and alterations to cervical mucus.

contracted pelvis, a pelvis is contracted if any diameter is shorter than normal (*see* DIAMETERS and CONJUGATE). May cause problems during labour and delivery.

contractile, having the ability to contract, such as muscle fibres.

contraction, shortening, drawing together.

contracture, permanent contraction of a structure due to the formation of inelastic fibrous tissue. *Dupuytren's c.*: localized fibrosis of the palmar fascia causing flexion of the fingers towards the palm. *Volkmann's ischaemic c.*: flexion deformity of the wrist caused by lack of blood to the forearm muscles, such as may occur with tourniquet use or brachial artery compression following a supracondylar fracture of the elbow.

contralateral, on the opposite side.

contrast medium, radiopaque substance used in radiography, e.g. barium sulphate, to outline or visualize structures under examination.

contrecoup, (kon-tr-koo) injury through transmission of the force of a blow, remote from the original point of contact, such as damage to the brain as it hits the inside of the skull on the opposite side to the blow.

control, 1. a standard against which the validity of test or experiment results are measured. **2.** in research, a subject who does not receive the research intervention (for example a new drug) but whose condition is compared with the subjects who received the intervention.

controlled cord traction, a method of delivering the placenta and membranes.

controlled drugs (CD), a group of drugs subject to statutory control. *See* MISUSE OF DRUGS.

contusion, a bruise.

convalescence, period of recovery following illness, surgery or injury.

convection, the heat of gases and liquids transferred by the circulation of heated particles.

convergence, moving together, such as the eyes moving to focus on a close object.

conversion, 1. mental defence mechanism where an intense emotional conflict is converted into a physical manifestation *C. disorder*: psychological disorder in which the conflict is converted into physical symptoms, e.g. blindness or loss of sensation. **2.** correcting fetal position during labour.

convex, with outline curved, like exterior of circle.

convolutions, folds and twists, such as the renal tubules or on the surface of the brain.

convulsions, fits or seizures. Violent spasms of alternate muscular contraction and relaxation. Caused by a variety of conditions, e.g. epilepsy. *Clonic c.*: associated with muscle contraction and relaxation. *Febrile c.*: occur in young children with pyrexia (high temperature). *Tonic c.*: associated with complete muscle rigidity.

convulsive therapy, electroplexy. *see* ELECTROCONVULSIVE THERAPY.

85

Cooley's anaemia, see THALASSAEMIA.

Coombs' test, used to detect antibodies to red blood cells. Direct and indirect versions are used in the diagnosis of various haemolytic conditions.

COPD, abbreviation for **chronic obstructive pulmonary disease.**

coping, protective behaviour which allows an individual to deal with stress and difficult situations. C. *strategies*: techniques which a person utilizes to maintain emotional well-being, e.g. relaxation.

copper (Cu), an element. Required in trace amounts for red cell formation and the synthesis of catecholamines, enkephalins and some enzymes.

copraphagy, *(kop-ra-fa'-ji),* eating of faeces.

coprolalia, *(kop-rō-la-li-a),* uncontrolled use of obscene words; may be due to cerebral disease. See TOURETTE'S SYNDROME.

copropraxia, obscene gesture. See TOURETTE'S SYNDROME.

copulation, sexual intercourse.

cor pulmonale, *(kor pul-mon-ah-le),* right heart failure resulting from chronic respiratory disease.

coracoid, *(kor'-a-koyd)* a process of bone on the scapula which resembles a crow's beak.

cord, thread or cord-like structure. *Spermatic c.*: runs through the inguinal canal where it encloses vessels and nerves supplying the testis, and the vas deferens. *Spinal c.*: part of the central nervous system continuous with the medulla oblongata and runs inside the vertebral canal to the level of the first/second lumbar vertebra in adults. *Umbilical c.*: links the fetus to the placenta, carries two arteries and one vein. *Vocal c.*: folds in the larynx which vibrate to produce sound.

cordotomy, see CHORDOTOMY.

core, at the centre. *C. temperature*: the temperature at the body core.

Cori cycle, a biochemical process whereby lactic acid is converted to glucose for cell use. It takes place in the liver when oxygen is available.

Cori's disease, a glycogen storage disease.

corium or dermis, internal layer of the skin. The true skin.

cornea, transparent, avascular membrane covering the front of the eye ball.

corneal, pertaining to the cornea. *C. graft*: replacement of opaque diseased cornea with the transplantation of healthy cornea.

cornu, horn-like.

corona, crown-like. *C. dentis*: crown of a tooth. *C. radiata*: cells surrounding an oöcyte.

coronal, pertaining to a crown-like structure. *C. suture*: suture joining the frontal and parietal skull bones.

coronary, *(kor-on-a-rē),* crown-like encircling, as a vessel. *C. arteries* supply blood to the myocardium (Figure 22). Narrowing by spasm or c. artery disease produces angina

22 Coronary arteries

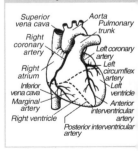

Superior vena cava

Aorta

Pulmonary trunk

Right coronary artery

Left coronary artery

Left circumflex artery

Right atrium

Left ventricle

Inferior vena cava

Marginal artery

Anterior interventricular artery

Right ventricle

Posterior interventricular artery

pectoris or myocardial infarction. Diseased vessels are cleared using laser, balloon angioplasty or replaced using vein grafts from the legs (c. artery bypass or c. artery vein graft). C. care unit (CCU): a unit providing specialist care for acutely ill patients with cardiac conditions, such as myocardial infarction, arrhythmias and unstable angina. C. heart disease (CHD): another name for ischaemic heart disease. C. sinus: vessel through which most venous blood from the myocardium returns to the right atrium. C. thrombosis: occlusion of coronary artery by blood clot.

coroner, in England and Wales a medically or legally qualified person appointed to investigate sudden, violent or unexplained deaths. In Scotland reports about such deaths are submitted to the Procurator Fiscal. The Scottish equivalent to a coroner's inquest is the Fatal Accident Enquiry.

coronoid, like a crow's beak, as with certain bony processes.

corpus, a body. C. albicans (white body): scar tissue remaining on the ovary, after degeneration of the c. luteum. C. callosum: band of white matter connecting the two cerebral hemispheres. C. cavernosa: two lateral columns of penile erectile tissue. C. luteum (yellow body): structure formed on the ovary after ovulation. It secretes hormones which maintain pregnancy, should fertilization occur, until the placenta is functional. Without fertilization it degenerates and menstruation occurs. C. spongiosum: single ventral column of penile erectile tissue. C. striatum: grouping of basal nuclei.

corpuscle, term applied to a small mass of tissue. Outdated term for blood cells.

corrective, drug modifying the effects of another.

Corrigan's pulse, waterhammer or collapsing pulse associated with aortic regurgitation. Characterized by arterial distension followed by sudden emptying.

cortex, outer layer of an organ or structure, such as in the adrenal glands, cerebrum and kidney.

Corti's organ, (kaw-tēz), contains the auditory receptor cells of the cochlear branch of the vestibulo-cochlear nerve (VIII) in the cochlea.

corticospinal, pertaining to the cerebral cortex and spinal cord. C. tracts: main voluntary motor pathways in the brain and spinal cord. Also called pyramidal tracts.

corticosteroids, (kor-ti-kō-ster-oyds), steroid hormones secreted by the adrenal cortex, e.g. cortisol or the synthetic forms available for therapeutic purposes, e.g. prednisolone.

corticotrophin, (kor-ti-kō-trō'-fin), see ADRENOCORTICOTROPHIC HORMONE (ACTH). C. releasing factor (CRF): a hypothalamic factor which stimulates pituitary secretion of corticotrophin/ACTH.

cortisone, one of the steroid hormones of the adrenal cortex. It is converted to cortisol before use in the body. Used therapeutically for replacement therapy in Addison's disease. See GLUCOCORTICOID.

Corynebacterium, (ko'-rin-ē-bak-tēr-ē-um), a genus of Gram-positive bacilli. C. diphtheriae: bacterium causing diphtheria.

coryza, (ko-rī'-za), acute viral infection of upper respiratory tract. Common cold.

COSHH, abbrevation for **control of substances hazardous to health**.

cosmetic, improving the appearance. C. operation: operation designed to

87

improve the appearance of disfigured or unsightly part.

costal, pertaining to the ribs. *C. cartilages*: join ribs to the sternum and each other.

cost-effectiveness analysis (CEA), an assessment of efficiency. The comparison of measurable health gains (outcomes) with the net cost of the healthcare intervention (input).

cot death, *see* SUDDEN INFANT DEATH SYNDROME.

cotyledon, *(kot-il-ē-don)*, one of several placental segments, seen on the maternal surface.

cough, forced expiration of air through the mouth. It is a protective mechanism, e.g. to expel foreign bodies, but is also associated with numerous respiratory diseases.

counselling, a process by which a person is helped to identify, accept or solve personal problems.

counterconditioning, a behavioural technique which seeks to replace a learned response with one that is more acceptable.

countercurrent, change of fluid flow directions, such as the heat exchange system in the blood vessels of the legs where cold venous blood is warmed by arterial blood before returning to the body core. *C. multiplication theory*: a hypothesis which can be used to explain osmolarity gradients, within the interstitial fluid surrounding the renal tubule, required for the production of urine of different concentrations.

counterextension, extension by means of holding back the upper part of a limb while the lower is pulled down.

countertraction, a force which counters the pull of traction, often the body weight of the person.

countertransference, the conscious or unconscious emotional reaction of therapist to client.

coupling, abnormal pulse where the normal beat is followed immediately by a ventricular extrasystole and then a pause. Associated with digitalis toxicity.

Cowper's glands, *(kow-perz)*, *see* BULBOURETHRAL.

cowpox, *see* VACCINIA.

coxa, the hip joint. *C. valga*: deformity in which the angle made by the neck and shaft of the femur is greater than normal. *C. vara*: in this case the angle is less than normal.

coxalgia, pain in the hip joint.

Coxiella, a genus closely related to *Rickettsia*.

coxsackie viruses, group of enteroviruses responsible for aseptic meningitis, epidemic pleurodynia (Bornholm disease), myocarditis and pericarditis.

CPAP, *see* CONTINUOUS POSITIVE AIRWAY PRESSURE.

CPD, abbreviation for **continuing professional development**.

CPN, abbreviation for **community psychiatric nurse**.

CPR, abbreviation for **cardiopulmonary resuscitation**.

CPU, in computing the abbreviation for **central processing unit**. The chip which ultimately controls the functioning of a PC. Term also used (erroneously) to describe the 'box' containing the main circuitry of the computer.

crab louse, the *Phthirus pubis* which infests the pubic region.

'crack', *see* COCAINE.

cradle, appliance used to support bedclothes away from an injured part or to ensure the free circulation of air.

cramp, sudden painful tonic contraction of the muscles.

ranial, (krā-nē-al), pertaining to the cranium. C. *cavity:* skull cavity, contains the brain. C. *nerves:* twelve pairs of peripheral nerves which originate from the brain. Identified by name and Roman numerals I–XII.

raniometry, (krā-nē-om'-et-ri), measurement of skulls.

raniosacral, (krā-nē-ō-sā-kral), pertaining to the cranium and sacrum. The parasympathetic nerves have a *c.* outflow.

raniostenosis, (krā-nē-ō-sten-ō'-sis), premature fusion of the skull sutures.

raniosynostosis, (krā-nē-ō-sin-os'-tō-sis), premature fusion of the skull sutures during the time just before or after birth.

raniotabes, (krā-nē-ō-tā'-bēz), thinning of the skull bones of an infant. Due to faulty mineralization such as might occur in rickets.

raniotomy, (krā-nē-ot'-ō-mi), operation in which the skull is opened.

ranium, the part of the skull enclosing the brain. It is formed from eight bones: occipital, two parietals, frontal, ethmoid, sphenoid and two temporals.

rash, in computing a sudden and serious malfunction or complete loss of program.

rash team, a specialist medical and nursing team organized in hospitals to attend emergencies such as cardiac arrest to perform advanced life support.

reatine, (krē'-at-in), important nitrogenous substance found in muscle where it combines with phosphate to form a high energy molecule; creatine phosphate. C. *kinase (CK):* enzyme which facilitates the release of energy (ATP) from creatine phosphate. Levels in the blood are raised following muscle damage such as

myocardial infarction. Occurs as three isoenzymes.

creatinine, (krē'-at-in-ēn), a nitrogenous waste product of protein and nucleic acid metabolism. C. *clearance:* see CLEARANCE.

crenation, reaction of red blood cells, which shrink when placed in a hypertonic solution.

crepitation, (krep-i-tā-shon), also called crepitus. **1.** grating of fractured bone ends. **2.** crackling sound in joints. **3.** crackling sounds heard via stethoscope. **4.** crackling sound heard when pressure is applied to air-filled tissue (surgical emphysema).

crepitus, noisy passage of flatus. See CREPITATION.

cresol, a phenolic disinfectant derived from coaltar.

cretinism, outdated term previously used to describe congenital hypothyroidism.

Creutzfeldt–Jakob disease (CJD), form of progressive dementia transmissible through prion protein. New variant CJD, found in young adults, is possibly linked with bovine prion of spongiform encephalopathy. It runs a rapid degenerative course and is usually fatal.

cribriform, perforated like a sieve. C. *plate:* part of the ethmoid bone, its perforations give passage to the olfactory nerve fibres.

cricoid cartilage, ring-shaped cartilage of the larynx.

cri du chat syndrome, (krē-dū-sha), a congenital condition caused by an anomaly of chromosome 5. It is characterized by a high-pitched cry like that of a kitten, micrognathia, low-set ears and severe learning disability.

Crigler–Najjar, a genetic disorder where the absence of a specific liver enzyme leads to high levels of unconjugated bilirubin in the blood, jaundice and problems of the central nervous system.

criminal law, law creating offences heard in the criminal courts. *C. wrong:* an act or omission which can be pursued in the criminal courts.

crisis, 1. a critical turning point in an acute illness, after which the patient either recovers or dies. **2.** sudden severe pain or other forms of deterioration associated with certain conditions. *See* THYROID CRISIS. *C. intervention:* in psychiatry when the therapeutic team intervenes to assist in solving an immediate crisis and its problems.

critical appraisal, technique for making an objective judgement regarding a research study in terms of research design, methodology, analysis, interpretation of results and how appropriate the study findings are to a particular area.

critical path analysis (CPA), a project management technique used where operations, tasks and actions are interdependent. The timing of each action or stage is crucial to the overall success of the project, i.e. some actions or stages must be completed before others can be started.

Crohn's disease, an inflammatory bowel disease. Commonly affects the terminal ileum, but lesions may occur elsewhere in the small bowel and in the colon and rectum. Causes pain, diarrhoea, malabsorption, weight loss and fever. Complications include: obstruction, fistula formation and perforation.

cross-infection, a hazard of hospitals where, for a variety of reasons, infections are transferred from one person to another.

crossmatching, testing for compatibility prior to transfusion by mixing donor red cells with recipient serum to observe for signs of agglutination. *See* BLOOD GROUPS, BLOOD TRANSFUSION

cross-over studies, a research study where participants experience both the experimental agent and the placebo one after another.

croup, laryngeal obstruction. Croupy breathing in a child is often called 'stridulous', meaning noisy or harsh-sounding. Narrowing of the airway, which gives rise to the typical attack with crowing inspiration may result from oedema or spasm or both. May be due to infection, allergy, foreign bodies, etc.

crowning, the stage of labour at which the fetal head is visibly distending the vaginal orifice.

cruciate, cross-shaped. *C. ligaments* strong ligaments which stabilize the knee joint.

crural, relating to the thigh.

crus, Latin for leg. A limb-like structure.

crush syndrome, seen after extensive crush injuries to muscle tissue. Shock and myoglobulin release into the circulation causing changes in renal blood flow with tubular necrosis and eventual renal failure.

crutch, the appliance used to facilitate walking and increase mobility. *C. paralysis:* arm paralysis caused by pressure on nerves from an improperly used crutch or one of the wrong height.

cryoanalgesia, relief of pain by ice packs or by the use of a cryosurgical probe to block peripheral nerve function.

cryoprecipitate, (krī-ō-prē-sip-it-āt) factor VIII obtained by rapidly freezing and thawing blood plasma. Used in the treatment of haemophilia.

cryosurgery, (krī-ō-ser-je-ri), surgery which utilizes very low temperatures to destroy tissue, such as during lens extraction in cataract operations.

Cryptococcus, *(krip-to-ko-kus),* a genus of fungi. *C. neoformans* is an occasional cause of disease in humans, the commonest form being subacute or chronic meningitis.

cryptomenorrhoea, *(krip-to-men-o-rē'-a),* hidden menstruation. Apparent amenorrhoea due to an obstruction to the menstrual flow, such as an imperforate hymen. *See* HAEMATO-COLPOS.

cryptorchism, *(krip-tor-kizm),* condition where one or both testes have failed to descend into the scrotum.

cryptosporidiosis, disease caused by *Cryptosporidium* species (protozoa). Infection can be asymptomatic but may result in profuse watery diarrhoea. Patients with AIDS and other causes of immunodeficiency may have serious effects: pain, anorexia, fever and weight loss.

crypts of Leiberkühn, *(lē-be-koon),* glands found in the mucosa of the small intestine. They produce a secretion containing several digestive enzymes.

crystalline lens, lens of the eye.

crystalloids, substances in solution that will diffuse through a selectively permeable membrane. Administered intravenously to maintain fluid and electrolyte balance. May be used in conjunction with colloids in seriously ill patients.

crystalluria, *(kris-tal-ūr-ē-ah),* urinary excretion of crystals.

CSF, abbreviation for **cerebrospinal fluid** and **colony-stimulating factors**

cubit, cubitus, 1. the forearm. **2.** the elbow.

cuboid, cube-shaped. One of the seven tarsal bones of the ankle.

culdoscopy, *(kul-dos'-ko-pi),* an endoscopic examination of the pelvic cavity. An instrument known as a culdoscope is passed into the vagina, through the posterior vaginal fornix and into the peritoneal cavity.

Cullen's sign, discoloration around the umbilicus, a sign seen in acute pancreatitis.

culture, 1. the cultivation of microorganisms or tissue cells in the laboratory using various culture media which meet their specific requirements. **2.** the attitudes, beliefs, ideas, practices, values, etc. which members of different groups hold about themselves, and which inform the behaviour of the group.

cumulative action, if the dose of a slowly excreted drug is repeated too frequently, an increasing action is obtained. This can be dangerous as, if the drug accumulates in the system, toxic symptoms may occur, such as with digoxin.

cuneiform, *(kū-nē-form),* wedge-shaped. Three of the tarsal bones.

curative, a treatment or therapy aimed at the restoration of health.

curettage, *(kū-re-tahj),* the scraping of a cavity with a curette.

curette, a spoon-shaped instrument with both blunt and sharp edges.

curie (Ci), *(kū-rē),* old unit of radioactivity, now replaced by the SI unit the becquerel (Bq).

Curling's ulcer, acute peptic ulceration associated with the physiological stress of extensive burns. *See* STRESS ULCER.

curriculum vitae (CV), literally 'the course of one's life'. A summary of personal details, education, professional qualifications and employment experience.

cursor, in computing a blinking line on screen showing the location at which information entered from the keyboard will appear.

Cusco's speculum, see SPECULUM.

Cushing's disease, pituitary adenoma or hyperplasia with hypersecretion of ACTH/corticotrophin resulting in adrenal cortical overactivity. See CUSHING'S SYNDROME for physical effects.

Cushing's syndrome, due to an elevated level of corticosteroids either through oversecretion or as a side-effect of therapeutic corticosteroids. Characterized by the typical cushingoid appearance of moon face, fat redistribution, muscle wastage and weakness, purpura, hirsutism, with hypertension, glycosuria, osteoporosis and mental disturbances, etc.

cusp, projection, especially on crown of tooth; also applied to part of heart valve.

cutaneous, *(kū-tā'-ne-us),* pertaining to the skin.

cutdown, incision into a vein to facilitate the insertion of an intravenous catheter, such as for hyperalimentation when a central vein is required.

cuticle, 1. epidermis. **2.** eponychium, thickened area at the base of a nail.

cutis, true skin or derma.

CVA, abbreviation for **cerebrovascular accident**.

CVP, abbreviation for **central venous pressure**.

CVS, abbreviation for **cardiovascular system** and **chorionic villus sampling**.

cyancobalamin, *(sī-an-ō-kō-bal-a-min),* commercially produced substance with vitamin B$_{12}$ activity. See COBALAMIN.

cyanosis, *(sī-an-ō'-sis),* blue discoloration of the skin and mucous membranes due to poor oxygenation of the blood. It may be observed

centrally or in peripheral structures such as the digits.

cycle, repeated series of events, e.g. cardiac cycle, menstrual cycle.

cyclic adenosine monophosphate (cAMP), an important metabolic molecule which acts as the 'second messenger' in the action of many hormones.

cyclical, occurring in cycles. *C. syndrome*: term used to describe the diverse effects seen in the premenstrual phase. *C. vomiting*: recurrent attacks of vomiting with ketosis seen in childhood.

cyclitis, *(sik-lī'-tis),* inflammation of ciliary body of the eye.

cyclodialysis, *(sī-klō-dī-al'-i-sis),* operation to improve drainage from the anterior chamber of the eye which aims to reduce intraocular pressure in glaucoma.

cyclodiathermy, *(sī-klō-dī-a-ther-mi),* use of diathermy to destroy part of the ciliary body as a treatment for glaucoma.

cycloplegia, *(sī-klō-plē'-jē-a),* paralysis of the ciliary muscle of the eye.

cyclosporin, a group of immunosuppressant agents used to reduce the risk of graft versus host (GvH) disease following tissue transplantation.

cyclothymia, *(sī-klō-thī'-mē-a),* a tendency to alternating, but relatively mild, mood swings between depression and elation.

cyclotomy, *(sī-klot-o-mē),* incision through the ciliary body of the eye.

cyesis, *(sī-ē-sis),* pregnancy. *Pseudo-c.*: false pregnancy.

cyst, *(sist),* **1.** enclosed area filled with fluid or semisolid material. **2.** a stage in the life cycle of some parasites (protozoa). See CHALAZION, CHOCOLATE CYST, DERMOID CYST, HYDATID CYST, THYROGLOSSAL CYST, OVARIAN CYST.

cystadenoma, *(sis-tad-en-ō-ma),* benign cystic growth of glandular tissue.

cystalgia, pain in the urinary bladder.

cystathionine, *(sis-ta-thī-o-neen),* an intermediate in methionine metabolism. Increased levels are excreted in the urine (cystathioninuria) in an inherited disorder of methionine metabolism.

cystectomy, *(sis-tek'-to-mi),* surgical removal of the urinary bladder, may be partial or total. *Ovarian c.:* excision of an ovarian cyst.

cysteine, *(sis-tēn),* a sulphur-containing amino acid.

cystic, *(sis-tik),* pertaining to a cyst. *C. duct:* the duct leading from the gallbladder to the common bile duct. *C. fibrosis (CF):* an autosomal recessive disorder affecting the exocrine glands; diagnosis may be confirmed by high levels of sodium in sweat. Meconium ileus may be an early physical effect. The affected glands produce viscous mucus which leads to blocked dilated ducts, stasis, infection and fibrosis. The lungs and pancreas are primarily affected giving rise to repeated chest infections, respiratory and cardiac deterioration and digestive problems. Current treatment centres upon physiotherapy, antimicrobial drugs and replacement of pancreatic enzymes, but advances in management include: heart/lung transplants, recent identification of the defective gene, antenatal testing, gene therapy and genetic counselling.

cysticercosis, *(sis-ti-ser-kō'-sis),* infection with the larval stage of various tapeworm, e.g. *Taenia solium* (pork tapeworm). May affect muscle, liver, lung and brain where it can cause epilepsy.

cystine, *(sis-tin),* a non-essential amino acid derived from cysteine.

cystinosis, *(sis-tin-ō-sis),* inherited disorder where cystine accumulates in the tissues. Causes renal damage with excretion of amino acids in the urine. *See* FANCONI'S SYNDROME.

cystinuria, *(sis-tin-ū-rē-a),* excretion of cystine in the urine associated with an inborn error of metabolism, where basic amino acids are not reabsorbed by the renal tubules. Stones containing cystine form in the kidney.

cystitis, *(sis-tī'-tis),* inflammation of the urinary bladder.

cystocele, *(sis'-to-sēl),* prolapse or herniation of the bladder into the vaginal wall.

cystodiathermy, *(sis-to-dī-a-ther-mē),* use of electrical current via a cystoscope to treat bladder conditions such as papilloma. *See* DIATHERMY.

cystography, radiographic examination of the urinary bladder following instillation of radiopaque contrast medium, when the urethra is also viewed the procedure is termed cystourethrography. *Micturating c.:* cystography whilst the patient passes urine.

cystolithiasis, *(sis-tō-li-thī'-a-sis),* stone in the bladder.

cystometry, *(sis-tom-et-ri),* measurement of bladder pressures and capacity. Results recorded graphically as a cystometrogram.

cystoscope, *(sis-to-skōp),* endoscope used for examination and treatment of the urinary bladder.

cystostomy, *(sis-tos'-to-mi),* operation of producing an opening from the bladder to the exterior.

cystotomy, *(sis-tot'-o-mi),* incision of the bladder.

cytochromes, series of iron or copper-containing proteins that are similar in structure to haemoglobin. They are involved in mitochondrial oxidation–reduction reactions of the electron transport chain which generate ATP.

cytogenetics, the study of cells with particular emphasis upon genes and chromosomes.

cytokines, general term for signalling molecules produced by immune cells. They include interleukins, interferons and tumour necrosis factors.

cytokinesis, (*sī-tō-kin-ē'-sis*), cytoplasmic division, process by which a cell divides into two following nuclear division.

cytology, (*sī-tol'-ō-je*), the study of cells. *Exfoliative c.:* the study of shed cells used in the diagnosis of premalignant disease.

cytolysis, (*sī-tol'-i-sis*), cell disintegration.

cytomegalovirus (CMV), (*sī-tō-meg'-al-ō-vī-rus*), a herpesvirus. May cause latent or asymptomatic infection. Virus particles are commonly transmitted to the fetus, where the virus may cause abortion, stillbirth or serious neonatal disease characterized by hepatosplenomegaly, purpura, encephalitis, microcephaly and learning disability and developmental delay, or death. The virus is a serious threat to immunocompromised individuals, such as those with AIDS.

cytometer, (*sī-tom'-et-er*), an instrument for counting cells, usually of the blood.

cytopheresis, (*sī-tō-fer-ē-sis*), the separation and removal of specific cellular components of blood. May be used therapeutically to remove abnormal components or to collect specific components required by patients.

cytoplasm, (*sī-tō-plazm*), the protoplasm excluding that surrounding the nucleus.

cytosine, (*sī-tō-sēn*), nitrogenous base derived from pyrimidine. A component of nucleic acids. *See* NUCLEIC ACIDS, DNA, RNA.

cytosol, the fluid part of the cytoplasm.

cytotoxic, (*sī-tō-tok-sik*), substance that causes cell damage and inhibits cell division. *C. drugs:* used to destroy malignant cells.

cytotoxin, (*sī-tō-tok-sin*), antibody inhibiting a cell's normal activity.

D

dacryadenitis, *(dak-ri-ad-en-ī-tis)*, inflammation of the lacrimal gland.

dacryocystitis, *(dak'-ri-ō-sis-tī-tis)*, inflammation of the lacrimal sac.

dacryocystorhinostomy, *(dak-ri-ō-sis-tō-rī-nos'-to-mi)*, operation to establish a communication between the lacrimal sac and the nose.

dacryocystotomy, *(dak-ri-ō-sis-tot-o-mi)*, incision into the lacrimal sac.

dacryolith, *(dak'-ri-ō-lith)*, stone in the lacrimal duct.

dacryoma, *(dak-ri-ō-mah)*, benign tumour arising from lacrimal epithelium.

dactyl, *(dak-til')*, a digit of the hand or foot.

dactylion, *(dak-til-i'-on)*, webbed fingers or toes.

dactylitis, *(dak-ti-lī-tis)* inflammation of fingers or toes.

dactylology, *(dak-til-ol-o-je)*, communication method using hands and fingers. *See* SIGNING.

Daltonism, a form of red–green colour blindness.

Dalton's law (of partial pressures), states that the pressure of a gas mixture is a sum of the partial pressures which each gas would exert if it completely filled the space.

dark adaptation, adjustments required by the eye to facilitate vision in poor light or darkness.

data, information, facts. *D. analysis*: stage in research where data are coded and classified. *D. collection*: stage in research during which information is gathered.

database, a computer file which stores information, e.g. a mailing list. The stored information can be accessed and sorted as required.

day case surgery, *see* AMBULATORY SURGERY.

day centre, facilities which provide nursing, medical care, treatment facilities and rehabilitation for older adults and those with mental health problems or learning difficulties.

dead space, any part of the respiratory tract where no gaseous exchange occurs; the conducting airways and any alveoli not involved in gas exchange. *Anatomical d.s.*: an area with a volume of around 150 ml formed by the conducting airways which contains air that does not reach the alveoli.

deafness, partial or complete loss of hearing. *Conductive d.*: due to impaired sound conduction, e.g. excess ear wax. *Mixed d.*: combination of both conductive and sensorineural deafness. *Sensorineural d.*: due to damage to hearing receptors, nerves or auditory cortex, e.g. maternal rubella during early pregnancy or occupational noise damage. *See* RINNE'S TEST, WEBER'S TEST.

deamination, *(dē-am-in-ā-shon)*, the removal of NH_2 groups from organic compounds. The liver removes the NH_2 group from excess amino acids and uses it to synthesize non-essential amino acids and urea.

death, permanent cessation of vital functions. *Brain d.*: see BRAIN DEATH. *D.*

certificate: official document issued by the registrar of deaths, to relatives or authorized person, which allows for the disposal of the body. It is issued after a notification of probable cause of death is completed by the medical officer in attendance upon the deceased or with the appropriate documentation from the coroner. *D. rate*: *see* MORTALITY RATE.

debility, weakness, loss of power.

debridement, thorough surgical cleansing of a wound with removal of foreign bodies, devitalized or infected tissue and cell debris. *chemical/medical d.*: is accomplished by use of external applications to the wound.

decalcification, loss or removal of calcium salts from bone or teeth.

decapsulation, removal of the capsule of an organ.

decay, breakdown of organic material. *Radioactive d.*: disintegration of an unstable atom with the emission of radioactive particles.

decerebrate, (*dē-se-re-brāt*), being without cerebral function. Associated with severe brain damage, has a characteristic posture where all limbs are spastic.

decibel (dB), unit of sound intensity or loudness.

decidua, (*dē-sid-ū-a*), the thickened uterine lining (endometrium) formed to receive the fertilized ovum. It is shed at the end of pregnancy.

deciduous, temporary, a structure which is shed, e.g. the first teeth or the decidua.

decompensation, failure of compensation, as of the heart.

decomposition, 1. putrefaction. 2. breakdown of substances by hydrolytic enzymes.

decompression, the relief of internal pressure, e.g. trephining the skull. *D. sickness*: *see* CAISSON DISEASE.

deconditioning, the elimination of a unwanted response to a particular stimulus.

decubitus, (*dē-kū'-bi-tus*), a recumbent or horizontal position. *D. ulcer*: *see* PRESSURE ULCER.

decussation, an intersection; crossing over of nerve fibres at a point beyond their origin, e.g. optic and pyramidal tracts.

deep vein thrombosis (DVT), thrombosis occurring mainly in the deep veins of the legs or the pelvis. Associated with immobility leading to venous stasis, injury to vessel walls, and where blood coagulation has been altered, e.g. contraceptive pill. Material may become detached to form an embolus. *See* EMBOLUS.

defecation, the act of evacuating the bowel.

defence mechanism, in general the body's ability to defend itself; most commonly applied to immunity. The immune response may be non-specific (innate), e.g. intact skin, and phagocytosis, or specific (adaptive) e.g. cell-mediated or humoral immunity. *See* MENTAL DEFENCE MECHANISMS.

defibrillation, conversion of ventricular or atrial fibrillation and some tachycardias to normal sinus rhythm. A defibrillator is used to deliver an electric shock to the heart.

defibrination, removal of fibrin from plasma, prevents clotting in a sample of blood.

degeneration, deterioration in structure and function of tissue. When the structural changes are marked descriptive terms are sometimes used, e.g. colloid, fatty, hyaline, etc.

deglutition, act of swallowing.

dehiscence, (*dē-hīs-ens*), bursting or splitting open, as of a wound.

dehydration, loss of water with varying degrees of electrolyte depletion.

7-dehydrocholesterol, sterol present in the skin, converted to vitamin D by sunlight.

dehydrogenases, *(dē-hī-dro-jen-āz-es),* enzymes which facilitate the removal of hydrogen from a compound.

déjà vu phenomenon, *(dā-ja-vū),* illusion of familiarity when experiencing something new.

deliquescent, *(de-li-kwe-sent),* able to absorb moisture and become fluid.

delirium, abnormal mental state based on hallucinations or illusion. May be due to high temperature, toxic states or some mental health problems. *D. tremens*: acute psychosis usually associated with chronic alcohol misuse. There is disorientation, terror, hallucinations and tremor.

delivery, parturition, childbirth.

Delphi technique, a research method where a consensus of expert opinion is obtained by using a seven-step process with the chosen group of contributors who are asked to rate a number of items, e.g. areas for research, in order of importance.

delta (δ), fourth letter of the Greek alphabet. *D. cells*: see ISLETS OF LANGERHANS. *D. waves (rhythm)*: high-amplitude brain waves with a frequency of less than 4 Hz, recorded during deep sleep and when the reticular activating system is inhibited.

deltoid, *(del'-toyd),* triangular. Muscle of the shoulder.

delusion, a false idea, entirely without foundation, which cannot be altered by reasoning. Associated with psychotic conditions.

demarcation, the marking of a boundary. *Line of d.*: red line which forms between dead and living tissue in gangrene.

dementia, organic brain syndrome; a deterioration in mental functioning resulting from brain changes from a variety of causes which include: Alzheimer's disease, arteriosclerosis, multi-infarcts, toxins and trauma. It is characterized by personality changes, memory loss, poor judgement and a decline in intellectual function. *See* ALZHEIMER'S DISEASE, PICK'S DISEASE.

demineralization, see DECALCIFICATION.

demography, the study of populations. Demographic indices such as age distribution, birth and mortality rates, occupation, geographical distribution are used to provide a profile of a given population and plan services.

demulcents, agents which protect sensitive surfaces from irritation.

demyelination, a degenerative process where the myelin sheath is lost from nerve fibres; occurs in multiple sclerosis.

dendron, dendrite, branching processes of the neurone. They receive nerve impulses from other neurones and transmit them towards the cell body.

denervated, *(de-ner-vā-ted),* deprived of nerve supply.

dengue, *(deng'-ge),* a virus disease of the tropics, transmitted by mosquitoes and characterized by fever, headache, pains in the limbs, and a rash. A haemorrhagic form has a high mortality rate from disseminated intravascular coagulation and acute circulatory collapse.

denial, a mental defence mechanism where difficult situations or painful facts are not acknowledged in order to avoid conflict or distress.

Denis Browne splints, see BROWNE, DENIS.

dens, a tooth.

density, the mass of matter contained in a unit of volume.

dental, pertaining to teeth. *D. calculus*: mineralized dental plaque deposited on the tooth surface. *D. hygienist*: a person qualified to provide dental services under the supervision of a dentist. They are primarily concerned with dental hygiene and the promotion of dental health. *D. plaque*: soft mass of bacteria and cellular debris which rapidly coats the teeth when effective oral hygiene is absent.

dentine, bone-like substance forming the body of a tooth. *See* TOOTH.

dentition, teething. *See* TEETH.

deodorant, deodorizer, a substance that masks or destroys an unpleasant odour, e.g. charcoal dressings.

deontology, an ethical theory supporting the view that there is a duty to act within certain universal rules of morality. An approach associated with the work of Immanuel Kant: *See* UTILITARIANISM.

deoxygenation, the removal of oxygen from a substance.

deoxyribonucleic acid (DNA), *(dē-ok-sē-rī-bō-nū-klā-ik)*, a nucleic acid found in the chromosomes, it has a complex helical structure which carries the genetic code (Figure 23).

dependence, 1. state of being dependent upon others. **2.** a psychophysical addiction to substances such as drugs or alcohol where intake must continually increase to avoid withdrawal symptoms.

dependency, state of needing the help of others to meet physical and emotional needs. *D. studies*: a method of calculating patient dependency levels and required staffing ratios.

depersonalization, a state occurring with some mental health problems where individuals may feel that they no longer exist. There are feelings of unreality and the person may view his or her own behaviour and

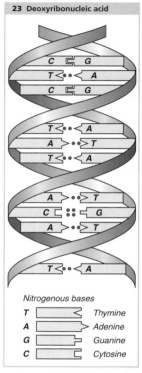

23 Deoxyribonucleic acid

Nitrogenous bases

T	Thymine
A	Adenine
G	Guanine
C	Cytosine

actions as if through the eyes of an onlooker.

depilatory, *(de-pil'-ā-to-ri)*, an agent for removing superfluous hairs from the body.

depolarization, the inside of a membrane becomes electrically positive in respect to the outside, such as occurs during the transmission of a nerve impulse.

depressant, an agent reducing functional activity.

depression, 1. in anatomy a hollow or fossa 2. a decrease in some activity. 3. common psychiatric disorder. It may be bipolar, where it coexists with hypomania, or unipolar when it is characterized only by feelings of depression. *Endogenous d.:* occurring without an obvious reason. *Reactive d.:* due to a life event such as bereavement. *Seasonal d.:* associated with low light levels during the winter months, it is known as seasonal affective disorder (SAD).

depressor, a drug, muscle or instrument that depresses a structure or function.

deprivation, the withholding or absence of some factor that is needed or is considered valuable. *D. indices:* set of census variables and weightings used to assess levels of deprivation within a population.

Derbyshire neck, *see* GOITRE.

derealization, a feeling that the world is unreal and strange.

dereism, a fantasy which continues undisturbed by outside events or logic.

derma, dermis, the true skin.

dermal, pertaining to the skin.

dermatitis, inflammation of the skin. The numerous causes may be of external or internal origin. Some common external irritants are dyes, metals, disinfectants, flowers. A term used synonymously with eczema.

dermatology, the science of the skin and its diseases.

dermatome, 1. instrument for cutting a skin graft. 2. an area of the body surface or a segment of skin that receives sensory innervation from the cutaneous branches of a particular spinal nerve.

dermatomycosis, *(der-mat-ō-mī-kō-sis),* a skin disease caused by a fungus.

dermatomyositis, *(der-mat-ō-mī-ō-sī'-tis),* rare connective tissue disease characterized by inflammation and breakdown of skin and progressive weakness of muscles.

dermatophyte, *(der-mat-ō-fīt),* the three genera of fungi which cause superficial infections of the skin, nails and hair such as athlete's foot.

dermatosis, any skin disease.

dermis, the true skin which lies below the epidermis.

dermographism, the production of wheals on the skin, resembling urticaria, after a blunt instrument or fingernail has been lightly drawn over it.

dermoid, resembling the skin. *D. cyst:* benign cystic teratoma of the ovary containing a variety of tissue: skin, neural tissue, teeth and bone.

Descemet's membrane, *(des-e-mā),* posterior membrane of the cornea.

descriptive statistics, that which describes or summarizes the observations of a sample. *See INFERENTIAL STATISTICS.*

desensitization, to remove sensitivity. 1. for allergies: resistance to the allergen is achieved by repeated exposure to small doses. 2. behavioural therapy used to help phobic people overcome their irrational fears. The person is exposed to the fear through imagining the objects, looking at pictures or by confronting the real object or situation.

desiccation, drying out.

desmoid, like a bundle. Fibrous tissue.

desquamation, peeling of the skin.

detoxification, a process by which toxic substances are rendered harmless.

detrusor, expelling muscle. *Urinary d.:* muscle of the urinary bladder.

development, maturation with an increase in complexity, differentiation and skills.

developmental, pertaining to development. *D. dysplasia of the hip*: also known as congenital dislocation of the hip. Poor development of the acetabulum, allowing dislocation of the femoral head, is present at birth. Early diagnosis and treatment (splinting, or possibly surgery) are important. *See* BARLOW'S SIGN, or TOLANI'S TEST. *D. milestones*: important events or behaviours used to mark developmental progress, such as walking.

deviance, a departure from the accepted norm, such as behaviour. A feature that is different.

deviation, any feature that is different to the normal.

dexter, right. Upon the right side.

dextran, a colloid solution previously used for replacing fluids in hypovolaemia.

dextrin, an intermediate product in the conversion of starch into sugar.

dextrocardia, transposition of the heart to the right side of the chest.

dextrose, glucose. Used in many solutions for intravenous infusion.

dhobie itch, *see* TINEA CRURIS.

diabetes insipidus, deficient secretion of antidiuretic hormone (ADH) from the pituitary gland causes a syndrome characterized by the passage of large quantities of pale low specific gravity urine and polydipsia. *nephrogenic D.I.*: where the renal tubules become insensitive to ADH.

diabetes mellitus, *(mel-ĭ-tus)*, common condition caused by an absolute or relative deficiency of insulin. The body is unable to use glucose, resulting in hyperglycaemia, polyuria, glycosuria with high specific gravity, polydipsia and abnormal fat and protein metabolism. Distinct forms of the disease are: insulin-dependent diabetes mellitis (IDDM) or type I, usually diagnosed in people aged under 40 years, and non-insulin-dependent diabetes mellitus (NIDDM) or type II, which is usually seen in people over 50 years, but can occur in much younger people. *See* HYPERGLYCAEMIA, HYPEROSMOLAR, HYPOGLYCAEMIA, KETOACIDOSIS.

diagnosis, to identify the disease or condition. *Clinical d.*: one based on examination and consideration of the signs and symptoms. *Differential d.*: a diagnosis made after comparing the features of two or more similar diseases. *Laboratory d.*: one based on the result of laboratory tests. *Nursing d.*: a process by which the nurse identifies actual or potential health problems requiring nursing interventions which the nurse is qualified and competent to deliver. Used throughout the United States. *See* NURSING.

dialysate, *(dī-al-is-āt)*, the fluid used in dialysis.

dialyser, machine or equipment used for dialysis.

dialysis, *(dī-al-is-is)*, the separation in solution of small molecular weight substances such as electrolytes, from a mixture containing colloids, using a selectively permeable membrane. A technique employed to remove waste products from the blood in renal failure and reduce high levels of toxic substances such as drugs. *See* HAEMODIALYSIS, PERITONEAL DIALYSIS.

diamorphine, heroin, An alkaloid of morphine with many medicinal uses including relief of severe pain. Controlled by the Misuse of Drugs Act and Regulations, it is addictive and subject to considerable criminal misuse.

diapedesis, *(dī-a-ped-ē'-sis)*, the passage of blood cells through the vessel walls. Usually refers to the movement of leucocytes in inflammation.

diaphoresis, *(di-a-fo-rē'-sis),* perspiration.

diaphoretics, *(di-a-for-et'-iks),* agents which increase perspiration.

diaphragm, 1. the muscular septum separating the chest and abdomen. It is the main respiratory muscle (Figure 24). **2.** a contraceptive device worn over the cervix. Very effective if fitted properly and used correctly in conjunction with a spermicidal cream (Figure 25).

diaphragmatic, pertaining to the diaphragm. *D. breathing*: breathing mostly achieved by the diaphragm. *D. hernia*: herniation of the abdominal viscera through the diaphragm into the chest. Due to a congenital defect of the diaphragm. *See* HIATUS HERNIA.

diaphysis, the middle part of long bones; the shaft, *cf.* EPIPHYSIS.

diarrhoea, frequent loose stools.

diarthrosis, *(di-arthrō'-sis),* a synovial or freely movable joint.

25 Contraceptive diaphragm in position

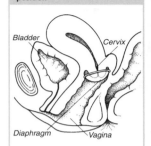

Bladder
Cervix
Diaphragm
Vagina

24 The undersurface of the diaphragm

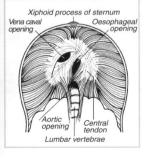

Xiphoid process of sternum
Vena caval opening
Oesophageal opening
Aortic opening
Central tendon
Lumbar vertebrae

diastasis, *(di-as'-tā-sis),* forcible separation of bones without fracture; dislocation.

diastole, *(di-as'-tō-lē)* that part of cardiac cycle when the ventricles fill with blood, *cf.* SYSTOLE.

diastolic, *(di-as'-tol-ik),* pertaining to diastole. *D. murmur*: heart murmur heard during diastole. *D. pressure*: the lowest pressure reached during the relaxation stage of the cardiac cycle. *See* BLOOD PRESSURE.

diathermy, the passage of a high frequency electrical current through tissue. The heat produced is used to: stop bleeding during surgery, destroy superficial tumours, cut through tissue and to treat inflammation by using large electrodes to spread the heat.

DIC, abbreviation for **disseminated intravascular coagulation.**

dichotomy, *(di-kot'-o-mi),* division into two parts.

dichromatopsia, *(di-krō-ma-top'-si-ah),* a form of colour blindness where the individual can see only two of the three primary colours.

dicrotic, *(dī-krot'-ik),* having two beats *D. pulse:* presence of a small secondary wave of distention in the artery.

diencephalon, *(dī-en-kef'-al-on),* the part of the brain between the telencephalon and mesencephalon; includes the thalamus, hypothalamus, epithalmus and the third ventricle.

diet, pattern of food intake developed according to physiological needs, cultural and religious factors, availability, cost and individual preferences. The many therapeutic diets prescribed for the management of disease include: diabetic, low fat, high protein and low salt.

dietary, relating to diet. *D. fibre:* nonstarch polysaccharides. *D. reference values (DRV):* values that provide a range of intakes for most nutrients. *See* EAR, LRNI, RNI.

dietetics, *(dī-e-tet'-iks),* the study of nutritional values and the use of diets to maintain health and manage illness.

dietitian, a person qualified in the principles of nutrition and dietetics.

Dietl's crisis, *(dē'-tl),* sudden, severe loin pain due to an obstruction in the renal pelvis which causes it to distend with urine.

differential, a difference. *D. blood count: see* BLOOD COUNT. *D. diagnosis: see* DIAGNOSIS.

differentiation, the changes that occur in cells and tissues as they develop the ability to perform specialized functions; these changes distinguish one cell type from another. Cancers are graded by their degree of differentiation: well-differentiated cancer cells resemble their tissue of origin but poorly differentiated cancer cells are more primitive, usually with poorer prognosis. *See* GRADING, STAGING.

diffuse, 1. to scatter or disperse. 2. widespread not localized.

diffusion, the process by which gases and liquids of different concentrations mix when brought into contact, until their concentration is equal throughout.

digestion, mechanical and chemical processes which convert food into simple substances which can be absorbed in the blood or lymph.

digestive, pertaining to digestion. *D. system/tract:* the structures of the gastrointestinal tract plus the accessory glands.

digit, a finger or toe.

digitalis, the foxglove; containing glycosides such as digoxin used in the treatment of heart disease.

1, 25-dihydroxycholecalciferol, *see* CALCITRIOL.

dilatation, stretching or opening. *D. and curettage (D & C):* where the cervix is dilated and the endometrium scraped or curetted.

dilator, 1. an instrument for dilating any narrow passage, such as the rectum, urethra or cervix. 2. a drug which dilates a passage, e.g. bronchodilator. 3. a muscle which dilates.

Diogenes syndrome, a state where the person, usually elderly, lives in the most appalling conditions of squalor, often with many companion animals. The person concerned strenuously opposes any efforts to change his or her environment.

dioptre, *(dī-op'-ter),* the unit of refractive power of lens. A lens of 1 dioptre has a focal length of 1 metre.

dioxide, a compound containing two atoms of oxygen, e.g. carbon dioxide (CO_2).

dipeptidases, intestinal enzymes which split dipeptides into amino acids.

dipeptide, a pair of linked amino acids.

diphasic, having two phases.

2, 3-diphosphoglycerate (2, 3-DPG), *(dī-fos-fo'-glis-er-āt),* substance present in red blood cells which decreases the affinity of haemoglobin for oxygen and enhances oxygen release to the tissues.

diphtheria, a serious, notifiable infectious disease caused by *Corynebacterium diphtheriae.* It affects the respiratory mucosa with the production of thick exudate and laryngeal obstruction. Production of an exotoxin causes serious systemic effects which include heart and nervous system damage. Immunization is available as part of the routine programme at 2, 3 and 4 months with a preschool and school leaving booster.

Diphyllobothrium, *(dī-fil-ō-both'-rē-um),* a genus of tapeworm. Occurs from eating uncooked fish.

diplegia, *(dī-plē-ji-ah),* paralysis of both sides of the body.

diplococcus, a coccus usually occurring in twos, e.g. pneumococcus.

diploë, *(dip'-lō-ē),* cancellous bone found between the two layers of compact bone in the skull.

diploid (2n), a cell containing a set of paired chromosomes, seen in all cells apart from the gametes. *See* HAPLOID.

diplopia, *(dī-plō'-pi-a),* double vision.

dipsomania, *(dip-sō-mā-ni-a),* pathological craving for alcohol, occurs in bouts.

disability, any condition or physical defect which limits the person's ability to learn or perform activities of living.

disaccharide, *(dī-sak-ar-īd),* a carbohydrate formed from two monosaccharides, e.g. sucrose from glucose and fructose.

disarticulation, amputation or separation at a joint.

disc, a circular plate or surface. *Intervertebral d.:* pad of cartilage between the vertebrae. Damage may cause a slipped d. *Optic d.:* the point on the retina where the optic nerve leaves the eye and can be viewed with an ophthalmoscope.

discharge, 1. emission of material, e.g. fluid, pus. **2.** leaving a healthcare facility or finishing outpatient care received from a health professional.

discission, *(dis-sish'-on),* also called **needling,** Surgical rupture of the lens capsule of the eye.

discrimination, 1. prejudice or bias by virtue of gender, age, religion or racial group. **2.** ability to distinguish between certain characteristics, such as sounds.

disease, any deviation from or interruption of the normal structure and function of a body part. It is manifested by a characteristic set of signs and symptoms and in most cases the aetiology, pathology and prognosis are known. May be acute or chronic.

disinfectants, agents which destroy pathogenic microorganisms, such as heat, sunlight and chemicals. Generally the term is used for chemicals too toxic or corrosive to be applied to tissues.

disinfection, removal or destruction of harmful microorganisms but not usually bacterial spores. It is commonly achieved by using heat or chemicals.

disinfestation, riddance of animal parasites, e.g. lice.

disk, in computing a generic term describing different types of storage medium which permanently store computer data files. Most work by recording data by magnetic means, but some such as CD-ROM operate optically. *Floppy d.:* so called because it uses flexible magnetic material. It is removable from the computer allowing the physical transfer of data (maximum around 2 megabytes or Mb) to another location.

Hard d.: so called because it uses several metal platters. It is usually a fixed device in the computer and is capable of storing very large amounts of data. Often referred to as C drive. See BYTE, CD-ROM, DRIVE.

dislocation, displacement of the articular surfaces of the bones at a joint. See DEVELOPMENTAL DYSPLASIA OF THE HIP, SUBLUXATION.

disorientation, loss of orientation. An inability to locate oneself in terms of person, time and place. Occurs in toxic states, trauma and many mental health problems.

displacement, 1. moved from the normal position. **2.** a mental defence mechanism where a distressing emotion is transferred to a person or situation which produces less anxiety.

disproportion, see CEPHALOPELVIC DISPROPORTION.

dissection, a separation by cutting parts of the body.

disseminated, scattered throughout an organ or body. *D. intravascular coagulation (DIC)*: a pathological overstimulation of the coagulation processes, characterized by a rapid consumption of clotting factors which leads to microvascular thrombi and bleeding. It occurs in situations where there is inadequate organ perfusion, such as hypovolaemia and/or sepsis.

dissociation, 1. separation of complex substances into their components. **2.** ionization, when ionic compounds dissolve in water they dissociate or ionize into their ions. **3.** an abnormal mental process by which the mind achieves non-recognition and isolation of certain unpalatable facts. Seen in an exaggerated form in delusional psychoses.

dissolution, breaking up or decomposition.

distal, situated away from the centre or point of attachment, *cf.* PROXIMAL.

distichiasis, *(dis-ti-kī-a-sis),* a double row of eyelashes, causing irritation and inflammation.

district nurse, a registered nurse with specialist qualifications who is responsible and accountable for the planning and provision of nursing services within a person's home or other community setting.

diuresis, *(dī-ū-rē-sis),* an increased secretion of urine.

diuretic, *(dī-ū-ret-ik),* substance that increases the production of urine by the kidney.

diurnal, *(dī-er-nal),* daily or occurring during the day.

divalent, bivalent, having a valence of two.

divergence, drawing apart, as when the eyes turn outwards.

diverticulitis, *(dī-ver-tik-ū-lī'-tis),* inflammation of diverticula. Specially applied to those diverticula occurring in the colon.

diverticulosis, *(dī-ver-tik-ū-lō'-sis),* presence of large numbers of diverticula, especially in the pelvic colon.

diverticulum, *(dī-ver-tik-ū-lum),* a pouch-like process from a hollow organ or tube, e.g. colon, urinary bladder and oesophagus. See MECKEL'S DIVERTICULUM.

dizygotic, *(dī-zī-got-ik),* pertaining to two zygotes. Twins arising from two zygotes. Non-identical twins who are genetically no more alike than siblings born at separate times.

DNA, abbreviation for **deoxyribonucleic acid**.

Döderlein's bacillus, *(der-der-lins),* non-pathogenic bacterium which is normally part of the vaginal flora in women of reproductive age. Contributes to the protective acidic environment by the production of lactic acid. See LACTOBACILLI.

doll's eye reflex, a reflex present in the newborn where the eyes remain still when the head is moved from side to side. Normally disappears as development occurs.

dolor, pain.

dominant gene, a gene which produces its characteristic whether inherited from one or both parents, either in the heterozygous or homozygous state. Examples include: freckles, Huntington's disease, etc. *See* RECESSIVE GENE.

dominant hemisphere, on the opposite side of the brain to the preferred hand. The dominant hemisphere for language is the left in 90% of right-handed and 30% of left-handed people.

donor, individual from whom tissue is removed or collected for transfer to another, e.g. blood, bone marrow, semen, oöcytes and organs.

dopamine, a monoamine neurotransmitter found in the central nervous system, especially the basal nuclei where its lack is linked to the development of parkinsonism. Used therapeutically to increase cardiac output and renal blood flow in the treatment of shock. It is the precursor of noradrenaline and adrenaline.

Doppler, *D. effect:* an observed change in the frequency of sound, light and radio waves as the source of that emission moves relative to the operator. *D. ultrasound scanning:* a method of assessing blood flow or blood pressure using equipment which emits ultrasonic sound waves.

dorsal, relating to the back or the posterior part of an organ.

dorsiflexion, bending backwards or in a dorsal direction.

dorsum, the back, or upper surface of a body structure, e.g. the foot.

dosimeter, small monitoring device worn by staff who may be exposed to ionizing radiation.

double-blind, a trial, usually for a drug, where neither the subjects nor the researchers know the identity of those chosen as controls or those being given the actual substance being tested. *See* CONTROL.

douche, *(doosh),* irrigation of a body cavity with water.

Douglas' pouch, peritoneal pouch between the vagina/uterus and rectum. *See* RECTOVAGINAL, RECTOUTERINE.

Down's syndrome, a chromosomal abnormality, usually of chromosome 21, which fails to separate during meiosis resulting in an individual with 47 chromosomes, also called **trisomy 21**; it increases with maternal age. It may also be due to a problem between chromosomes of groups 13–15 and 21–22 which may occur at a younger maternal age. The affected individual has a typical facial appearance with low-set ears, slanted eyes, epicanthic folds, broad hands with a single palmar crease and some degree of learning disability. Congenital anomalies such as heart defects are more common, as are thyroid disease and acute lymphatic leukaemia. *See* BRUSHFIELD'S SPOTS.

dracontiasis, *(dra-kon-ti-a-sis),* infestation with the Guinea worm *Dracunculus medinensis.* Found in parts of Africa, Asia, South America and the Middle East where it is spread through contaminated drinking water.

drainage tubes, tubes made of various materials which are inserted into cavities and surgical wounds to allow the drainage of blood, pus, serum, air and urine.

dressing, *see* WOUND DRESSINGS.

Dressler's syndrome, pyrexia pericarditis, pleurisy and effusion seen post myocardial infarction.

drive, 1. in psychology, an urge to satisfy a basic need, such as hunger. **2.** in computing that part of the computer that writes to and reads from a disk. *See* DISK.

droplet infection, transmission of pathogens via moisture droplets produced by sneezing, coughing and talking.

drug, substance used as a medicine. *D. dependence*: psychological or physical dependence on a particular drug. *D. interactions*: the interference of one drug on the action of another or the interaction of a drug with a particular food or beverage. *D. misuse*: improper or non-therapeutic use of a drug. *D. reaction*: an adverse or unexpected effect associated with the administration of a drug, e.g. a rash. *D. resistance*: bacterial strains may become resistant to the action of certain antimicrobial drugs. *See* MRSA. *D. tolerance*: where the therapeutic effects of a drug reduce over time requiring an increase in dosage.

DRV, abbreviation for **dietary reference value**.

DTPer, diphtheria, tetanus and pertussis vaccine. Injectable, vaccine offered to infants at 2, 3 and 4 months; the triple vaccine.

Dubin–Johnson syndrome, rare genetic condition where bile transport is abnormal, it is characterized by conjugated hyperbilirubinaemia and mild jaundice.

Duchenne-type muscular dystrophy, a degenerative myopathy inherited as a sex-linked recessive condition where a female carrier passes the abnormal gene to her male offspring. It is characterized by progressive muscle weakness and wasting which lead ultimately to death from infection, respiratory cardiac failure in early adulthood.

duct, a tube or channel conveying secretions or excretions.

ductless glands, *see* ENDOCRINE.

ductus, a duct; small canal. *D. arteriosus*: vessel which bypasses the fetal lungs by shunting blood from the pulmonary trunk to the aorta. Occasionally it remains patent after birth, a problem which may require surgical intervention. *D. venosus*: vessel which bypasses the fetal liver by shunting blood from the umbilical vein to the inferior vena cava.

dumping syndrome, a condition affecting people after gastrectomy, it is characterized by epigastric fullness weakness, palpitations, flushing, dizziness, sweating and nausea following a meal. It results from the rapid movement of hypertonic stomach contents into the duodenum where fluid from the blood moves into the lumen of the intestine.

duodenal, (dū-ō-dē′-nal), relating to the duodenum. *D. ulcer*: a type of peptic ulcer occurring in the duodenum, often associated with the presence of the bacterium *Helicobacter pylori* in the upper gastrointestinal tract. *See* PEPTIC ULCER.

duodenectomy, (dū-ō-de-nek′-to-mi), partial or total excision of the duodenum.

duodenoenterostomy, (dū-ō-dē′-nō-en-ter-os′-to-mi), operation to establish an anastomosis between the duodenum and another part of the small intestine.

duodenopancreatectomy, (dū-ō-dē′-nō-pan-krē-a-tek′-to-mi), excision of the duodenum and head of pancreas. *See* WHIPPLE'S OPERATION.

duodenoscopy, endoscopic examination of the duodenum.

duodenostomy, operation to establish an anastomosis between the duodenum and another structure.

duodenum, first part of the small intestine, it connects the stomach and jejunum. Contains the opening for the pancreatic and bile ducts (Figure 26).

Dupuytren's contracture, (dū-pwē'-trenz), see CONTRACTURE.

dura mater, outer fibrous meningeal membrane. See FALX CEREBRI, MENINGES, TENTORIUM CEREBELLI.

duty of care, the legal obligation in the law of negligence that a person must take reasonable care to avoid causing harm.

DVT, abbreviation for **deep vein thrombosis.**

dwarf, individual with dwarfism, growth is stunted for a variety of reasons, e.g. pituitary hyposecretion.

dynamometer, device for testing the strength of grip.

dysaesthesia, (dis-es-thē-zi-a), abnormality of sense of touch.

dysarthria, (dis-ar'-thri-a), speech disorders resulting from disturbance in muscular control of speech mechanism due to damage to the nervous system (central and/or peripheral).

dyschezia, (dis-che-si-a), painful defecation.

dyschondroplasia, (dis-kon-drō-plā-si-a), multiple enchondromas, developmental problem where cartilage is deposited within bones or on the cortical surface.

dyschromatopsia, (dis-krō-mat-op'-si-a), loss of colour vision.

dyscoria, (dis-ko-ri-a), abnormality in the shape of the pupil.

dyscrasia, an abnormality of component parts such as blood or bone marrow cells.

dysentry, acute inflammation of the colon. Types include: **1.** amoebic due to *Entamoeba histolytica*; **2.** bacillary due to a bacteria of the genus *Shigella*.

dysfunction, (dis'-funk-shon), abnormal or impaired function.

dysgammaglobulinaemia, (dis-gam'-ma-glob'-ūl-in-ēm-i-ah), an inherited immunodeficieny due to a failure to produce certain classes of immunoglobulins.

dysgenesis, abnormal development.

dysgraphia, acquired disorder of written language due to brain injury.

dyshidrosis, (dis-hīd-rō-sis), abnormal sweat production.

dyskinesia, (dis-kīn-ē'-zi-a), (clumsy child syndrome), impairment of voluntary movement.

dyslalia, (dis-lā'-li-a), mechanical speech defect, cf. DYSPHASIA.

dyslexia, (dis-lek-si-a), difficulty in reading and with spelling.

dysmaturity, signs and symptoms of growth retardation at birth.

dysmenorrhoea, (dis-men-o-rē'-a), painful or difficult menstruation, may be primary (spasmodic) or secondary (congestive).

dysorexia, (dis-o-rek-si-a), an unnatural appetite.

dysosmia, (dis-oz-mi-a), abnormal sense of smell.

dysostosis, (dis-os-tō-sis), abnormal bone formation.

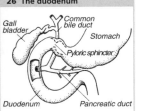

26 The duodenum

Gall bladder
Common bile duct
Stomach
Pyloric sphincter
Duodenum
Pancreatic duct

dyspareunia, *(dis-par-ū´-ni-a)*, painful coitus.

dyspepsia, *(dis-pep´-si-a)*, indigestion.

dysphagia, *(dis-fā-si-a)*, difficulty in swallowing.

dysphasia, *(dis-fā-si-a)*, disorder of language. A common cause is the occurrence of a left-sided stroke. Also called aphasia.

dysphonia, disorder of voice due to organic, neurological, behavioural or psychogenic causes.

dysphoria, *(dis-for-i-a)*, opposite to euphoria. Restless mood with depression and anguish.

dysplasia, changes in epithelial cell size and shape, resulting from chronic irritants or inflammation.

dyspnoea, *(disp-ne´-a)*, difficult breathing.

dyspraxia, *(dis-prak´-si-a)*, difficulty in performing coordinated movements.

dysreflexia, abnormal reflexes. Associated with some types of spinal injury, it is characterized by headache, hypertension, sweating and fits.

dysrhythmia, abnormal rhythm.

dystaxia, *(dis-tak-si-a)*, difficulty in controlling voluntary movements. Mild ataxia. *See also* ATAXIA.

dystocia, *(dis-tō´-ki-a* or *dis-tō´-si-a)*, a difficult labour (obstetric).

dystrophy, *(dis´-trō-fē)*, abnormality of a structure due to shortage of an essential factor. Often applied to muscles. *See* DUCHENNE-TYPE MUSCULAR DYSTROPHY.

dysuria, *(dis-ū´-ri-a)*, painful micturition.

ear, the organ of hearing and balance. It consists of external (outer), middle, and internal (inner) ear (Figure 27). *External e.*: comprises the pinna (auricle) and external auditory canal, the tympanic membrane separates it from the middle ear. *Middle e.*: air-filled cavity which communicates with the mastoid air cells and the nasopharynx via the pharyngotympanic (eustachian) tube. It contains three tiny bones or ossicles: malleus, incus and stapes which transmit sound waves from the tympanic membrane to the internal ear via the oval window. *Internal e.*: the

fluid-filled internal ear comprises the organ of hearing; the cochlea, and the semicircular canals which are concerned with balance. These structures contain nerve endings of the cochlear and vestibular branches of the vestibulocochlear nerves (VIIIth cranial, also called auditory). *E. drum*: tympanic membrane. *E. wax*: see CERUMEN.

EAR, abbreviation for **estimated average requirement**.

eating disorders, a group of disorders that include anorexia nervosa, bulimia nervosa.

Ebola virus disease, a serious viral haemorrhagic fever which occurs

---

27 The ear

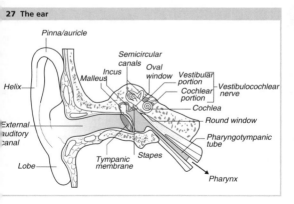

sporadically in Africa. It is spread via body fluids and mortality rates may be as high as 90% depending on the quality of medical care available. *See* MARBURG DISEASE.

EBV, abbreviation for **Epstein–Barr virus.**

ecbolic, an agent that stimulates contraction of the gravid uterus.

eccentric, 1. off centre. **2.** describing behaviour that is idiosyncratic, odd, peculiar or bizarre.

ecchondroma, *(ek-on-drō'-ma),* a tumour of cartilage arising from the bone surface.

ecchymosis, *(ek-i-mō'-sis),* a bruise; an effusion of blood under the skin.

eccrine, *(ek-rīn),* the sweat glands located generally on the body, very numerous on the feet and hands. *See* APOCRINE.

ECF, abbreviation for **extracellular fluid.**

ECG, *see* ELECTROCARDIOGRAM.

Echinococcus, *(e-kī-nō-kok'-us),* a genus of tapeworm which infests dogs and other carnivores. Its larval stage infests humans to produce hydatid cysts.

echocardiography, *(ek-kō-kar-dē-og-ra-fi),* a non-invasive cardiac investigation which utilizes ultrasound, useful for the identification of structural changes such as valve deformities.

echoencephalography, *(ek-kō-en-kef-al-og-ra-fi),* an ultrasound investigation of the brain. Used to demonstrate blood clot, abscess, tumour or injury.

echolalia, *(ek-kō-lal'-i-a),* repetition of everything said.

echopraxia, involuntary repetition of acts originally performed by others.

echovirus, enteric cytopathic human orphan virus. A member of the enterovirus group, it causes meningitis; gastroenteritis and respiratory tract infections, etc.

eclampsia, severe manifestation of pregnancy-induced hypertension, associated with fits and coma. *See* PRE-ECLAMPSIA.

ecmnesia, *(ek-nē'-zē-a),* memory impairment for recent events with normal recollection of the more distant past.

ECMO, abbreviation for **extracorporeal membrane oxygenation**.

ecological study, research study where a group of people, e.g. villages, universities, etc., are the observation unit.

ectasy, 1. state of extreme exaltation, elation or delight. **2.** popular name for the illegal stimulant 3, 4 methylene-dioxymethamphetamine. Also called 'E'.

ECT, *see* ELECTROCONVULSIVE THERAPY.

ectasia, dilatation of a hollow structure.

ecthyma, *(ek-thī-ma),* a pustular skin disease, a form of impetigo.

ectoderm, a primary germ layer of the early embryo which gives rise to some epithelium and nervous tissue. *See* ENDODERM, MESODERM.

ectogenous, *(ek-toj'-en-us),* originating outside the body.

ectoparasite, parasite living on the surface of its host.

ectopia, *(ek-tō'-pi-a),* not in the usual place.

ectopic, outside the normal place or time. *E.* beat: a heart beat not initiated by cells of the sinoatrial node. *E. gestation:* a pregnancy outside the uterus. Usually refers to one developing within a uterine tube which results in tubal rupture with severe haemorrhage and shock, tubal abortion or mole. Those occurring in the abdominal cavity are extremely rare but some have progressed to term.

ectrodactylia, *(ek-trō-dak-til'-i-a)* absence from birth of one or more toes or fingers.

ectropion, *(ek-tro-pē-on).* eversion or turning outward, especially of the lower eyelid.

eczema, *(ek-ze-ma),* acute or chronic inflammation of the skin. Characterized by redness, irritation, vesicles which weep, crusts, scales and thickened areas.

edentulous, *(ē-den'-tū-lus),* without teeth.

Edward's syndrome, trisomy 18, an abnormality affecting chromosomes in group E; 17–18, the individual has an extra chromosome 18 which results in the person having 47 chromosomes. It is characterized by micrognathia, 'rocker bottom' feet, multiple congenital anomalies and severe learning disability, but few babies survive more than a few months.

EEG, see ELECTROENCEPHALOGRAPHY.

EFAs, abbreviation for **essential fatty acids.**

effacement, shortening of the cervical canal prior to dilatation during labour.

effector, nerve endings found in muscles, glands, etc., which effect a response to a stimulus.

efferent, conveying, carrying, conducting away from the centre. See AFFERENT.

effleurage, *(ef-fler-arj),* a massage manipulation used in physiotherapy.

effort syndrome, neurotic anxiety regarding the heart; the person complains of palpitations, chest pain, breathlessness with sweating and dizziness, etc.

effusion, escape of fluid into a body cavity or tissues from another part.

ego, refers to the conscious self, the 'I' which, according to Freud, deals with reality, is influenced by social forces and controls instinctual urges (the id).

egocentric, self-centred.

ejaculation, forcible, sudden expulsion, especially of semen. *Retrograde e.:* occurs when semen is transported backwards into the bladder, a complication of diabetes mellitus or prostate surgery.

ejaculatory duct, duct carrying semen from the seminal vesicle to the urethra.

elastic, capable of stretching and returning to original length or position. *E. bandage or stocking:* contains elastic material, used for support and compression and graduated compression. See ANTIEMBOLISM HOSE. *E. tissue:* a connective tissue with the ability to stretch and recoil due to the presence of many elastic fibres within the matrix. It is found in structures required to distend and change shape, such as large arteries.

elastin, protein component of elastic fibres.

elation, ecstatic, excited state of mind. May be abnormally marked in some mental health problems, e.g. mania.

elbow, hinge joint between the arm and forearm.

elective, planned treatment or surgery rather than as an emergency.

Electra complex, excessive emotional attachment of daughter to father. See OEDIPUS COMPLEX.

electrocardiogram (ECG), *(e-lek-trō-kar-dē-ō-gram),* a graphic record of the electrical events occurring in the heart muscle during the cardiac cycle. This graphical display may be in the form of a paper tracing or on an oscilloscope. The normal heart produces a typical waveform, sinus rhythm, which consists of five deflection waves, known universally as PQRST.

electrocardiography, *(e-lek-trō-kar-dē-og'-ra-fi),* technique which records the electrical events occurring in the

111

heart muscle. The electrical impulses are picked up by using an electrocardiograph and electrodes placed on the skin. Used in the diagnosis of heart diseases such as myocardial infarction.

electroconvulsive therapy (ECT), a treatment for severe depression. An electric current is passed through the brain (frontal lobe) by means of electrodes placed on either side of the head. The convulsion produced is modified by a general anaesthetic and muscle relaxant drugs.

electrocorticography, *(e-lek-trō-kaw-ti-kog'-ra-fi),* a form of electroencephalography where the electrodes are placed directly on the brain during surgery.

electrode, in medicine, a conductor through which an electric current enters or leaves the battery or the body of the patient.

electroencephalogram (EEG), *(e-lek-trō-in-kef'-al-ō-gram),* a graphic recording of the electrical activity occurring in the brain.

electroencephalography, *(e-lek-trō-en-kef-al-og'-ra-fi),* technique which records the electrical activity of the brain by use of an electroencephalograph connected to electrodes placed on the scalp. Used in the diagnosis of conditions such as epilepsy.

electrolysis, *(e-lek-trol'-i-sis),* **1.** separation of ions by placing them in an electric field. **2.** destruction of hair follicles by the passage of an electric current.

electrolyte, *(e-lek-trō-līt),* any substance, such as sodium chloride, which when dissolved in water dissociates into electrically charged ions and will conduct electricity. *See* ANION, CATION. *E. balance:* balance of relative amounts of electrolytes, such as sodium, potassium, chlo-

ride, hydrogen carbonate and phosphates in body fluids and tissues. Balance between positive and negative ions ensures overall electrical neutrality within the fluid compartments of the body.

electromechanical dissociation (EMD), a form of cardiac arrest characterized by an ineffective cardiac output where electrical activity is normal or nearly so.

electromotive force (EMF), a measure of the force required for an electric current to flow between two points. Unit used is the volt (V), a derived SI unit.

electromyography (EMG), *(e-lek-trō-mī-og'-ra-fi),* technique which records the electrical events occurring in muscle contraction.

electron, a negatively charged subatomic particle. *E. microscopy:* uses a beam of electrons rather than light to visualize extremely small objects, such as viruses. *E. transfer chain:* a series of oxidation–reduction reactions occurring in the mitochondria that generate energy as ATP.

electrophoresis, *(e-lek-trō-faw-rē'-sis),* an analytical technique. Separation of a mixture of substances by their different rates of movement in any charged field. Used to measure plasma protein levels.

electroplexy, *(e-lek-trō-plek'-si),* *see* ELECTROCONVULSIVE THERAPY.

electroretinogram (ERG), *(e-lek-trō-ret'-in-ō-gram),* a graphic recording of the electrical responses of the retina on exposure to light.

electroretinography, *(e-lek-trō-ret-in-og'-ra-fi),* technique which records the electrical responses of the retina to light. Used in the diagnosis of eye problems.

element, a primary part. In chemistry, elements are the primary substances which, in pure form, or combined into compounds, constitute all matter. They cannot be broken down by ordinary chemical processes.

elephantiasis, (el-e-fan-fi'-a-sis), the swelling of a limb, usually the leg, as a result of lymphatic obstruction caused by filarial infestation. The skin and subcutaneous tissues are thickened (pachydermia), coarsened and fissured. See FILARIASIS.

elevator, a muscle or instrument which raises a part.

elimination, the expulsion of poisons or waste products from the body.

ELISA, abbreviation for **enzyme-linked immunosorbent assay**.

elliptocytosis, (e-lip-to-sī-tō-sis), an inherited defect of the red cells which are elliptical in shape. Increased haemolysis causes haemolytic anaemia.

emaciation, extreme body wasting with severe weight loss.

e-mail, electronic mail. A communication system where messages are stored centrally prior to their dispatch via networks or modem to other computers.

emanation, the act of flowing out. Applied especially to the rays given out by radioactive substances.

emasculation, castration of the male.

embolectomy, (em-bol-ek'-to-mi), removal of an embolus.

embolism, obstruction of a blood vessel by a body of undissolved material. Most commonly due to thrombus but other causes include: fat, malignant cells, amniotic fluid, gases, bacteria and parasites. *Pulmonary e.*: arises when a thrombus from the leg or pelvic veins becomes detached and travels to the heart. This causes sudden death if large enough to block a heart valve or the pulmonary artery. Smaller thrombi pass into the pulmonary

circulation where they eventually block a small vessel and cause infarction of lung tissue. See DEEP VEIN THROMBOSIS. *Arterial e.*: arising from the left side of the heart or a diseased artery may travel to various sites including brain, bowel or limb; the effects depend on the size of vessel occluded and location. See CEREBROVASCULAR ACCIDENT. Rarer emboli such as fat may follow long bone fractures, air may enter the circulation via a penetrating chest wound and amniotic fluid during labour.

embolus, (em'-bō-lus), a blood clot or other foreign body in the blood stream.

embrocation, a lotion for rubbing on the skin.

embryo, early developmental stage from gastrulation until the eighth week of gestation. See GASTRULATION.

embryology, (em-brē-ol'-o-ji), science of the development of the embryo.

embryonic, (em-brē-on-ik), pertaining to the embryo.

embryoma, (em-brē-ō-ma), see TERATOMA.

embryotomy, (em-brē-ōt'-ō-mi), describes an obsolete procedure that involves destruction of the fetus to facilitate delivery.

EMD, abbreviation for **electromechanical dissociation**.

emergency protection order (EPO), replaces a place of safety order. An order issued by the court when they believe that a child may suffer significant harm. It transfers parental responsibility rights and allows for the child's removal to a safe place.

emesis, (em'-e-sis), vomiting.

emetic, any agent or means used to induce vomiting.

emission, discharge, especially of semen.

EMLA, abbreviation for **eutectic mixture of local anaesthetics**.

emmetropia, *(em-e-trō'-pi-a),* normal sight.

emollients, *(e-mol'-li-ents),* softening and soothing applications or liniments.

emotion, feelings such as fear, joy or anger that produce physical changes and typical behaviour.

empathy, an ability to identify with and show an understanding of the feelings and situation of another person.

emphysema, *(em-fi-se'-ma),* gaseous distension of tissues. *Pulmonary e.:* the overdistention and destruction of the alveoli; often accompanies chronic bronchitis. A cause of chronic pulmonary disease. *See* CHRONIC OBSTRUCTIVE PULMONARY DISEASE. *Surgical e.:* air in the subcutaneous tissues caused by trauma or surgery.

empirical, based on experience and observation and not on scientific reasoning.

employment law, the law, common and statute, relating to the relationship between employer and employee.

empowerment, the enabling process by which individuals gain power and control over decisions which affect their lives. May occur when individuals with learning disabilities acquire the ability to live independently in the community, or when a group of professionals who share the same goals are able to take collective control or responsibility for the decisions which affect their practice.

empyema, *(em-pī-ē-ma),* a collection of pus within a cavity, most commonly referring to the pleural cavity.

emulsion, fluid containing two immiscible fluids, the particles of one suspended in the other, e.g. milk which is an emulsion of fat in an aqueous solution.

enamel, extremely hard substance covering the exposed areas of a tooth. *See* TOOTH.

enarthrosis, *(en-ar-thrō'-sis),* a ball-and-socket joint.

encanthis, small tumour occurring at the inner canthus of the eye.

encapsulated, contained within a capsule.

encephalin, *see* ENKEPHALIN.

encephalitis, *(en-kef-al-ī'-tis),* inflamation of the brain, due to viral or bacterial infection.

encephalocele, *(en-kef'-a-lō-sēl),* protrusion of the brain through the skull.

encephalography, *(en-kef-a-log-ra-fi),* a technique to examine the brain, to produce a visible or printed record of the findings. *See* ECHOENCEPHANOGRAPHY, ELECTROENCEPHALOGRAPHY PNEUMOENCEPHALOGRAPHY.

encephaloid, *(en-kef'-a-loyd),* brain-like.

encephalomalacia, *(en-kef'-a-lō-mal-ā-she-a),* softening of the brain.

encephalomyelitis, *(en-kef'-a-lō-mi-e-lī'-tis),* inflammation of the brain and spinal cord.

encephalon, *(en-kef'-a-lon),* the brain.

encephalopathy, *(en-kef-a-lop-a-thi),* disease of the brain. Generally applied to those conditions caused by: toxins, e.g. lead poisoning; nutritional diseases, e.g. lack of the B vitamin thiamine; and metabolic disorders, e.g. hepatic failure. *See* WERNICKE'S ENCEPHALOPATHY.

enchondroma, *(en-kon-drō'-ma),* a tumour of cartilage occurring within a bone.

encopresis, *(en-ko-prē-sis),* faecal incontinence not linked to organic defect or disease.

encounter groups, in psychology a type of therapy where people meet in a group to improve their interpersonal skills, self esteem and awareness.

encysted, (en-sis'-ted), enclosed in a sac or cyst.

endarterectomy, (en-dar-ter-ek'-to-mi), an operation which 'rebores' an artery narrowed by disease. Also called disobliteration.

endarteritis, (en-dar-te-rī'-tis), inflammation of the lining of an artery or tunica intima. *E. obliterans*: inflammation with partial occlusion of the arterial lumen.

end-diastolic volume (EDV), the volume of blood in the ventricles at the end of diastole.

endemic, (en-dem-ik), occurring frequently in a locality. Applied to a disease prevalent in a particular area.

endemiology, study of endemic diseases.

endocarditis, (en-dō-kar-dī-tis), inflammation of the endocardium and heart valves. It may complicate rheumatic fever leading to valve damage. Common causative microorganisms in the infective type include: *Streptococcus viridans*, *S. pneumoniae*, *Staphylococcus aureus* and, less commonly, rickettsiae, *Chlamydia* and fungi. It may be acute, as in staphylococcal septicaemia, or subacute where the onset is insidious. Both normal and abnormal hearts and all ages may be affected. Prophylactic antimicrobial drugs are used to cover dental treatment and surgical procedures, where microorganisms may enter the blood, to protect people with existing heart lesions.

endocardium, smooth endothelial tissue lining the heart and covering the valves.

endocervicitis, (en-dō-ser-vi-sī'-tis), inflammation of the mucous membrane lining the canal of the cervix uteri.

endocervix, lining membrane of the cervical canal.

endocolpitis, (en-dō-kol-pī'-tis), inflammation of the vaginal lining.

endocrine, (en-dō-krīn), applied to those ductless glandular structures that discharge their hormone secretions directly into the blood or lymph. Examples include: hypothalamus, pituitary gland, thyroid gland, parathyroid glands, adrenal glands, pancreas, gonads, thymus and pineal body (gland). Other structures also produce hormones, such as the placenta, kidney, gastrointestinal tract and heart. Endocrine structures function with the nervous system to regulate the body and maintain homeostasis. *See* HORMONES.

endocrinology, (en-dō'-krin-ol-ō-ji), science of the endocrine glands.

endocytosis, (en-dō'-sī'-t ō-sis), general term for the bulk transport processes by which large molecules enter the cell. *See* PHAGOCYTOSIS, PINOCYTOSIS.

endoderm, a primary germ layer of the early embryo which gives rise to some epithelial tissue. *See* ECTODERM, MESODERM.

endogenous, (en-doj-en-us), produced within the body, e.g. *e. infection*, or *e. depression*.

endolymph, (en-dō-limf), fluid of the membranous labyrinth of the ear.

endometriosis, (en-dō-me-tri'-ō'-sis), a condition where functional endometrium is found in ectopic sites, e.g. myometrium, ovaries (chocolate cyst), bowel, bladder and peritoneum. Clinical features depend upon the site involved. A tumour consisting of ectopic endometrium is known as an endometrioma.

endometritis, (en-dō-mē-trī'-tis), inflammation of the endometrium.

endometrium, the lining mucosa, of the uterus.

115

endomysium, thin connective tissue around individual muscle fibres.

endoneurium, (en-dō-nū-ri-um), delicate connective tissue surrounding individual nerve fibres.

endoparasite, a parasite living within the host.

endoplasmic reticulum, subcellular organelle concerned with the production and movement of various substances within the cell, e.g. proteins, lipids. The rough endoplasmic reticulum has ribosomes on its surface, whereas the smooth variety has none.

endorphins, (en-dor-finz), neuropeptides found in the central nervous system and pituitary gland. They have opiate-like properties and modulate pain interpretation. See ENKEPHALIN.

endoscope, lighted instrument used to visualize the inside of hollow structures. Most are now flexible fibreoptic, e.g. gastroscope, but rigid metal instruments are used in some situations, e.g. sigmoidoscope.

endoscopic retrograde cholangiopancreatography (ERCP), (en-do-skop-ik ret-rō-grād ko-lan-jē-ō-pan-krē-a-tog-ra-fi), introduction of radiopaque contrast medium via a catheter from an endoscope located in the duodenum.

endoscopy, (en-dos'-ko-pi), visualization of hollow structures and organs using an endoscope, e.g. bronchoscopy, cystoscopy, laparoscopy and oesophagoscopy.

endospore, the resting structure formed by some bacteria, e.g. Clostridium, in response to unfavourable environmental conditions.

endosteoma, (en-dos-tē-ō'-ma), tumour arising in the medullary canal of a bone.

endosteum, (en-dos'-tē-um), membrane lining the medullary cavity of long bones.

endothelioma, (en-dō-thē-li-ō-ma), a malignant growth originating in endothelium.

endothelium, (en-dō-thē'-lē-um), lining membrane of serous cavities, blood and lymph vessels.

endotoxin, an intracellular toxin released only when bacteria (mainly Gram-negative, e.g. Salmonella typhi are destroyed.

endotracheal, (en-dō-tra-ke-al), within the trachea. E. tube: used to establish or maintain an airway and facilitate ventilation, e.g. during anaesthesia.

endplate, see MOTOR END PLATE.

end-systolic volume (ESV), the volume of blood remaining in the ventricles following systole.

enema, introduction of fluid into the rectum. Used to evacuate the bowel, administer drugs (e.g. corticosteroids) and to introduce radiopaque contrast medium (barium sulphate) prior to large bowel radiography.

enervation, (en-er-vā-shon), 1. weakness. 2. removal of a nerve.

engagement, descent of the presenting part, usually the fetal head, into the pelvic cavity during the late stages of pregnancy.

engorgement, vascular congestion.

enkephalin, peptide neurotransmitters found in the central nervous system and pituitary gland and the gastrointestinal tract. They have opiate-like properties and act as natural painkillers. Also known as encephalins. See ENDORPHINS.

enophthalmos, (en-of-thal-mos), recession of the eyeball into the socket.

ensiform cartilage, the sword-shaped process of the lower end of the sternum.

Entamoeba histolytica, (ent-am-ē-ba his-to-lit-i-ka), the protozoal parasite which causes amoebic dysentery.

enteral, within the gastrointestinal tract. *E. nutrition:* method of providing nutrition when the gastrointestinal tract is functioning. Includes orally, via nasogastric and nasoduodenal tubes or via gastrostomy and jejunostomy tubes.

enterectomy, (en-ter-ek'-to-mi), excision of part of the intestine.

enteric, pertaining to the intestine. *E. coated:* a coating applied to a tablet or pill which prevents release of the drug until it enters the intestine. *E. fevers:* typhoid and the paratyphoid fevers.

enteritis, (en-ter-ī'-tis), inflammation of the small intestine.

Enterobacteriaceae, (en-ter-ō-bak-teer-i-ā'-se-e), a family of bacteria (Gram-negative) many of which are found in the human bowel. Includes the genera: *Proteus, Escherichia, Salmonella, Shigella* and *Klebsiella.*

enterobius, (en-te-rō-bi-us), genus of nematode worm. *E. vermicularis:* threadworm. Infestation with threadworms is called **enterobiasis.**

enterocele, (en'-ter-ō-sēl), hernia containing a piece of bowel. Also describes a prolapse of intestine through the vaginal wall.

enterococcus, (en-ter-ō-kok-us), a genus of Gram-positive cocci commensal in the bowel, e.g. *Enterococcus faecalis.* They cause wound and urinary tract infection and many strains are developing antibiotic resistance. *See* VANCOMYCIN-RESISTANT ENTEROCOCCI.

enterocolitis, (en-ter-ō-kol-ī-tis), inflammation of small intestine and colon. *See* NECROTIZING ENTEROCOLITIS.

enterokinase, (en-ter-ō-ki-nāz), intestinal enzyme which converts inactive trypsinogen into the active form trypsin. Also called **enteropeptidase.**

enterolith, (en'-ter-ō-lith), stone in the intestines.

enteropathy, (en'-ter-op-a-thi), disease of the small intestine.

enteropeptidase, (en'-ter-ō-pep-ti-dāz), *see* ENTEROKINASE.

enterostomy, (en-ter-os'-to-mi), an opening into the small intestine. It may be to connect it to another structure, e.g. gastroenterostomy, or opened on to the abdominal wall as an ileostomy.

enterotomy, (en-ter-ot'-o-mi), incision into the small intestine.

enterotoxin, toxins which have their effects on the gastrointestinal tract, causing diarrhoea, vomiting and pain.

enterovirus, a group of picornaviruses that enter the body via the alimentary tract. They include the polioviruses, coxsackie virus and the ECHO viruses.

entropion, (en-tro'-pi-on), inversion of the margin of the eyelid.

enucleation, (e-nū-klē-ā-shon), the entire removal of a structure such as the eye or a tumour.

enuresis, (en-ū-rē'-sis), incontinence of urine in the absence of disease. *Noctural e.:* bedwetting at night.

environment, the outside physical conditions which surround and influence all living organisms.

enzymatic agent, used for wound debridement, e.g. streptokinase.

enzyme, organic compound, usually a protein, which catalyses a specific biochemical reaction. Types include: proteolytic, dehydrogenases and aminotransferases. *See* CATALYST.

enzyme-linked immunosorbent assay (ELISA), a test for the presence of antibodies, including HIV, and antigens. The test is not highly specific for HIV and if positive it is usually repeated and followed up with more specific tests, e.g. Western blot.

eosin, (ē-o-sin), a red acid dye used for staining histological and other biological specimens.

eosinophil, (ē-ō-sin-ō-fil), a polymorphonuclear leucocyte with an affinity for acid dyes. It is concerned with immune processes involving immunoglobulin (IgE) and allergic reactions. *See* BLOOD, BLOOD COUNT.

eosinophilia, (ē-ō-sin-ō-fi-li-a), increase in the number of eosinophils in the blood, seen in parasitic and allergic conditions, e.g. asthma.

ependymal cell, a neurological cell found lining the fluid-filled cavities of the CNS.

ependymoma, (ep-en-di-mō′-ma), a tumour arising from ependymal cells.

ephelis, (ef-e-lis), a freckle.

epiblepharon, (ep-i-blef′-a-ron), a congential condition where an excessive amount of skin in the eyelid folds causes the eyelashes to press upon the eyeball.

epicanthus, a fold of skin, either side of the nose, which may cover the inner canthus of the eye. Characteristic in certain groups of people, such as Chinese.

epicardium, (ep-i-kar′-di-um), visceral layer of the pericardium.

epicondyle, (ep-i-kon′-dil), bony eminence as upon the femoral condyles.

epicranium, (ep-i-krā-nē-um), the integuments lying over the cranium. The scalp.

epicritic, (ep-i-krit-ik), describes the somatic sensations of fine touch, vibration, two-point discrimination and proprioception.

epidemic, (ep-i dem′ik), a particular illness affecting a large number of people (more than normally expected) in the same group or geographical area at the same time.

epidemiology, (ep-i-dē-mē-ol′-o-ji) study of disease distribution within a population.

epidermis, the outer layer of the skin, also called the **cuticle.**

epidermophytosis, (ep-i-der-mō-fi-tō′-sis), fungal infection of the skin or nails, e.g. ringworm. Caused by fungi of the genus *Epidermophyton*.

epididymis, (ep-i-did-i-mis), small oblong body attached to the posterior or aspect of each testis. It consists of the seminiferous tubules which convey spermatozoa from the testis to the vas deferens.

epididymitis, (ep′-i-did-i-mī′-tis), inflammation of the epididymis.

epididymo-orchitis, (ep-i-did-i-mō-or-ki′-tis), inflammation of the epididymis and the testis.

epidural, (ep-i-dū-ral), outside the dura. *E. analgesia:* injection of local anaesthetic agents into the epidural space, usually at lumbar level. Very commonly used in labour and increasingly used to control pain in other situations, e.g. following major surgery.

epigastrium, (ep-i-gas′-tri-um), region of abdomen situated over the stomach. *See* ABDOMEN.

epiglottis, leaf-shaped cartilage which covers the entrance to the larynx during swallowing.

epilation, removal of hair with destruction of the hair follicle.

epilepsy, a disorder of cerebral function due to abnormal electrical discharges, characterized by convulsions, altered consciousness and other manifestations such as warning aura. It may be primary (idiopathic) where the cause is unknown or secondary to some cerebral disorder such as infection, tumours, vascular problems and trauma. *Generalized e.:* grand mal (tonic-clonic) with major fits and unconsciousness or petit mal (absences) with short-duration alterations in consciousness without fits. *Focal/partial e.*: Jacksonian. Characterized by a local spasm which may spread to become generalized or temporal lobe epilepsy with hallucinations, memory problems and disturbances of consciousness and behaviour. *See* ELECTROENCEPHALOGRAPHY, STATUS EPILEPTICUS.

epileptiform, *(ep-i-lep′-ti-form)*, like the convulsions of epilepsy.

epiloia, *(ep-i-loy′-a)*, tuberous sclerosis. An inherited condition characterized by multiple tumours of the brain with progressive deterioration in mental functioning, facial adenomas and tumours of the retina and kidneys. Fits are an early sign of the disease.

epimenorrhoea, *(ep-i-men-or-rē′-a)*, frequent menstruation caused by a reduction in the length of the menstrual cycle.

epimysium, *(ep-i-miz-ē-um)*, fibrous connective tissue which encloses the whole muscle.

epinephrine, *see* ADRENALINE.

epineurium, *(ep-i-nūr′-ē-um)*, fibrous connective tissue around a nerve trunk.

epiphora, *(ep-if′-or-a)*, an excessive flow of tears.

epiphysis, *(ep-if′-i-sis)*, the separately ossified end of growing bone separated from the shaft (diaphysis) by a cartilaginous plate (epiphyseal plate). When growth is completed the epiphysis and diaphysis fuse.

epiphysitis, *(ep-if-is-ī-tis)*, inflammation of an epiphysis.

episcleritis, *(ep-i-skler-ī-tis)*, inflammation of the outer layers of the sclera. *See* EYE.

episiotomy, *(ep-is-ē-ot′-o-mi)*, incision of the perineum during the second stage of labour to prevent perineal tears or to facilitate delivery (Figure 28).

epispadias, *(ep-is-pa′-di-as)*, a congenital malformation in which the urethra opens on the dorsum of the penis.

epistasis, in genetics the suppression of a gene by one at another locus.

epistaxis, *(ep-is-taks′-is)*, bleeding from the nose.

epistemology, discussion and debate about knowledge and 'truth' and how it varies between different disciplines.

epithalamus, part of the brain above and behind the thalamus. It contains the pineal body and forms part of the third ventricle.

epithelial, *(ep-ith-ēl′-ē-al)*, pertaining to epithelium. *E. cast: see* CAST.

epithelialization, *(ep-ith-ēl-ē-al-īs-ā-shon)* migration of epithelial cells over the raw area of a wound. It occurs during the proliferative phase of wound healing.

epithelioma, *(ep-ith-ēl-i′-ō-ma)*, tumour of epithelium. *See* BASAL CELL CARCINOMA.

28 Episiotomy

Fetal head distending the vulva

Perineum

Medio-lateral episiotomy incision

epithelium, (*ep-ith-ēl-i-um*), one of the basic tissues, it covers the body, lines cavities and form glands. Types include: simple, single layer which may be squamous, cuboidal or columnar, and stratified which has several layers, e.g. stratified squamous or transitional.

EPO, abbreviation for **emergency protection order**.

eponym, (*ep-ō-nim*), a disease or anatomical structure, etc., named after a place or person, e.g. Malta fever, circle of Willis.

Epstein–Barr virus, a herpesvirus, the causative agent of infectious mononucleosis (glandular fever). Also linked with the formation of some malignant tumours. *See* BURKITT'S LYMPHOMA.

epulis, (*ep-ū'-lis*), tumour on the gums.

equinus, condition where the toes point down and the person walks on tiptoe.

equity, fairness of the distribution of resources. Access to resources according to need and ability to benefit.

erasion, scraping.

Erb's palsy or paralysis, paralysis of the arm due to brachial plexus damage usually resulting from a birth injury.

erectile tissue, specialized vascular tissue which becomes rigid when filled with blood, e.g. penis.

erection, the rigid enlargement of the penis during sexual arousal. The clitoris undergoes a similar change.

erector, a muscle which raises a part.

ergocalciferol, (*er-gō-kal-si'-fer-ol*), vitamin D₂ obtained from the diet. It is formed by the action of ultraviolet light on ergosterol, a plant sterol.

ergograph, an instrument for recording the amount of work done by a muscular action.

ergonomics, the scientific study o human working environments and efficient use of energy.

ergosterol, plant sterol provitami converted to ergocalciferol by ultra violet light.

erogenous, (*e-roj'-en-us*), giving rise t sexual arousal. *E. zones*: areas of th body which cause sexual arousa when stimulated.

erosion, ulceration. *Cervical e.*: th squamous epithelium of the vagina part of the cervix is replaced b columnar epithelium from the cer vical canal.

erotic, pertaining to sexual arousal o desire.

eructation, (*e-ruk-tā'-shon*), flatulenc with passage of gas from stomac through mouth.

eruption, a breaking out on the ski Or the process by which a toot emerges through the gum.

erysipelas, (*e-ri-sip'-e-las*), acute strep tococcal infection of the skin.

erythema, (*e-ri-thē-ma*), redness of th skin. *E. multiforme*: raised red lesior of varying size and shape whic may be associated with allergies an drug sensitivities. *See* STEVENS–JOHN SON SYNDROME. *E. nodosum*: red ter der skin nodules which may occu in conditions such as tuberculos: and sarcoidosis.

erythroblast, (*e-rith-rō-blast*), a nucle ated cell found in the bone marrov a stage in the development of re cells.

erythroblastosis fetalis, (*e-rith-rō blas-tō-sis fe-ta-lis*), *see* HAEMOLYTI DISEASE OF THE NEWBORN.

erythrocyte, (*e-rith'-rō-s īt*), red bloo cell. Non-nucleated biconcave dis which contains haemoglobir Concerned with the carriage of oxy gen, buffering pH changes and ca rying some carbon dioxide. *Se* BLOOD, BLOOD COUNT, HAEMOGLOBIN.

erythrocyte sedimentation rate (ESR), the rate at which erythrocytes settle to the bottom of a test tube in a given time (1 hour). Increases may indicate the presence of a disease process such as inflammation.

erythrocythaemia, *(e-rith-rō-sī-thē-mi-a)*, an overproduction of erythrocytes which may be physiological or pathological. See ERYTHROCYTOSIS, POLYCYTHAEMIA.

erythrocytopenia, *(e-rith-rō'-sī-tō-pē-ni-a)*, diminished number of red blood cells.

erythrocytosis, *(e-rith-rō'-s ī-tō'-sis)*, an abnormal increase in erythrocytes where the cause is known. See ERYTHROCYTHAEMIA, POLYCYTHAEMIA.

erythropoiesis, *(e-rith-rō-poi-ē'-sis)*, formation of erythrocytes by the bone marrow. Stimulated by the growth factor (hormone) erythropoietin.

erythropoietin, *(e-rith-rō-poi-ē-tin)*, a hormone which stimulates red cell production. It is formed from renal erythropoietic factor (REF) within the kidney and in the liver.

erythropsia, *(e-ri-throp-sē-a)*, a visual defect where all objects appear to be red.

eschar, *(es'-kar)*, a dry-healing scab on a wound; generally the result of caustics or burns.

Escherichia *(esh-er-ik'-ē-a)*, a genus of Gram-negative bacilli belonging to the family Enterobacteriaceae. *E. coli*: part of the bowel flora. Common cause of wound and urinary infections. See ENTEROBACTERIACEAE.

Esmarch's bandage, *(es-mar-ches)*, special bandage which may be used to reduce the vascularity of a limb to provide a bloodless field during surgery.

ESR, see ERYTHROCYTE SEDIMENTATION RATE.

essential, an indispensable substance. *E. amino acid*: see AMINO ACID. *E. fatty acid*: see FATTY ACID. *E. hypertension*: high blood pressure of unknown aetiology. *E. oil*: undiluted oil extracted from plants, commonly diluted in a carrier oil prior to use by aromatherapists.

ester, an organic compound formed by the reaction between an organic acid and an alcohol.

estimated average requirement (EAR), a dietary reference value. It is an estimate of the average requirement of a group of individuals. This means that 50% of the group will need less and 50% will need more.

ethanol, ethyl alcohol.

ethics, the study of the code of moral principles derived from a system of values and beliefs and concerned with rights and obligations. *E. committees*: bodies set up by universities, NHS Trusts and Health Authorities, etc. to consider proposals for research projects.

ethmoid, a complex bone of the cranium which lies between the nasal and sphenoid bones and forms part of the nasal cavity and orbit. See CRIBRIFORM PLATE.

ethnic, pertaining to a social group who share customs and culture.

ethnocentrism, *(eth-nō-sen-trizm)*, the belief that one's own ethnic group or life-style is superior to others.

ethnography, a study of people in their usual surroundings. Used in qualitative research to describe culture, customs and social life through observation and informal interview.

ethology, study of animal behaviour within their natural environment.

ethylene oxide, gas used to sterilize some types of delicate medical equipment.

121

eugenics, (ū-jen'-iks), the study of genetic characteristics aimed at improving future generations.

eukaryote, a cell that has the genetic material contained in a nuclear membrane. Found in all higher animals and some microorganisms. *See* PROKARYOTE.

eunuch, (ū-nuk), a castrated human male.

euphoria, sense of well-being, may be exaggerated in some mental health problems.

eustachian tube, (ū-stā-shan), *see* PHARYNGOTYMPANIC TUBE.

eutectic mixture of local anaesthetics, a cream for anaesthetizing the skin, e.g. for venepuncture of a child.

euthanasia, 1. a painless and easy death. **2.** the act of causing a painless and planned death.

euthyroid, (ū-thī-royd), having normal thyroid function.

eutocia, (ū-tō'-sē-a), easy labour (obstetric).

evacuation, emptying of the contents of an organ, e.g. stomach, bowel. The uterus is emptied following a miscarriage by an ERPC (evacuation of retained products of conception).

evaluation, a stage of the nursing process where the extent to which goals have been achieved is assessed and the need to modify goals or nursing interventions is determined.

eventration, (ē-ven-trā-shon), protrusion of the intestines.

eversion, folding outwards.

evidence-based practice, describes the delivery of healthcare interventions based on systematic analysis of information available about their effectiveness in relation to cost-effective health outcomes.

evisceration, (ē'-vis-ser-ā'-shon), **1.** removal of the abdominal organs.

2. protrusion of viscera through a wound or surgical incision.

evulsion, (ē-vul'-shon), a tearing apart

Ewing's tumour, malignant tumour of bone occurring in young adults.

exacerbation, an increase in the severity of symptoms.

examination under anaesthetic (EUA), commonly gynaecological.

exanthema, a skin eruption.

exchange transfusion, replacement of part of blood volume with compatible donor blood. Uses include severe haemolytic disease of the newborn due to rhesus or, rarely ABO incompatibility. Routine use of anti-D immunoglobulin for rhesus negative women has reduced the incidence of rhesus incompatibility and the need for exchange transfusions. *See* BLOOD GROUPS, ANTI-D, HAEMOLYTIC DISEASE OF THE NEWBORN.

excipient, (ek-sip'-i-ent), the substance used as a medium for giving a medicament.

excision, (ek-siz'-zhon), a cutting out.

excitability, (ek-sī-ta-bi-li-ti), rapid response to stimuli; a state of being easily irritated.

excitable cells, those cells that are able to produce an action potential by reversibly altering the potential difference across their membrane, such as muscle and nerve cells.

excoriation, (eks-ko-rē-ā'-shon), abrasions of the skin.

excrement, faecal matter.

excrescence, (eks-kres'-sens), abnormal growth or protuberance of tissues.

excreta, the natural discharges from the body: urine, faeces, sweat.

excrete, discharge waste from the body.

exenteration, (eks-en-ter-ā'-shon), removal of contents. *E. of the orbit:* removal of the contents of the bony orbit. *Pelvic e.:* removal of pelvic contents, usually performed for malignancy.

exercise, physical activity designed to improve or maintain health, increase mobility and to enhance physical performance. *See* ACTIVE MOVEMENTS, AEROBIC EXERCISE, ANAEROBIC EXERCISE, PASSIVE MOVEMENTS, RANGE OF MOTION.

exfoliation, (eks-fō-lē-ā-shon), excessive loss of superficial layers of skin in thin flakes. Also applies to the shedding of the primary (deciduous) teeth.

exfoliative cytology, (eks-fōl-ē-a-tiv-sī-tol-ō-jē), diagnostic examination of cells shed from the surface of an organ or structure. Examples include: smear from uterine cervix, bladder cells in urine and bronchial cells in sputum. *See* CERVICAL INTRAEPITHELIAL NEOPLASIA, PAPANICOLAOU SMEAR.

exhalation, breathing out.

exhibitionism, extravagant behaviour aimed at attracting attention; includes acts such as indecent exposure.

exocrine, (eks-ō-krīn), a gland which has a duct through which its secretions are discharged, e.g. salivary, sweat and pancreas which is also ENDOCRINE, *cf.*

exocytosis, (eks-ō-sī-tō-sis), process by which some molecules, e.g. hormones, mucus, leave the cell.

exogenous, (eks-oj'-en-us), due to an external cause.

exomphalos, (eks-om'-fal-os), umbilical hernia of congenital origin causing a protrusion of intestines through gap in abdominal wall.

exophthalmos, (eks-of-thal-mos), protrusion of the eyeball. *See* HYPERTHYROIDISM.

exostosis, (eks-os-tō'-sis), a bony tumour growing from the bone.

exotoxin, toxin released from the exterior of a living microorganism, usually Gram-positive such as *Clostridium tetani.*

expanded role of the nurse, nurses are increasingly taking on additional roles and responsibilities, traditionally regarded as belonging to doctors and other professionals. These include specific skills, such as intravenous cannulation, and roles, such as nurse-led clinics. The UKCC has set out the professional framework in which such practice may develop in its document 'Scope of Professional Practice'.

expected date of delivery (EDD), date predicted for a pregnant woman's delivery. Calculated from the first day of the last menstrual period (LMP). *See* NÄGELE'S RULE.

expectorant, a drug which increases expectoration.

expectoration, the coughing up of sputum.

experiential learning, learning through experience of the actual situation, role play or simulation. *See* ROLE PLAY, SIMULATION.

experimental method, *see* RESEARCH METHODS.

expiration, 1. dying. **2.** breathing out.

expiratory, pertaining to expiration. *E. reserve volume (ERV):* the volume of air that can be forcibly expelled after a normal expiration.

expression, 1. act of expulsion. **2.** facial appearance. **3.** in genetics the appearance of a particular trait or characteristic.

exsanguinate, (ek-san'-gwin-āt), to make bloodless.

extended, expanded, comprehensive. *E. family:* see FAMILY.

extension, 1. straightening of a flexed limb. **2.** the pull exerted on a limb as part of treatment following fracture or dislocation. *See* TRACTION.

extensor, a muscle which extends a part.

external, outer. *E. conjugate.* see CONJUGATE. *E. os:* junction between the cervical canal and vagina. *E. respiration:* the exchange of gases between the alveolar air and the pulmonary capillary blood. *E. version:* method of changing the lie or presentation of a fetus by manipulation through the abdominal wall.

extirpate, to remove completely.

extracapsular, outside a capsule.

extracellular, outside the cell. *E. fluid (ECF):* includes interstitial (tissue) fluid, plasma, cerebrospinal fluid, lymph and gastrointestinal secretions.

extracorporeal, outside the body, such as the circulation in open heart surgery and haemodialysis. *See* BYPASS, HAEMODIALYSIS. *E. membrane oxygenation (ECMO):* the ECMO circuit is a cardiopulmonary bypass device which uses a membrane oxygenator or artificial lung.

extract, concentrated form of a drug.

extraction, 1. pulling out. **2.** making an extract. *Lens e.:* removing the lens of the eye. *Vacuum e.:* using a vacuum to remove the uterine contents such as in an assisted delivery.

extradural, outside the dura, such as an *e. haematoma* where blood collects outside the dura.

extrahepatic, outside the liver.

extramural, outside the wall of a structure such as bowel or blood vessel.

extraocular, outside the eyeball. *E. muscles (intrinsic):* the muscles which move the eyeball.

extraperitoneal, (eks-tra-per-i-to-nē′-al), outside the peritoneal cavity.

extrapyramidal, outside the pyramidal tracts. *E. effects:* include the tremor and rigidity seen in parkinsonism and the side-effects of some

drugs, e.g. phenothiazine neuroleptics. *E. motor tracts:* motor pathways which pass outside the internal capsule. They modify the motor functions of the pyramidal tracts that connect the cerebral cortex to other parts of the brain, muscles and sensory receptors. They influence coarse voluntary movements and affect balance, posture and coordination. *See* PARKINSONISM.

extrasensory, outside the normally accepted senses. *E. perception (ESP):* a knowledge of future events or the thoughts of others in the absence of normal communication.

extrasystoles, (ek-stra-sis-tō-lēz), ectopic beats. Premature contraction of the heart stimulated by an impulse arising from outside the sinoatrial node. They may affect the atria or the ventricles. *See* VENTRICULAR ECTOPICS.

extrauterine gestation, (ek-stra-ū′-te-rin), pregnancy outside the uterus. *See* ECTOPIC GESTATION.

extravasation, (eks-trav-a-sā′-shon), escape of fluid from its proper channel into surrounding tissue.

extremity, (eks-trem-i-ti), the end part of any organ. A limb.

extrinsic, external, from without. *E. factor:* vitamin B_{12}. *See* COBALAMIN, INTRINSIC FACTOR. *E. muscles:* see EXTRAOCULAR. *E. sugars:* those such as fructose in honey, lactose in milk and sucrose, not contained in cell walls.

extrovert, an outgoing, sociable personality, having interests outside oneself. Opposite to introvert.

extubation, removing a tube, such as an endotracheal tube.

exudation, oozing; slow escape of fluid (the exudate) through vessel walls in response to the inflammatory process. Or the sweat through the skin pores.

29 Sagittal section through the eye

eye, organ of vision. Consists of three layers: sclera (outer), pigmented choroid and the light-sensitive retina (Figure 29). Light rays entering the eye are focused on to the retina by the lens. Specialized nerve endings in the retina convert the images for transmission to the brain, via the optic nerves (cranial nerves II), for interpretation. *See* CONES, RODS.

F

F, abbreviation for **Fahrenheit.**

face, anterior part of the head. *F. presentation*: fetus presents face first into the pelvis during labour.

facet, one side of a many-sided body, applied to the small, smooth, articulating surface of a bone.

facial, pertaining to the face. *F. nerve*: VIIth cranial nerve, it supplies part of the tongue, facial muscles and various glands; salivary, nasal and lacrimal. Damage may result in facial paralysis. *See* BELL'S PARALYSIS.

facies, *(fa-sēs)*, surface of a structure, the face or its expression, e.g. abdominal f., adenoidal f. or moon f.

facilitated diffusion, a process by which larger molecules (e.g. glucose), that are not fat-soluble, diffuse through the plasma membrane by using a protein carrier molecule. The process does not use energy, but does need a concentration gradient.

facultative, *(fa-kul-ta-tiv)*, able to live under varying conditions.

faecal, *(fē-kal)*, pertaining to faeces. *F. impaction*: build-up of hard faeces within the rectum and colon.

faeces, *(fē-sēs)*, waste discharged from the bowel. Contains water, epithelial cells, mucus, bacteria, undigested cellulose, electrolytes, stercobilin and chemicals causing odour.

faecolith, *(fē-kō-lith)*, hard mass in the bowel formed from faeces.

Fahrenheit, thermometric scale, now replaced by Celsius.

faint, *see* SYNCOPE.

falciform, *(fal-si-form)*, sickle-shaped. *F. ligament*: peritoneal fold separating right and left lobes of the liver.

fallopian tube, *see* UTERINE TUBE.

Fallot's tetralogy, *(fa-lōz)*, congenital heart defect consisting of overriding of the aorta, ventricular septal defect, pulmonary stenosis and right ventricular hypertrophy.

falx, *(falks)*, sickle-shaped. *F. cerebelli*: fold of dura between the cerebellar hemispheres. *F. cerebri*: fold of dura between the cerebral hemispheres.

familial, affecting several members of one family.

family, 1. a group of related people. **2.** a category used in taxonomy. *Extended f.*: one that consists of the nuclear family plus other relatives such as grandparents. *F. planning*: methods used for limiting or spacing the number of children and for enhancing conception. *F. therapy*: in psychiatry, the involvement of several members of the family in therapy based on the idea that psychological problems may arise from the way family members interact. *Nuclear f.*: one that consists of a couple and their children. *One-parent f.*: consists of one parent with his or her child/children.

Fanconi's syndrome, an inherited disorder where the renal tubules are unable to reabsorb amino acids, glucose, uric acid and phosphates. Proximal renal tubular acidosis.

fanaticism, zeal for some belief or cause carried to excess.

fantasy, a world of imagination controlled by the whim of the individual.

farinaceous, *(far-i-nā'-shius),* starchy. Containing flour or cereals.

farmer's lung, see ALVEOLITIS.

FAS, see FETAL ALCOHOL SYNDROME.

fascia, *(fa-shi-a),* fibrous connective tissue such as that around muscles or between body compartments.

fascicle, *(fas'-i-kl),* a small bundle of fibres (nerve or muscle). **A fasciculus.**

fasciculation, *(fas-ik-ū-lā'-shon),* an isolated visible muscle twitching, such as the flickering of an eyelid.

fastigium, *(fas-tij-ē-um),* the summit or height, e.g. of a fever.

fat (neutral), 1. organic compound consisting of fatty acids and glycerol, a triglyceride (triacylglycerol). Fats and oils. **2.** fatty deposits of the body. *F. embolus:* see EMBOLISM. *See also* ADIPOSE, FATTY ACIDS, GLYCEROL, LIPIDS, TRIGLYCERIDE.

Fatal Accident Enquiry, see: CORONER.

fatty acids, hydrocarbon constituent of lipids. Classified as saturated or unsaturated (monounsaturated or polyunsaturated) according to the number of double bonds in their structure. *Essential f. a. (EFA):* linoleic, linolenic acids, and in certain situations arachidonic acid is also essential. Required in the diet for prostaglandin synthesis and cell membranes.

fatty degeneration, a degenerative process where fat is deposited within damaged cells, especially those of the liver, heart and kidney.

fauces, *(faw'-sēs),* opening between the mouth and pharynx.

favism, inherited deficiency in the red cell of the enzyme glucose-6-phosphate dehydrogenase (G6PD). Affected individuals develop haemolytic anaemia if they eat fava beans (broad beans) or inhale the pollen. Seen in Mediterranean and Middle Eastern countries.

favus, a type of ringworm infection.

febrile, relating to fever. *F. convulsions:* see CONVULSIONS.

fecundation, *(fe-kund-dā'-shon),* impregnation. Fertilization.

fecundity, *(fe-kun-di-ti),* fertility. Power of reproduction.

feedback, homeostatic control mechanism where the process product regulates the rate at which the physiological process proceeds. It may be negative where high product levels turn off the process or positive (rarely) where high levels stimulate further activity.

Felty's syndrome, adult rheumatoid arthritis, leucopenia and splenomegaly.

feminism, a sociological doctrine that puts forward the idea that women have been disadvantaged in every area of society. It supports the idea of equal opportunities for women and men.

feminization, 1. normal development of female characteristics in females. **2.** abnormal development of female characteristics in males.

femoral, relating to the femur or thigh. Applied to the artery, vein, nerve and canal. *See* HERNIA.

femur, bone of the thigh. It is the largest and strongest bone of the body.

fenestra, a window, applied to certain apertures, e.g. fenestra ovalis.

fenestration, 1. making a window or opening surgically. **2.** a perforation, pore or opening. The capillaries in the glomerulus have fenestrations which facilitate filtration.

fermentation, the process by which enzymes in yeasts and bacteria break down sugars and other organic substances. Used in the production of alcohol, vinegar, cheese and bread.

ferning, microscopic pattern seen in dried cervical mucus around ovulation.

ferric, pertaining to trivalent iron and its salts.

ferritin, an iron storage complex formed by the combination of iron and a protein.

ferrous, pertaining to bivalent (divalent) iron and its salts.

fertility, ability to produce young. *F. control: see* CONTRACEPTION, FAMILY PLANNING. *F. rate:* the number of live births occurring per 1000 women aged 15–44.

fertilization, impregnation of an oöcyte by a spermatozoon and the fusion of their nuclei to form the diploid zygote.

fester, superficial inflammation with suppuration.

festination, increasingly rapid gait as in parkinsonism.

fetal, pertaining to the fetus. *F. alcohol syndrome:* physical and mental syndrome seen in neonates where maternal alcohol intake is high during pregnancy. It is characterized by poor growth, facial, heart and limb defects. *F. assessment:* various methods used to assess fetal wellbeing, including physical examination, ultrasound scan, chorionic villus sampling, blood tests, amniocentesis, kick charts and checks on placental function. *F. circulation:* circulation adapted for intrauterine life. Extra vessels and shunts allow blood largely to bypass the lungs, liver and gastrointestinal tract as their functions are dealt with by maternal systems and the placenta.

fetishism, a condition where a particular object is regarded with irrational awe or has strong emotional attachment. May have a psychosex-

ual dimension in which such an object is repeatedly used to achieve sexual excitement and gratification.

fetor, a very unpleasant odour. *F. hepaticus:* foul breath odour associated with hepatic encephalopathy.

fetoscopy, *(fe-tos-ko-pi),* endoscopic examination of the fetus.

fetus, developmental stage from the eighth week of gestation until birth. The unborn child.

fever, a rise in body temperature above normal.

fibre, 1. thread-like structure. **2.** non-starch polysaccharide (NSP). Indigestible plant material which adds bulk to faeces, reduces bowel transit times and helps to ensure that nutrients such as glucose are absorbed at a constant rate. Inadequate dietary intake is linked with conditions which include bowel cancer and diverticular disease. *See* NUTRITION, APPENDIX.

fibreoptics, *(fi-ber-op-tiks),* transmission of light via very fine glass or plastic fibres enclosed in a flexible tube. The technology utilized in endoscopic equipment.

fibrillation, uncoordinated contraction of muscle, usually of the myocardium (Figure 30). *See* ATRIAL FIBRILLATION, CARDIAC ARREST, VENTRICULAR FIBRILLATION.

30 Atrial (B) and ventricular (E) fibrillation

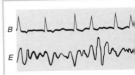

fibrin, insoluble substance formed by the action of thrombin upon fibrinogen. *F. stabilizing factor*: factor XIII in blood clotting. *See* BLOOD CLOTTING.

fibrinogen, a plasma protein produced by the liver. Factor I in the blood coagulation mechanism. *See* BLOOD CLOTTING.

fibrinolysin, enzyme which dissolves fibrin. Also called **plasmin**.

fibrinolysis, *(fi-brin-ol´-i-sis),* one of the four overlapping processes of haemostasis. The process by which enzymes remove clots from vessels when healing is complete.

fibrinolytic, dissolving fibrin clots. *F. therapy*: drugs, e.g., alteplase, given to dissolve clots following myocardial infarction and other thromboembolic conditions. Also called thrombolytic therapy.

fibroadenoma, a benign tumour composed of mixed fibrous and glandular elements.

fibroblast, the immature blast cell which forms some connective tissue. Active during tissue development and repair.

fibrocartilage, cartilage with fibrous tissue.

fibrochondritis, inflamed fibrocartilage.

fibrocystic disease, *(fi-brō-sis-tik),* see CYSTIC FIBROSIS.

fibrocyte, *see* FIBROBLAST.

fibroid, *(fi´-broyd),* a tumour composed of fibrous and muscular tissue. *See also* FIBROMYOMA.

fibroma, *(fi-brō-ma),* benign tumour of fibrous tissue.

fibromyoma, *(fi-brō-mī-ō-ma),* fibroids. A tumour of muscle and fibrous tissue, especially common in the uterus.

fibroplasia, *(fi-brō-plā-zē-a),* formation of fibrous tissue which is part of normal healing. *See* RETROLENTAL FIBROPLASIA.

fibrosarcoma, *(fi-brō-sar-kō-ma),* malignant tumour of fibrous tissue.

fibrosis, *(fi-brō-sis),* formation of fibrous tissue in areas of cell damage, often as a result of inflammation. *Pulmonary f.*: may be caused by serious lung diseases such as pneumoconiosis, radiation to the chest, or the use of certain drugs, e.g. some cytotoxic drugs.

fibrositis, *(fi-brō-sī´-tis),* inflammation of fibrous tissue.

fibula, *(fib-ū-la),* the small bone on the outer side of the leg.

field of vision, the area which can be seen without movement of the eyes.

fight or flight mechanism, extreme physiological response to an immediate stressor or as perceived danger. The release of adrenaline (epinephrine) and nonadrenaline (norepinephrine) stimulates an increase in heart rate, rise in blood pressure, increased blood glucose and diversion of blood to vital organs and skeletal muscles. These changes allow the body to deal with the stressor or remove itself from immediate danger.

filament, a thread-like structure.

Filaria, a genus of thread-like nematode worms, e.g. *Wuchereria bancrofti, Loa Loa,* etc.

filariasis, *(fil-ar-ī´-a-sis),* infestation with *Filaria*. The adult worms live in the lymphatics, connective tissue or mesentery, where they may cause obstruction, but microfilariae migrate to bloodstream and some invade the skin, eye or pulmonary capillaries. *See* ELEPHANTIASIS, LOIASIS, ONCHOCERCIASIS.

file, in computing a discrete set of characters stored on a disk. Files may hold information in a variety of forms which include: database, program, document or graphic image. Individual files and their

129

contents are identified by a specific filename.

filiform, thread-like. *F. papillae*: projections on the tongue.

filipuncture, insertion of a thin wire into an aneurysm to clot the blood contained in its sac.

filoviruses, family of RNA viruses that include Ebola and Marburg viruses.

filter, device used to remove certain substances, particles or electromagnetic rays of a particular wavelength while allowing others to pass through, e.g. optical filters, fluid filters.

filterable, filtrable, able to pass through a filter.

filtration, passage through a filter.

filum, *(fē-lum)*, any thread-like structure. *F. terminale*: modified pia matter securing the end of the spinal cord to the coccyx.

fimbria, a fringe, especially those at the end of the uterine tube.

first aid, immediate care given after injury or sudden illness. Aims to preserve life, prevent deterioration and promote recovery.

first pass metabolism, where drugs given orally are absorbed in the gastrointestinal tract and pass to the liver where they are rapidly metabolized. This results in a situation where insufficient amounts of active drug reach the systemic circulation. It can be overcome by use of other delivery methods, e.g. transdermally or sublingual.

first intention, primary union. Healing seen in clean surgical wounds where the edges are in apposition.

fission, division into two or more parts. *Binary f.*: a mode of reproduction for bacteria and protozoa.

fissure, split or cleft. *F. in ano*: anal fissure. Ulcerated cleft in the anal mucosa. *F. of Rolando*: central sulcus, separates frontal and parietal cerebral lobes. *F. of Sylvius*: lateral sulcus, separates the frontal and temporal cerebral lobes.

fistula, an abnormal passage connecting two organs or an organ and the outside. *Anal f.*: a sinus leading from the anal canal to the skin surface which discharges faeces. Associated with bowel disease and ischiorectal abscess. *Biliary f.*: opening between gallbladder and bowel or the external leakage of bile after surgery. *Faecal f.*: communication between the bowel and the surface. Seen after bowel surgery where faeces discharges via the wound or drain site. *Gastrocolic f.*: communication between stomach and colon. A complication of malignancy. *Rectovaginal f.*: opening between rectum and vagina. May follow perineal lacerations. *Tracheo-oesophageal f.*: congenital abnormality. Opening between trachea and oesophagus. *Vesicointestinal f.*: opening between bladder and intestine, may result from diverticular disease. *Vesicovaginal f.*: opening between the bladder and vagina. Causes include: cervical tumours, radiotherapy and damage during surgery or labour.

fit, convulsion, often with altered consciousness. *See* EPILEPSY.

Fitness for Practice, report prepared by the Commission for Education established by the UKCC to look at preregistration nursing and midwifery education and propose education that 'enabled fitness for practice based on healthcare need' (UKCC 1999).

fixation, 1. focusing the eyes on an object so the image falls on the retina. **2.** arrested psychological development. **3.** technique used to preserve specimens for microscopy.

4. securing a part in a fixed position. *Complement f.:* see COMPLEMENT FIXATION TEST.

flaccid, *(flas-sid),* soft, lacking rigidity.

flagellum, *(fla-jel-um),* thread-like projection from the surface of some cells: human spermatozoa, some bacteria and protozoa. Used for movement.

flail chest, *see* CHEST, PARADOXICAL RESPIRATION.

flap, tissue used to repair defects in an adjacent or distant part of the body, e.g. a piece of skin cut to fold over the stump in operation for amputation.

flat foot, flattening or total loss of foot arches.

flat or flattened pelvis, *see* CONTRACTED PELVIS.

flatulence, distention of gastrointestinal tract with gas. Causes belching and discomfort.

flatus, gas present in the gastrointestinal tract. Usually applied to that passed rectally.

flea, wingless, parasitic, blood-sucking insect. *Pulex irritans* is the human flea. The rat flea, *Xenopsylla cheopis,* spreads plague.

flexion, being bent; the opposite of extension.

Flexner bacilli, *see* SHIGELLA.

flexor, a muscle which causes flexion.

flexure, a bend. A curvature of an organ, e.g. *hepatic f.:* bend of the colon beneath the liver.

flight of ideas, state seen in some mental health problems where the person talks continually with constant changes of topic.

floating ribs, the two lower pairs of ribs not articulating with the sternum.

floccilation, *(flok-si-lā-shon),* picking at the bedclothes, seen in delirium.

flocculation, *(flok-kū-lā-shon),* the process where colloidal particles in suspension clump together to form a visible aggregation.

flooding, 1. popular term for excessive uterine bleeding. **2.** a behaviour therapy in the treatment of phobias and avoidance behaviour where the person is imaginary or real exposure to the feared stimulus.

flow chart, 1. a computer program sequence in graphical format. **2.** a chronological record of several changing features, e.g. vital signs, treatment and drugs, in a tabular or graphical format. Also called a **flow sheet.**

flow meter, instrument used to measure the flow rate of gases or liquids.

fluctuation, a wave-like motion felt on palpation of an abscess or a cyst containing fluid.

fluid, 1. a substance which flows (either liquid or gaseous). **2.** body fluids which may be intracellular or extracellular (Figure 31). *See* AMNIOTIC FLUID, CEREBROSPINAL FLUID, EXTRACELLULAR FLUID, INTRACELLULAR FLUID, LYMPH, PLASMA.

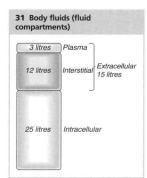

31 Body fluids (fluid compartments)

3 litres	Plasma	
12 litres	Interstitial	Extracellular 15 litres
25 litres	Intracellular	

fluke, any of the trematode class of worm.

fluorescein, *(flo-re-sēn),* substance which stains the cornea a vivid green in areas where there is damage, e.g. in an abrasion or ulcer.

fluorescence, emission of light at a wavelength which is different from that of the incident light. The emitted light has a lower energy, i.e. is of longer wavelength, from the incident irradiation which is absorbed.

fluorescent, producing fluorescence. *F. screen:* in radiology a screen which will fluoresce when exposed to X-rays.

fluoridation, the addition of fluoride, such as when added to drinking water.

fluorine (F), halogen element. Its salts are added to drinking water and toothpaste to reduce dental caries. See NUTRITION APPENDIX.

fluoroscopy, X-ray examination of movement in the body, observed by means of a fluorescent screen and TV system.

flush, sudden redness of the skin of the neck and face. *Hot f.:* caused by vasomotor instability during the climacteric. Accompanied by feeling hot and sweating.

flutter, an abnormal heart rhythm. See ATRIAL FLUTTER.

foam dressing, wound dressing available as sheets, or as cavity dressings. Used for a wide range of wounds to provide a moist wound environment with varying degrees of absorption.

focus, 1. point of maximum intensity. **2.** point where light rays or sound waves converge. *F. groups:* a research method where data are collected by interviewing people in small interacting groups.

foetus, see FETUS.

folates, collective name for the B vitamin compounds derived from folic acid. Folates occur naturally in foods such as liver, yeast and leafy green vegetables. They are coenzymes involved in many biochemical reactions in the body, e.g. purine synthesis, and adequate amounts are required for normal red cells. Deficiencies have been linked with fetal neural tube defects and poor growth in children, and megaloblastic anaemia.

folic acid, *(fō-lik),* the molecule that gives rise to a large group of molecules called folates that form part of the vitamin B complex. See FOLATE.

folie à deux, delusion shared by two persons.

follicle, small sac or gland containing a secretion. See GRAAFIAN FOLLICLE, HAIR FOLLICLE, PRIMORDIAL FOLLICLE. *F. stimulating hormone (FSH):* a gonadotrophin hormone secreted by the anterior part of the pituitary gland. In the female it stimulates the growth of ovarian follicles and the production of oestrogens. In the male it promotes the development of spermatozoa in the testis.

follicular, *(fo-lik'-ū-lar),* relating to a follicle. *F. phase:* days 1–14 of the ovarian cycle which includes ovulation. *F. tonsillitis:* tonsillitis caused by infection of the tonsil follicles.

folliculitis, inflammation of the hair follicles.

fomites, *(fō-mīts),* articles of bedding or other equipment which have been in contact with infection and may transmit that infection.

font, describes the design, size and style of a particular typeface.

fontanelle, 'soft spots' or membranous spaces between the skull bones of an infant prior to complete ossification. The anterior fontanelle or bregma is at the junction of the frontal and two parietal bones and is usually closed by 18 months. The posterior fontanelle is at the junction of the occipital and two parietal bones and closes within a few weeks of birth (Figure 32). *See* SUTURES.

food allergy, allergic reactions to substances in foods, such as peanuts, shellfish, eggs and strawberries. The reactions occur immediately on contact with the food and can be very severe, leading to life-threatening anaphylaxis. Those at risk of severe attacks carry pre-filled devices of adrenaline (epinephrine) for injection.

food poisoning, a group of notifiable diseases characterized by diarrhoea and/or vomiting caused through eating food contaminated with live microorganisms (bacteria and viruses), bacterial toxins or by chemical toxins. Bacterial food poisoning may be produced by the multiplication of the microorganisms within the food, e.g. *Campylobacter jejuni*, *Salmonella typhimurium*, or from toxins produced by bacteria such as *Staphylococcus aureus*, *Clostridium perfringens* and *Escherichia coli* 0157.

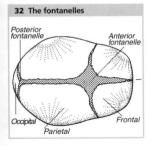

32 The fontanelles

Posterior fontanelle

Anterior fontanelle

Occipital

Frontal

Parietal

Food Standards Agency, a UK body set up by the government to oversee food standards and safety.

foot, that part of the leg below the ankle. *F. drop*: inability to keep foot bent at right angles with the leg. The toes and foot drop and walking becomes difficult. Caused by pressure of bedclothes, or inadequate support to underside of foot when leg is in a splint for a long time, or from paralysis of the muscles which produce dorsiflexion of the ankle.

foramen, an opening. *F. magnum*: opening in the occipital bone through which the spinal cord passes. *F. ovale*: opening between the right and left atria in the fetus which allows blood to bypass the pulmonary circulation. It is occluded by a flap after the infant's first breath but takes some months to close completely. *Obturator f.*: opening in the innominate bone which gives passage to nerves and vessels. *Optic f.*: opening through which the optic nerves enter the skull.

forced expiratory volume (FEV), volume of air exhaled during a given time (usually the first second) whilst performing a forced vital capacity.

forced vital capacity (FVC), volume of air expired forcefully soon after a maximal inspiratory effort.

forceps, surgical instruments made of metal or plastic used for holding, moving and clamping etc. *F. delivery*: the use of obstetric forceps to deliver the infant during the second stage of labour.

forebrain, *see* PROSENCEPHALON.

forensic medicine, also called legal medicine. The application of medical knowledge to questions of law.

forensic mental health services, those services concerned with the relevant laws, e.g. current Mental Health Act, and with legal

133

matters/problems. They include: hospitals/clinics providing secure environments; the mental health nurses designated to work closely with the criminal justice system, such as court diversion schemes for offenders with mental health problems and nurses working with Youth Offending Teams.

foreskin, fold of skin covering the glans penis in the male. The **prepuce.**

formal operations, according to Piaget a stage in cognitive development occurring from 12 years of age and continuing throughout life, characterized by the ability to deal with abstract concepts.

formaldehyde, toxic, pungent-smelling gas used as a disinfectant. Dissolved in water (formalin) it is used to preserve histological specimens and for disinfection.

format, in computing 1. *see* FORMATTING. 2. the structure which determines the way in which data is stored in a file. In order to read or write files a program which recognizes the structure is required.

formative evaluation, ongoing assessment or judgement about performance, such as nursing actions.

formatting, in computing the procedure by which a new disk is prepared to store data in the manner required by the operating system of the computer. *See* FORMAT, OPERATING SYSTEM.

formication, the sensation of insects such as ants creeping over the body. Occurs in nerve lesions, particularly in the regenerative phase.

formula, 1. a prescription. 2. symbols representing chemical substances. 3. ingredients for a milk-based infant food.

formulary, a collection of formulae (*pl.* of formula). The *British National Formulary* (BNF) description of licensed pharmaceutical preparations available in the UK. A *Nurse Prescribers' Formulary* (NPF) containing a limited range of preparations is available to suitably qualified nurses who have completed an approved course and demonstrated competence.

fornix (*pl.* **fornices**), an arch. Applied to various anatomical structures, but especially to the roof of the vagina.

fossa (*pl.* **fossae**), a depression in a structure. *Olecranon f.:* in the humerus it receives the ulnar process during elbow extension. *Pituitary f.:* in the sphenoid bone it accommodates the pituitary gland, the **sella turcica.**

Fothergill's operation, operation to correct a uterine prolapse. Also called a Manchester repair.

fourchette, posterior fusion of the labia minora in front of the perineum.

fovea, (*fŏ-vea*), fossa or cup. *F. centralis:* a depression on the retina containing many cones, it is important for clear colour vision.

fractionation, 1. in radiotherapy the division of the total dose of radiation prescribed into smaller portions to be given over a period of time. 2. in chemistry the division of a substance into its constituent parts.

fracture, a break in the continuity of a bone, characterized by pain, swelling, deformity, loss of function, shortening and crepitus (Figure 33). A fracture may be: 1. simple or closed. 2. open, communicating with the surface via a wound. 3. complicated, where the fracture is associated with injury to another structure such as nerve, artery or organ, e.g. bladder damage from fractured pelvis. 4. comminuted, where the bone is broken into two or more

33 Types of fracture

Transverse   Oblique   Greenstick

Comminuted   Open   Impacted

Spiral   Depressed fracture of skull

fragments. **5.** impacted, where one fragment is driven into the other. **6.** pathological, fracture associated with existing bone disease, e.g. metastatic malignancy. **7.** greenstick, where the bone is fractured half through on the convex side of the bend (as in a green twig); seen only in children. The type of break in the bone may be: **1.** transverse, due to direct violence at the point of fracture. **2.** oblique, due to indirect violence, when a force applied at some distance causes the bone to break at its weakest point. **3.** spiral, when a limb is violently rotated. **4.** depressed, e.g. the skull, when the bone is driven inwards.

fragile X syndrome, genetic condition caused by a defective X chromosome. It causes learning disability which usually, but not exclusively, affects men. In many cases the condition is passed from a female carrier to an affected son. Physical features include: enlarged testes and ears, a long narrow face, and sometimes a smooth skin, flat feet and heart valve problems. Learning disability ranges from mild to severe.

fragilitas ossium, *(fraj-il-it-as os-ē-um),* a congenital abnormality with brittle bones, otosclerosis and blue sclerae. *See* OSTEOGENESIS IMPERFECTA.

framboesia, *(fram-bē-zia), see* YAWS.

Frank–Starling, *see* STARLING'S LAW.

free radical, activated oxygen species such as superoxide ions (O_2^-) and hydroxyl radicals. They are extremely reactive chemicals produced during normal cell metabolism. They are usually dealt with by complex antioxidant enzymes, but will cause oxidative damage to cells where defences are overwhelmed. *See:* ANTIOXIDANT.

Frei test, a skin test used as an aid in the diagnosis of lymphogranuloma venereum.

frenulum, small fold of mucous membrane. *Lingual f.:* attaches the tongue to the floor of the mouth.

frequency, 1. rate at which an action/event is repeated. **2.** the need to pass urine more often than is acceptable to the person. The person passes small amounts of urine. It may be a sign of infection. **3.** rate of vibration or cycles per second, such as sound waves, measured in hertz (Hz).

frequency distribution, in research the number of times (frequency) that each value in a variable is observed.

Freud Sigmund, a famous Austrian psychoanalyst (1856–1939).

Freudian, psychoanalysis and the psychoanalytical theory of the causation of neuroses, according to the teachings of Freud.

friction, 1. rubbing together. **2.** a circular movement used in the massage of deep tissues. **3.** a type of injury caused by rubbing the skin. **4.** a sound heard on auscultation when two dry surfaces rub together, such as the pleura in pleurisy. *See* PLEURAL RUB.

Friedreich's ataxia, *(frēd-rīks ā-taks-i-a),* inherited degenerative disease of the nervous system. The onset is in childhood and is progressive. There is clumsiness, unsteady gait, weakness, dysarthria and other neurological disturbances.

frigidity, diminished sexual desire.

Fröhlich's syndrome, *(frer-liks),* **adiposogenital dystrophy.** A disorder with obesity, sexual infantilism, somnolence, disturbance of temperature regulation and diabetes insipidus due to damage of the pituitary gland and hypothalamus.

frontal, relating to the front of the body or the forehead. *F. bone:* one of the cranial bones, the forehead. *F. sinus: see* SINUS.

frostbite, injury to the skin or a part from extreme cold. There is redness, swelling and pain and necrosis may result.

frozen shoulder, a chronic condition where the shoulder joint is stiff and painful.

fructose, *(fruk-tōz),* fruit sugar. A monosaccharide found in fruit and vegetables and in honey, which combines with glucose to form sucrose.

FSH, see FOLLICLE-STIMULATING HORMONE.

fugue, (*fūg*), a state of altered consciousness in which the person has no recollection of his actions during this time.

full term or **term,** mature fetus, when the pregnancy has lasted 40 weeks.

fulminant, fulminating, sudden, severe, rapid in course, as in fulminant glaucoma.

fumigation, sterilization of rooms by disinfectant vapour.

functional, pertaining to function. *F. disorder.* malfunction of an organ when organic disease is absent. In psychiatry a mental health problem with a neurotic basis, where organic disease is absent. *F. endoscopic sinus surgery (FESS):* minimally invasive surgery performed on the sinuses via a nasal endoscope. *F. residual capacity (FRC):* volume of air in the lungs after normal expiration.

fundal, pertaining to the fundus of an organ. *F. height:* palpation of the top of the uterus or measuring the distance from the symphysis pubis to the fundus to assess the period of gestation.

fundoplication, surgical folding of the fundus of the stomach to prevent reflux of gastric contents into the oesophagus.

fundus, the enlarged part of an organ furthest removed from the opening. *F. of the eye:* the back of the eye viewed through the pupil with an ophthalmoscope. *F. of the stomach:* at the top of the greater curvature. *F. of the uterus:* the top of the uterus.

fungate, (*fun-gāt*), very rapid growth of fungus-like tumour, seen in the

later stages of some cancers where the growth has involved the skin, e.g. breast.

fungating wounds, may occur when cancer has involved the epithelium and has ulcerated through the skin. Most commonly seen in breast cancer, melanoma, head and neck cancers and cancers involving the vulva, vagina and cervix. They present with pain, exudate, infection causing malodour and haemorrhage, and cause considerable distress. Management includes: specialist wound care and dressings, topical antibiotics and local radiotherapy.

fungi, simple plants. Mycophyta which include mushrooms, yeasts, moulds and rusts. Used in wine making, brewing, baking, pharmaceutical industry and as a food source. Some fungi are pathogenic in humans. See ASPERGILLOSIS, CANDIDIASIS, TINEA.

fungicide, any substance used for the destruction of fungi.

funic, pertaining to the umbilical cord. *F. soufflé:* the blowing sound heard as blood passes through the umbilical vessels.

funiculitis, (*fū-nik-ū-lī'-tis*), inflammation of the spermatic cord.

funnel chest, also called **pectus excavatum.** A developmental deformity in which the sternum is depressed towards the spine.

furuncle, (*fū'-rung-kl*), a boil.

furunculosis, (*fū-run-kū-lō'-sis*), the appearance of one or more boils.

fusiform, (*fū'-zi-form*), spindle-shaped. Can describe a bacillus. See ANEURYSM.

fusion, joining together.

G

GABA, abbreviation for **gamma-aminobutyric acid.**

gag, instrument used to keep the mouth open. *G. reflex*: reflex contraction of the pharyngeal muscles and elevation of the palate when the soft palate or posterior pharynx is touched.

gait, manner of walking.

galactagogue, (*ga-lak'-to-gog*), an agent that causes an increased flow of breast milk.

galactocele, (*ga-lak'-tō-sēl*), a cyst of the breast containing milk.

galactorrhoea, (*ga-lak-to-re'-a*), excessive flow of milk. Usually reserved for abnormal or inappropriate milk secretion.

galactosaemia, (*ga-lak-to-sē'-mē-a*), an inherited autosomal recessive error of metabolism where enzymes required to convert galactose to glucose are absent. High blood levels of galactose cause diarrhoea, failure to thrive, jaundice, cataracts and learning disability.

galactose, a monosaccharide which combines with glucose to form lactose.

galactosuria, (*gal-ak-tos-ūr-i-a*), galactose in the urine.

gall, *see* BILE.

gallbladder, the sac where bile is concentrated and stored; it is attached to the posterior surface of the liver. *See* BILE, BILIARY, CHOLECYSTOKININ.

gallipot, small pot for lotions.

gallows traction, *see* BRYANTS' 'GALLOWS' TRACTION.

gallstone, a calculus in the gallbladder frequently associated with infection; cholecystitis. May be formed from cholesterol, bile pigments or a mixture of these. The stone may move into the ducts giving rise to very severe pain (*see* COLIC) or become impacted in the common bile duct causing obstruction to the flow of bile and jaundice.

galvanometer, instrument used to measure the magnitude of an electric current.

gamete, reproductive cell having the haploid (n) number of chromosomes, an oöcyte or spermatozoon. *G. intrafallopian transfer (GIFT)*: an assisted fertilty/conception technique where female and male gametes are introduced directly into the uterine tube.

gametogenesis, (*gam-et-ō-jen-ē-sis*), formation of gametes in the ovary or testis. *See* OÖGENESIS, SPERMATOGENESIS.

gamma (γ), third letter of the Greek alphabet. *G.-aminobutyric acid (GABA)*: an inhibitory neurotransmitter found in the central nervous system and in other locations. *See* HUNTINGTON'S DISEASE. *G. camera*: a device used in radionuclide imaging. Following the introduction of radioactive isotopes into the body it is able to detect the amount of radioactivity in a specific area. *See* NUCLEAR MEDICINE, RADIONUCLIDE IMAGING. *G. globulins. see* GLOBULINS, IMMUNOGLOBULINS. *G. radiation*: used in diagnostic studies, for treatment and to sterilize items such as plastic syringes. *G. rays*: electromagnetic radiation of extremely short wavelength emitted by certain radioactive isotopes.

gammaglobulinopathy, *(gam-a-glob-ū-lin-op-a-thi)*, an abnormality of gamma globulin.

gamma-glutamyl transferase (γGT), enzyme present in many tissues. Increased levels may indicate liver disease.

ganglion, *(gang-lē-on)*, **1.** a collection of nerve cell bodies in the peripheral nervous system, such as those containing the cell bodies of the autonomic nervous system and the dorsal root ganglia which contain the cell bodies of sensory nerves. **2.** synovial cyst generally connected with a tendon sheath; most common site is on the back of the hand near the wrist.

ganglionectomy, *(gang-lē-ō-nek-to-mi)*, excision of a ganglion.

ganglioside, *(gang-lē-ō-sīd)*, a carbohydrate-rich lipid substance found in the brain. Accumulation may occur in certain inherited disorders. *See* TAY–SACH'S DISEASE.

gangrene, massive tissue necrosis resulting from ischaemia. Causes include: vessel disease, embolus, frostbite, infection, external pressure such as from a tourniquet or trauma. Lower limb gangrene is a complication of diabetes mellitus and is also seen in heavy smokers. *Dry g.*: seen in a limb where the arterial supply is gradually occluded, such as with arterial disease. Infection and oedema are usually absent. *Gas g.*: seen in contused wounds infected with anaerobes such as *Clostridium perfringens*. It is characterized by local swelling, discoloration, foul discharge, gas formation which crack-

les when the tissue is touched and severe systemic effects including circulatory collapse. *Moist/wet g.*: seen in a limb or the bowel when the arterial supply is suddenly occluded, often with impaired venous return. Infection and oedema usually present.

Gardnerella vaginalis, bacterium that causes bacterial vaginosis. There is a grey frothy discharge and a fishy odour. It has been linked to late miscarriage and preterm delivery.

gargoylism, inherited mucopolysaccharide disorder which causes defects in skeletal development, enlarged liver, spleen and heart and learning disability. *See* HUNTER'S SYNDROME, HURLER'S SYNDROME.

gas, matter in a form where it has mobility and no defined shape. *G. chromatography. See* CHROMATOGRAPHY. *G. embolus: see* CAISSON DISEASE, EMBOLUS. *G. gangrene: see* GANGRENE. *G. laws: see* BOYLE'S LAW, CHARLES' LAW, DALTON'S LAW, HENRY'S LAW.

gastrectomy, *(gas-trek-to-mi)*, removal of the stomach. *See* BILLROTH'S GASTRECTOMY.

gastric, pertaining to the stomach. *G. aspiration* or *suction*: the aspiration of stomach contents via a nasogastric tube, may be used to obtain samples for analysis, where the bowel is obstructed and following gastrointestinal surgery. *G.-inhibitory peptide (GIP)*: regulatory peptide hormone which inhibits gastric secretion and stimulates insulin secretion by the pancreas. *G. juice*: fluid produced by the stomach, contains enzymes, hydrochloric acid, mucus and the intrinsic factor. *G. lavage*: washing out the stomach, may be used preoperatively where there are emptying problems, and following some cases of poisoning *G. partitioning*: surgical procedure to reduce gastric capacity, may be used in severe obesity. *G. ulcer*: a type of peptic ulcer where the gastric mucosa is ulcerated. May be acute or chronic. *See* PEPTIC ULCER.

gastrin, a hormone produced by cells in the gastric antrum which acts locally by stimulating further gastric secretion. *See* OXYNTIC CELLS. Abnormal production of gastrin may occur. *See* ZOLLINGER–ELLISON SYNDROME.

gastritis, inflammation of the epithelium lining the stomach.

gastrocele, *(gas'-trō-sēl)*, hernia of the stomach.

gastrocnemius, *(gas-trŏk-nē-me-us)*, a large muscle of the calf of the leg.

gastrocolic, *(gas-trō-ko-lik)*, pertaining to stomach and colon. *G. reflex*: reflex colonic peristalsis occurring as food fills the stomach.

gastroduodenoscopy, *(gas-trō-dū-ō-de-nos'-ko-pi)*, endoscopic examination of the stomach and duodenum.

gastroduodenostomy, *(gas-trō-dū-ō-de-nos'-to-mi)*, operation to establish an anastomosis between the stomach and duodenum.

gastroenteritis, *(gas'-trō-en-ter-ī-tis)*, inflammation of the stomach and intestines.

gastroenterology, *(gas'-trō-en-ter-ol-o-ji)*, the study of disease affecting the gastrointestinal tract.

gastroenterostomy, *(gas'-trō-en-ter-os'-to-mi)*, operation to establish an anastomosis between the stomach and small intestine.

gastrointestinal tract, the alimentary tract/canal including the mouth, oesophagus, stomach, small and large intestine, rectum and anus and the associated structures.

gastrojejunostomy, *(gas-trō-je-jūn-os'-to-mi)*, operation to establish an anastomosis between the stomach and jejunum.

gastro-oesophageal, pertaining to the stomach and oesophagus. *G. reflux*: reflux of gastric acid contents into the oesophagus. *G. sphincter*: physiological sphincter between the oesophagus and the stomach (also called cardiac sphincter).

gastropexy, fixing a displaced stomach to the abdominal wall by surgery.

gastroplasty, an operation to correct a deformity of the stomach.

gastroscopy, endoscopic examination of the stomach using a fibreoptic gastroscope; with this type of instrument various treatments can also be performed, e.g. laser coagulation of bleeding vessels. Usually the oesophagus (oesophagoscopy) and duodenum (duodenoscopy) are examined at the same time.

gastrostomy, an opening into the stomach via the abdominal wall. May be used for feeding in situations where the oesophagus is blocked, e.g. cancer, trauma and following surgery. *See* PERCUTANEOUS ENDOSCOPIC GASTROSTOMY.

gastrotomy, incision into the stomach.

gastrulation, the complex cellular movements in the embryo as those cells destined to become tissues and organs migrate to the inside to form the three primary germ layers. *See* ECTODERM, ENDODERM, MESODERM.

gate control theory, a theory that seeks to explain how the transmission of pain impulses is modulated by gates operating at spinal cord level.

Gaucher's disease, *(gow-cherz)*, very rare inherited disorder of fat metabolism. Results in hepatosplenomegaly, enlarged lymph nodes and bone marrow malfunction.

gauze, open-meshed material used in surgical procedures to dry the operative field and facilitate the procedure.

GCS, abbreviation for **Glasgow coma scale**.

Geiger-Muller counter, machine which detects and registers radioactivity.

gelatin, *(je-lat-in)*, a protein found in various connective tissues, used in capsules and suppositories, culture medium and in food preparation.

gemellus, *(je-mel'-lus)*, two muscles of the buttock.

gender, different from biological sex. The term includes the concept of socially constructed views of feminine and masculine behaviour in individual social groups.

gene, hereditary factors located at a specific place (locus) on a specific chromosome; consisting of DNA they are responsible for the transmission of various characteristics and the precise replication of proteins. The genetic code. *See* DOMINANT, RECESSIVE.

general adaptation syndrome (GAS), proposed by Seyle, a triphasic (three-phase) response of the body to stressors. The three stages are: alarm, resistance/adaptation, exhaustion. *See* STRESSORS.

general sales list, in the UK drugs on sale to the public through a variety of retail outlets, e.g. mild analgesics.

generation, 1. reproduction, the begetting of children. 2. specific group of individuals resulting from a mating.

genetic, pertaining to genetics. Term applied to the inherited characteristics of an individual which are due to genes. *G. code*: information carried on DNA molecules which codes for the precise replication of all cell proteins. *G. counselling*: specialized service available to couples with a history of genetic disease, where the risk of producing affected children may be assessed and discussed.

genetics, study of heredity and its variations.

genital, pertaining to the generative or reproductive structures. *G. stage*: final stage of psychosexual development, commencing during puberty and resulting in adult sexuality. *G. warts*: warts on the genitalia and anal area. They are caused by the human papilloma virus.

genitalia, *(jen-it-ā'-li-a)*, the generative organs. Divided into external and internal structures.

genitourinary, *(jen-it-ō-ū'-rin-a-ri)*, referring to the genital and urinary tracts. *G. medicine (GUM)*: branch of medicine dealing with sexually transmitted infections in specialist GUM clinics.

genome, the complete gene complement of each chromosome of a species.

genotype, *(jen-ō-tīp)*, the genetic make-up of an individual, i.e. the set of alleles inherited by the individual.

genu, the knee. *G. valgum*: knock-knees, where the knees are bent inwards. *G. varum*: bowlegged.

genupectoral position, the knee–chest position – the person rests on knees and chest (Figure 34).

geriatrics, *(je-rē-at-riks)*, the study of disease among the elderly.

German measles, *see* RUBELLA.

34 The genupectoral position

germicide, agent which destroys microorganisms.

gerontology, *(je-ron-tol-o-ji)*, the study of ageing.

Gessel's development charts, *(je-sels)*, charts which show expected motor activity, manipulative skills, adaptive behaviour, language, play and social skills in children at certain ages.

gestaltism, *(ges-talt'-izm)*, a holistic theory of behaviour which concludes that ideas and mental processes are part of the whole and cannot be sub-divided.

gestation, *(jes-tā'-shon)*, pregnancy. *G. sac*: the fetus with its enveloping membranes, decidua, etc. The contents of a pregnant uterus.

gestational age, the age of the fetus or neonate, in weeks, calculated from the first day of its mother's last menstrual period.

Ghon's focus, *(gōns fō-kus)*, *see* PRIMARY FOCUS.

giardiasis, *(gi-ar-dē-ā-sis)*, infestation of the bowel with the protozoon *Giardia intestinalis*. May cause diarrhoea and malabsorption.

gigantism, abnormal growth in height due to an oversecretion of growth hormone prior to ossification of the epiphyses. *See* ACROMEGALY.

Gillick competence, In Gillick *v*. West Norfolk and Wisbech Area Health Authority (1985) 3 all ER 402 the House of Lords ruled that children under 16 can give legally effective consent to medical treatment providing they can demonstrate 'sufficient maturity and intelligence to understand'.

gingiva, the gum.

gingival, *(jin-ji-val)*, pertaining to the gum. *G. hyperplasia*: overgrowth of gum tissue associated with certain drugs, e.g. phenytoin.

gingivectomy, excision of part of the gum.

gingivitis, *(jin-ji-vī-tis)*, inflammation of the gums.

gland, an organ composed of specialized cells which produce substance which are secreted or excreted vi ducts or directly into the blood o lymph. *See* ENDOCRINE, EXOCRINE.

glanders, a bacterial disease of horses mules, etc. which may be transmit ted to humans.

glandular fever, *see* INFECTIOU MONONUCLEOSIS.

glans, bulbous extremity of the peni and clitoris.

Glasgow coma scale (GCS), a stand ardized evaluation technique use to assess changes in the state of con sciousness. Criteria used are: verba response, eye opening and moto response combined with vital signs such as blood pressure, to provide comprehensive neurological assess ment.

glaucoma, *(glaw-kō-ma)*, a conditio where intraocular pressure is raised There are several different type which cause eye pain, loss of visua field, visual disturbances such a halos around lights, nausea and vom iting and eventual blindness if th optic nerve is damaged. Treatmen may be medical or surgical.

glenoid, a socket, a term applied t the cavity in the scapula in whic the head of the humerus articulate at the shoulder joint.

glia, *(glī-a)*, *see* NEUROGLIA, SCHWAN CELLS.

glioma, *(glī-ō-ma)*, tumour, usuall malignant, arising in the neuroglia *See* ASTROCYTOMA.

gliomyoma, *(glī-ō-mī-ō'-ma)*, a tumou composed of nerve and muscle tissue

globin, *(glō-bin)*, a protein, it combine with haem to form the haemoglobi molecule.

globulins, *(glob-ū-lins)*, a group of pro teins widely distributed in the body

Those in the plasma are classified as alpha, beta and gamma; their functions include transport of substances (alpha, beta) and protection against infection (gamma). *See* ANTIBODIES, IMMUNOGLOBULINS.

globus, a globe. *G. hystericus*: a subjective feeling of neurotic origin of a lump in the throat. Can cause difficulty in swallowing. *G. pallidus*: part of the tissue masses comprising the basal nuclei.

glomerular, pertaining to the glomerulus. *G. filtration rate (GFR)*: the rate at which the kidneys (glomeruli) can filter blood. Usually around 120 ml/min.

glomerulonephritis, (*glo-mer-ū-lō-nef-rī-tis*), a group of conditions characterized by inflammation of the renal glomeruli with the presence of antibodies and immune complexes; it may be acute or chronic. May be idiopathic but many cases are associated with other conditions such as streptococcal infections and systemic lupus erythematosus. Progression to chronic renal disease and eventual failure may occur.

glomerulus, (*glo-mer-ū-lus*), knot of capillaries which lie within the invaginated blind end of the renal tubule, together they comprise the nephron.

glossal, relating to the tongue.

glossectomy, surgical removal of the tongue.

glossitis, inflammation of the tongue.

glossodynia, (*glos-ō-di-ni-a*), pain in the tongue.

glossopharyngeal, (*glos-ō-fa-rin-jē-al*), pertaining to the tongue and pharynx. *G. nerves*: the ninth pair of cranial nerves. They innervate the tongue and pharynx and are concerned with taste, salivation, swallowing and gag reflex.

glossoplegia, (*glos-ō-plē'-ji-a*), paralysis of the tongue.

glottis, the aperture between the vocal cords in the larynx.

glucagon, (*gloo-ka-gon*), a hormone produced by the alpha cells of the pancreas. It raises blood glucose levels by stimulating the release of liver glycogen. *Cf.* INSULIN.

glucocorticoids, (*gloo-kō-kaw-ti-koydz*), large group of steroid hormones produced by the adrenal cortex, e.g. cortisol. Essential to life, they are concerned with many metabolic processes, such as gluconeogenesis and stress reactions.

glucogenesis, synthesis of glucose

gluconeogenesis, (*gloo-kō-nē-ō-jen-ē-sis*), the process by which the liver and, to a limited extent, the kidney synthesize glucose from non-carbohydrate sources such as amino acids, glycerol and lactate.

glucose, dextrose. A monosaccharide present in some foods, but produced for cellular energetic needs by the digestion of complex carbohydrates. *G. tolerance test*: serial estimation of blood and urine glucose levels following the administration of a standard dose of glucose. Used in the diagnosis of diabetes mellitus and other conditions. *G-6-phosphate dehydrogenase (G6PD)*: enzyme of the pentose phosphate pathway. Deficiencies occurring in the red blood cell may be inherited. It affects Africans, their descendants elsewhere, and people living in Mediterranean and Middle Eastern areas. People lacking G6PD develop haemolytic anaemia when exposed to certain foods or drugs. *See* FAVISM.

glucuronic acid, (*gloo-ku-rŏn-ik*), carbohydrate derivative used in the liver for the conjugation of bile pigments.

glutamate, glutamic acid, an amino acid.

glutamine, an amino acid.

glutathione, a tripeptide important in maintaining red cell structure and for conjugation in the liver. Liver stores are seriously depleted by paracetamol overdose.

gluteal, pertaining to the buttock.

gluten, a protein constituent of certain cereals: wheat, oats, rye and barley. *G. induced/sensitive enteropathy*: bowel disease caused by a component of gluten. *See* COELIAC DISEASE.

gluteus, *g. maximus, g. medius, g. minimus* – the three large muscles of the buttock.

glycaemic index, classification of foods according to their acute effect on blood glucose level.

glycerin, colourless liquid used as an emollient and in suppositories and mouthwashes.

glycerol, a sugar alcohol which combines with fatty acids to form phospholipids and triglycerides (triacylglycerols).

glycine, an amino acid.

glycogen, *(glī-kō-jen),* storage carbohydrate, a polysaccharide formed from many glucose units. It is stored in the liver and skeletal muscles by a process called glycogenesis. The conversion of liver glycogen back to glucose is termed glycogenolysis. *See* GLYCOGENESIS, GLYCOGENOLYSIS. *G. storage diseases*: a group of inherited disorders where enzyme deficiencies lead to the accumulation of glycogen in organs and tissues.

glycogenesis, *(glī-kō-jen-ē-sis),* the conversion of glucose (in excess of immediate needs) to glycogen for storage. It is stimulated by insulin.

glycogenolysis, *(glī-kō-jen-ol'-i-sis),* reconversion of liver glycogen to glucose, a process stimulated by glucagon and adrenaline (epinephrine).

glycolysis, *(glī-kol-i-sis),* a metabolic pathway consisting of a series of reversible reactions where glucose is broken down to produce pyruvic acid and small amounts of energy (ATP).

glycoprotein, *(glī-kō),* a protein conjugated with a carbohydrate, e.g. collagen.

glycoside, *(glī-kō-sīd),* complex substance containing a sugar found in some plants. May contain pharmacologically active substances, such as digitalis from foxgloves.

glycosuria, *(glī-kō-sū-ri-a),* presence of glucose in the urine. May indicate a low renal threshold for glucose, diabetes mellitus, or occur after a high carbohydrate meal.

glycosylated haemoglobin (HbA₁), *(glī-kō-sil-ā-ted),* haemoglobin plus glucose, the amount reflects blood sugar levels over a period of some months and can be used to assess the degree of control in diabetes mellitus.

gnathic, *(nath-ik),* relating to the jaw or cheek.

goal setting, establishment of desired outcomes, such as for nursing interventions or treatment.

goblet cells, mucus-secreting cells situated in the mucosal lining of the respiratory and gastrointestinal tracts (Figure 35).

goitre, *(goy-ter),* thyroid enlargement. Types include: *simple g.*: may occur during puberty and pregnancy. It is also associated with a lack of iodine

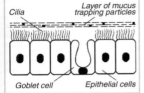

35 A goblet cell in the respiratory tract

Cilia

Layer of mucus trapping particles

Goblet cell   Epithelial cells

in the diet. In regions where this occurs frequently it is termed endemic goitre. In the UK it was previously common in Derbyshire hence the term 'Derbyshire neck'. *toxic g.*: where there is oversecretion of thyroid hormones *See* HYPERTHYROIDISM. Enlargement may be due to cysts benign and malignant growths, or result from infection or autoimmune disorder. *See* HASHIMOTO'S DISEASE.

gold (Au), metallic element used as a treatment for rheumatoid arthritis. Its radioactive isotope ^{198}Au is used in certain malignant diseases.

Golgi organs, specialized receptors in tendons and muscle spindles which provide information about body position. *See* PROPRIOCEPTION.

Golgi region (body) or complex, cell organelle consisting of a network of membranes within the cytoplasm. Involved in the synthesis of glycoproteins and lipoproteins. They are larger and more extensive in secretory cells.

gomphiasis, *(gom-fi-a-sis),* looseness of teeth.

gomphosis, *(gom-fō-sis),* a type of fibrous joint where very slight movement is possible, e.g. teeth in their sockets.

gonad, *(gō-nad),* the primary reproductive structure, ovary (female) and testis (male).

gonadotrophic, *(gon-ad-ō-tro-fik),* stimulating or influencing the gonads.

gonadotrophins, hormones which stimulate the gonads – follicle-stimulating hormone (FSH) and luteinizing hormone (LH). *See* CHORIONIC GONADOTROPHIN.

goniometer, instrument used to measure angles or the range of movement at a joint.

gonioscopy, *(gon-ē-os'-ko-pi),* an examination of the angle of the anterior chamber of the eye using a gonioscope.

goniotomy, incision into the canal of Schlemm for glaucoma.

Gonococcus, *(go-nō-kok-us),* Neisseria gonorrhoeae. The Gram-negative diplococcus causing gonorrhoea.

gonorrhoea, *(go-no-re-a),* a sexually transmitted infection caused by gonococcus. It is notifiable and classified legally as venereal. An acute inflammation affecting the genital tract, urinary tract and the mucosa of the throat and anus. Usual sites are the cervix and urethra in females and the urethra in males. It presents with dysuria and discharge but it may be asymptomatic in females, and may lead to sterility if the uterine tubes or epididymis become involved. Rare systemic effects include arthritis and septicaemia. Non-sexual spread may occur, e.g. an infant's eyes infected during birth (*see* OPHTHALMIA NEONATORUM), and vulvovaginitis in prepubertal girls.

Goodpasture's syndrome, haemorrhagic lung disease associated with glomerulonephritis.

gouge, a grooved instrument of steel used to scoop out dead bone.

gout, group of metabolic disorders where serum uric acid levels are elevated. It may be due to abnormal purine metabolism or increased intake, increased uric acid production and reduced renal excretion of uric acid. Urate crystals are deposited within joints leading to swelling and pain.

Graafian follicle, the mature ovarian follicle. It contains fluid and an oöcyte which is released when it ruptures at ovulation. One primordial ovarian follicle per menstrual cycle will develop into a g. follicle under the influence of gonadotrophic hormones. *See* CORPUS LUTEUM.

grading, a method of classifying a cancer based on certain histopathological characteristics, such as amount of abnormal cells compared with normal cells in the tissue. *See* STAGING.

graft, transplanted living tissue, e.g. skin, bone, bone marrow, cornea and organs such as kidney, heart, lungs, pancreas and liver. They may be autografts when tissue is moved from one site to another; isografts between genetically identical individuals; allografts (homografts) where tissue is obtained from a suitable donor or xenografts (heterografts) between different species. *G.-versus-host (GvHD) disease:* may follow a successful transplant, especially bone marrow, where the graft 'attacks' the tissues of the immunologically compromised host causing rashes, liver problems and diarrhoea.

gram (g), a unit of mass. 1000th part of a kilogram.

Gram's stain, a bacteriological stain for the identification and classification of some bacteria. They may be either Gram-positive (staining violet) or Gram-negative (staining pink).

grand mal, *see* EPILEPSY.

granular, composed of grains; having granules or granulations.

granulation, the growth of fibroblasts and blood vessels in wounds healing by secondary intention, such as pressure ulcers and leg ulcers. It occurs during the proliferative phase of wound healing. *G. tissue:* the new, soft tissue formed by the process of granulation.

granule, small particle or grain.

granulocytes, *(gran-ū-lō-sītz),* cells containing granules in their cytoplasm, such as polymorphonuclear leucocytes.

granulocytopenia, *(gran-ū-lō-sī-to-pe'-ne-a),* decrease in the number of granulocytes in the blood.

granuloma, tumour of granulation tissue.

graphics, in computing any output (screen display or printout) which includes pictures made up of small dots or pixels.

grasp reflex, primitive reflex normally present in neonates – when the sole or palm is stroked the digits flex.

Graves' disease, *see* HYPERTHYROIDISM.

gravid, pregnant.

gravitational ulcer, *see* VENOUS ULCER.

gravity, weight. *See* SPECIFIC GRAVITY.

Grawitz tumour, *see* HYPERNEPHROMA.

gray (Gy), derived SI unit of absorbed dose of radiation, replaced the rad.

greenstick fracture, *see* FRACTURE.

grey matter, nerve cell bodies and unmyelinated nerve fibres within the central nervous system. *See* WHITE MATTER.

Grey Turner's sign, discoloration of the skin of the loin in acute pancreatitis.

grief, normal emotional and physical responses to bereavement or loss.

Griffith's typing, a subdivision of *Streptococcus pyogenes* (Lancefield group A) which uses differences in their antigenic structure.

grounded theory, research where the hypothesis is derived from the data obtained.

group, people or objects which form a well-defined unit, e.g. control g. in research or a family g.

group C meningococcal disease, serious infection caused by *Neisseria meningitidis* of the serological group C. It causes meningococcal meningitis and life-threatening septicaemia in children and young adults. Effective immunization is available and is included in the routine programme.

growth, increase in size. *G. hormone (GH)*: a protein hormone with widespread effects on body tissues. Its secretion, by the anterior pituitary, is regulated by two hypothalamic hormones: growth hormone-releasing hormone (GHRH) and growth hormone-inhibiting hormone (GHIH) or somatostatin. GH stimulates growth of bone etc., and influences the metabolism of proteins, fats and carbohydrates.

guaiac test, *(gwi-ak),* a test for faecal occult blood.

guanine, *(gwa-nēn),* a nitrogenous base derived from purine. A component of the nucleic acids DNA and RNA. *See* NUCLEIC ACIDS, DNA, RNA.

Guillain–Barré syndrome, *(gwē-ān-ba-re),* acute demyelinating peripheral polyneuropathy which may follow a viral or bacterial infection, or immunization. It results in pain, weakness, paralysis and possibly respiratory problems.

guillotine, an instrument for excising the tonsils.

guinea worm, a genus of nematode worm which may infest humans. *See* DRACONTIASIS.

gullet, the oesophagus.

gumma, localized granuloma with fibrosis, necrosis and ulceration which develops in the later (tertiary) stages of syphilis. They may affect any organ and have a characteristic 'punched out' appearance.

gustatory, pertaining to taste.

gut, the intestine.

Guthrie test, a screening blood test used in the diagnosis of phenylketonuria (PKU).

gynaecoid pelvis, *(gī-ne-koyd),* the normal female pelvis, with shallow cavity and round brim, it is suited to childbearing.

gynaecology, *(gī-ne-kol-o-ji),* the science dealing with disorders of the female genital tract.

gynaecomastia, *(gī-ne-ko-mas'-tē-a),* enlargement of the male breast.

gypsum, *(jip-sum),* calcium sulphate (plaster of Paris).

gyrus *(pl.* **gyri),** *(ji-rus),* a convolution, such as the convolutions of the brain.

H

H₂-receptor antagonists, agents that selectively block the H_2 histamine receptors that normally stimulate gastric secretion and thereby decrease the secretion of gastric juice, e.g. ranitidine. They are used in the management of peptic ulcer, hyperacidity and gastro-oesophageal reflux, and in the prophylaxis of gastrointestinal ulceration and bleeding in critically ill patients.

habilitation, usually applied to the process by which individuals with learning disabilities, mental health problems or physical disabilities are equipped to achieve maximum levels of independence with the activities of daily living.

habit, 1. constant and often involuntary action established by frequent repetition. **2.** regular and repeated use of addictive substances.

habituation, 1. the process by which a person becomes used to his or her environment and repeated stimuli. **2.** psychological dependence on a substance, e.g. drugs. *See* ADDICTION.

haem, iron-containing pigment of haemoglobin.

haemangioma, *(hē-man-jē-ō-ma)*, a malformation of blood vessel, e.g. naevi and portwine stain birthmarks.

haemarthrosis, *(hē-mar-thrō'-sis),* effusion of blood into a joint cavity.

haematemesis, *(hē-ma-te-mē-sis),* vomiting blood. It may be bright red or dark brown with the appearance of 'coffee grounds'. Bleeding is usually gastrointestinal and causes include: peptic ulcer, varices, neoplasms, drug erosions and coagulation defects, but blood swallowed from elsewhere may also be vomited.

haematin, *(hē-ma-tin),* a ferric iron derivative of haemoglobin. Produced during haemolysis, such as in malaria.

haematinic, *(hē-ma-tin'-ik),* a substance required for the production of red blood cells and constituents, e.g. iron.

haematocele, *(hē-ma-to-sēl),* a swelling containing extravasated blood, such as around a testis or in the pelvis.

haematocolpos, *(hē-ma-to-kol-pos),* collection of menstrual blood in the vagina due to an imperforate hymen or septum. *See* CRYPTOMENORRHOEA.

haematocrit, *(hē-mat-o-krit),* see PACKED CELL VOLUME.

haematology, *(hē-ma-tol'-o-ji),* the science of the blood.

haematoma, *(hē-ma-tō'-ma),* a collection of clotted blood, such as an extradural or subdural h.

haematometra, *(hē-ma-to-me'-tra),* accumulation of blood in the uterus.

haematomyelia, *(hē-ma-tō-mī-e-li-a),* haemorrhage into the spinal cord.

haematoporphyrins, *(hē-ma-to-paw-fi-rinz),* see PORPHYRINS.

haematosalpinx, *(hē-ma-to-sal-pinks),* collection of blood within the uterine tube.

haematozoa, *(hē-ma-to-zō'-a),* parasites in the blood stream.

haematuria, (*hē-ma-tū-ri-a*), blood in the urine. It may be gross; bright red, dark red or smoky in appearance or may only be detected by testing or microscopy. Causes include: tumours, calculi, infection, trauma and coagulation defects.

haemochromatosis, (*hē-mō-krō-ma-tō-sis*), condition caused by excess iron in the body. Iron is deposited in organs such as the liver and pancreas, and in the skin causing bronze pigmentation. Causes include: defect of iron metabolism or high intake, excessive haemolysis and frequent blood transfusion.

haemoconcentration, concentration of the blood. An increase in the proportion of red cells relative to the amount of plasma.

haemocytoblast, (*hē-mō-sī-to-blast*), primitive stem cell found in the marrow which gives rise to all blood cells.

haemocytometer, (*hē-mō-sī-tom-et-er*), device used to count blood cells in a sample.

haemodiafiltration, a form of renal replacement therapy similar to haemofiltration, but with the addition of dialysate fluid, thus allowing diffusion to occur, which enhances the removal of molecules.

haemodialysis, (*hē-mō-dī-al-i-sis*), removal of waste products, electrolytes, other toxic substances and excess water from the body by dialysis, which is achieved by putting the selectively permeable membrane between the blood and a rising solution (dialysate) within a dialyse (artificial kidney). Used in the management of end-stage renal failure, acute renal failure or after poisoning, such as drugs overdose. *see* HAEMODIAFILTRATION, HAEMOFILTRATION, PERITONEAL DIALYSIS.

haemodilution, dilution of the blood. A decrease in the proportion of red cells relative to the amount of plasma.

haemofiltration, a continuous form of renal replacement therapy similar to haemodialysis, but utilizing ultrafiltration to remove molecules.

haemoglobin (Hb), (*hē-mo-glō-bin*), red iron-containing pigment – protein complex contained in red blood cells. A molecule has four haem groups containing ferrous iron and four globin chains. Several forms exist: fetal type (HbF) and two major forms of adult haemoglobin (HbA, HbA$_2$). It carries oxygen, some carbon dioxide and buffers pH changes. *See* GLYCOSYLATED HAEMOGLOBIN.

haemoglobinometer, (*hē-mo-glō-bin-om'-e-ter*), an instrument for estimating the amount of haemoglobin in the blood.

haemoglobinopathies, (*hē-mo-glō-bin-o'-pa-thez*), inherited disorders of haemoglobin structure. *See* SICKLE CELL DISEASE, THALASSAEMIA.

haemoglobinuria, (*hē-mo-glob-in-ū'-ri-a*), haemoglobin in the urine.

haemolysin, (*hē-mol'-i-sin*), agent causing the breakdown of the red cell membrane.

haemolysis, (*hē-mol-i-sis*), disruption of red blood cells. *See* HAEMOLYTIC.

haemolytic, (*hē-mo-lit'-ik*), pertaining to haemolysis or the power to disrupt red blood cells. Causes include: red cell defects, infections, antibodies, incompatible transfusion, drugs, chemicals and hypersplenism. *H. anaemia*: due to excessive breakdown of red cells, may be accompanied by mild jaundice. *H. disease of the newborn*: haemolysis, usually due to rhesus or rarely ABO incompatibility, causes jaundice, anaemia and hyperbilirubinaemia which may damage the brain. *See* ANTI-D, BLOOD GROUPS, EXCHANGE TRANSFUSION, KERNICTERUS.

haemolytic uraemic syndrome (HUS), potentially fatal intravascular haemolysis and acute renal failure occurring secondary to another condition such as food poisoning with enterohaemorrhagic *Escherichia coli* type 0157. Those affected may need renal replacement therapy.

haemoperfusion, technique where blood is perfused through an absorbent substance, such as charcoal, to remove poisons and metabolites. Used in cases of poisoning and liver and kidney failure.

haemopericardium, *(hē-mō-per-ē-kar-dē-um),* blood in the pericardial sac.

haemoperitoneum, *(hē-mō-per-ē-ton-ē-um),* blood in the peritoneal cavity.

haemophillas, *(hē-mō-fil-i-a),* a group of inherited blood coagulation defects. Either factor VIII is deficient to cause haemophilia A or factor IX to cause haemophilia B (Christmas disease). Both are recessive sex-linked conditions carried by females and affecting 50% of their male offspring.

Haemophilus, *(hē-mō-fil-us),* a genus of bacteria. Gram-negative rods *H. ducreyi:* causes chancroid. *H. influenzae type B:* causes respiratory tract infection and a type of meningitis against which the Hib vaccine is offered.

haemophobia, fear of blood.

haemopneumothorax, the presence of blood and air in the pleural cavity.

haemopoiesis, *(hē-mō-poy-ē-sis),* the formation of blood cells.

haemoptysis, *(hē-mop´-ti-sis),* coughing up blood or blood-stained mucus from the respiratory tract. Causes include: cancer, infection and pulmonary infarction, left heart failure coagulation defects and anticoagulant drugs.

haemorrhage, *(hem-or-aj),* loss of blood from the vessels, usually refers to rapid and considerable loss. It is classified in a variety of ways. **1.** by type of vessel – arterial, venous or capillary. **2.** by the time since surgery or injury – *primary,* at the time of surgery or injury; *reactionary,* within 24 hours as blood pressure rises; or *secondary,* around 7–10 days after the event, associated with sepsis. **3.** haemorrhage may be external (revealed) or internal (concealed). is also named for the site of bleeding, e.g. subarachnoid haemorrhage. *Severe h.:* leads to hypovolaemic shock characterized by tachycardia, hypotension, pallor, sweating, restlessness, air hunger, oliguria and eventual loss of consciousness.

haemorrhagic disease of the newborn, *(he-mo-ra´-jik),* lack of vitamin K causing a deficiency of clotting factors in neonates. There is an increased risk of intracranial and gastrointestinal haemorrhage.

haemorrhoidectomy, *(hem-o-royd-ek´to-mi),* surgical removal of haemorrhoids.

haemorrhoids, *(hem-o-roydz),* piles. Enlarged anal veins which may prolapse or become thrombosed. These can be associated with colon malignancy or serious liver disease.

haemosiderin, *(hē-mō-sid-er-in),* an iron storage complex stored in the liver and spleen.

haemosiderosis, *(hē-mō-sid-er-ō´-sis),* an accumulation of haemosiderin and iron in organs and tissue. Associated with excessive red cell breakdown.

haemostasis, *(hē-mō-s'tā-sis),* **1.** stasis of blood flow. **2.** physiological process by which bleeding from small vessels is controlled. It involves four overlapping stages: vasoconstriction, platelet plug formation, coagulation and fibrinolysis. Also describes the measures to prevent or control haemorrhage.

haemostatic, (hē-mō-sta′-tik), an agent used to arrest a flow of blood.

haemothorax, (hē-mō-tho′-raks), collection of blood in the pleural cavity.

Hageman factor, factor XII in coagulation (clotting).

hair follicle, a structure derived from skin, it contains a hair which consists of keratinized cells.

halal, describes meat obtained from animals killed according to Islamic law.

half-life ($t \frac{1}{2}$), **1.** time taken for a radioactive isotope to decay to half its original activity. A constant for each isotope, e.g. ^{131}iodine = 8 days. **2.** time taken for plasma levels of a drug to fall to half the initial level.

halitosis, (ha-li-tō-sis), foul breath.

hallucination, (hal-lū-si-nā-shon), a false perception occurring without any true sensory stimulus. A common symptom in severe psychoses, including schizophrenia. cf. DELUSION.

hallucinogenic, pertaining to hallucinogens.

hallucinogens, (hal-lū-si-nō-jens), an agent or drug such as LSD which causes hallucinations.

hallux, great toe. H. valgus: lateral displacement of the great toe. Associated with a bunion.

halo, circle of light such as that seen around lights by people with glaucoma. Or a ring splint which encircles the head.

halogens, (hal-ō-jens), non-metallic elements including fluorine, chlorine, bromine and iodine.

halopelvic traction, a means of applying traction to the spine, between two fixed points.

hamate, a carpal or wrist bone.

hammer toe, permanent dorsal flexion of the first phalanx and plantar flexion of the second and third phalanges.

hamstrings, three flexor muscles of the posterior thigh.

hand-arm vibration syndrome (HAVS), occupational hazard of certain machine or tool operators. Effects include vascular blanching and neurological numbness and tingling.

hand, foot and mouth disease, infectious disease of children. It is caused by a coxsackie virus and characterized by vesicles on hands, feet and mouth.

haploid, having a set of unpaired chromosomes in the nucleus, seen in the gametes following meiosis. See DIPLOID.

hapten, incomplete antigens. Small molecules, such as peptides, which combine with a body protein to become antigenic. Alone they cause no immunological response.

haptoglobin, an alpha globulin which combines with free haemoglobin in the plasma.

hardware, a computer and its associated peripherals such as monitor, printer and modem.

Hardy–Weinberg equilibrium equation, in genetics the relationship between gene frequency and genotypes occurring in a given population.

harelip, see CLEFT LIP.

Hartmann's solution, sodium lactate and chloride, potassium chloride and calcium chloride solution for infusion.

Hartnap disease, an inborn error in the metabolism of neutral amino acids such as tryptophan from which nicotinamide is synthesized. This results in a condition similar to pellagra with skin and neurological problems.

Hashimoto's thyroiditis, an autoimmune condition affecting the thyroid. Antithyroid antibodies are produced in response to antigens and the gland is infiltrated by immune cells such as lymphocytes. It causes goitre with or without hypothyroidism.

hashish or **hash,** *see* CANNABIS.

Hassal's corpuscles, small bodies of the thymus.

haustrations, sacculations of the colon.

HAV, abbreviation for **hepatitis A virus.**

haversian system, the basic unit of bone tissue (also known as an osteon).

hay fever, allergic rhinitis caused by exposure of sensitized respiratory mucosa and conjunctiva to various antigens, such as pollen.

HBV, abbreviation for **hepatitis B virus.**

HCV, abbreviation for **hepatitis C virus.**

HDL, abbreviation for **high-density lipoprotein.** *See* LIPOPROTEIN.

HDV, abbreviation for **hepatitis D virus.**

headache, pain in the head. Causes include: tension, migraine, intracranial disorders and diseases of the sinuses and eyes.

Heaf test, a multiple puncture test with tuberculin, used pre-BCG and in the diagnosis of tuberculosis.

healing, a procedure that cures. The repair of damaged tissue. *See* FIRST INTENTION, GRANULATION.

health, generally understood to identify a state to which we all aspire. Commonly defined as the absence of disease or illness, the opposite to being sick. This is negative and a more positive definition is that of

the World Health Organization in 1948: 'a state of complete physical, mental and social well-being.'

health and safety legislation, the law, common law and statute covering health and safety duties. Health and Safety and Welfare at Work Act 1974 sets out the responsibilities of the employer in relation to the workforce, work environment, equipment and substances, and those of individual employees to themselves and others.

Health Authority, a body that administers the NHS at local level. Recent changes have resulted in fewer, many of which have common boundaries with local government authorities, e.g. Norfolk Health Authority covers the whole county of Norfolk.

Health Board, in Scotland, the equivalent of a Health Authority.

health care system, the way in which a government organizes the finance and administration of its healthcare policies.

Health Development Agency, a statutory body set up to improve standards in public health. It is concerned with the need for evidence and commissioning research. Other roles include: standard setting, health promotion campaigns and distributing examples of good practice.

health education, aims to help people to make and sustain healthy actions and equip them with the skills to exercise choice.

health improvement programme (HImP), a focused action plan aimed at improving health and healthcare at a local level. The lead organization is the Health Authority, in collaboration with Primary Care Trusts, health professionals, local government and other groups with an interest.

health promotion, an inclusive term used to describe any measure aimed at health improvement in individuals, communities or the population as a whole.

health visitor, a nurse with a specialist qualification in health visiting who is concerned with preventive care, mainly with the under 5s, school-aged children, mothers and older people.

hearing, audition, the ability to perceive sound. *H. loss. see* DEAFNESS. *H. test: see* AUDIOMETRY, RINNE'S TEST, WEBER'S TEST.

heart, a hollow muscular organ which pumps blood around the general and pulmonary circulations. Situated in the mediastinum behind the sternum, it is about the size of the owner's fist. It is divided into a right and left side by a septum and has four chambers: two small upper receiving chambers

– the atria – and two large lower pumping chambers – the ventricles. The heart has three layers: the outer serous pericardium, a middle of cardiac muscle (myocardium) and a lining (endocardium). Valves control blood flow between the atria and ventricles – tricuspid on the right and bicuspid on the left – and semilunar valves prevent backflow from aorta and pulmonary artery (Figure 36). As these valves close during the cardiac cycle, they produce the heart sounds 'lubb dupp'. *H. failure. see* CARDIAC FAILURE. *H. murmur. see* CARDIAC MURMUR. *See* CARDIAC, CIRCULATION.

heart block, a partial or complete block to the passage of impulses through the conducting system. May require cardiac pacing. *See* PACEMAKER.

36 The heart

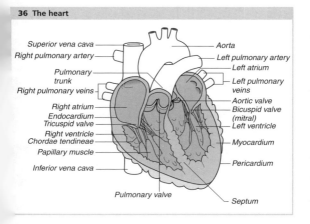

Superior vena cava
Right pulmonary artery
Pulmonary trunk
Right pulmonary veins
Right atrium
Endocardium
Tricuspid valve
Right ventricle
Chordae tendineae
Papillary muscle
Inferior vena cava
Pulmonary valve

Aorta
Left pulmonary artery
Left atrium
Left pulmonary veins
Aortic valve
Bicuspid valve (mitral)
Left ventricle
Myocardium
Pericardium
Septum

heartburn, burning sensation at the lower end of the oesophagus, due to reflux of acidic gastric contents.

heart lung machine, see CARDIOPULMONARY BYPASS.

heat, 1. a form of energy. **2.** to increase temperature. *H. exhaustion*: caused by extreme heat. Considerable loss of water and electrolytes through sweating causes headache, cramp, nausea, tachycardia, cold clammy skin and hypotension. *H. stroke*: hyperpyrexia with cessation of sweating which develops in conditions of high temperature and humidity. A life-threatening condition which may follow h. exhaustion.

hebephrenia, a form of schizophrenia sometimes found in young adults.

Heberden's nodes, small bony swellings forming over the terminal phalangeal joints in many types of arthritis.

hedonism, excessive devotion to pleasure.

Hegar's sign, spongy feel of the cervix in early pregnancy.

Heimlich manoeuvre, *(hēm-lik)*, abdominal thrusts. Emergency technique for removing a foreign body in the larynx. Achieved by a forceful compression of the upper abdomen.

Helicobacter pylori, bacterium that causes gastric inflammation. The presence of bacteria is associated with gastritis, peptic ulceration and possibly gastric cancer. It is transmitted by the oral–faecal and oral–oral routes and many people are asymptomatic carriers.

helium, inert gas used medically to dilute other gases and in pulmonary function tests.

helix, spiral. Used to describe the configuration of certain molecules, e.g. DNA, and also the outer rim of the external ear.

Heller's operation, cardiomyotomy. Used to relieve difficulty in swallowing caused by achalasia.

helminthiasis, *(hel-min-thī-a-sis)*, infestation with parasitic worms.

helminthology, study of parasitic worms.

hemeralopia, *(hem-er-al-ō'pi-a)*, day blindness, poor vision in bright light which improves in dim light.

hemianopia, *(hem-i-an-ō'-pi-a)*, loss of sight in half of the visual field of one or both eyes.

hemiatrophy, *(hem-i-at'-ro-fi)*, atrophy of one side of the body only.

hemiballismus, violent, involuntary jerky movements on one side of the body.

hemicolectomy, *(hem-i-ko-lek'-tō-mi)*, surgical removal of half colon.

hemicrania, *(hem-i-kra-ni-a)*, headache on one side of the head. Migraine.

hemiparesis, *(hem-i-par-rē-sis)*, weakness or slight paralysis on one side of the body.

hemiplegia, *(hem-i-plē'-ji-a)*, paralysis of one side the body. The lesion is in the opposite side of the brain.

hemispheres, *(hem'-i-sfērs)*, half spheres. *Cerebral h.*: the two sides of the cerebrum.

Henderson–Hasselbach equation, the equation that explains how the ratio between the concentration of a weak acid and an alkali will influence the pH, e.g. of the blood.

blood pH = 6.1 +

$$\log \frac{[hydrogen\ carbonate]}{[carbon\ dioxide\ in\ solution]}$$

Henle's loop, part of the renal tubule, important in the production of urine of variable concentration.

Henoch–Schönlein purpura, anaphylactoid purpura, small-vessel vasculitis mainly affecting children. A hypersensitivity disorder which may follow streptococcal respiratory tract infections. Immune complexes may damage capillaries, joints, gut and kidney, resulting in a purpuric rash, abdominal pain, rectal bleeding, joint involvement and glomerulonephritis, nephrotic syndrome and acute renal failure.

Henry's law, states that the amount of gas dissolving in a fluid is proportional to its partial pressure and solubility at a constant temperature.

hepadnaviruses, a family of DNA viruses that include the hepatitis B virus.

hepar, the liver.

heparin, anticoagulant formed in the liver. Used therapeutically in thromboembolic conditions.

hepatectomy, *(hep-a-tek´-to-mi),* partial or total removal of the liver.

hepatic, *(he-pat´-ik),* pertaining to the liver. *H. ducts:* two bile ducts which carry bile from the liver. *H. encephalopathy:* brain disease associated with the severe metabolic distrubances of liver failure. *H. flexure:* 90° angle formed by the colon under the liver. *H. portal circulation:* that of venous blood from the gastrointestinal tract, pancreas and spleen to the liver before returning to the heart. *H. portal vein:* conveys blood to the liver. It is formed by the union of the superior mesenteric and splenic veins.

hepaticostomy, *(he-pat-i-kos´-to-mi),* an opening into the hepatic duct.

hepatitis, *(hep-a-tī-tis),* inflammation of the liver. Causes include: alcohol, drugs, chemicals, several viruses (A, B, C, D, E, F and G) and other microorganisms and metabolic disorders such as Wilson's disease. The effects may range from a mild illness caused by the hepatitis A virus (HAV) to cirrhosis and hepatic failure following alcohol misuse and viruses such as hepatitis B (HBV). *See* AUSTRALIA ANTIGEN.

hepatocellular, *(hep-at-ō-sel-ū-lar),* pertaining to liver cells.

hepatocyte, *(hep-at-ō-sīt),* parenchymal or functional liver cell.

hepatoma, *(hep-at-ō-ma),* primary neoplasm of the liver.

hepatomegaly, *(hep-a-tō-meg-a-li),* an enlarged liver.

hepatopancreatic, *(hep-at-ō-pan-krē-ik),* pertaining to the liver and pancreas. *H. ampulla: see* VATER'S AMPULLA.

hepatorenal syndrome, *(hep-at-ō-rē-nal),* renal failure resulting from cirrhosis and hepatic failure.

hepatosplenomegaly, enlarged liver and spleen.

herbalism, the therapeutic use of herbs or mineral remedies.

hereditary, *(he-red´-i-ta-ri),* inherited; capable of being inherited.

heredity, *(he-red´-i-ta-ri),* transmission of genetic characteristics and traits.

Hering–Breuer reflex, stretch reflex that prevents lung overinflation.

hermaphrodite, a person who has both ovarian and testicular tissue. Associated with an ambiguity of secondary sexual characteristics.

hernia, rupture. Protrusion of an organ through a defect in the structures which normally support and enclose; commonly it is the protrusion of the abdominal contents through a defect in the abdominal muscles. Types include: inguinal, femoral, umbilical, diaphragmatic (*see* HIATUS HERNIA), incisional. Rarely at other sites, e.g. cerebral. A hernia may be reducible by manipulation or irreducible when it cannot be returned to the correct position. If the blood supply becomes impaired the hernia is said to be strangulated; this leads to necrosis, gangrene and acute intestinal obstruction.

hernioplasty, operation for hernia when the weak structures are repaired.

herniorrhaphy, operation to repair a hernia.

herniotomy, operation for a hernia where the hernia sac is removed and the protruding structures are returned to a normal position.

heroin, diamorphine. It is addictive and subject to considerable criminal misuse. *See* CONTROLLED DRUG, MISUSE OF DRUGS.

herpes, *(her-pēz)* infection caused by herpesvirus. *H. simplex (HSV-1)*: causes skin ulceration usually around the mouth. *H. genitalis (HSV-2)*: a related virus which infects the genitalia, it produces genital lesions, dysuria and systemic illness. Spread is usually through sexual contact, but infants born to infected women may be affected. The presence of HSV-2 correlates with cervical cancer, but the link remains unproven. *H. zoster*: caused by varicella zoster virus, which also causes chickenpox. Affects the sensory nerves causing pain and skin eruption along the course of the nerve (shingles).

herpesviruses, group of viruses which include: herpes simplex virus (HSV) type 1 and 2, varicella zoster virus (VZV), Epstein–Barr virus, human herpesvirus 6 (HHV6) and cytomegalovirus (CMV).

hertz (Hz), derived SI unit of frequency.

heterogeneous, *(het-er-ō-jē-ne-us)*, differing in kind or in nature.

heterograft, xenograft. *See* GRAFT.

heterologous, *(het-er-ol-o-gus)*, derived from a different species.

heteroplasty, in plastic surgery when the graft is taken from another person and not from another part of the patient's body.

heterosexual, attracted to a person of the opposite gender.

heterotropia, *(het-er-ō-trō'-pi-a)*, squint.

heterozygous, *(het-er-ō-zī-gus)*, having different alleles or genes at the same locus on both chromosomes of a pair

(one of maternal and the other paternal origin).

HEV, abbreviation for **hepatitis E virus.**

hexose, a six carbon monosaccharide, e.g. glucose.

hiatus, *(hī-ā-tus)*, an opening or space. *H hernia*: hernia of the stomach through the diaphragm at the oesophageal opening.

Hib vaccine, vaccine used to immunize against *Haemophilus influenzae* type B. Offered to infants at 2, 3 and 4 months by injection.

hiccup, hiccough, repeated spasmodic inspiration associated with sudden closure of the glottis and contraction of the diaphragm.

Hickman line, a type of central line catheter commonly used to deliver chemotherapy or total parenteral nutrition.

hydrosis, *(hī-drō'-sis)*, sweating.

high dependency unit (HDU), a unit providing specialist monitoring and care to patients who require more care than is available on general wards, but who do not need intensive care.

hilar, relating to the hilum.

hilum, the point at which structures enter and leave an organ, e.g. blood and lymphatic vessels, nerves and ducts.

HImP, abbreviation for **Health Improvement Programme.**

hindbrain, *see* RHOMBENCEPHALON.

hip, upper part of thigh where it joins the pelvis. *H. joint*: ball and socket joint between the head of the femur and the acetabulum. *H. replacement*: *see* ARTHROPLASTY. *See also* DEVELOPMENTAL DYSPLASIA OF THE HIP.

hippocampus, *(hip-pō-kam'-pus)*, part of the brain involved in limbic system function.

Hippocrates, *(hip-pok'-ra-tēz)*, Greek physician who lived around 400 BC, the 'father of medicine'.

Hirschsprung's disease, congenital megacolon. Defective innervation to the terminal colon causes hypertrophy, massive dilatation and obstruction.

hirsute, hairy.

hirsutism, excessive hair growth.

Hirudo, leech.

His, bundle of, *see* ATRIOVENTRICULAR BUNDLE.

histamine, an amine released in a variety of tissues where it causes smooth muscle constriction, gastric secretion and vasodilation. Its release from mast cells as part of the inflammatory response leads to capillary dilatation and increased vessel permeability.

histidine, an essential amino acid during childhood.

histiocyte, *(his-ti-ō-sīt)* macrophage. Phagocytic tissue cells involved in the inflammatory process.

histocompatibility antigens, genetically determined antigens present on the cell surface. They are responsible for the immune response which results in transplant rejection. The presence of certain antigens also increases the susceptibility to specific diseases, e.g. insulin-dependent diabetes, rheumatoid arthritis. *See* HUMAN LEUCOCYTE ANTIGEN, MAJOR HISTOCOMPATIBILITY COMPLEX.

histiocytosis X, rare disorder of the monocyte–macrophage system in which there is an abnormal increase in histiocytes and a local inflammatory reaction. Types include: Hand–Schüller–Christian disease and Letterer–Siwe disease.

histogram, a bar chart. Graphical representation of variables plotted against frequency or time.

histology, the morphological study of tissues.

histolysis, *(his-to-li-sis)* disintegration of organic tissue.

histones, proteins associated with chromosomal DNA.

histoplasmosis, infection caused by the fungus *Histoplasma capsulatum.*

HIV, abbreviation for **human immunodeficiency virus,** *see* ACQUIRED IMMUNE DEFICIENCY SYNDROME, ARC.

hives, urticaria.

HLA, abbreviation for **human leucocyte antigens.**

Hodge's pessary, *see* PESSARY.

Hodgkin's disease, *see* LYMPHOMA.

holandric inheritance, expression of a trait transmitted by a gene carried on the Y chromosome.

holistic, relating to the theory of holism. This considers that individuals function as a whole rather than as separate parts or systems.

Homan's sign, physical sign of deep vein thrombosis in the leg. Pain is felt in the calf when toes are dorsiflexed.

homeostasis, *(hō-mē-ō-stā-sis),* body equilibrium. The autoregulatory processes that maintain a stable internal body environment. Controls functions such as blood pressure, temperature and electrolytes, which are maintained within set parameters.

homeothermic, an animal able to maintain a constant body temperature regardless of environmental temperatures.

homicide, the act of killing a person. Manslaughter (culpable homicide in Scotland) if accidental, murder if intentional.

homocysteine, an intermediate which reacts with serine to form cysteine. Also involved in reactions requiring folates and cobalamins. A deficiency in folates is associated with increased homocysteine levels in the blood and an increased risk of coronary heart disease.

homoeopathy, a branch of medicine based on the theory of 'like cures like'. Treatment involves the use of small doses of substances capable of producing symptoms similar to those of the disease.

homogeneous, (hō-mō-jē'-ne-us), of the same kind. Uniform.

homogenized, term applied to a substance which has a uniform consistency throughout.

homograft, allograft, see GRAFT.

homolateral, relating to the same side.

homologous, (hō-mol-ŏ-gus), of the same type. Identical in structure.

homosexual, attracted to a person of the same gender.

homozygous, (hō-mō-zī'-gus), having identical genes or alleles in the same locus on both chromosomes of a pair (one of maternal and the other of paternal origin).

hookworm, see ANCYLOSTOMA.

hoop traction, fixed skin traction used for fractures of the femur in children, and in the management of developmental dysplasia of the hip.

hordeolum, (hor-dē-ō-lum), a stye on the eyelid.

hormone, a chemical substance which affects the functioning of structures distant from its source, e.g. thyroxine. See ENDOCRINE. Some hormones have a local influence on structures in which they are produced, e.g. gastrin. *H. replacement therapy (HRT):* the replacement of any deficient hormone, but generally applied to the oestrogen hormones (usually with progestogens) administered to reduce the effects of the climacteric.

Horner's syndrome, unilateral constriction of the pupil, ptosis and vasodilation of the face with absence of sweating. Due to paralysis of the cervical sympathetic fibres caused by apical bronchial tumours and brain stem lesions.

horseshoe kidney, a congenital abnormality where the two kidneys are united, usually at the lower pole.

Horton's syndrome, release of histamine in the body causing severe headache.

hospice, system of care given to the chronically or terminally ill person and family. It is designed specially for the purpose of family-centred care and may involve care at home, in a day unit and in the actual hospice (terminal care unit) premises.

hospital-acquired infection (HAI), new infection occurring in a patient who has been in hospital more than 48 hours. Around 10% of patients develop such infections. They include: urinary tract, skin, respiratory and wound infections.

host, organism on which a parasite lives.

hourglass contracture, caused by a constriction in the middle of an organ. Occurs in the stomach and uterus.

housemaid's knee, inflammation of prepatellar bursa, caused by kneeling.

HPV, abbreviation for **human papilloma viruses**

HSV, abbreviation for **herpes simplex virus.**

HTLV, abbreviation for **human T-cell lymphotrophic viruses.**

human chorionic gonadotrophin (hCG), (kor-i-on-ik go-na'-dō-trō-fin), see CHORIONIC GONADOTROPHIN.

human immunodeficiency viruses (HIV), retroviruses. Currently designates the AIDS virus. These are two types: HIV-1 and HIV-2. See ACQUIRED IMMUNODEFICIENCY SYNDROME.

human leucocyte antigens (HLA), major histocompatibility complexes, so called because they were first described on leucocytes.

human papillomavirus (HPV), a wart virus associated with the development of genital warts and cervical malignancy. *See* CERVICAL INTRAEPITHELIAL NEOPLASIA.

human T-cell lymphotrophic viruses (HTLV), retroviruses. There are two types: HTLV-1 and HTLV-2, both of which are associated with some forms of leukaemia.

humanism, a philosophy based on human values, needs, interests and rational problem solving. Frequently seen as an underlying theme in nursing models.

humerus, the bone of the upper arm.

humidifier, appliance which adds moisture to room air or to gases being administered to a patient.

humidity, moisture. The amount of moisture in the atmosphere.

humoral immunity, that part of the immune response initiated by B lymphocytes and antibodies.

humor, a body fluid other than blood. *See* AQUEOUS HUMOR, VITREOUS HUMOR.

Hunter's syndrome, an inherited mucopolysaccharidosis. *See* GARGOYLISM.

Huntington's disease, an inherited disorder which usually appears in adult life (30s and 40s). It is characterized by choreiform movements, dementia and eventual death. It is associated with destruction of the basal nuclei and a lack of the neurotransmitter GABA.

Hurler's syndrome, an inherited mucopolysaccharidosis. *See* GARGOYLISM.

HUS, abbreviation for **haemolytic uraemic syndrome**.

Hutchinson's teeth, abnormality of the permanent teeth. Seen in congenital syphilis.

hyaline, (*hī'-a-lin*), transparent, glasslike. *H. cartilage*: smooth cartilage covering the articular surfaces of bones. *H. membrane disease*: see

NEONATAL RESPIRATORY DISTRESS SYNDROME, SURFACTANTS.

hyalitis, (*hī-al-ī-tis*), inflammation of the vitreous humour or the hyaloid membrane of the eye.

hyaloid membrane, (*hī'-a-loyd*), membrane enclosing the vitreous humour.

hyaluronic acid, a mucopolysaccharide which acts as an intercellular 'cement'. A constituent of synovial fluid.

hyaluronidase, (*hī-al-yur-on-i-dāz*), an enzyme present in spermatozoa that allows penetration of the oöcyte. Used medically to aid the absorption of drugs or fluids administered by the intramuscular or subcutaneous route.

hybrid, (*hī-brid*), offspring resulting from gametes which are genetically unlike.

hydatid cyst, (*hī-dat-id*), cysts occurring in the liver, lungs and brain, caused by the tapeworm *Echinococcus granulosus* which infests dogs. The larval stage takes place in sheep and cattle.

hydatidiform mole, (*hī-dat-id-i-form*), a condition characterized by the abnormal development of the chorionic villi which form grape-like vesicles within the uterus and the secretion of high levels of human chorionic gonadotrophin. May become malignant. *See* CHORIOCARCINOMA.

hydramnios, (*hī-dram'-nē-os*), excess of amniotic fluid.

hydrarthrosis, (*hī-drar-thrō-sis*), accumulation of watery fluid within a joint cavity.

hydrate, 1. a chemical compound formed from the addition of water. **2.** to add or take up water.

hydroa, (*hī-drō-a*), a skin condition characterized by vesicles or bullae.

hydrocarbon, (*hī-drō-kar'-bon*), a compound formed of hydrogen and carbon.

159

hydrocele, (hī-drō-sēl), swelling containing clear fluid. Most often applied to that occurring in tunica vaginalis of the testis.

hydrocephalus, (hī-drō-kef-a-lus), obstruction to the circulation of cerebrospinal fluid resulting in an accumulation of fluid around the brain, 'water on the brain'. It may be: **1.** congenital when it is often associated with spina bifida, or **2.** acquired following infection, trauma or tumours. Treatment is usually based on diverting the excess fluid back to the circulation via various types of shunt. *See* SPITZ–HOLTER VALVE.

hydrochloric acid, an acid formed from hydrogen and chlorine. The acid produced by the parietal (oxyntic) cells of the stomach.

hydrocolloid dressings, absorbent dressings available in sheets or shaped for use on heels or the sacral area. They reduce pain, rehydrate wounds, encourage autolytic debridement and can be used at all phases of wound healing, and on wounds with low to moderate exudate.

hydrocortisone, (hī-drō-kaw'-ti-zōn), cortisol. A steroid hormone produced by the adrenal cortex. Therapeutic uses include: replacement in adrenal insufficiency and the suppression of inflammatory and allergic conditions. *See* GLUCO-CORTICOIDS.

hydrogel dressings, sheets or gels (for cavities) used to rehydrate necrotic tissue, reduce pain. They can be used at all phases of healing in dehydrated wounds or those with moderate exudate.

hydrogen (H), a gaseous element. A constituent of all organic compounds. *H. ion concentration* (pH): a measure of acidity (concentration of hydrogen ions) or alkalinity (concentration of hydroxyl ions) of a solution. The pH is measured on logarithmic scale (0–14) and represents the indices of the concentration rather than the actual number of hydrogen ions. A pH below 7 is acid having an excess of hydrogen ions, 7 is neutral and a pH above 7 is alkaline having an excess of hydroxyl ions. *H. peroxide*: an oxidizing agent, used in suitable dilution as a mouth wash.

hydrogenation, (hī-droj-ēn-ā'-shon), addition of hydrogen to substance. *See* REDUCTION.

hydrolysis, (hī-drol'-i-sis), breakdown of complex substance(s) with the addition of water to give simpler substances.

hydrometer, (hī-drom'-e-ter), an instrument for determining the specific gravity of liquids.

hydronephrosis, (hī-drō-nef-rō'-sis), collection of urine in the renal pelvis and calyces due to an obstruction to the flow of urine. Causes include: calculi, tumours and prostatic hypertrophy. Unrelieved it causes renal damage.

hydropericardium, (hī-drō-pe-ri-kar'-dē-um), fluid in the pericardial sac, i.e. pericardial effusion.

hydroperitoneum, (hī-drō-pe-ri-tō-nē'-um), peritoneal effusion, i.e. ascites.

hydrophilic, (hī-drō-fi-lik), having an affinity for water.

hydrophobia, (hī-drō-fō'-bē-a), an aversion to water. *See* RABIES.

hydropneumothorax, (hī-drō-nū'-mō-thor-aks), fluid and air in the pleural cavity.

hydrops, (hī-drops), oedema. *H. fetalis*: generalized oedema associated with severe haemolytic anaemia in the fetus or newborn due to rhesus incompatibility. Severe form of haemolytic disease of the newborn.

hydrorrhachis, (hī-dror'-a-kis), abnormal accumulation of cerebrospinal fluid in the spinal canal.

hydrosalpinx, (hī-drō-sal'-pinks), distension of the uterine tube by clear fluid.

hydrostatic pressure, that pressure exerted by fluids on the walls of their container, e.g. blood on the vessel walls.

hydrotherapy, treatment of disease using water, such as exercises in water.

hydrothorax, fluid in the pleural cavity.

hydroxyapatites, (hī-drok-si-ap'-at-ites), see APATITES.

hydroxybutyric acid, (hī-drok-si-bū-ti-rik), a ketone formed from the incomplete oxidation of fatty acids.

5-hydroxyindoleacetic acid (5-HIAA), (hī-drok-si-in-dol-as-et-ik), a breakdown product of 5-hydroxytryptamine. High levels in the urine confirm the diagnosis of carcinoid tumour.

hydroxyl, (hī-drok-sīl), OH. Chemical group with one oxygen and one hydrogen atom. See pH.

4-hydroxy, 3-methoxymandelic acid (HMMA), (hī-drok-si,meth-ok-si-man-del-ik), see VANILLYLMANDELIC ACID (VMA).

5-hydroxytryptamine (5-HT), (hī-drok-si-trip'-ta-mēn), serotonin. A monoamine neurotransmitter. Also present in high concentration in platelets and the gastrointestinal tract.

hygiene, the science of the maintenance of health by promoting cleanliness.

hygrometer, an instrument for measuring the moisture in the atmosphere.

hygroscopic, having the property of absorbing moisture, e.g. glycerin.

hymen, a normally perforated membrane at the vaginal entrance.

hymenotomy, (hī-men-ot'-o-mi), incision of the hymen.

hyoid, (hī-oyd), shaped like a V; the name of a bone at the root of the tongue.

hypalgesia, (hī-pal-jē'-zi-a), diminished sensitivity to pain impulses.

hypamnios, (hī-pam-ne-os), less amniotic fluid than normal.

hyperacidity, abnormal concentration of acid. See HYPERCHLORHYDRIA.

hyperactivity, overactivity.

hyperaemia, (hī-per-ē-mi-a), excess blood in a part, it may be active or passive.

hyperaesthesia, (hī-per-es-thē-zi-a), excessive sensitivity to touch and other sensations.

hyperalgesia, (hī-per-al-jē'-zi-a), excessive sensibility to pain.

hyperalimentation, an excess of nutrients. Usually refers to total parenteral nutrition. See ENTERAL NUTRITION, TOTAL PARENTERAL NUTRITION.

hyperbaric, term applied to a gas at greater pressure than normal, e.g.h. oxygen chamber.

hyperbilirubinaemia, (hī-per-bi-li-rū-bi-nē-mi-a), elevated levels of bilirubin in the blood.

hypercalcaemia, (hī-per-kal-sē-mi-a), an increase in the serum calcium levels.

hypercalciuria, (hī-per-kal-sē-ū-ri-a), increased excretion of calcium in the urine.

hypercapnia, (hī-per-kap'-ni-a), raised CO_2 tension in the blood (arterial); $Pa\ CO_2$.

hypercatabolism, excessive breakdown of body proteins. Seen in situations where there are increased nutritional requirements, e.g. major trauma, burns and sepsis.

hyperchloraemia, (hī-per-klor-ī-mi-a), excess chloride in the blood.

hyperchlorhydria, (hī-per-klor-hī-dri-a), excess of hydrochloric acid in the gastric juice.

hypercholesterolaemia, (hī-per-ko-les-ter-ol-ē-mi-a), excess cholesterol in the blood.

hyperchromia, (hī-per-krō-mi-a), excessively coloured.

hyperemesis, (hī-per-em'-e-sis), excessive vomiting. *H. gravidarum*: of pregnancy.

hyperextension, overextension, e.g. of a joint.

hyperflexion, overflexion.

hypergammaglobulinaemia, (hī-per-gam-a-glob-ū-lin-ē'-mi-a), excess gammaglobulins in the blood.

hyperglycaemia, (hī-per-glī-sē-mi-a), abnormally high levels of glucose in the blood; seen in diabetes mellitus. *See* HYPEROSMOLAR DIABETIC COMA, KETOACIDOSIS.

hyperhidrosis, (hī-per-hī-drō-sis), excess of perspiration.

hyperimmune, high levels of antibodies.

hyperinsulinism, high levels of insulin, may be intrinsic or extrinsic.

hyperkalaemia, (hī-per-ka-lē-mi-a), elevated levels of potassium in the blood. Very high levels cause arrhythmias and cardiac arrest.

hyperkeratosis, (hī-per-ke-ra-tō-sis), excess growth of the horny layer of the skin.

hyperkinesis, (hī-per-kī-nē-sis), excessive movement.

hyperlipidaemia, (hī-per-lip-i-dē-mi-a), high levels of lipids (fats) in the blood. May be due to an inherited disorder or secondary to dietary intake of saturated fats and diseases such as diabetes.

hypermagnesaemia, excess magnesium in the blood.

hypermetropia, (hī-per-me-trō-pē-a), long sight, a visual defect (Figure 37). Opposite to myopia.

hypermnesia, an exaggerated memory involving minute detail.

37 Hypermetropia (long sight) and its correction

Hypermetropia long sight

Corrected

Biconvex lens

hypermotility, increased smooth muscle activity, e.g. peristalsis.

hypermyotonia, (hī-per-mī-ō-tō-ni-a), increase in muscle tone.

hypernatraemia, (hī-per-na-trē-mi-a), excessive levels of sodium in the blood.

hypernephroma, (hī-per-ne-frō'-ma), malignant tumour of kidney, also called **Grawitz's tumour**.

hyperonychia, (hī-per-ō-ni-ki-a), thickening of the nails.

hyperosmolar, (hī-per-os-mō-la), higher than normal osmolarity (osmotic pressure). *H. coma*: seen in diabetes mellitus, it is characterized by hyperglycaemia and dehydration without ketoacidosis.

hyperostosis, (hī-per-os-tō'-sis), overgrowth of bone tissue.

hyperparathyroidism, excessive secretion from the parathyroid glands due to adenoma, hyperplasia or hypertropy.

hyperphagia, (hī-per-fā-ji-a), eating to excess.

hyperphasia, talking excessively.

hyperphoria, (hī-per-fo-ri-a), elevation of one visual axis above the other.

hyperphosphataemia, (hī-per-fos-fa-tē'-mi-a), high levels of phosphates in the blood.

hyperpituitarism, (hī-per-pit-ū-it-ar-izm), excessive secretion from the anterior lobe of the pituitary gland. See ACROMEGALY, CUSHING'S DISEASE/SYNDROME, GIGANTISM, HYPERPROLACTNAEMIA.

hyperplasia, (hī-per-pla-zē-a), an increase in the number of cells, such as bone marrow hyperplasia in some types of anaemia, or prostatic hyperplasia cells; c.f. HYPERTROPHY.

hyperpnoea, (hī-per-pnē-a), increased depth and rate of respiration.

hyperprolactinaemia, (hī-per-prō-lak-tin-ē-mi-a), high levels of prolactin in the blood. Normal in lactating women, but may be due to pituitary tumours and some drugs.

hyperpyrexia, (hī-per-pī-rek'-sē-a), very high body temperature, usually above 40–41°C. Malignant h.: inherited condition which presents in response to certain drugs used during general anaesthesia and neuroleptic drugs; the temperature rises progressively and, if untreated, may be fatal.

hyperreflexia, an abnormally exaggerated tendon reflex.

hypersensitive, abnormally sensitive, e.g. to certain foodstuffs.

hypersensitivity, abnormally intense reactions to an allergen or other stimulus. H. reactions: may be classified by the timing and whether it involves antibodies or is cell-mediated: (a) antibody-mediated type I reaction (anaphylaxis) occurs when IgE binds to an allergen such as pollen. (b) antibody-mediated type II reaction (cytotoxic) involves IgG or IgM. An example would be the agglutination of donated red cells

occurring after a mismatched blood transfusion. (c) antibody-mediated type III reaction (immune complex) involves antibodies and complement activation, such as in extrinsic allergic alveolitis or the Arthus reaction. (d) cell-mediated type IV reaction which occurs 24–48 hours after exposure to the antigen. Examples include chronic skin inflammation caused by exposure to nickel, cosmetics and plants, such as poison ivy. It is also seen in the local reaction to skin testing with tuberculin. (e) mixed antibody/cell-mediated type V reaction involving antibodies, T lymphocytes and phagocytes, such as may be seen in some autoimmune diseases.

hypersplenism, overactivity of the enlarged spleen, especially haemolytic activity.

hypertension, a blood pressure sustained above the accepted normal level for age. It may be essential, when no cause can be found, or secondary to conditions such as coarctation of the aorta, renal disease and endocrine problems. See PORTAL HYPERTENSION, PULMONARY HYPERTENSION.

hyperthermia, raised body temperature.

hyperthyroidism, (hī-per-thī-royd-izm), oversecretion of the thyroid hormones T_3 and T_4. Also called thyrotoxicosis. Results in an increased metabolic rate with tachycardia, raised temperature, heat intolerance, weight loss with good appetite, diarrhoea, tremor and anxiety. Eye signs may be present, e.g. lid lag and exophthalmos and some people have a goitre. Graves' disease is an autoimmune hyperthyroidism where antibodies stimulate thyroid activity; it is accompanied by lid lag and exophthalmos.

hypertonia, excessive tonicity, as in a muscle or an artery.

hypertonic, high tone. 1. increased tone of muscle. 2. having a higher osmotic pressure in relation to the fluid with which it is being compared. *See* HYPOTONIC, ISOTONIC.

hypertrichosis, (*hī-per-tri-kō'-sis*), excessive growth of hair, or growth of hair in unusual places.

hypertrophy, increase in tissue size due to individual cells enlarging; *cf.* HYPERPLASIA.

hyperuricaemia, (*hī-per-ū-ri-sē'-mi-a*), high levels of uric acid in the blood. *See* GOUT.

hyperventilation, overbreathing.

hypervitaminosis, (*hī-per-vi-ta-min-ō-sis*), abnormally high levels of vitamins, especially the fat-soluble vitamins A and D.

hyphaema, (*hī-fē-ma*), bleeding into the anterior chamber of the eye.

hypnagogic hallucination, occurs in the stage between being awake and asleep.

hypnosis, condition resembling sleep in which the conscious control of behaviour is reduced and the person responds more easily to suggestion. Used in pain relief, relaxation and in psychotherapy.

hypnotic, 1. relating to hypnotism. 2. drug producing sleep, e.g. temazepam.

hypnotism, practice of hypnosis.

hypoacidity, reduced acidity. *See* HYPOCHLORHYDRIA.

hypoaesthesia, (*hī-pō-ēs-thē-zi-a*), diminished sense of feeling in a part.

hypoalbuminaemia, (*hī-pō-al-bū-min-ē'-mi-a*), low levels of albumin in the blood.

hypobaric, gas at a lower than normal pressure.

hypocalcaemia, (*hī-pō-kal-sē-mi-a*), decrease in serum calcium levels. *See* TETANY.

hypocalciuria, (*hī-pō-kal-sē-ū'-ri-a*), decreased levels of calcium in the urine.

hypocapnia, (*hī-pō-kap-ni-a*), reduced CO_2 tension in arterial blood; Pa CO_2. Can be caused by hyperventilation.

hypochloraemia, (*hī-pō-klor-ē'-mi-a*), low levels of chloride in the blood.

hypochlorhydria, (*hī-pō-klor-hī'-dri-a*), deficiency of hydrochloric acid in the gastric juice.

hypochlorite, (*hī-pō-klor-īt*), a salt of hypochlorous acid. Sodium hypochlorite used as a disinfectant.

hypochondria, (*hī-pō-kon'-dri-a*), excessive anxiety about one's health. Common in anxiety states and depression.

hypochondrium, (*hī-pō-kon-dri-um*), abdominal region situated under the ribs, right and left lateral areas either side of the epigastrium. *See* ABDOMEN.

hypochromic, (*hī-pō-krō'-mik*), decreased colour or pigmentation.

hypodermic, (*hī-pō-der'-mik*), below the skin; subcutaneous.

hypofibrinogenaemia, (*hī-pō-fi-brin-ō-je-nē-mi-a*), *see* AFIBRINOGENAEMIA.

hypogammaglobulinaemia, (*hī-pō-gam-a-glob-ū-lin-ē-mi-a*), *see* AGAMMA-GLOBULINAEMIA.

hypogastric, (*hī-pō-gas'-trik*), pertaining to the hypogastrium.

hypogastrium, (*hī-pō-gas'-tri-um*), central abdominal region below the umbilicus. *See* ABDOMEN.

hypoglossal, (*hī-pō-glos-sal*), under the tongue. *H. nerves:* twelfth pair of cranial nerves; they innervate the tongue movements required for moving food, swallowing and speaking.

hypoglycaemia, (*hī-pō-glī-sē-mi-a*), abnormally low level of glucose in the blood. May happen in diabetes mellitus when the person has too much insulin, misses a meal or exercises strenuously, but can occur in non-diabetics.

hypoglycaemic drugs, (hī-pō-glī-sē'-mĭk), oral drugs that reduce blood glucose levels in some types of diabetes mellitus. They include: sulphonylureas, e.g. glipizide; biguanides, e.g. metformin; alpha-glucosidase inhibitors, e.g. acarbose. Rosiglitazone may be used in conjunction with other hypoglycaemics where blood sugar control is difficult in people with type 2 diabetes.

hypogonadism, (hī-pō-gō-nad-izm), undersecretion of testes or ovaries.

hypokalaemia, (hī-pō-ka-lē-mi-a), low level of potassium in the blood. Leads to muscle weakness, arrhythmias and cardiac arrest.

hypokinesis, diminished movement.

hypomania, milder form of the affective disorder mania, in which there is abnormal elation of mood and great energy.

hypomotility, decreased movement.

hypomyotonia, (hī-pō-mī-ō-to'-ni-a), decrease in muscle tone.

hyponatraemia, (hī-pō-na-trē-mi-a), low level of sodium in the blood.

hypoparathyroidism, (hī-pō-pa-ra-thī-royd-izm), undersecretion of the parathyroid glands. Causes include damage to the glands during thyroid surgery. See HYPOCALCAEMIA, TETANY.

hypophoria, (hī-pō-for-ē-a), depression of one visual axis below the other.

hypophosphataemia, (hī-pō-fos-fa-tē'-mi-a), low levels of phosphates in the blood.

hypophysectomy, (hī-pof-i-sek-to-mi), operation to remove the pituitary gland.

hypophysis, (hī-pof-i-sis), outgrowth. H. cerebri: pituitary gland.

hypopituitarism, (hī-pō-pi-tū-i-tar-izm), undersecretion of the pituitary

hormones, especially of the anterior lobe. There is a general reduction in the functioning of the gonads, adrenal glands, thyroid gland and lack of growth hormone.

hypoplasia, failure of organs to grow to full size.

hypoproteinaemia, (hī-pō-prō-ti-nē-mi-a), reduced amounts of the serum proteins.

hypopyon, (hī-pō'-pi-on), pus in the anterior chamber of the eye.

hyporeflexia, diminished reflexes.

hyposecretion, too little secretion.

hyposensitivity, diminished response to a stimulus.

hyposmia, diminished sense of smell.

hypospadias, (hī-pō-spa'-dē-as), a malformation in which the urethra opens on to the ventral surface of the penis, or in the perineum.

hypostasis, (hī-pō-stā-sis), deposit, passive congestion.

hypostatic, pertaining to hypostasis. H. pneumonia: associated with lung congestion and immobility.

hypotension, abnormally low blood pressure. Postural h.: temporary low blood pressure experienced when standing up suddenly.

hypotensive drug, a drug which reduces high blood pressure, e.g. captopril.

hypothalamus, (hī-pō-thal-a-mus), an area of grey matter at the base of the brain which has links with other parts of the nervous system and pituitary gland. Its many functions include: production of factors/hormones which control anterior pituitary hormone secretion; neurosecretory production of ADH and oxytocin; control of temperature, appetite, thirst, sleep, and emotions such as rage.

hypothenar eminence, prominence on the palm below the little finger.

hypothermia, a core body temperature below 35°C. Accidental hypothermia with very low temperatures is seen in older people, associated with hypothyroidism, babies and individuals inappropriately prepared for severe climatic conditions. Hypothermia may be artificially induced to reduce the metabolic rate and hence oxygen demands, e.g. during cardiac surgery.

hypothesis, a statement that can be tested by a statistical test (inferential). It is a prediction based on the relationship between the dependent and independent variables.

hypothetico-deductive method, theories are considered and hypotheses for testing are derived in a deductive manner. The research study tests the hypotheses by data analysis that either supports or rejects the original theory.

hypothyroidism, *(hī-pō-thī-royd-izm),* undersecretion of the thyroid hormones T_3 and T_4. Also called **myxoedema.** Results in decreased metabolic rate with bradycardia, low temperature and cold intolerance, weight gain, constipation, thin hair, skin changes, facial swelling and slow speech. *Congenital h.:* can be detected by blood testing soon after birth and treated successfully with thyroxine. Untreated it leads to impaired mental and physical development with a failure to achieve normal milestones. It is characterized by coarse facies and protruding tongue. Previously known as cretinism.

hypotonia, deficient muscle tone.

hypotonic, 1. lacking in tone. **2.** having a lower osmotic pressure than the fluid to which it is being compared. *See* HYPERTONIC, ISOTONIC.

hypoventilation, decreased ventilation of the lungs.

hypovitaminosis, *(hī-pō-vi-ta-min-ō'-sis),* a lack of vitamins in the body due to deficient intake or a failure in absorption.

hypovolaemia, *(hī-pō-vo-lē-mi-a),* a severe reduction in the volume of circulating blood which results in shock. Causes include haemorrhage and loss of other body fluids, or increased vessel permeability due to sepsis or anaphylaxis.

hypoxaemia, *(hī-pok-sē-mi-a),* lack of oxygen in the blood.

hypoxia, *(hī-pok-si-a),* insufficient tissue oxygenation or poor utilization of oxygen. May be anaemic, hypoxic, histotoxic or stagnant.

hysterectomy, *(his-ter-ek-to-mi),* removal of the uterus. *Subtotal h.:* removal of the body of the uterus. *Total h.:* removal of the body and cervix. *Vaginal h.:* removal of the uterus via the vagina. *See* WERTHEIM'S OPERATION.

hysteria, previously used to describe conversion disorder. Describes the loss of emotional control characterized by laughing, crying and intense activity.

hysterical, relating to hysteria.

hysteromyomectomy, *(his-ter-ō-mī-ō-mek'-to-mi),* surgical removal of a uterine fibroid.

hysterosalpingectomy, *(his-ter-ō-sal-pin-gek'-to-mi),* surgical removal of the uterus and uterine tube(s).

hysterosalpingography, *(his-ter-ō-sal-pin-gog'-ra-fi),* radiographic examination of the uterus and tubes following the instillation of radiopaque contrast medium.

hysterosalpingostomy, *(his-ter-ō-sal-pin-gos'-to-mi),* an anastomosis between the uterus and uterine tube.

hysteroscopy, endoscopic examination of the uterine cavity. It provides a direct view and the opportunity to biopsy abnormal areas.

hysterotomy, *(his-ter-ot'-o-mi)*, incision into the uterus. The term usually excludes caesarean section.

hysterotrachelorrhaphy, *(his-ter-ō-trak-el-or'-a-fi)*, repair of a lacerated cervix uteri.

I

IAA, abbreviation for **indispensable amino acid**.

iatrogenic, (*i-at′-rō-jen-ĭk*), a condition or disease caused by medical or surgical intervention, e.g. drug side-effects.

IBD, abbreviation for **inflammatory bowel disease**.

IBS, abbreviation for **irritable bowel syndrome**.

ICD, abbreviation for **International Classification of Diseases**.

ice, water at or below 0°C (freezing point). *Dry i.:* carbon dioxide snow, used in some skin conditions. Also an acronym for ice, compress and elevation. Used in the treatment of bruises and swelling of limbs.

ichthyosis, (*ik-thi-ō′-sis*), inherited defect of keratinization in which the skin is dry and scaly. The so-called acquired i. is similar in appearance but due to defective nutrition.

ICSH, abbreviation for **interstitial cell stimulating hormone**.

icterus, jaundice. *I. gravis neonatorum:* see HAEMOLYTIC DISEASE OF THE NEWBORN.

id, unconscious part of the mind, containing the primitive, instinctive urges.

IDDM, abbreviation for **insulin dependent diabetes mellitus**.

ideation, process concerned with the highest function of awareness, the formation of ideas. Memory and intellect.

identical twins, uniovular. Twins of the same gender which develop from a single zygote. They are genetically identical. *See* MONOZYGOTIC.

identification, 1. recognition. **2.** an emotional attachment to an individual resulting in the transposition of behaviour characteristics, values and beliefs, role modelling. Also a mental defence mechanism where people adopt the characteristics of the admired role model figure.

identity, a concept of self image; existing as a unique personality separate from other people.

ideomotor, (*id-ē-ō-mō′-tor*), association of spontaneous movement with an idea.

idiopathic, without apparent cause.

idiosyncrasy, (*id-ē-ō-sin-kra-si*), individual character or property. It may relate to an unusual response to a particular food or drug.

IHD, abbreviation for **ischaemic heart disease**.

ileal, (*il-ē-al*), referring to the ileum. *I. conduit/bladder:* an operation where the ureters are anastomosed to an isolated portion of ileum; this is brought out on to the surface of the abdomen where it discharges urine into a bag. Also known as ileoureterostomy.

ileitis, (*il-ē-I-tis*), inflammation of the ileum. Regional ileitis. *See* CROHN'S DISEASE.

ileocaecal, (*il-ē-ō-sē′-kal*), pertaining to the ileum and caecum. *I. valve:* sphincter valve between the ileum (small bowel) and caecum (large bowel).

ileocolitis, *(il-ē-ō-ko-lī'-tis),* inflammation of the ileum and colon.

ileocolostomy, *(il-ē-ō-ko-los'-to-mi),* surgical anastomosis between the ileum and the colon.

ileoproctostomy, *(il-ē-ō-prok-tos-to-mi),* surgical anastomosis between ileum and rectum.

ileorectal, pertaining to the ileum and the rectum.

ileosigmoidostomy, *(il-ē-ō-sig-moy-dos'-to-mi),* surgical anastomosis between ileum and sigmoid colon.

ileostomy, *(il-ē-os-to-mi),* the ileum is brought out on to the surface of the abdomen as a stoma where it discharges faecal material into a bag. It may be performed to bypass the large bowel or where a colectomy has been necessary.

ileoureterostomy, *see* ILEAL CONDUIT/ BLADDER.

ileum, *(il-ē-um),* last part of the small intestine. Important for the absorption of vitamin B_{12} and other substances.

ileus, *(il-ē-us),* obstruction of the intestine. Usually applied to paralytic ileus rather than a mechanical obstruction. Causes include: peritonitis, following bowel surgery, spinal injuries, and hypokalaemia. Peristalsis ceases, there is stasis of intestinal contents, toxin absorption, vomiting, distension, pain and constipation. *Meconium i.:* seen in newborns, it is associated with cystic fibrosis.

iliac, pertaining to the ilium. *I. arteries:* supply blood to the pelvis and legs. *I. crest:* highest part of the ilium. *I. region:* abdominal region situated near the iliac bones, right and left lateral areas either side of the hypogastrium. *See* ABDOMEN. *I. veins:* drain venous blood from the legs and pelvis.

iliococcygeal, *(il-ē-ō-kok-si-jē-al),* pertaining to the ilium and coccyx.

iliofemoral, *(il-ē-ō-fem-or-al),* pertaining to the ilium and femur.

iliopectineal, pertaining to the ilium and pubis. *I. line:* bony ridge which marks the division between the false pelvis and true pelvis.

iliopsoas, *(il-ē-ō-sō-as),* the psoas and iliacus muscles.

ilium, *(il'-i-um),* the upper part of the innominate bone.

illness, disease or disorder causing a health deficiency which adversely affects the physical, mental or social functioning of an individual.

illusion, a deceptive appearance. The misinterpretation of a sensory image.

image, 1. a mental picture. **2.** the optical reproduction of an object formed on the retina as light is focused through the eye. **3.** an accurate reproduction of an object or person.

IM&T, abbreviation for **information management and technology**.

imagery, vivid mental pictures, imagination. *Guided i.* is used as a pain/symptom relief strategy.

imaging techniques, the diagnostic techniques used to investigate the state and functioning of body structures, e.g. radiography, radionuclide scans, ultrasonography, computed tomography, magnetic resonance and positron emission tomography.

imago, *(i-mah-gō),* in psychology a fantasy concerning a person from childhood, usually a parent.

imbalance, lack of balance, e.g. electrolytes and water balance.

immobility, state of being fixed; movement not possible.

immune, having immunity. Protected against a particular disease. *I. complexes:* antigen–antibody complexes. *I. response:* the antigen-specific defences provided by humoral immunity (B lymphocytes) and cell-mediated immunity (T lymphocytes). *I. system*: a functional system which is able to recognize antigens (foreign substances) and use various methods of preventing them from causing damage in the body, e.g. antigen destruction.

immunity, state of resistance to infection conferred by the presence of antibodies capable of combining with antigens, or antitoxins which neutralize toxins or other chemicals. *See* CELL-MEDIATED IMMUNITY, HUMORAL IMMUNITY. Immunity may be: **1.** natural. This may be inborn (passive), acquired by the transfer of maternal antibodies via the placenta and in colostrum and breast milk; or active, where the person produces his or her own antibodies in response to having the disease or being exposed to the microorganism over time. **2.** artificial. Immunity acquired by immunization, it can be active or passive (Figure 38). *See* IMMUNIZATION.

immunization, artificial means by which immunity is initiated or augmented. *Active i.*: achieved by using vaccines containing attenuated microorganisms or inactive microorganisms or bacterial products such as toxins. This results in antibody production and is generally long-lasting. *Passive i.*: achieved by injection of antibodies, it is generally of short duration and affords only temporary protection. *I. programme*: a routine programme of immunization offered during childhood and at other times, and to special groups such as healthcare workers.

immunoassay, an assay technique which utilizes an antibody.

immunocompetence, the ability to initiate a specific immune response following exposure to an antigen.

immunocompromised patient, a person with defective immune responses or where their immune system is prevented from functioning normally, often produced by drugs, irradiation and AIDS. Patients having invasive procedures, those with cancer and other conditions affecting the immune response may also be affected. Patients are liable to develop opportunistic infections such as those caused by *Pneumocystis carinii* and *Candida albicans*.

immunodeficiency, an impairment of humoral or cell-mediated mechanisms. Causes include: deficiency

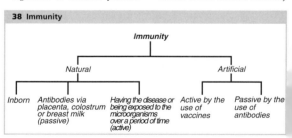

38 Immunity

Immunity
— Natural
— Artificial

Natural:
- Inborn
- Antibodies via placenta, colostrum or breast milk (passive)
- Having the disease or being exposed to the microorganisms over a period of time (active)

Artificial:
- Active by the use of vaccines
- Passive by the use of antibodies

of immunoglobulin synthesis, AIDS.

immunoglobulins, antibodies. A group of proteins present in the blood, interstitial fluid and body fluids such as saliva, intestinal secretions and respiratory secretions. The groups are IgG, IgM, IgA, IgD and IgE, each with different properties and functions within the immunological system.

immunology, the study of immunity.

immunosuppression, deliberate inhibition of the immune response with drugs, e.g. ciclosporin, radiation or antilymphocyte immunoglobulin to prevent rejection of transplanted tissue.

immunotherapy, term that describes immunization and specific treatments aimed at the immune system, e.g. interferons and anti-tumour necrosis factor (TNF) monoclonal antibody.

impacted, wedged or jammed together. *I. fracture:* one where the broken ends are jammed together. *I. faeces:* hard immobile mass of faeces in the rectum.

impalpable, not capable of being felt.

imperforate, completely closed. *See* ANUS.

impermeable, material which prevents the passage of substances.

impetigo, *(im-pe-ti′-gō),* a skin rash of an acute kind, generally a streptococcal and staphylococcal infection. It is contagious.

implantation, the act of planting or setting in; grafting. **1.** the fertilized ovum embedding into the decidua. **2.** a drug, substance or object inserted into the tissues. **3.** healthy tissue replacing damaged tissue.

implants, drugs, devices or tissue implanted into the body, e.g. drug pellets inserted under the skin. May be used to replace hormones.

implementation, a stage of the nursing process where planned nursing interventions are initiated.

impotence, inability of the male to achieve or maintain erection or premature ejaculation. May have physical or psychological causes.

impregnate, 1. to permeate or saturate. **2.** to make pregnant.

impulse, sudden irrational driving force or urge. *Nerve i.:* the transmission of electrochemical energy occurring along nerve fibres as electrical and concentration gradients result from the movement of ions.

in extremis, *(in eks-trē-mis),* at the point of death.

in situ, in position.

in utero, *(in ū-te-rō),* within the uterus.

in vitro, *(in vē-trō),* literally, in glass. *I. v. fertilization (IVF):* an assisted fertility technique where oöcytes collected from the ovaries are fertilized by spermatozoa outside the body prior to their introduction into the uterus.

in vivo, *(in vē-vō),* in the living body.

inaccessibility, unresponsiveness seen in some mental health problems.

inborn, occurring before birth, both normal inherited characteristics and abnormal traits or developmental anomalies.

incarcerated, imprisoned. Term applied to a hernia which cannot be reduced, or to a gravid uterus which cannot rise from the pelvis.

incest, sexual intercourse between near relatives, whose marriage would not be legal.

incidence, occurrence rate. The number of new cases of a disease seen in a population over a given period of time.

incipient, beginning.

incision, a wound produced by a sharp instrument, such as during surgery.

incisors, *(in-sī-sers),* eight chisel-shaped cutting teeth at the front of the jaw.

inclusion bodies, intracellular bodies seen in certain viral infections, e.g. Negri bodies in rabies.

incompatible, not capable of association, lacking compatibility. Usually applied to drugs or the transfusion of blood, or transplanted tissue.

incompetence, incapable of functioning normally, e.g. a heart valve.

incontinence, inability to control the passage of urine and/or, less commonly, faeces. *Faecal i.:* loss of anal sphincter control may be due to faecal impaction, neurological problems, rectal prolapse, drugs causing diarrhoea and certain bowel diseases. *Urinary i.:* several types exist—functional, neurological, overflow, stress and urge (due to detrusor instability).

incoordination, inability to perform harmonious muscular movements.

incubation, hatching. *I. period:* time between infection and the appearance of signs and symptoms of an infectious disease.

incubator, 1. apparatus used to provide optimum conditions for the growth of microorganisms in the laboratory. **2.** apparatus in which pre-term or sick infants can be provided with a controlled temperature and oxygen concentration environment.

incus, a small anvil-shaped bone of the middle ear. *See* EAR.

index, 1. the forefinger. **2.** the ratio of measurement of any quantity in comparison with a fixed standard.

Indian hemp, *see* CANNABIS.

indicanuria, *(in-di-kan-ū-ri-a),* excess indican in the urine, associated with increased bacterial breakdown of tryptophan in the bowel, as in blind loop syndrome. *See* INDOLE.

indicator, substance showing a chemical reaction by its change in colour.

indigenous, *(in-dij'-en-ūs),* native to a particular place.

indigestion, dyspepsia. Difficulty with the digestive processes.

indole, substance formed in the bowel by bacterial action on certain amino acids. Excreted in the urine as indican. *See* INDICANURIA.

indolent, a term applied to a painless sore which is slow to heal.

induction, the act of bringing on or causing to occur, as applied to anaesthesia and labour.

induration, abnormal hardening of tissues or organs.

industrial disease, occupational disease, a disease associated with an individual's occupation, e.g. asbestosis and back injuries.

inert, without action. *I. gases:* gases such as neon which form part of the atmosphere.

inertia, sluggishness. **1.** resistance to change in motion. **2.** in psychiatry, extreme apathy. **3.** *uterine i.:* sluggish contraction of the uterus during labour.

inevitable haemorrhage, bleeding due to a placenta praevia. *See* ANTEPARTUM HAEMORRHAGE, PLACENTA PRAEVIA.

infant, a child during the first year of life. In legal terms a person under the legal age of maturity. *I. mortality: see* MORTALITY.

infanticide, the killing of an infant by its mother within the first year of its life.

infantilism, persistence of childish characteristics in an adult.

infarct, an area of necrosis within an organ. Due to an occlusion of the artery supplying that part, usually by thrombosis or embolus.

infarction, formation of an infarct. *See* EMBOLISM, MYOCARDIAL INFARCTION, PULMONARY INFARCTION.

infection, the successful invasion, establishment and multiplication of microorganisms in the host tissues. May be chronic or acute. *See* CROSS-INFECTION, HOSPITAL-ACQUIRED INFECTION, OPPORTUNISTIC INFECTION.

infection control, the policies and protocols determined by a healthcare institution or community which seek to reduce the spread of infection, operate effective surveillance and increase awareness through education programmes. *I.c. nurse:* a nurse with specialist knowledge and qualifications who is concerned with implementing and monitoring infection control policies and protocols.

infectious disease, 1. a communicable disease. **2.** a disease caused by infection.

infectious mononucleosis, (mon-ō-nū-klē-ō'-sis), **glandular fever.** Caused by the Epstein–Barr virus, it commonly affects adolescents and young adults. It is characterized by extreme lethargy, enlarged lymph nodes, splenomegaly, pyrexia and sore throat. Occasionally causes hepatomegaly and jaundice.

inferential statistics, also called inductive statistics. That which uses the observations of a sample to make a prediction about other samples. It generalizes from the sample. *See* DESCRIPTIVE STATISTICS.

inferior, lower or below. *I. vena cava:* large vein which returns blood from the trunk and legs to the heart.

inferiority complex, feelings of inferiority compensated for by aggressive extrovert behaviour.

infertility, an inability to reproduce. May be due to problems with either partner and may be primary or secondary.

infestation, the invasion of the body by parasites such as lice.

infibulation, extreme form of female circumcision where the clitoris, labia minora and part of the labia majora are removed.

infiltration, the entry into cells, tissues and organs of abnormal cells or substances, e.g. fat.

inflammation, a non-specific local defence mechanism initiated by tissue injury. It is characterized by heat, redness, swelling, pain and loss of function. The inflammatory response involves the tissue changes of inflammation, caused by chemical mediators, blood cells, vascular changes and the production of exudate.

inflammatory bowel disease (IBD), non-specific inflammatory conditions affecting the alimentary canal. *See* CROHN'S DISEASE, ULCERATIVE COLITIS.

influenza, an acute illness caused by a group of myxoviruses of which there are several strains. It causes pyrexia, limb pains, headache, cough, anorexia and sometimes nausea. Epidemics occur and occasionally pandemics.

informatics, information management and technology (IM&T).

informed consent, *see* CONSENT.

infrared, long-wavelength, invisible rays of the electromagnetic spectrum.

infundibulum, (in-fun-dib'-ū-lum), **1.** funnel-shaped structure, such as the end of the uterine tube. **2.** the stalk which connects the pituitary gland to the hypothalamus.

infusion, 1. crude extract of a substance using boiling water; tea is an infusion. **2.** the introduction of fluid or drugs into the body by gravity flow, either intravenously or subcutaneously.

ingestion, the taking in of food or other substances into the body. Or the

173

means by which a phagocytic cell engulfs surrounding solid material.

ingrowing toenail, lateral extension of the nail bed.

inguinal, *(in-gwi-nal),* pertaining to the groin. *I. canal:* an intermuscular canal running obliquely through the abdominal muscles at the level of the inguinal ligament, it carries the round ligament in females and the spermatic cord in males. A 'weak spot' where herniation occurs. *See* HERNIA.

inhalation, act of breathing in air, fumes or vapour. A method of administering drugs, especially those used in the treatment of respiratory conditions.

inhaler, apparatus used to administer a drug or vapour by inhalation.

inherent, inborn.

inheritance, 1. obtaining traits or characteristics by the transmission of genes from parent to offspring. **2.** the actual characteristics obtained in this way.

inhibin, protein hormone which inhibits the release of follicle-stimulating hormone.

inhibition, restraint. The term is used ubiquitously to imply the prevention of some activity; thus psychological i., enzymatic i., etc.

injected, 1. congested. **2.** administered by injection.

injection, 1. the introduction of fluid material into the body under pressure, usually by syringe. It may be: intra-arterial, intra-articular, intradermal, intramuscular, intrathecal, intravenous, subcutaneous or into a hollow structure (Figure 39). **2.** the substance to be injected.

innate, congenital, inborn.

innervation, the nerve supply to a particular part.

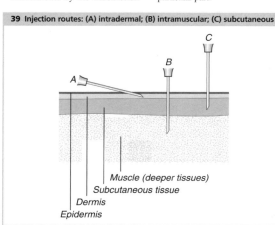

39 Injection routes: (A) intradermal; (B) intramuscular; (C) subcutaneous

Muscle (deeper tissues)
Subcutaneous tissue
Dermis
Epidermis

innocuous, harmless.

innominate, nameless or unnamed. *I. artery*: large artery arising from the aortic arch which forms the right common carotid and right subclavian arteries. Usually called **brachiocephalic**. *I. bone*: one of two bones forming the front and sides of the pelvis. Formed from the ilium, ischium and pubis. *I. veins*: formed from the jugular and subclavian veins. Usually called **brachiocephalic**.

inoculation, 1. insertion of microorganisms into culture medium. **2.** introduction of antigenic material into tissues to augment immunity.

inorganic, a compound that generally contains no carbon or hydrogen.

inositol, *(in-ō′-sit-ol)*, a substance found in certain animal and plant tissues.

inotropes, substances that have an effect on myocardial contractility. Those increasing contractility are termed positive inotropes, e.g. dobutamine, and those that decrease contractility, e.g. atenolol and nifedipine, are negative inotropes.

inquest, in England and Wales, a legal enquiry held by a coroner into the cause of sudden or unexpected death.

insecticide, a preparation for destroying insects.

insemination, introduction of semen into the vagina. *Artificial i.*: injection of semen into the vagina or uterus.

insertion, the attachment of a muscle to the part it moves.

insidious, proceeding in a concealed or subtle manner.

insight, an awareness of one's own mental state and behaviour.

insolation, exposure to the sun's rays.

insomnia, sleeplessness.

inspiration, breathing in.

inspiratory, pertaining to inspiration. *I. capacity (IC)*: maximum amount of air inspired after a normal expiratory effort.

inspissated, thickened by evaporation.

instep, arch on the dorsal surface of the foot.

instillation, pouring in drop by drop, e.g. into eye.

instinct, an inborn organization of perception, feeling and action, e.g. the sight of something which threatens life arouses the emotion of fear and the instinct of flight.

institutionalization, the dependence, apathy and lack of motivation which may accompany prolonged residence, or working in long-stay institutions, where routines are rigid and residents and staff are not involved in making decisions.

insufflation, blowing powder, air or gas into a body cavity.

insula, *(in-sū-la)*, an island of cerebral hemisphere surrounded by the lateral sulcus.

insulation, non-conducting material which prevents loss of heat, electrical or sound energy. The myelin sheath insulates some nerve fibres to facilitate rapid transmission of nerve impulses. *See* DEMYELINATION, MYELIN.

insulator, a substance which does not conduct electricity.

insulin, polypeptide hormone produced by the beta cells of the pancreas. It lowers the blood glucose in various ways, e.g. by facilitating the passage of glucose into cells, and influences the metabolism of fats and amino acids. *I. dependent diabetes mellitus (IDDM)*: *see* DIABETES MELLITUS; *cf.* GLUCAGON.

insulinoma, *(in-sū-lin-ō-ma)*, *see* ISLET CELL TUMOUR.

integrated medicine, a term ascribed to complementary medicine to reflect a harmonious integration of

175

particular complementary therapies within orthodox healthcare practice.

integration, the processes by which an individual with learning disabilities is able to function as an equal member of the community, e.g. attend mainstream schools or live and work within the community.

integument, (in-teg-ū'-ment), the skin.

intellect, reasoning power, thinking faculty.

intelligence, intellect. Inborn mental ability. *I. quotient (IQ)*: the ratio of mental age to chronological age. *I. test*: test designed to assess intellectual ability, usually expressed as IQ.

intensive therapy unit (ITU), unit where highly specialized monitoring equipment, resuscitation and therapeutic techniques are used to support critically ill patients. *See* HIGH DEPENDENCY UNIT.

intention, healing process. *See* FIRST INTENTION, GRANULATION, HEALING. *I. tremor*: one increasing during a voluntary movement, symptomatic of parkinsonism.

interarticular, (in-ter-ar-tik'-ū-la), between joints.

intercellular, (in-ter-sel-ū-la), between cells.

intercostal, between the ribs. *I. muscles*: respiratory muscles between the ribs.

intercourse, communication. *Sexual i.*: coitus.

intercurrent, occurring at the same time. *I. infection*: one that occurs while the person has some other infection or disease.

interferons (IFNs), (in-ter-fēr-onz), protein mediators that enhance cellular resistance to viruses. Interferons also act as cytokines to modulate the immune response. Interferon has caused the regression of some tumours and is used in the management of some types of multiple sclerosis.

interleukins, (in-ter-lū-kins), a group of signalling molecules or cytokines. They are non-specific immune chemicals produced by macrophages and activated T-lymphocytes. They also act with other cytokines in the regulation of haemopoiesis.

interlobular, between lobules.

intermenstrual, between one menstruation and another.

intermittent, occurring at intervals. *I. claudication*: see CLAUDICATION. *I. peritoneal dialysis*: see PERITONEAL DIALYSIS. *I. pneumatic compression*: a stocking worn to prevent deep vein thrombosis of upper or lower limb. *I. positive pressure ventilation (IPPV)*: assisted ventilation via an endotracheal tube or tracheostomy to support breathing in respiratory failure. This may be required for patients with acute lung disease, chest injuries, neurological conditions or during anaesthesia.

internal, inside. *I. capsule*: area in the brain between the basal nuclei and the thalamus, it is formed by the efferent and afferent fibres that connect the cerebral cortex with other parts of the brain, muscles and sensory receptors. *I. ear*: see EAR. *I. environment*: the extracellular fluids surrounding cells. Homeostatic mechanisms maintain its physical and chemical conditions. *I. os*: junction between cervical canal and uterus.

International Classification of Diseases (ICD), a list of disease categories compiled by the World Health Organization (WHO).

International System of Units (SI), Système International d'Unités, a system of measurement used for medical, technical and scientific purposes. It is based upon seven base units, which include: kilogram, metre, second and mole, and several derived units. *See* APPENDIX 4: UNITS OF MEASUREMENT.

internet, in computing a large world-wide network providing access to information sources and the transmission of electronic mail. *See* LAN, NETWORK, WAN.

interneurone, a connecting or linking neurone.

interphase, phase between mitotic divisions during which the cell performs its normal metabolic processes and prepares for mitosis.

interpretive approach, a research approach used by social scientists that includes the meaning and significance people attach to situations and behaviour.

intersex, imperfect sexual differentiation of an individual into either male or female.

interstitial, *(in-ter-sti-shal),* between. *I. cell-stimulating hormone (ICSH)*: synonym for luteinizing hormone which in the male causes the testis to produce testosterone. *See* LUTEINIZING HORMONE. *I. fluid* or *tissue fluid*: the fluid which surrounds the cells. This plus the plasma forms the extracellular fluid. *I. keratitis*: see KERATITIS.

intertrigo, *(in-ter-trī-go),* inflammatory skin eruption seen where moist skin folds are in contact, e.g. groin, under the breasts.

intertrochanteric, *(in-ter-trō-kan-te-rik),* between the trochanters.

interval cancer, a cancer diagnosed in the interval between screening appointments.

interval data, measurement data with a numerical score, e.g. temperature, that has an arbitrary zero. The intervals between successive values are the same, e.g. a one-degree increase from 36 to 37 is the same as from 37 to 38. *See* RATIO DATA.

interventions, a planned course of action, such as nursing actions

which alleviate or prevent a health problem. They may be proactive or reactive.

interventricular, between the ventricles.

intervertebral, between the vertebrae. *I. disc*: pad of fibrocartilage between the vertebrae. Prolapse of a disc causes severe pain from pressure on nerve root.

intestinal, pertaining to the intestine. *I. obstruction*: obstruction to the passage of the intestinal contents. May be mechanical, e.g. strangulated hernia, or due to the absence of peristalsis. *See* PARALYTIC ILEUS.

intestine, the alimentary canal from the duodenum to the anus. *See* BOWEL.

intima, inner coat of an artery or vein. Consists of very smooth endothelium.

intolerance, being unable to endure. Usually applied to drugs and certain foods.

intoxication, poisoning; drunkenness.

intra-abdominal, within the abdominal cavity.

intra-amniotic, within the amniotic fluid.

intra-aortic, within the aorta, such as an i. balloon pump (IABP) used to enhance the cardiac output in ventricular failure.

intra-arterial, within an artery.

intra-articular, within a joint cavity.

intracardiac, within the heart.

intracellular, *(in-tra-sel-ū-la),* within a cell. *I. fluid*: the fluid and electrolytes within the cell.

intracerebral, *(in-tra-ser-e-bral),* within the cerebrum. *I. haemorrhage*: bleeding into the substance of the brain.

intracranial, *(in-tra-krā-nē-al),* within the skull. *I. pressure (ICP)*: the pressure within the skull which may be raised in certain conditions such as tumours, haemorrhage and head injury.

intracytoplasmic sperm injection (ICSI), an assisted conception technique which involves the direct insertion in vitro of a single chosen spermatozoon into an oöcyte. The fertilized oöcyte is then placed inside the uterus.

intradermal, within the skin.

intradural, (*in-tra-dū'-ral*), within the dura mater.

intragastric, (*in-tra-gas-trik*), within the stomach.

intrahepatic, (*in-tra-hep-a'-tik*), within the liver.

intralobular, (*in-tra-lo'-bū-la*), within a lobule.

intramedullary, (*in-tra-me-dū-la-ri*), within the medullary cavity of a bone. *I. nail*: used for the fixation of certain fractures.

intramural, within the wall of an organ or hollow tube.

intramuscular, within a muscle. Frequently used route for the injection of drugs.

intranasal, (*in-tra-nā'-sal*), within the nasal cavity.

intranet, connection of computer networks within an organization, such as the NHS.

intraocular, (*i-tra-ok-ū-la*), within the eyeball.

intraoperative, during an operation.

intraosseous, (*in-tra-os-ē-us*), within a bone. A route for the administration of fluids when rapid establishment of systemic access is vital and venous access is impossible. It provides an alternative route for the administration of drugs and fluids.

intraperitoneal, (*in-tra-per-i-to-nē-al*), within the peritoneal cavity.

intrathecal, (*in-tra-thē-kal*), pertaining to the lumen of a sheath or canal. Most often means within the meninges usually the subarachnoid

space. Drugs may be administered via this route, e.g. antimicrobial drugs for meningitis.

intratracheal, (*in-tra-trak-ē-al*), endo-tracheal. Within the trachea. *I. anaesthetic*: administration of anaesthetic gases via an endotracheal tube.

intrauterine, (*in-tra-ū-ter-ln*), within the uterus. *I. contraceptive device (IUCD)*: a device of plastic and metal which is placed inside the uterus to prevent conception. *I. death*: the fetus dies while still in the uterus.

intravenous (IV), (*in-tra-vē-nus*), within the lumen of a vein. *I. cholangiography*: see CHOLANGIOGRAPHY. *I. pyelography/urography*: see PYELOGRAPHY, UROGRAPHY. See also INFUSION, INJECTION.

intrinsic, inherent, peculiar to a part. *I. factor*: glycoprotein produced by the gastric mucosa, it facilitates the absorption of vitamin B_{12} in the ileum. *I. sugars*: those found in the cell walls of various plant foods.

introitus, (*in-trō'-it-us*), an entrance, applied to the inlets of the pelvis and vagina.

introjection, a mental defence mechanism where the person takes on the values and standards of another person or group.

introspection, looking inwards. State of mental self-examination.

introversion, 1. directing thoughts or interests inwards. **2.** a hollow structure which invaginates or turns in on itself.

introvert, an individual whose attention centres upon self rather than outside activities. Opposite to extrovert.

intubation, insertion of tube into a passage or organ, especially tracheal intubation.

intumescence, (*in-tū-mes'-sens*), swelling, increase in size.

intussusception, (*in-tus-sus-sep-shon*), telescoping (invagination) of one bowel segment into another. Occurs in infants, often around weaning. It is characterized by severe colic, obstruction, vomiting and the passage of blood and mucus rectally ('redcurrant jelly' stools). It may be reduced by a non-surgical hydrostatic reduction, usually by barium enema, but surgery may be required (Figure 40).

inulin, *(in-ū-lin),* a sugar used to assess renal function. As it is filtered but not reabsorbed or secreted, its clearance rate will be the same as the glomerular filtration rate (GFR).

invagination, *(in-vaj-i-nā´-shon),* turning inwards to form double-layered pouch.

invasion, onset, especially of a disease. Entry of microorganisms or the spread of malignant cells.

inversion, turning upside down or inside out.

involucrum, *(in-vo-lū-krum),* layer of new bone ensheathing a sequestrum.

involuntary, independent of the will. *I. muscle:* smooth muscle. Innervated by the autonomic nervous system.

involute, rolled inward from the edges; becoming smaller.

involution, 1. the normal shrinkage of an organ after fulfilling its functional purpose, e.g. the uterus after childbirth. *See* SUBINVOLUTION. **2.** period of progressive decline occurring after midlife when tissues and organs reduce in size and functional ability declines.

iodine (I), an element essential for the production of the thyroid hormones. Used as a skin antiseptic prior to invasive techniques. Its radioactive isotopes, e.g. ^{131}I, are used for the diagnosis and treatment of thyroid conditions.

ion, an atom or radical with an electrical charge: cations which have a positive charge or anions which are negatively charged.

ionization, the dissociation of a substance in solution into electrically charged ions.

ionizing radiation, a form of radiation which destabilizes an atom, forming an ion. X-rays, gamma-rays and particle radiation are all examples. Has the ability to cause tissue damage.

iontophoresis, treatment whereby ions of various soluble salts are introduced into the tissues by means of a constant electrical current. The drug pilocarpine can be introduced into the skin by this method during a sweat test for cystic fibrosis.

40 Intussusception

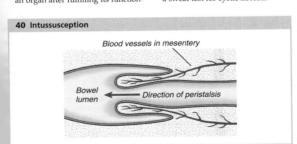

Blood vessels in mesentery

Bowel lumen ← Direction of peristalsis

IPPV, abbreviation for intermittent positive pressure ventilation.

ipsilateral, on the same side.

IQ, abbreviation for intelligence quotient. *See* INTELLIGENCE.

iridectomy, (ir-i-dek-to-mi), excision of part of the iris.

iridencleisis, (ir-i-den-klē-sis), an older type of operation which reduces intraocular pressure. Used in glaucoma.

iridium (Ir), (ir-id'-ē-um), a metallic element. Its radioactive isotope ^{192}Ir is implanted (in pins and wires) into certain tumours as brachytherapy.

iridocele, (ī-ri-do-sēl), protrusion of a portion of iris through a wound in the cornea.

iridocyclitis, (ir-id-ō-sī-klī'-tis), inflammation of the iris and ciliary body.

iridodialysis, (i-ri-do-dī-al-i-sis), a condition where the border of the iris has become separated from its ciliary attachment, often as a result of trauma.

iridoplegia, (ī-ri-dō-plē'-ji-a), paralysis of the muscle which constricts or dilates the pupil.

iridotomy, (ī-rid-ot-o-mi), an incision into the iris.

iris, (ī'-ris), coloured circular structure, containing muscle fibres, which surrounds and controls the size of the pupil. Situated behind the cornea and in front of the lens it forms a division between the anterior and posterior chambers.

iritis, (ī-rī'-tis), inflammation of the iris.

iron (Fe), a metallic element essential for the production of haemoglobin and several enzymes. *I. deficiency anaemia*: a very common anaemia which may be due to iron loss through acute or chronic haemorrhage, inadequate intake in the diet or a failure to absorb iron.

irradiation, exposure to any form of radiant energy, e.g. heat, light or X-ray.

irreducible, incapable of being returned to its proper place by manipulation; term usually applied to a hernia.

irrigation, washing out.

irritable, reacting to a stimulus. *I. bowel syndrome*: a common condition of bowel dysfunction for which no organic cause can be found. Characterized by pain and passage of mucus rectally, with alternating diarrhoea and constipation.

irritant, agent causing irritation.

ischaemia, (is-kē'-mi-a), diminished blood supply to a part.

ischaemic contracture, (is-kē'-mik), permanent damage and shortening of muscle fibres by fibrosis resulting from an impaired blood supply. *See* CONTRACTURE, VOLKMANN'S ISCHAEMIC CONTRACTURE.

ischaemic heart disease, insufficient blood supply to the myocardium, causing central chest pain which may radiate to the arms, neck and jaw. *See* ANGINA PECTORIS, MYOCARDIAL INFARCTION.

ischiofemoral, (is-kē-o-fem'-or-al), pertaining to ischium and femur. *I. ligament*: strong ligament which runs posteriorly from ischium to the greater trochanter of the femur.

ischiorectal, (is-kē-o-rek'-tal), pertaining to ischium and rectum. *I. abscess*: collection of pus in the ischiorectal connective tissue.

ischium, (is-kē'-um), the lower and hind part of the innominate bone.

Ishihara chart, colour chart used to test for colour blindness.

islet cell tumour, tumour of the beta cells of the pancreas which secrete insulin, resulting in hypoglycaemia. More rarely a tumour which secretes

gastrin. *See* ZOLLINGER-ELLISON SYN-
DROME.

islets of Langerhans, *see* LANGERHANS'
ISLETS

isoenzyme, an enzyme which has several forms, may be produced in different sites, but catalyses the same
reactions, such as alkaline phosphatase.

isograft, graft with material obtained
from a donor of identical genotype –
an identical twin. *See* GRAFT.

isoimmunization, *(i-sō-im-mūn-i-sā-
shon),* the formation of antibodies
following exposure to an antigen
from an individual of the same
species, such as anti D formation
when a rhesus (Rh)-negative person
is exposed to Rh-positive blood.

isolation, the act of setting apart. A
measure taken to contain an infectious condition. *See* BARRIER NURSING,
CONTAINMENT ISOLATION, PROTECTIVE
ISOLATION, SOURCE ISOLATION.

isoleuceine, *(i-so-lū-sēn),* an essential
(indispensable) amino acid.

isomers, compounds made up of the
same elements, but a different atomic
structure confers different properties.

isometric, *(i-sō-met-rik),* of equal measure. *I. muscle contraction*: tension
increases in the muscle without
shortening. Occurs when you push
against a fixed object or hold a posture. *I. exercises*: static exercises without movement occurring.

isotonic, *(i-sō-ton-ik),* of equal tension.
1. having the same osmotic pressure
as the fluid with which it is being
compared. *See* HYPERTONIC, HYPO-
TONIC. 2. muscle contraction where
the tension is constant. Here the
fibres shorten to produce movement
as the load tension is overcome,
such as during lifting. 3. exercises that involve movement. Those
that increase muscle strength and
endurance.

isotope, two or more forms of the
same element having identical
chemical properties and the same
atomic number but different mass
numbers, e.g. hydrogen which has
three forms. *Radioactive i.*: some elements produce heavy unstable isotopes which emit radiation (alpha,
beta and gamma) as the nucleus disintegrates, e.g. ^{131}I, ^{137}Cs and ^{99m}Tc.
Used in diagnosis and treatment of
disease. *See* RADIOISOTOPE, RADIONU-
CLIDE, RADIOTHERAPY.

isthmus, *(is'-mus),* the neck or constricted part of an organ.

IT, abbreviation for **information technology.**

ITU, abbreviation for **intensive therapy unit.**

IUCD, *see* INTRAUTERINE.

IVF, *see* IN VITRO FERTILIZATION.

IVP, IVU, intravenous pyelography,
intravenous urography.

J

Jacksonian epilepsy, see EPILEPSY.

Jacquemier's sign, *(jak-mē-āz)*, blueness of the vaginal walls seen in early pregnancy.

jactitation, restlessness with tossing and turning associated with pyrexia.

Jarisch–Herxheimer reaction, a situation where the symptoms of a disease are initially worsened by drug treatment, e.g. pencillin for syphilis.

jaundice, yellow discoloration of the skin, sclerae and mucosae due to an increase in serum bilirubin; pruritus occurs as bile salts also accumulate in the blood. Jaundice can be classified as: **1.** prehepatic or haemolytic, where excessive breakdown of red blood cells releases bilirubin into the blood, such as with physiological jaundice of the newborn and haemolytic anaemia. See HAEMOLYSIS, HAEMOLYTIC DISEASE OF THE NEWBORN. **2.** hepatocellular; arises when liver cell function is impaired, such as with hepatitis. See HEPATITIS. **3.** obstructive or cholestatic where the flow of bile is obstructed either within the liver or in the bile ducts. Causes include: cirrhosis, tumours, parasites and gallstones (Figure 41). See CIRRHOSIS, GALLSTONES.

jaw bone, either the maxilla (upper jaw) or mandible (lower jaw).

jejunectomy, *(jē-jū-nek-to-mi)*, excision of part of the jejunum.

jejunostomy, *(je-jū-nos'-to-mi)*, an artificial opening in the jejunum which can be used for feeding.

jejunum, *(je-jū- num)*, middle portion of the small intestine between the duodenum and ileum. See BOWEL.

jet lag, distruption of body processes which normally follow diurnal rhythms, occurs after travel through different time zones. There are problems with sleep, appetite, concentration and memory. Similar effects are reported in people whose work involves different shift patterns.

jigger, tropical sand flea which is parasitic to humans, burrowing into the skin of the feet.

joint, point of contact between two or more bones. An articulation. They may be synovial: diarthroses (freely movable), cartilaginous: amphiarthroses (slightly movable) or fibrous: synarthroses (immovable).

joule (J), derived SI unit for energy/quantity of heat/work.

jugular, pertaining to the neck. *J. veins*: two large neck veins which carry most blood from the head. *J. venous pressure (JVP)*: pressure in the jugular veins—a guide to the pressure in the right side of the heart.

Jung, a Swiss psychiatrist/psychologist (1875–1961).

Jungian, in psychology the theories of psychoanalysis and 'collective unconscious' according to Jung.

jurisprudence, medical, see MEDICAL JURISPRUDENCE.

41 Types and causes of jaundice

Prehepatic or haemolytic	Hepatocellular	Obstructive (cholestatic)
Haemolysis and release of haem		
Causes	**Causes**	**Causes**
Haemolytic anaemia	Hepatitis	Intrahepatic
Overactive spleen	• drugs	• cirrhosis
Rhesus incompatibility	• alcohol	• drugs
ABO mismatch	• viruses	• metastatic cancer
Abnormal RBCs		
Drugs	Conjugation problems	Extrahepatic
Infections	• in the newborn	• gallstone in CBD
Physiological jaundice in newborns	• Gilbert's syndrome	• cancer in head of pancreas
		• other tumours
		• parasites
Results	**Results**	**Results**
Mild jaundice (lemon)	Jaundice variable	Jaundice severe (green)
Urine contains increased urobilinogen but no bilirubin (acholuric)	Urine may have bilirubin and urobilinogen varies	Urine contains bilirubin but no urobilinogen
Stools: dark due to increased stercobilin	Stools: normal or paler	Stools: pale (clay coloured)

justice, ethical principle involving concepts of fairness and justness.

juvenile chronic arthritis (JCA), inflammatory arthritis occurring in children. There are varying degress of inflammation in joints with loss of articular cartilage and premature ossification of the epiphyseal growing plates.

juxtaglomerular, *(juk-sta-glo-mer-ū-la),* near to the glomerulus. *J. apparatus (JGA)* or *cells*: specialized cells in the nephron. Concerned with monitoring pressure changes and sodium levels in the blood and initiating the release of renin that converts a precursor to angiotension when pressure falls, or when sodium levels fall; or blood flow is slow.

juxtaposition, placed alongside or next to.

K

Kahn test, obsolete serological test for syphilis.

kala-azar, *(ka-la-ā'-za)*, generalized leishmaniasis occurring in the tropics. Transmitted to humans by sand flies and caused by the protozoan parasite *Leishmania donovani*. There is splenomegaly, fever and anaemia.

kaolin, natural aluminium silicate. Various forms are used for poultices and in antidiarrhoeals.

Kaposi's disease, *see* XERODERMA PIGMENTOSUM.

Kaposi's sarcoma, *(ka-pō'-sēs sar-kō-ma)*, a viral-induced malignant disease of the skin where new blood vessels develop to produce firm blue/brown nodules in the skin. It is usually seen in tropical Africa and in individuals who are immunocompromised, such as those with AIDS.

Kaposi's spots, skin eruptions seen in a form of herpesvirus-induced eczema.

karaya, *(kar-rē-ā)*, plant gum used to protect the skin around a stoma.

karyon, *(kar-ē-on)*, cell nucleus.

karyotype, *(ka-rē-ō-tīp)*, **1.** number and structure of chromosomes for an individual. **2.** a diagrammatic representation of a set of chromosomes; autosomes groups A–G and the sex chromosomes.

katal, *(kā-tal)*, the amount of enzyme needed to catalyse one mole of the substrate per second under defined physical conditions.

Kayser–Fleischer rings, *(kā-ser-flī-sher)*, brownish pigmented rings seen in the cornea of patients with Wilson's disease.

Kegel's exercises, pelvic floor-strengthening exercises used to overcome stress incontinence.

Keller's operation, surgical correction of hallux valgus.

keloid, hard, raised overgrowth of scar tissue during the healing of burns or other skin wounds. A common feature of pigmented skin.

keratectasia, *(ker-a-tek-tā'-si-a)*, protrusion of the cornea.

keratectomy, *(ker-a-tek'-to-mi)*, excision of part of the cornea.

keratin, a fibrous protein found in tissues such as the outer layer of the skin, nails, horn and hooves.

keratinization, the process by which tissue is converted to keratin. Occurs pathologically in vitamin A deficiency.

keratitis, *(ker-a-ti-tis)*, inflammation of the cornea. *Interstitial k.:* inflammation of the deeper layers of the cornea may be associated with syphilis.

keratocele, *(ker-a-tō-seel)*, protrusion of Descemet's membrane of the cornea.

keratoconjunctivitis, inflammation of cornea and conjunctiva.

keratoiritis, inflammation of cornea and iris.

keratolytics, *(ker-a-tō-li-tiks)*, agents which break down keratin.

keratoma, *(ker-a-tō'-ma)*, a callosity or horny overgrowth.

keratomalacia, *(ker-at-ō-ma-la-she-a)*, softening of the cornea. May be caused by a deficiency of vitamin A.

keratome, knife used in corneal surgery.

keratometer, ophthalmometer, for measuring corneal astigmatism.

keratoplasty, *(ker-a-tō-pla-sti)*, corneal graft.

keratosis, *(ker-a-tō-sis)*, skin disease with excess of horny tissue.

keratotomy, *(ker-a-tot-o-mi)*, incision into the cornea.

kerion, inflammed area with swelling and suppuration seen with scalp ringworm.

kernicterus, *(ker-nik-te-rus)*, staining of brain cells, especially the basal nuclei with bilirubin. A complication of jaundice in pre-term infants and in haemolytic disease of the newborn.

Kernig's sign, a sign of meningeal irritation such as with meningitis. There is an inability to extend the knee when the thigh is flexed at 90° to the abdomen.

ketoacidosis, *(kē-tō-as-i-dō-sis)*, acidosis with an excess of ketone bodies in the blood. A complication of diabetes mellitus but also seen in starvation and pregnancy. *Diabetic k.*: ketones are formed as fatty acids are incompletely oxidized when glucose is unavailable as an energy source. There is acidosis and dehydration occurring with hyperglycaemia.

ketogenic diet, *(kē-tō-jen-ik)*, a diet high in fat which produces ketosis.

ketonaemia, *(kē-tō-nē-mi-a)*, ketone bodies in the blood.

ketones, *(kē-t ōnz)*, an organic compound containing a keto group. *K. bodies*: acetoacetic acid, acetone and beta-hydroxybutyric acid, substances formed when fat is oxidized. Small amounts can be used as metabolic fuel but excess formation leads to ketoacidosis.

ketonuria, *(kē-to-nū-ri-a)*, ketone bodies in the urine.

ketosis, *(kē-tō-sis)*, excess formation of ketones in the body such as in diabetes mellitus or starvation. *See* KETOACIDOSIS.

17-ketosteroids, *(kē-to-ste-roydz)*, steroid hormones containing a keto group and an additional oxygen molecule. They are produced by the adrenal cortex and to a lesser extent the gonads. Normally excreted in urine, its measurement can be used to diagnose adrenal or gonadal malfunction.

khat, leaves containing two psychostimulants similar to amfetamine (amphetamine). Increasingly available in the UK.

kick chart, *see* FETAL ASSESSMENT.

kidneys, paired retroperitoneal organs situated on the posterior abdominal wall in the lumbar region. Concerned with homeostasis, they produce urine to excrete waste such as urea, control water and electrolyte balance and blood pH. They also produce renin and erythropoietin and are involved in vitamin D metabolism (Figure 42). *Artificial k.*: *see* HAEMODIALYSIS.

killer cell, cytotoxic cell, a T lymphocyte, part of cell-mediated immunity. They lyse cells carrying antigens to which they are sensitized and provide mobile immune surveillance.

kilocalorie (kcal), *see* CALORIE.

kilogram (kg), SI unit of mass. A thousand grams.

kilojoule (kJ), a unit equal to 1000 joules, used for measuring large amounts of energy. It replaces the kilocalorie (kcal) which is still in use (1kcal = 4.2 kJ).

Kimmelstiel–Wilson syndrome, *(kimmel-stēl)*, diabetic nephropathy, a glomerulosclerosis caused by dam-

42 Section through a kidney

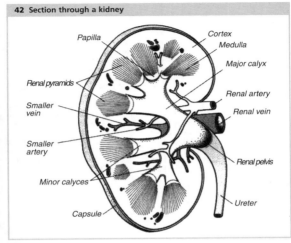

Papilla
Cortex
Medulla
Major calyx
Renal pyramids
Renal artery
Smaller vein
Renal vein
Smaller artery
Renal pelvis
Minor calyces
Ureter
Capsule

age to the glomerular capillaries. Characterized by proteinuria, hypertension and the nephrotic syndrome progressing to renal failure.

kinaesthesia, *(kin-es-thē'-zē-a),* perception of body weight, position and muscular movement.

kinase, enzyme that catalyses the transfer of a high-energy group of a donor, usually adenosine triphosphate, to some acceptor, usually named after the acceptor (e.g. fructokinase).

kinematics, *(kin'-e-mat-iks),* the study of motion.

kineplasty, *(kin'-e-plas-ti),* a plastic amputation with the object of making the stump useful for locomotion.

kinesis, *(kī-nē-sis),* movement.

kinetics, *(kīn-et-iks),* the study of movement or change.

kinins, *(kī-ninz),* biologically active polypeptides, e.g. bradykinin, which initiate vasodilation, vessel permeability and pain.

kinship, relationships linking people genetically, by marriage or adoption.

Kirschner wire, *(ker-shner),* wire used in orthopaedic surgery to apply skeletal traction to fractured bone.

Klebsiella, *(kleb-si-el-la),* a genus of anaerobic Gram-negative bacteria of the family Enterobacteriaceae. They form part of the bowel flora. A common cause of respiratory, urinary and wound infections. *See* ENTEROBACTERIACEAE, FRIEDLÄNDER'S BACILLUS.

kleptomania, obsessional neurosis manifested by compulsive stealing.

Klinefelter's syndrome, *(klīn-fel-terz),* a chromosomal abnormality of males – XXY. The person has male external genitalia, but the testes remain small. There is obesity, gynaecomastia, female body hair distribution, eunuchoid build and infertility.

Klumpke's paralysis, *(kloomp-kerz)*, paralysis of the hand and arm which may be caused by a birth injury to the lower brachial plexus.

knee, joint between the femur and tibia. K. *cap*: patella. K. *jerk*: a deep tendon reflex where the quadriceps muscle contracts when the patellar tendon is tapped when the knee is flexed. Absent in lower motor neurone disease and exaggerated in upper motor neurone conditions.

Koch's bacillus, *see* MYCOBACTERIUM TUBERCULOSIS.

Köhler's disease, osteochondritis of the tarsal navicular bone. Confined to children of 3–5 years.

koilonychia, *(koy-lō-ni-ki-a)*, spoon-shaped nails found in iron deficiency anaemia.

Koplik's spots, small white spots to be found on the inner surface of the cheeks in measles, often before the skin rash appears.

Korotkoff's (Korotkov) sounds, the sounds heard whilst recording arterial blood pressure. The phases are: 1. a sharp thud which represents systolic pressure; 2. a swishing sound; 3. a soft thud; 4. a soft blowing becoming muffled; 5. silence. In practice opinion is divided as to whether phase 4 or 5 should represent diastolic pressure.

Korsakoff's syndrome or **psychosis,** a confusional state characterized by memory changes and confabulation. Associated with the thiamine (vitamin B_1) deficiency which may occur in malnutrition or chronic alcohol misuse. *See* WERNICKE'S ENCEPHALOPATHY.

kosher, food which conforms to and is prepared according to the laws of Judaism.

kraurosis, *(kraw-rō-sis)*, skin changes with atrophy and shrinking. K. *vulvae*: itching and dryness affecting the vulva post climacteric. Due to reduced oestrogen levels it may be premalignant. *See* LEUCOPLAKIA.

Krebs' cycle, final common pathway for the oxidation of fuel molecules: glucose, fatty acids, glycerol and amino acids. Most enter the cycle as acetyl CoA and are oxidized to liberate energy (ATP), carbon dioxide and water. Various intermediates of these reactions are converted to other molecules. Also called **citric acid cycle** and **tricarboxylic acid cycle**.

Krukenberg's tumour, *(kroo-ken-bergs)*, a secondary tumour occurring in the ovary, the primary growth being usually in the stomach or large bowel.

krypton (kr), an inert gas. Its radioactive isotope is used in lung ventilation scans.

Küntscher nail, an intramedullary nail used in the fixation of fractures, such as those of the femur.

Kupffer's cells, *(koop-ferz)*, large phagocytic cells of the liver. Part of the monocyte–macrophage system (reticuloendothelial), they are concerned with the phagocytosis of bacteria and 'spent' erythrocytes.

Kussmaul's respiration, deep sighing respirations associated with diabetic ketoacidosis.

Kveim test, *(kvēm)*, a skin test for sarcoidosis.

kwashiorkor, *(kwa-shi-aw-kor)*, a form of protein-energy malnutrition seen when children are weaned on to a low-protein diet with a relatively adequate amount of calories from carbohydrate sources. It is characterized

by a thin miserable child who fails to
thrive. There is generalized oedema,
hair and skin colour changes, diarrhoea and hepatomegaly.

kypholordosis, coexistence of kyphosis and lordosis.

kyphoscoliosis, *(kī-fō-skō-li-ō-sis)*,
combined anteroposterior and lateral deformity of the spine. May
lead to difficulties with lung expansion and respiratory problems.

kyphosis, *(kī-fō-sis)*, an anteroposterior
deformity of the thoracic spine with
the formation of a hump (Figure 43).
May be caused by osteoporosis.

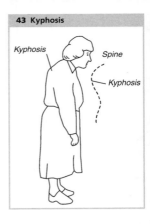

43 Kyphosis

L

labelling, 1. provision of data regarding the composition of food, drugs and other items. **2.** using a term to describe a person in terms of a characteristic or type of behaviour.

labia, *(sing.* **labium***)*, lips. *L. majora*: two large outer skin folds of the vulva. *L. minora*: two smaller skin folds within the l. majora.

labial, *(lā-bi-al)*, pertaining to the lips or labia.

labile, *(lā-bīl)*, unstable. *L. factor* (proaccelerin): factor V in blood coagulation.

labioglossopharyngeal, *(la-bē-ō-glos-ō-fa-rin'-jē-al)*, pertaining to the lips, tongue and pharynx. *L. paralysis: see* BULBAR PALSY.

labour, parturition or childbirth. There are three stages: **1.** dilatation of the cervix. **2.** full dilatation until the infant is expelled. **3.** expulsion of the placenta and membranes. *Induced l.:* one that has been initiated by drugs and/or rupture of the fetal membranes artificially. *Precipitate l.:* very rapid labour. *Premature l.:* occuring before term, usually before the 37th week of pregnancy.

labyrinth, structures of the inner ear – bony and membranous. *See* EAR.

labyrinthitis, *(lab'-i-rin-thī'-tis)*, inflammation of the inner ear labyrinth.

laceration, a lacerated wound with torn or irregular edges; not clean cut.

lacrimal, *(lak'-ri-mal)*, relating to tears. *L. apparatus* the glands, ducts, sacs and canaliculi that produce and convey tears (Figure 44).

44 The lacrimal apparatus

Lacrimal gland — *Outline of orbit* — *Ducts of gland* — *Lacrimal sac* — *Nasal duct* — *Upper and lower canaliculi*

lacrimation, *(lak-ri-mā'-shon)*, flow of tears.

lactagogue, *(lak'-ta-gog)*, *see* GALACTAGOGUE.

lactalbumin, *(lak'-tal-bū-min)*, one of the proteins of milk.

lactase, enzyme which converts lactose to glucose and galactose.

lactate, 1. salt of lactic acid. **2.** to produce milk. *L. dehydrogenase (LD, LDH):* an enzyme found in many tissues, including liver, skeletal muscle and myocardium. Its level in the blood is elevated in muscle disease and after myocardial infarction.

lactation, 1. the process of milk production. **2.** the period during which an infant is breast-fed.

lacteals, *(lak-tē-alz)*, lymphatic vessels in the intestinal villi which absorb digested fats.

lactic, pertaining to milk. *L. acid:* an organic acid formed from the fermentation of lactose. It is produced in the body during the anaerobic breakdown of glucose in strenuously contracting skeletal muscle. *L. acidosis*: acidosis resulting from a buildup of lactic acid in the blood. Occurs in conditions causing tissue hypoxia, such as shock and respiratory failure, and diabetes mellitus, liver failure, some drugs (e.g. biguanides) and toxins, such as alcohol.

lactiferous ducts, (lak-tif′-er-us), channels draining milk from a breast lobule.

Lactobacillus, (lak-tō-ba-si-lus), a genus of non-pathogenic Gram-positive bacteria of the family Lactobacillaceae which form part of the normal flora of the body. *See* DÖDERLEIN'S BACILLUS. They ferment sugars and are important in the production of yoghurt and other foods.

lactoferrin, an acute-phase protein involved in non-specific body defences, it is found in many body fluids.

lactogenic, (lak-tō-je-nik), promoting the flow of milk. *L. hormone: see* PROLACTIN.

lacto-ovovegetarian, an individual whose diet consists of milk, milk products, eggs, vegetables, fruits and grain, but with no meat, poultry or fish.

lactose, a disaccharide present in milk, it consists of glucose and galactose. *L. intolerance*: due to lactase deficiency. Characterized by colic and diarrhoea following the intake of milk or milk products.

lactovegetarian, an individual whose diet consists of milk, milk products, vegetables, fruits and grain, but with no eggs, meat, poultry or fish.

lacuna, a space.

Laennec's cirrhosis, (lā-neks), a type of liver cirrhosis associated with alcohol misuse. *See* CIRRHOSIS.

laevulose, (lē-vū-lōs), obsolete term for fructose.

lalling, repetitive sounds made by infants, individuals with severe learning disabilities and in some mental health problems. Often substituting the letter 'l' or 'r'.

lambdoid, (lam′-doyd), like Greek letter λ, chiefly applied to the suture between the occipital and parietal bones.

lambliasis, (lam-bli-ā-sis), *see* GIARDIASIS.

lamella (*pl.* **lamellae**), **1.** thin sheet of tissue, such as bone in haversian systems. **2.** drug-impregnated gelatin sheet placed under the eyelid, used to administer eye drugs.

lamina, (lam′-i-na), thin layer.

laminar flow, a method of controlling airflow as part of reducing infection risk in special units, e.g. those for immunosuppressed individuals.

laminectomy, (lam-in-ek′-to-mi), excision of some of the vertebral laminae to gain access to the spinal cord, or to relieve pressure on nerve roots as in prolapsed intervertebral disc.

LAN, in computing abbreviation for **local area network**. A single-site network where all the participating computers are linked directly together to share files and resources.

Lancefield's groups, a serological classification of streptococci into groups A–S according to their antigenic characteristics.

lancet, a sharp-pointed two-edged surgical knife.

lancinating, (lan-si-nā′-ting), cutting or tearing, often applied to pain.

Landrey's disease, *see* GUILLAIN–BARRÉ SYNDROME.

Landsteiner's groups, (lan-stī-nerz), the ABO blood group system. *See* BLOOD GROUPS.

Langerhans' cells, dendritic cells. Antigen presenting cells found in the epidermis. They are part of the biological barrier formed by the skin and are concerned with protecting the body from microorganisms that breach the chemical and physical barriers.

Langerhans' islets, small areas of specialized cells in the pancreas, concerned with its endocrine function. The four types of cells are: **1.** alpha which produce glucagon; **2.** beta which produce insulin and amylin; **3.** delta which produce somatostatin or growth hormone inhibiting hormone. **4.** other cells which produce regulatory pancreatic polypeptide.

language, 1. words and their use in communication. *Body l.*: non-verbal communication by posture, gesture and expression. **2.** the form in which computer programs are written. There are many different programming languages, e.g. BASIC.

lanolin, purified wool-fat. Used as the basis for various ointments.

lanugo, *(lan-ū'-go),* fine downy hair that covers the fetus from around the fifth month of gestation, it has mostly disappeared by term.

laparoscopy, *(lap-ar-os-ko-pi),* endoscopic examination of, or surgery to, the abdominal/pelvic organs using a laparoscope passed via small incisions in the abdominal wall. A variety of surgical procedures can be performed; biopsy, aspiration of cysts, division of adhesions, tubal ligation, assisted conception procedures, appendicectomy, cholecystectomy, etc. The technique minimizes the trauma of access and reduces morbidity and the length of hospital stay.

laparotomy, *(lap-ar-ot'-o-mi),* opening the abdominal cavity. Usually for investigation.

laryngeal, *(la-rin-jē-al),* relating to the larynx. *L. mask*: increasingly used in place of an endotracheal tube during a general anaesthetic.

laryngectomy, *(lar-in-jek'-to-mi),* removal of the larynx.

laryngismus stridulus, *(lar-in-jiz-mus stri-du-lus),* sudden laryngeal spasm with closure of the glottis. It is characterized by crowing sounds, respiratory distress and a period of apnoea. Associated with inflammation, foreign bodies and hypocalcaemia of childhood rickets.

laryngitis, *(la-rin-jī-tis),* inflammation of the larynx, it may be acute or chronic. Associated with a cold, smoking and irritating fumes.

laryngology, *(la-rin-gol-o-ji),* science of anatomy and diseases of the larynx.

laryngopharynx, *(la-rin-gō-fa-rinks),* the lower part of the pharynx.

laryngoscopy, *(la-rin-gos-ko-pi),* examination of the larynx, either indirectly with a mirror or with a laryngoscope which is also used to facilitate endotracheal intubation.

laryngospasm, *(la-rin'-gō-spazm),* muscular contraction of the larynx causing an obstruction to air flow.

laryngostenosis, *(la-rin'-gō-ste-nō'-sis),* narrowing of the glottic aperture.

laryngotomy, *(la-rin-got-o-mi),* opening into the larynx. *See* TRACHEOSTOMY.

laryngotracheitis, *(la-rin-gō-trā-ke-ī-tis),* inflammation of the larynx and trachea.

laryngotracheobronchitis, *(la-rin'-gō-tra'-ke-ō-bron-kī'-tis),* croup. An acute viral infection of the upper respiratory tract which may be complicated by secondary bacterial infection. Particularly serious when it occurs in small children.

larynx, *(la-rinks),* muscular cartilaginous structure situated at the upper end of the trachea containing the vocal cords. The organ of the voice.

LASER, acronym for **light amplification by stimulated emission of**

radiation. A device which produces an extremely intense beam of light used in the treatment of conditions as diverse as detached retina and cervical intraepithelial neoplasia.

Lassa fever, a serious viral haemorrhagic fever occurring in West Africa and elsewhere. Mortality is as high as 50%.

Lasser's paste, ointment containing zinc oxide, salicylic acid, starch and soft paraffin. Used in the treatment of hyperkeratotic and scaling skin conditions.

latency stage, a psychosexual developmental stage lasting from childhood to puberty. The need for sexual gratification is minimal.

latent, not visible, lying hidden for a time. *L. heat*: the heat absorbed or released in a change of state without an alteration in temperature, e.g. water into steam and vice versa. *L. period*: incubation time.

lateral, 1. on one side. **2.** a position removed from the midline.

latex sensitivity, an allergy to latex, present in some medical gloves and other items, such as urinary catheters. A particular problem for healthcare workers.

laughing gas, nitrous oxide.

lavage, *(lav-ahj),* washing out, such as gastric or peritoneal.

laxative, an aperient. Used to prevent or treat constipation.

lead (Pb), a soft heavy metal whose salts are poisonous. *L. poisoning*: may be due to exposure to high levels of lead in water or food (from lead pipes and cooking pots), and in children as a result of eating lead paint. It causes colic, anaemia, neuropathy, encephalopathy and a characteristic blue line in the gum. Abnormally high levels of lead have been linked to the discharges of lead into the environment by vehicle exhaust.

learning, 1. process of increasing skills and knowledge by experience or study. **2.** the actual skill or knowledge gained through study. *L. disability*: reduced ability to understand new or complicated material, experiencing problems with learning new skills, and in some instances being unable to function independently. The disability is present during childhood and affects development on a permanent basis.

lecithins, *(les'-i-thin),* a group of phospholipids found mainly in cell membranes. They are also present in surfactant.

leech, *Hirudo medicinalis,* an aquatic, bloodsucking worm used to suck blood from localized areas.

left ventricular assist device (LVAD), mechanical pump used to augment the output of blood from the left side of the heart. Used short-term to support critically ill patients, those waiting for transplant, or to allow the heart to recover.

leg, the lower limb from ankle to knee. *L. ulcer: see* ARTERIAL ULCER, VENOUS ULCER. *White l.*: condition caused by venous thrombosis. *See* PHLEGMASIA.

Legionella pneumophila, *(lē-ji-on-el-a nū-mō-fil-a),* small Gram-negative bacterium which causes Legionnaires' disease.

Legionnaires' disease, a serious pneumonia caused by *Legionella pneumophila*. It tends to occur in epidemics, often associated with an infected water supply in hotels, hospitals and other public buildings, but isolated cases also occur. Apart from the respiratory illness there may be gastrointestinal problems, electrolyte imbalance and renal involvement.

legumes, pulse vegetables; peas, beans, lentils. A major source of protein.

leiomyoma, *(li-ō-mī-ō´-ma),* benign tumour of smooth muscle, such as in the stomach or uterus.

Leishman–Donovanbodies, intracellular parasites (*Leishmania donovani*) found in the monocyte–macrophage system of individuals with leishmaniasis.

Leishmania, genus of flagellated protozoon *Leishmania donovani* responsible for several types of leishmaniasis.

leishmaniasis, *(lēsh-ma-nē-a-sis),* infection caused by one of the *Leishmania* parasites (protozoa) such as kala-azar or oriental sore.

lens, 1. avascular, biconvex, transparent structure of the eye which alters shape to focus light on to the retina. **2.** transparent material; glass or plastic used in optical equipment or to correct refractive errors in spectacles or contact lenses.

lenticular, 1. pertaining to a lens. **2.** lens-shaped.

lentigo, a freckle. *L. maligna*: a skin neoplasm, a type of melanoma.

leontiasis ossea, *(lē-on-tē-ā-sis os-sē-a),* lion face, enlargement and deformity of the face in conditions such as leprosy.

leproma (*pl.* **lepromata**), *(lep-rō-ma),* granulomatous cutaneous eruption of leprosy.

leprosy, an infection caused by the acid-fast bacillus *Mycobacterium leprae*. It affects the skin, nerves, mucous membranes and bone to cause tissue destruction and deformity. Common in tropical areas, but is seen in cooler regions such as Europe. Spread occurs through prolonged intimate contact and treatment is with specific antimicrobial drugs.

leptomeningitis, *(lep-tō-men-in-jī-tis),* inflammation of the inner meninges.

Leptospira, *(lep-tō-spī-ra),* a genus of spirochaete bacteria which cause leptospirosis. *L. interrogans* serotype *icterohaemorrhagiae* causes Weil's disease in humans and *L. interrogans* serotype *canicola* infects dogs and pigs. *See* CANICOLA FEVER, WEIL'S DISEASE.

leptospirosis, *(lep-tō-spī-rō´-sis),* the group of diseases caused by bacteria of the *Leptospira* genus.

lesbianism, sexual attraction between women.

Lesch–Nyhan disease, X-linked recessive genetic disorder of purine metabolism which leads to poor physical development, learning disabilities, self-mutilation of fingers and lips and impaired kidney function.

lesion, any injury or morbid change in the structure or function of a tissue/organ.

lethargy, drowsiness, apathy, indifference or sluggishness.

leucine, *(lū-sēn),* an essential (indispensable) amino acid.

leucocyte, *(lū-kō-sīt),* general name for white blood cells. *See* BLOOD, BLOOD COUNT.

leucocytolysis, *(lū-kō-sī-tol-i-sis),* destruction of leucocytes.

leucocytosis, *(lū-kō-sī-tō-sis),* an increase in the number of white cells in the peripheral blood, usually neutrophils.

leucodepleted, describes donated blood from which the leucocytes have been removed.

leucoderma, *(lū-kō-der-ma),* see VITILIGO.

leucoerythroblastosis, *(lū-kō-e-rith´-rō-blas-tō´-sis),* a condition where immature red cells and granulocytes appear in the blood; causes include neoplastic infiltration of the bone marrow and myelofibrosis.

leucoma, *(lū-kō-ma)*, a white spot present on the cornea.

leuconychia, *(lū-kō-nik-i-a)*, white marks on the finger nails.

leucopenia, *(lū-kō-pē-ni-a)*, decrease in the number of white cells in the peripheral blood.

leucopheresis, *(lū-kō-fe-rē-sis)*, separation and collection of white cells from donated blood (remaining blood is returned to the donor). The white cells so obtained are given by transfusion to severely neutropenic patients.

leucopoiesis, *(lū-kō-poy-ē-sis)*, formation of white blood cells. Regulated by several cytokines and colony-stimulating factors.

leucorrhoea, *(lū-kō-rē-a)*, white vaginal discharge. Normal unless it becomes copious, malodorous or abnormal in colour. May be caused by infection.

leucotomy, *(lū-kot-o-mi)*, transection of nerve fibres within the brain.

leukaemia, *(lū-kē-mi-a)*, a neoplastic disease of haemopoietic tissue characterized by an abnormal proliferation of immature white cells. This results in disruption of haemopoiesis with anaemia, thrombocytopenia with bleeding and neutropenia with infection. Factors associated with the development of leukaemia include: ionizing radiation, cytotoxic chemotherapy, retroviruses, chemicals and genetic predisposition, such as Down's syndrome. Leukaemias are classified by the cell type involved, its course and duration. *Acute l.:* onset is rapid and early immature cells are produced (blast cells), commonly of the lymphoid and myeloid series. Acute leukaemias include acute lymphoblastic L. (ALL) in children and acute myeloblastic L. (AML) in adults. *Chronic l.:* here the onset is insidious and the cells produced are more mature, commonly lymphocytes and granulocytes. Chronic forms can become acute with blast cell proliferation. Chronic leukaemias include chronic lymphocytic L. and chronic granulocytic (myeloid) L., both of which affect adults. Less common leukaemias include: monocytic, eosinophilic, basophilic and hairy cell. Management depends upon the type of cell involved, whether it is acute or chronic, and the aim of treatment, which may be remission or palliation. Treatments include: bone marrow transplant, chemotherapy, interferon-alpha radiotherapy, corticosteroids and supportive measures such as antimicrobial drugs, blood component transfusion and protective isolation.

leukoplakia, hyperplasia of squamous epithelium. Thick raised white patches occur on the tongue, vulva and in other sites. Considered to be premalignant.

leukotrienes, regulatory lipids derived from arachidonic acid. They act as signalling molecules and mediators of the inflammatory response and are involved in some allergic conditions.

levator, *(le-vā'-tur)*, an instrument or muscle which lifts a part. *L. ani:* muscle of the pelvic floor which supports the pelvic viscera.

Leydig cells, *(lā-dig)*, interstitial cells in the testes which produce androgens, e.g. testosterone. *See* INTERSTITIAL.

libido, *(li-bē-dō)*, drive or impulses which result in some action, usually applied to sexual desires.

lice, pl. of louse.

lichen, *(lī-ken),* a group of skin diseases characterized by aggregations of papular skin lesions.

lichenification, the abnormal process which produces irregular areas of thickened skin.

lid lag, jerky movement of the upper eyelid, may be a feature of exophthalmos.

lien, *(lĕ-en),* the spleen.

lienculus, *(lĕ-en'-kū-lus),* an accessory spleen.

life events, sociological term for the major and other important events in an individual's life, e.g. death of a spouse, marriage or job loss.

ligament, band of tough fibrous tissue which connects bones or other structures together. Provides strength and support at joints.

ligand, specific signalling chemicals, such as hormones, cytokines or neurotransmitters, that bind to cell membrane receptors to influence cell function in a variety of ways. Many drugs are designed to mimic the naturally occurring ligand.

ligation, *(li-gā'-shon),* application of a ligature. *Tubal l.:* female sterilization.

ligatures, *(lig'-a-tūrs),* various materials; silk, catgut, synthetics, fascia and wire, used to tie off vessels and stitch tissues. *See* SUTURE.

light adaptation, adjustments required by the eye to facilitate vision in bright light, e.g. chemical changes to photosensitive retinal pigments. The pupils constrict, the breakdown of rhodopsin reduces retinal sensitivity and cone activity increases.

lightening, relief of upper abdominal pressure experienced in the last weeks of pregnancy when the fetal presenting part enters the pelvis.

lightning pains, shooting, cutting pains felt in some cases of tabes dorsalis.

Likert scale, scale used in a questionnaire where participants are asked to indicate their level of agreement of a statement: strongly agree, agree, unsure, disagree and strongly disagree.

limbic system, a diffuse collection of nuclei and fibres in the cerebral hemispheres. Part of the 'primitive' brain, they influence feelings and emotions.

limbus, a border. Junction of cornea and sclera.

lime, calcium oxide. *L. water:* a solution of calcium hydroxide in water.

liminal, *(lim-i-nal),* the lowest threshold at which stimuli can be perceived.

linctus, a syrup-based medicine, e.g. cough linctus.

linea, *(lin-e-a),* a line. *L. alba:* the white line down the centre of the abdomen. *L. albicantes:* white streaks on the abdominal skin due to distension from pregnancy or new growth. *See* STRIAE GRAVIDARUM. *L. nigra:* dark pigmented line on the lower abdomen seen in some pregnant women.

linear, pertaining to a line. *L. accelerator:* a mega-voltage machine used to accelerate electrons and produce high-energy X-rays. May be used in radiotherapy to treat deep-seated tumours.

lingual, relating to the tongue.

liniment, a liquid preparation for application to the skin with friction.

linoleic acid, *(lin-ō-lay-ik),* a polyunsaturated essential fatty acid.

linolenic acid, *(lin-ō-len-ik),* a polyunsaturated essential fatty acid.

lipaemia, excess fat (especially cholesterol) in the blood.

lipases, *(lī-pā-zes),* enzymes which split fats into glycerol and fatty acids.

lipids, a large group of fat-like organic molecules which include: steroids (e.g. cholesterol), triglycerides (triacylglycerols), phospholipids, lipoproteins, fat soluble vitamins and prostaglandins, etc.

lipoatrophy, (*li-pō-a-trō-fi*), loss of subcutaneous fat. A complication which may arise at sites of insulin injections.

lipochondrodystrophy, (*li-pō-kon-drō-dis-tro-fi*), see GARGOYLISM.

lipogenesis, (*lip-ō-jen-ē-sis*), a process stimulated by insulin, by which glucose and amino acids are converted to triglycerides (triacylglycerols) prior to storage in adipose tissue.

lipolysis, (*li-pō-li-sis*), a process stimulated by hormones such as cortisol, by which stored triglycerides (triacylglycerols) are released from adipose tissue to provide energy.

lipoma, (*li-pō-ma*), a benign tumour of fat cells.

lipoprotein, (*li-pō-prō-tēn*), lipids combined with an apoprotein in the liver prior to release into the blood where they transport triglycerides (triacylglycerols) around the body. *Very low density l.* (VLDL) and *low density l.* (LDL): increased levels are associated with arterial disease. *See* HYPERLIPIDAEMIA. *High density l.* (HDL): considered to have a protective role.

liposarcoma, (*li-pō-sah-kō-ma*), a rare malignant tumour of fat cells.

liquor, (*li-kor*), watery fluid. *L. amnii:* see AMNIOTIC FLUID.

Listeria, a genus of bacteria. *L. monocytogenes:* causes septicaemia, intrauterine or perinatal infections and meningitis.

listeriosis, (*lis-ter-i-ō-sis*), infection with *Listeria.* It may be transmitted via contaminated soil, contact with infected animals, or by the consumption of unpasteurized foods such as soft cheeses which may be infected. Those particularly suscept-

ible to infection include: young infants, older people, debilitated people, pregnant women and the immunosuppressed. Infection during pregnancy may cause a flu-like illness in the woman, miscarriage, stillbirth, premature labour and septicaemia and meningitis in the neonate with a high mortality rate.

literature review, thorough and comprehensive examination of the papers relevant to a topic. Research methods and results are analysed and presented critically. The review should state how the search was undertaken, e.g. bibliographical databases such as CINAHL.

lithiasis, (*lith-ī-a-sis*), formation of stone.

lithium (Li), (*lith-ē-um*), a metallic element. *L. carbonate:* used in the treatment of bipolar disorders.

litholapaxy, (*lith-ol-a-paks'-ē*), operation for crushing a stone in the bladder and removing the fragments at the same time.

lithopaedion, (*lith-ō-pēd-ion*), a fetus that has died and been retained becomes calcified.

lithotomy, (*lith-ot'-o-mi*), opening the bladder to remove stones. *L. position:* the patient is supine with hips and knees flexed. The hips are abducted with the feet supported. To prevent injury it is essential that the legs are raised and lowered together. Maintaining privacy and patient dignity is a vital nursing role.

lithotripsy, (*lith-ō-trip-si*), technique which utilizes shock waves to disintegrate renal and biliary calculi without the need for surgery.

lithotripter, (*lith-ō-trip-ter*), a machine which produces shock waves. *See* LITHOTRIPSY.

lithotrite, (*lith-ō-trīt*), an instrument passed via the urethra which is used to crush stones in the bladder.

lithotrity, (lith-ŏ-trĭ-ti), operation of crushing a stone in the bladder.

litigation, civil proceedings.

litmus, a pigment used as an indicator for acidity/alkalinity. L. paper: blue paper turns red in acid, and red paper turns blue in alkali.

litre (l/L), a unit of volume. Based on the volume of a cube (10 cm × 10 cm × 10 cm) it can be divided into a smaller unit of volume, the millilitre (ml).

Little's disease, spastic diplegia present at birth. Congenital disease caused by cerebral atrophy or agenesis.

liver, largest gland of the body it weighs 1.2–1.5 kg and occupies the right upper abdomen. It is vital to homeostasis and its functions include: metabolism of nutrients, protein synthesis, detoxification, storage of vitamins and minerals and breakdown of red cells with the production of bile. With all these functions occurring the liver is the site of considerable heat generation. L. function tests (LFTs): a series of blood tests used to assess liver function which include: serum bilirubin, alkaline phosphatase, alanine aminotransferase, aspartate aminotransferase, gamma glutamyl transferase and serum proteins.

livid, blue-grey in colour.

living will, see ADVANCE DIRECTIVE.

LMP, abbreviation for last menstrual period.

Loa loa, one of the nematode parasites causing loiasis (filariasis).

lobar, pertaining to a lobe.

lobe, rounded division of an organ.

lobectomy, (lŏ-bek'-tŏ-mi), excision of a lobe.

lobule, subdivision of a lobe, such as in the liver or a small lobe.

localize, 1. contain disease process within an area. **2.** determine the site of the disease process.

localized, limited to a certain area; not widespread.

lochia, (lo-kē-a), vaginal discharge following childbirth or abortion. It has three stages; 1. rubra (red/brown), 1. serosa (pink) and 1. alba (white).

locomotor, pertaining to movement, such as muscles. L. ataxia: abnormal gait and loss of proprioception occurring in tabes dorsalis. See TABES DORSALIS.

loculated, divided into many cavities.

locus (pl. loci), specific site, such as a gene on a chromosome.

loiasis, (lō-i-as-is), infestation with the parasitic nematode Loa loa. A form of filariasis.

loin, the lateral portion of the back between the thorax and pelvis.

long sight, hypermetropia.

long-term care, health and social care required over a period of time by a person with a chronic condition.

long-term memory, the part of memory that deals with retention of information for longer periods. It is potentially permanent and has a greater capacity than short-term memory.

longtitudinal study, research study that collects data on more than one occasion, e.g. may study a cohort of people over many years.

lordosis, (lor-dō-sis), an exaggerated forward, convex curve of the lumbar spine. (Figure 45).

lotion, a medicinal solution for external use.

loupe, magnifying lens used in ophthalmology.

louse, see PEDICULUS.

low birth weight, birth weight below 2.5 kg regardless of gestation period. Either small-for-dates or pre-term.

lower motor neurone, that part of the descending pyramidal motor tract from the anterior horn of the spinal cord to the neuromuscular junction

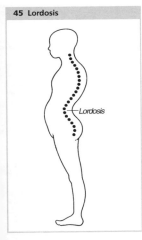

45 Lordosis

Lordosis

of the voluntary muscle fibres. *L. m. n. disease*: any disease affecting lower motor fibres. Characterized by flaccid paralysis and muscle wasting.

lower reference nutrient intake (LRNI), the amount of a nutrient (protein, mineral or vitamin) which is sufficient for only a few individuals, with low requirements, within a group.

lower uterine segment, area developed from the uterine isthmus during pregnancy. It thins and dilates during labour as it is stretched by the strong muscular contractions of the upper segment.

lozenge, a sweetened medicated tablet of various shapes which is kept in the mouth until dissolved.

LRNI, abbreviation for **lower reference nutrient intake**.

LSD, lysergic acid diethylamide. It has hallucinogenic properties and is subject to criminal misuse.

lubb-dupp, describe the heart sounds. The first is heard when the atrioventricular valves close, and the second on closure of the aortic and pulmonary valves.

lubricant, any substance which reduces friction, such as an oil. Also describe faecal softenerss (laxatives).

Ludwig's angina, *see* ANGINA.

lumbago (*lum-bā-go*), pain in the lumbar region. May be muscular in origin or due to a prolapsed intervertebral disc.

lumbar, pertaining to the region of the loins. *L. nerves*: five pairs of spinal nerves (L1–L5). *L. plexus*: the spinal nerves L1–L3 and part of L4. *L. puncture*: a diagnostic procedure where a needle is introduced into the subarachnoid space (between lumbar vertebrae 3, 4 or 5) to obtain samples of CSF and to record pressure using a manometer. *L. sympathectomy*: operation to remove the sympathetic chain in the lumbar region. *L. vertebrae*: five bones. They are the largest of the vertebrae, a fact that reflects their weight-bearing role.

lumbosacral, pertaining to the lumbar vertebrae and sacrum.

lumen, (*lū-men*), the cavity inside a tube.

lumpectomy, removal of a lump, usually refers to a breast cancer where the surrounding breast tissue is preserved, only the lump being removed.

lunate, a carpal or wrist bone.

Lund and Browder's chart, a chart for calculating the percentage of body surface area affected by a burn in infants and children. *See* WALLACE'S RULE OF NINES.

lungs, two conical organs of respiration situated in the thorax.

Arranged in lobes they receive air via the trachea, main bronchi and smaller airways which communicate with tiny air sacs or alveoli where gaseous exchange occurs (Figure 46).

lunula, (lū'-nū-la), white crescent at the root of the nail.

lupus erythematosus, (e-rith-em-a-tō-sus), see SYSTEMIC LUPUS ERYTHEMATOSUS.

lupus vulgaris, (lū-pus vul-ga-ris), tuberculosis affecting the skin.

luteal, pertaining to the corpus luteum. *L. phase*: that part of the ovarian cycle occurring after ovulation. Days 14–28 in a 28-day cycle, its length remains constant at around 14 days irrespective of overall cycle length.

luteinizing hormone (LH), (lū-ti-nī-zing), a gonadotrophin secreted by the anterior pituitary. In females high levels midway through the menstrual cycle cause ovulation and formation of the corpus luteum. In males the same hormone, known as interstitial cell-stimulating hormone (ICSH), stimulates Leydig cells in the testes to produce testosterone.

luteotrophin, (lū-tē-ō-trō-fin), see PROLACTIN.

luteus, (lū'-tē-us), Latin word for yellow. See MACULA LUTEA and CORPUS LUTEUM.

luxation, dislocation of a joint.

lying-in, old term for the early postnatal period or puerperium.

Lyme disease, infection caused by the spirochaete *Borrelia burgdorferi*. It is transmitted to humans by tick bites and is characterized by rash, joint pains, headache, pyrexia and occasionally meningitis. First identified in Lyme USA.

lymph, fluid in the lymphatic vessels derived from tissue fluid, similar in composition to blood plasma. *L. node*: small collections of lymphoid tissue situated at intervals along the lymphatic vessels with aggregations at strategic points, e.g. axilla. They filter the lymph and remove extraneous particles such as microorganisms and malignant cells. In addition they are a site for T and B lymphocyte proliferation and antibody production.

lymphadenitis, (lim-fad-en-ī-tis), inflammation of the lymph nodes.

lymphadenopathy, (lim-fad-en-o'-pathi), a disease of lymph nodes. See PERSISTENT GENERALIZED LYMPHADENOPATHY.

lymphangiectasis, (lim-fan-jē-ek'-ta-sis), dilated state of lymphatic vessels.

lymphangiography, (lim-fan-jē-og'-raf-ē), See LYMPHOGRAPHY.

lymphangioma, (lim-fan-jē-ō'-ma), tumour composed of lymphatic vessels.

lymphangioplasty, (lim-fan-jē-ō-pla'-sti), an operation for the relief of lymphatic obstruction.

lymphangitis, (lim-fan-jī-tis), inflammation of lymphatic vessels.

lymphatic, (lim-fat-ik), pertaining to lymph. *L. system*: the lymph vessels, nodes, tissues and organs, e.g. the spleen.

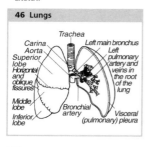

46 Lungs

Trachea

Carina
Aorta
Superior lobe
Horizontal and oblique fissures

Left main bronchus
Left pulmonary artery and veins in the root of the lung

Middle lobe
Inferior lobe

Bronchial artery
Visceral (pulmonary) pleura

lymphoblasts, *(lim-fō-blasts),* immature cells present in the blood and marrow in acute lymphoblastic leukaemia. *See* LEUKAEMIA.

lymphocytes, *(lim-fō-sīts),* a group of white blood cells found in the blood and lymphoid tissues, such as the spleen. They may be large or small. *Bl.*: part of humoral immunity, they become plasma cells which produce antibodies (immunoglobulins). *Tl.*: involved in cell-mediated immune responses such as transplant rejection.

lymphocytopenia, *(lim-fō-sī-tō-pē'-nē-a),* reduction in lymphocyte numbers in the blood.

lymphocytosis, *(lim-fō-sī-tō-sis),* increase in the number of lymphocytes in the blood.

lymphoedema, *(lim-fō-dē-ma),* oedema associated with an obstruction to lymphatic drainage. May be structural (primary) or secondary obstruction, e.g. following surgery for breast cancer.

lymphogranuloma venereum, *(limf-ō-gran-ū-lō-ma ven-ēr-ē-um),* sexually transmitted infection caused by *Chlamydia trachomatis.* It is characterized by genital ulcers and lymph node enlargement. Occurs worldwide but mainly in tropical regions. *See* CHLAMYDIA.

lymphography, X-ray examination of the lymphatic system. Largely replaced by computed tomography.

lymphoid, *(lim-foyd),* relating to the lymph. *L. tissue:* collections of tissue similar in structure to lymph nodes but found in sites other than the lymphatics, e.g. spleen, tonsils, thymus, bone marrow, liver, small bowel and appendix.

lymphokines, general term for cytokines produced by activated T lymphocytes. They function during the immune response as intercellular mediators.

lymphoma, *(lim-fō-ma),* a group of malignant tumours arising from lymphoid tissue. They are classified as either Hodgkin's disease or non-Hodgkin's lymphoma (NHL) which is classified as an AIDS–defining condition. The presenting features include: lymph node enlargement, splenomegaly, hepatomegaly and systemic effects, such as weight loss, night sweats and fever, etc. Treatment depends on the type and stage but includes radiotherapy, chemotherapy, interferon-alpha, bone marrow transplant and supportive measures, such as blood product transfusion and antibiotics. *See* BURKITT'S LYMPHOMA.

lymphosarcoma, *(lim-fō-sah-kō-ma),* old term for some types of non-Hodgkin's lymphoma.

lysergic acid, *(lī-ser-jik), see* LSD.

lysine, *(lī-sēn),* an essential (indispensable) amino acid.

lysins, *(lī-sins),* a substance which causes cell lysis.

lysis, *(lī-sis),* **1.** dissolution or breakdown of cells. **2.** decline of a fever.

lysosome, *(lī-sō-sōm),* cellular organelle containing lytic enzymes.

lysozyme, *(lī-sō-zīm),* antibacterial enzyme found in tears, nasal mucus and other secretions.

M

m, abbreviation for **metre.**

maceration, *(mas-er-ā-shon),* the process of softening which occurs when tissues/solids are immersed in liquid.

Mackenrodt's ligaments, *(ma-ken-rotz),* transverse cervical ligaments, a uterine support. *See* CARDINAL LIGAMENTS.

Macmillan nurse, nurses with specialist skills and qualifications in symptom control who provide support for people with cancer, their family and friends in a variety of settings. They also provide specialist information, advice and support for colleagues in the multidisciplinary team.

macrocephalous, *(mak-rō-kef'-a-lus),* having a large head.

macrocheilia, *(mak-rō-kī-li-a),* excessively large lips.

macrocytes, *(mak-rō-sīts),* abnormally large red blood cells.

macrocytic, *(mak-rō-si-tik),* describes a cell which is larger than normal. *M. anaemia:* a type of anaemia characterized by the presence of macrocytes in the peripheral blood. Associated with a deficiency of vitamin B_{12} or folate. *See* MEGALOBLAST.

macrodactyly, *(mak-rō-dak'-ti-li),* enlargement of the fingers or toes.

macroglobulinaemia, *(mak-rō-glob-ū-li-nē-mi-a),* condition where there are large amounts of macroglobulins (high-molecular-weight globulins) in the blood. *Waldenström's m.:* overproduction of monoclonal IgM which results in increased blood viscosity.

macroglossia, *(mak-rō-glos'-i-a),* abnormally large tongue.

macromastia, abnormally developed breasts.

macronutrient, nutrients, such as protein, carbohydrate and fats, required by the body in relatively large amounts.

macrophage, *(ma-kro-fāj),* cells forming part of the monocyte–macrophage system (reticuloendothelial). They are derived from monocytes and have an important defensive role which includes phagocytosis and the immune response. *See* MONOCYTES.

macroscopic, visible to the naked eye.

macula, *(mak-ū-la),* a spot discolouring the skin. *M. densa:* specialized cells of the distal convoluted tubule, part of juxtaglomerular apparatus. *M. lutea:* yellow spot on the retina where vision is most acute. *See* FOVEA.

macular degeneration, loss of retinal pigment cells and damage to the macula. It occurs with ageing and results in loss of colour vision and progressive visual impairment.

macule, *(ma-kūl),* a spot discolouring the skin but not raised above the surface.

maculopapular, *(mak-ū-lō-pap-ū-la),* a rash having both macules and papules.

Madura foot, see MYCOTEMA.

Magendie, foramen of, *(maj-en-di)*, an opening in the roof of the fourth ventricle through which the cere-brospinal fluid passes into the sub-arachnoid space.

magnesium (Mg), a metallic element. Required by the body as a cofactor for many enzyme reactions. Found in bone and as an intracellular cation, its metabolism is closely linked to that of calcium. *M. salts*: used therapeutically as antacids and laxatives.

magnetic resonance imaging (MRI), a non-invasive imaging technique that does not use ionizing radiation. It uses radiofrequency radiation in the presence of a powerful magnetic field to produce high-quality images of the body in any plane.

major histocompatibility complex (MHC), collection of genes that code for the MHC proteins (anti-gens) found as cell surface mol-ecules. These proteins act as 'self' markers and normally the T lym-phocytes learn to recognize them as belonging to the body. They are involved in the rejection of grafted tissue. *See* HUMAN LEUCOCYTE ANTI-GENS.

Makaton, a type of sign language.

mal, sickness. *M. de mer*: sea sickness.

malabsorption, an inability to absorb nutrients in sufficient quantities from the small intestine. Causes include: enzyme deficiency of cystic fibrosis, coeliac disease and Crohn's disease.

malacia, *(mal-ā-she-a),* pathological softening.

maladaptation, an abnormal response to a situation or change. It may re-late to social interactions or to a response to stress which results in ill health, e.g. tension headaches, alter-ations in blood chemistry.

maladjustment, not in line, as with a badly set bone. In psychology, poor-ly adapted to circumstances.

malaise, a general feeling of illness or discomfort.

malar, *(mā′-lar),* relating to the cheek-bone.

malaria, a serious disease caused by a protozoa of the genus *Plasmodium*, e.g. *P. falciparum*, which is spread by the bite of the anopheline mosquito. It is generally a disease of the tropics but does occur in other areas.

malformation, a deformity of struc-ture.

malignant, virulent and dangerous. *M. tumour*: a cancerous growth, which in the absence of effective treatment will spread locally and to distant sites (metastatic spread) eventually killing the individual. *M. hypertension*: a form of accelerated severe hypertension associated with renal failure, headaches and papill-oedema. *M. pustule*: skin lesion seen in anthrax.

malingering, shamming sickness.

malleolus, *(mal-le′-ō-lus),* the projec-tion of the ankle-bone. The internal malleolus is at the lower extremity of the tibia. The external one is at the lower extremity of the fibula.

mallet finger, deformed finger with flexion of distal phalanx.

malleus, a hammer-shaped bone of the middle ear. *See* EAR.

Mallory–Weiss syndrome, unusual cause of haematemesis where per-sistent vomiting causes small tears in the gastro-oesophageal mucosa.

malnutrition, any disorder caused by a diet which is defective in either quantity or content, malabsorption or an inability to utilize nutrients.

malocclusion, *(mal-o-klū-shon),* bad contact between the masticating sur-faces of the upper and lower teeth.

malpractice, improper or injurious medical or nursing treatment. Professional practice which falls short of accepted standards and causes harm. It may involve unethical behaviour, negligence, abuse or criminal activities.

malpresentation, any presentation, other than the vertex, of the fetus at the onset of labour.

Malta fever, see BRUCELLA.

maltase, an enzyme present in the intestine which converts maltose to glucose.

maltose, a disaccharide consisting of two glucose molecules.

malunion, faulty union of divided tissue, usually applied to a fractured bone.

mammae, the breasts, or milk-supplying glands.

mammary, relating to the breasts.

mammography, radiographic examination of the breast. Used to screen for early breast cancers and as a diagnostic aid where physical signs are present.

mammoplasty, plastic surgery of the breasts. May reduce breast size, alter shape or augment size.

mammothermography, (mam-ō-therm-og-ra-fi), breast examination where thermography apparatus is used to detect temperature changes which may indicate the presence of metabolically active new growths.

Manchester repair, see FOTHERGILL'S OPERATION.

mandatory minute volume, in respiratory support that uses mechanical means to impose breaths to augment spontaneous respiration to produce a minimum pre-set minute volume.

mandible, the lower jaw.

manganese (Mn), metallic element required by the body for various enzyme reactions.

mania, pathological combination of elation and energy. Flight of ideas and grandiose delusions are common.

manic-depressive psychosis, (sī-kō-sis), a mental illness when intense excitement alternates with depression. Also known as bipolar depression or bipolar affective disorders.

manipulation, skilled use of the hands to bring about a positive change, e.g. reducing a hernia.

Mann–Whitney test, in statistics, a non-parametric alternative to Student's t-test for independent groups.

mannitol, a carbohydrate which is not metabolized by the body. Used as an osmotic diuretic for forced diuresis or to reduce cerebral oedema.

manometer, an instrument for measuring the pressure of gases and liquids.

Mantoux test, (man-too), a skin test used pre-BCG or for the diagnosis of tuberculosis in which old tuberculin or PPD is injected intradermally; cf. HEAF TEST.

manual handling, the moving, lifting or supporting a load subject to legal regulations.

manubrium sterni, (man-ū'-bri-um ster'-nē), the uppermost part of the sternum.

manus, Latin for hand.

maple syrup disease, an inherited error of metabolism where an enzyme, required for the breakdown of certain amino acids, is deficient. They are excreted in the urine, giving rise to a characteristic odour of maple syrup. Leads to neurological problems and learning disability.

marasmus, a severe protein-energy malnutrition, caused by insufficient protein and calories in the diet. It affects young children who become very thin with muscle wasting and have a distended abdomen and diarrhoea. Cf. KWASHIORKOR.

marble bone disease, see OSTEOPETROSIS.

Marburg virus disease, a serious viral haemorrhagic fever usually occurring in Africa. It has a very high mortality rate. *See* EBOLA VIRUS DISEASE.

Marfan's syndrome, genetic disease affecting connective tissue. There is congenital heart disease, arachnodactyly with muscle hypotonia and lax ligaments, occasionally excessive height and abnormalities of the iris. *see* ARACHNODACTYLY.

marihuana, marijuana, *(ma-rū-ah-na)*, *see* CANNABIS.

marrow, *see* BONE MARROW. *M. puncture*: aspiration of haemopoietic tissue for examination.

Marshall–Marchetti–Krantz procedure, operation to relieve stress incontinence.

marsupialization, *(mar-sū-pē-al-ī-zā-shon)*, operative procedure where a cyst is drained and its edges sutured to form a patent opening.

masculinization, development of male secondary characteristics in the female.

Maslow's hierarchy of needs, a list (pyramid) of human needs which range from the basic physiological such as food and shelter to self-actualization (Figure 47).

masochism, *(mas-ō-kizm)*, deriving pleasure which is frequently of a sexual nature from experiencing physical or mental pain.

massage, 1. a technique of manipulation, rubbing and kneading, etc. which stimulates circulation and metabolism in the tissues. **2.** a complementary therapy. Gentle stroking, kneading or muscle manipulation to promote relaxation. *Cardiac m.: see* CARDIAC.

mass number, the total mass of protons and neutrons in an atom.

mass reflex, condition seen in individuals with spinal cord transection.

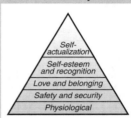

47 Maslow's hierarchy of needs

There is muscle contraction, sweating, bowel and bladder emptying and hypertension. Causes include: stress, overdistended bowel or skin stimulation.

mast cells, basophils which have migrated into the tissues. They bind to immunoglobulins (IgE) prior to releasing chemicals involved in anaphylactic reactions and inflammation.

mastalgia, *(mas-tal-ji-a)*, pain in the breast.

mastectomy, *(mas-tek-to-mi)*, surgical removal of the breast, usually for tumour. Various types include: radical, modified radical and simple. *See* LUMPECTOMY.

mastication, *(mas-tik-ā'-shon)*, chewing.

mastitis, *(mas-tī'-tis)*, inflammation of the breast.

mastodynia, *(mas-tō-din-i-a)*, pain in the breast.

mastoid, literally, breast-like. *M. process*: the projecting portion of the temporal bone behind the ear; it contains numerous air spaces (m. cells) which communicate with the m. antrum.

mastoidectomy, *(mas-toyd-ek'-to-mi)*, excision of the inflamed mastoid cells.

205

mastoiditis, *(mas-toyd-i'-tis),* inflammation of the mastoid antrum and cells.

masturbation, non-coital stimulation of the genitalia to produce orgasm.

materia medica, science dealing with the origin, action and dosage of drugs.

maternal, pertaining to the mother. *M. mortality: see* MORTALITY.

matriarchy, *(mai-tri-ah-ki),* a community or social structure where a female (wife, mother or daughter) inherits, dominates and controls.

matrix, foundation substance in which tissue cells are embedded.

matter, any substance. *Grey m.:* nerve cells and unmyelinated nerve fibres of the central nervous system. *White m.:* myelinated nerve fibres of the central nervous system.

maturation, ripening: the process of becoming fully developed. The last stage of wound healing; scar is reformed, the wound is strengthened and the scar gradually fades and shrinks.

maxilla, the upper jaw bone.

maxillary, pertaining to the maxilla, such as the m. sinus or antrum; a large paranasal sinus situated within the maxilla.

maxillofacial, *(maks-il-ō-fā'-shal),* pertaining to the maxilla and face.

McBurney's point, a point one-third of the way between the right anterior superior iliac spine and the umbilicus. The site of maximum tenderness in acute appendicitis.

Meals on Wheels, the provision of ready-cooked meals or frozen meals throughout the week for disabled and/or older clients in their own homes. An element of community care for which a charge is usually made.

mean, the midway point. *Arithmetic m.:* the figure calculated by dividing the total set of values by the number of items in that group. The average. *See* CENTRAL TENDENCY STATISTIC. *M. cell haemoglobin (MCH):* the amount of haemoglobin contained in an individual red cell. *M. cell haemoglobin concentration (MCHC):* an estimation of the amount of haemoglobin, in grams, contained in 100 ml of packed red cells. *M. cell volume (MCV):* the mean volume of a red cell.

measles, morbilli. An acute viral disease of children which is highly contagious. Spread by droplets, it has an incubation period of around 10 days. The disease presents with a cold-like illness, sore eyes, Koplik's spots and a maculopapular rash which becomes blotchy. It may be complicated by a secondary bacterial infection such as otitis media or pneumonia. Other effects include eye damage from corneal ulcers and fits. The mortality rate is very low in previously healthy and well-nourished individuals. Active immunity is offered as part of the routine immunization programme in conjunction with protection against mumps and rubella (MMR), and passive immunity is available in special cases. *German m.: see* RUBELLA.

meatus, *(mē-ā'-tus),* an opening into passage, such as the urinary m. a the urethral opening.

mechanical ventilation, describe the various mechanical method used to support patients when spontaneous respirations have ceased or are inadequate to main tain sufficient gas exchange of oxy gen and carbon dioxide, such a respiratory failure or during gene al anaesthesia.

mechanism of labour, the series forces which act upon the fetus force it through the birth canal an the resistance to these forces whi affects the attitude/position and movement of the fetus.

mechanoreceptors, receptors which are sensitive to mechanical forces. They include: proprioceptors, receptors in the ear, baroreceptors, pressure and touch receptors in the skin and stretch receptors in structures such as the bladder.

Meckel's diverticulum, *(me-kels dī-ver-tik-ū-lum),* a small blind protrusion occasionally found in the ileum. It is an embryonic remnant and may cause obstruction and intussusception or be a site of peptic ulceration (some contain ectopic gastric mucosa).

meconium, *(mē-kō-nē-um),* black-green, sticky material formed in the fetal bowel, it is discharged during the first day or two after birth. *M. aspiration:* aspiration of meconium into the respiratory passages before or during birth. *M. ileus:* bowel obstruction due to extremely viscous meconium associated with cystic fibrosis.

medial, *(mē-di-al),* relating to or close to the middle.

median, *(mē-di-an),* in the middle. In statistics the midway value in a series of scores. *See* CENTRAL TENDENCY STATISTIC. *M. line:* an imaginary longitudinal line running down the centre of the body *M. nerve:* a nerve of the arm. *M. plane:* vertical plane which divides the body into two equal halves.

mediastinal, pertaining to the mediastinum.

mediastinoscopy, *(mē-dé-as-tin-os-ko-pi),* endoscopic examination of the mediastinum and its contents.

mediastinum, *(mē-di-as-tī'-num),* space in the chest between the lungs. It contains the heart, great vessels and oesophagus.

medical, pertaining to medicine. *M. Devices Agency (MDA):* in the UK, a

government agency that works with government, users and manufacturers to ensure that medical devices meet the appropriate safety, quality and efficacy standards, and that they comply with European Union Directives. *M. jurisprudence:* situations where medicine has connections with the law. *See* FORENSIC MEDICINE. *M. model:* in a nursing context, the term signifies that the nursing focus is the medical diagnosis allocated by the doctor.

medicament, any medicinal drug or application.

medicated, impregnated with a medicament.

medication, a substance administered for therapeutic reasons. Taken orally or administered by injection (subcutaneously, intravenously, intramuscularly); also by inhalation, rectally, transdermally and topical application.

medicinal, pertaining to the science of medicine or to a drug.

medicine, 1. science and art of healing, especially as distinguished from surgery. 2. a therapeutic substance.

Medicines Control Agency (MCA), in the UK, a government agency that licenses new drugs. Decisions are based on safety, quality and efficacy.

medicochirurgical, *(me-di-kō-kī-rer-jik-al),* relating to both medicine and surgery.

medicosocial, pertaining to both medical and social factors, e.g. a medical condition caused by social conditions.

meditation, a technique used to reduce stress. The individual learns to modify his or her awareness of outside stimuli to produce a calm relaxed state.

Mediterranean fever, Malta fever, *see* BRUCELLA.

medium, material used to nourish cultures of cells, tissues and microorganisms.

Medline, computerized database of medical science literature.

medulla, Latin for marrow. Term also applied to central part of various organs, e.g. kidney, adrenal gland. *M. oblongata:* the lowest part of the brain stem where it passes through the foramen magnum to become the spinal cord. Contains nerve centres controlling various vital functions, e.g. respiratory and cardiac centres.

medullary, pertaining to the marrow or a medulla. *M. cavity:* marrow containing central cavity of a long bone.

medullated, with an enveloping sheath, such as a nerve fibre surrounded by a myelin sheath.

medulloblastoma, *(med-ūl-ō-blas-tō-ma),* a malignant tumour of the cerebellum, arising from the embryonic cells.

megacephaly, *(meg-a-ke'-fa-li),* an abnormally large head.

megacolon, *(meg-a-kō-lon),* a condition which presents with dilation of the colon and constipation. It may be congenital (*see* HIRSCHSPRUNG'S DISEASE), or acquired.

megakaryocytes, *(meg-a-ka-rē-ō-sīts),* large nucleated bone marrow cells, fragments of which break off to become non-nucleated platelets.

megaloblast, *(meg-a-lō-blast),* large, nucleated red blood cell formed when vitamin B_{12} is deficient.

megaloblastic anaemia, occurs when vitamin B_{12} or folate is deficient in the diet, and when B_{12} is not being absorbed through lack of an intrinsic factor (pernicious anaemia), with small bowel disease and following gastric or small bowel surgery.

megalomania, *(meg-al-ō-mā'-nia),* delusional ideas of personal greatness and grandeur.

Meibomian glands, *(mī-bō'-mi-an),* sebaceous glands of the eyelids. *M. cyst: see* CHALAZION.

Meig's syndrome, *(migs),* hydrothorax and ascites associated with an ovarian fibroma.

meiosis, *(mī-ō-sis),* **1.** the complex nuclear divisions by which a diploid (2n) cell undergoes two divisions to produce haploid (n) gametes. The gametes (oöcytes and spermatozoa) have half the number of chromosomes, so that on fertilization the zygote has the full diploid number. **2.** contraction of the pupil. *See* MIOSIS.

Meissner's corpuscles, *(mīz-nerz),* sensory receptors located in the skin which detect light pressure.

Meissner's plexus, *(mīz-nerz),* autonomic nerve fibres of the gastrointestinal tract. They facilitate communication between different parts and allow the tract to function as an integrated unit.

melaena, *(mel-ē-na),* black tar-like stools which contain altered blood. Bleeding is usually from the stomach or duodenum and is commonly due to peptic ulceration.

melancholia, *(mel-an-kō-li-a),* very severe depression. *See* DEPRESSION.

melanin, *(mel-a-nin),* a black or brown pigment derived from tyrosine. Found in skin, hair, the choroid of the eye and other sites. Pigmentation increases normally on exposure to sunlight and during pregnancy or abnormally in disease, e.g. Addison's disease.

melanocyte, *(mel-an-ō-sīt),* cells of the basal layer of the skin which produce melanin when stimulated by melanocyte-stimulating hormone (MSH) from the pituitary gland.

melanoma, *(mel-an-ō-ma),* a malignant tumour of melanocytes. It usually arises from a previously benign mole which becomes larger and darker with ulceration and eventual spread both local and distant. *M. coli*: pigmentation of the colonic mucosa.

melanosis, pigmented areas in the tissues. *M. coli*: pigmentation of the colonic mucosa.

melatonin, hormone produced by the pineal gland in response to the amount of light falling on the retina. It inhibits gonadotrophin release and is closely involved in reproductive function, mood, and various diurnal rhythms such as sleep and appetite.

membrane, a thin lining or covering substance, e.g. basement membrane, mucous membrane, cell membrane, etc.

memory, 1. the ability to store and recall information and events. It is a very complex process and types include: short- or long-term. **2.** the electronic storage areas which hold the data a computer is working on and the program which is running. Computers have two types of memory, *see* RAM and ROM. Powerful computers with considerable memory can use complex programs and handle data very quickly. Work must still be saved on to a disk before the computer is switched off as RAM memory holds material only whilst the computer is working.

menaquinones, a group of compounds with vitamin K activity that are synthesized by the intestinal bacteria.

menarche, *(men-ar-ke)*, commencement of menstrual cycles. The first menses.

Mendel's laws, first law (segregation) and second law (independent assortment) which are concerned with the fundamental theory of heredity and genetic inheritance. *See* DOMINANT, RECESSIVE.

Mendelson's syndrome, inhalation of regurgitated stomach contents, which can cause rapid death from anoxia, or may produce pulmonary oedema, severe bronchospasm and respiratory distress.

Ménière's syndrome, *(mā-nē-ers)*, distension of endolymphatic system (membranous labyrinth) of the inner ear from excess fluid. This results in nausea, tinnitus, vertigo and deafness.

meningeal, *(men-in-jē'-al)*, pertaining to the meninges.

meninges, *(men-in'-jeez)*, the membranes surrounding and covering the brain and spinal cord. They are, from without: the dura mater, the arachnoid, the pia mater.

meningioma, *(men-in-jē-ō'-ma)* tumour derived from the meninges.

meningism, *(men-in-jizm)*, meningeal irritation which produces signs and symptoms similar to meningitis but in the absence of infection.

meningitis, *(men-in-jī'-tis)*, inflammation of the meninges due to infection by microorganisms. Causes include: viral, e.g. coxsackievirus, bacterial, e.g. *Haemophilus influenzae*, *Streptococcus pneumoniae*, *Neisseria meningitidis* (meningococcal) and, less commonly, *Listeria monocytogenes*, *Cryptococcus neoformans*, *Staphylococcus aureus* and *Mycobacterium tuberculosis* where the onset is insidious. Acute infections are characterized by vague flu-like illness, headache, fever, neck stiffness, photophobia, altered consciousness, a positive Kernig's sign and changes in the CSF on lumbar puncture. Patients with meningococcal septicaemia will also have a dark purple /red petechial rash that does not disappear when pressure is applied.

209

meningocele, *(men-in-gō-sēl)*, protrusion of the meninges through a defect in the skull or spine, usually in the thoraco-lumbar region. *See* SPINA BIFIDA.

meningococcus, *(men-in-gō-kok-us)*, *Neisseria meningitidis*. A Gramnegative coccus which causes meningococcal meningitis and life-threatening septicaemia.

meningomyelocele, *(men-in-gō-mī-el-ō-sēl)*, protrusion of spinal cord and meninges through a defect in the spine, usually in the thoraco-lumbar region. *See* SPINA BIFIDA.

meniscectomy, *(men-i-sek-to-mi)*, removal of a semilunar cartilage from the knee joint.

meniscus, *(men-is-kus)*, **1.** a semilunar cartilage. **2.** a lens. **3.** the crescent-like surface of a liquid in a narrow tube.

menopause, cessation of menstruation, an event occurring during the climacteric. The mean age in the UK is 51 years. *See* CLIMACTERIC.

menorrhagia, *(men-o-rā'-ji-a)*, excessive menstrual bleeding.

menses, *(men-sēz)*, the menstrual flow.

menstrual, pertaining to the menses. *M. cycle*: (uterine cycle) the changes occurring in the uterus as the endometrium responds to the secretion of ovarian hormones. It corresponds to the ovarian cycle and is repeated every 28 days (range 21–35) or so, except during pregnancy, from the menarche to the menopause. It has three phases: proliferative, secretory and menstrual (Figure 48).

menstruation, the discharge of blood and endometrial debris from the uterus.

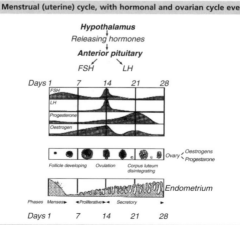

48 Menstrual (uterine) cycle, with hormonal and ovarian cycle events

mental, 1. pertaining to the chin. 2. pertaining to the mind. *M. age*: the age of a person with regard to his/her intellectual development which can be determined by intelligence tests. If a person aged 30 years can only pass the tests normally achieved by a child of 12 years, the person's mental age is said to be 12 years. *M. illness/disorder*: the definition in the English Mental Health Act is that 'mental illness, arrested or incomplete development of mind, psychopathic disorder and any other disorder or disability of mind, and "mentally disordered" shall be construed accordingly'. A patient can be detained in hospital only if, as one condition, he can be said to suffer from a 'mental disorder' in relation to this definition. The broader definition of mental distress includes any illness, developmental abnormality or personality disorder mentioned in the major classifications of mental distress. *M. health*: emotional and behavioural well-being. Coping is adequate and the individual is adjusted to their situation. *M. Health Acts*: various acts of parliament which regulate and control the rights, admission, treatment and subsequent stay in hospital for certain patients with mental health disorders. *M. Health Commission*: a body whose function is concerned with the care and welfare of those individuals detained under the provisions of the relevant part of the Mental Health Act. *M. Health Review Tribunal*: a body set up in each Regional Health Administration area to deal with patients' applications for discharge or alteration of their conditions of detention in hospital (in England and Wales, with a separate, similar system in Northern Ireland). In Scotland, the same function is performed by requests for review of detention to the Mental Welfare Commission, or appeal to the sheriff. *M. Health Welfare Officer*: an approved social worker (ASW) appointed by the Local Health Authority to deal with: (a) applications for compulsory or emergency admission to hospital, or for conveyance of patients there; (b) applications concerning guardianship, the functions of the nearest relative, or acting as nearest relative if so appointed; (c) returning patients absent without leave, or apprehending patients escaped from legal custody. In addition the ASW may have a wide range of functions in the care and aftercare of the mentally disordered in the community. This includes home visiting, training centres, clubs and general supervision of the discharged patient. The Scottish equivalent is the Mental Health Officer (MHO). The MHO is also a social worker with special experience in mental disorder (mental distress is the preferred term). MHOs can make application for admission of a patient under the Mental Health (Scotland) Act 1984, or for guardianship under the same Act. They have a duty to provide reports on the social circumstances of patients who are detained in hospital and of certain other functions under the Act.

mental defence mechanism, unconscious defence mechanism by which individuals attempt to cope with stressful, difficult or threatening emotions, e.g. projection, sublimation, etc.

mentor, an experienced professional who supports, guides and acts as a role model for a student or new practitioner.

mercurialism, *(mer-kū-ri-al-izm)*, chronic poisoning with mercury occurring in individuals whose work involves contact with the metal or through foods such as fish which contain high levels. May present with paraesthesia, ataxia, sore mouth, loose teeth and gastrointestinal problems, etc.

mercury (Hg), a poisnous liquid metallic element. Uses include: measuring instruments, disinfectants and dental fillings which are amalgams of several metals. *M. poisoning*: see MERCURIALISM.

meridians, conceptual channels running through and across the body through which Qi energy flows. *See* ACUPUNCTURE.

mesarteritis, *(mes-ar-ter-ī-tis)*, inflammation of the middle coating of an artery.

mesencephalon, *(mes-en-kef′-a-lon)*, the midbrain.

mesenchyme, *(me-sen-kīm)*, embryonic connective tissue which gives rise to all connective tissues.

mesenteric, *(mes-en-ter-ik)*, pertaining to the mesentery. *M. adenitis*: inflammation of lymph nodes in the mesentery. *M. arteries*: arteries supplying the bowel. *M. veins*: veins draining the bowel, they empty into the hepatic portal vein.

mesentery, *(mes-en-ter-i)*, fan-shaped fold of peritoneum which enfolds the small bowel and secures it to the posterior abdominal wall. It also carries vessels and nerves.

mesocolon, *(mes-ō-kō′-lon)*, double fold of peritoneum which secures the transverse colon to the abdominal wall.

mesoderm, *(mes′-ō-derm)*, a primary germ layer of the early embryo which gives rise to muscle, connective tissue and some epithelium, etc. It lies between the ectoderm and endoderm. *See* ECTODERM, ENDODERM.

mesonephros, *(mes-ō-nef-ros)*, a primitive structure occurring during embryonic development of the urinary tract.

mesothelioma, *(mes-ō-thē-lē-ō-ma)*, a tumour of serous membranes; pleura and peritoneum. *Malignant m.*: rapidly growing tumour of pleura or peritoneum which is usually associated with exposure to asbestos, especially blue asbestos.

mesothelium, *(mes-ō-thē-li-um)*, general term applied to the epithelium lining serous cavities.

messenger RNA (mRNA), the ribonucleic acid which carries the genetic information from DNA to the ribosomes. *See* TRANSCRIPTION.

meta-analysis, a statistical summary of many research studies using complex analysis of the primary data.

metabolic, *(met-a-bol′-ik)*, pertaining to metabolism. *Basal m. rate*: see BASAL METABOLISM. *M. acidosis*: excess acid in the blood which has a metabolic rather than a respiratory cause, e.g. diabetic ketoacidosis. *M. alkalosis*: excess alkali in the blood which has a metabolic rather than a respiratory cause, e.g. taking excessive alkali indigestion medicine.

metabolism, general term applied to all the biochemical processes occurring within an organism. The synthesis of new substances is known as anabolism and the breaking down of complex substances into simple ones is catabolism. *Basal m.*: see BASAL METABOLISM.

metacarpal, *(met-a-kar-pal)*, 1. pertaining to the metacarpus. 2. a bone of the metacarpus.

metacarpophalangeal, *(me-ta-kar-pō-fal-an-jē-al)*, relating to the metacarpus and the phalanges.

metacarpus, the five bones joining the carpus (wrist) and phalanges (fingers).

metaphase, (me-ta-fāz), second stage of nuclear division occurring during mitosis and meiosis.

metaphysis, (me-ta'-fi-sis), part between the shaft (diaphysis) and the end (epiphysis) of the long bones.

metaplasia, (me-ta-plā-zi-a), the change of cells to another type (usually less specialized – a reverse of differentiation). May occur in response to chronic inflammation, it is generally reversible but can progress to malignant changes.

metastasis, (met-as-tā'-sis), the spread of tumour cells from one part of the body to another, usually via the blood or lymph, but cancer cells may spread across serous membranes and may be 'seeded' during surgery. A secondary growth.

metatarsal, (met-a-tar'-sal), 1. pertaining to the metatarsus. 2. a bone of the metatarsus.

metatarsalgia, (met'-a-tar-sal'-ji-a), pain in the fore part of the foot.

metatarsus, the five bones joining the tarsus (ankle) and phalanges (toes).

metencephalon, (met-en-kef'-al-on), that part of the developing brain forming the pons and cerebellum.

methadone, synthetic opioid used to relieve unpleasant symptoms in people undertaking heroin withdrawal programmes.

meteorism, (mē-tē-or-izm), distension of the intestines by gas. *See* TYMPANITES.

ethaemoglobin, (met-hē-mō-glō-bin), haemoglobin in which the iron is oxidized to the ferric state, it cannot carry oxygen and may result in cyanosis. May be produced by certain drugs.

methaemoglobinuria, (met-hē-mō-glō-bin-ū'-ri-a), the presence of methaemoglobin in the urine.

methanol, methyl alcohol.

methicillin (multi)-resistant *Staphylococcus aureus*, (MRSA), strains of *S. aureus* which have become resistant to most antibacterial agents. Causes very serious and sometimes fatal infections in hospital. Increasingly encountered in community settings. Infection control measures include: hand washing, environmental cleaning and isolation or patient cohorting.

methionine, (me-thē-ō-nēn), an essential (indispensable) amino acid. Contains sulphur.

metra, the uterus.

metre (m), measurement of length. One of the seven base units of the International System of Units (SI). A thousand millimetres.

metric system, decimal system of measurement.

metritis, inflammation of the uterus.

metrocolpocele, (met-rō-kol'-pō-sēl), protrusion of the uterus into the vagina. Uterine prolapse.

metroptosis, (me-trop-tō-sis), uterine prolapse.

metrorrhagia, (met-rō-ra-ji-a), bleeding from the uterus, at a time other than during menstruation. It may follow coitus or examination and should always be investigated to exclude serious pathology. *See* POST-MENOPAUSAL BLEEDING.

MHC, abbreviation for **major histocompatibility complex.**

micelle, very small globules of lipids and bile salts formed during fat digestion. Micelles transport fatty acids and glycerol to the enterocytes where they are absorbed leaving the bile salts in the lumen of the bowel.

Michel's clips, metal clips used for wound closure.

microangiopathy, disease of small blood vessels, such as that occurring in diabetes and leading to renal failure.

microbe, microorganism, especially those causing disease. *See* BACTERIA, VIRUS.

microbiology, the study of microorganisms.

microcephalic, *(mī-krō-kef-al'-ik),* having an abnormally small head.

microcirculation, flow of blood through very small vessels; arterioles, capillaries and venules.

Micrococcus, *(mī-krō-kok'-us),* genus of Gram-positive cocci, generally nonpathogenic.

microcyte, *(mī-krō-sīt),* abnormally small red blood cell.

microcytic, *(mī-krō-si-tik),* describes a cell which is smaller than normal. *M. anaemia:* one where the red cells are small. The microcytosis is commonly associated with iron deficiency, which may be due to blood loss, insufficient iron in the diet, failure of iron absorption or chronic disease. *See* ANAEMIA.

microfilaria, immature *Filaria. See* FILARIA, FILARIASIS.

microglial cells, a type of macrophage found in the central nervous system. *See* NEUROGLIA.

micrognathia, *(mī-krō-nā-thē-a),* small chin. Poorly developed lower jaw.

microgram, (μg), a millionth of a gram.

micrometer, instrument for measuring very small distances or objects being observed under a microscope.

micrometre (μm), a millionth part of a metre. Often still called a micron.

micron, a millionth part of a metre.

micronutrient, a nutrient, such as vitamins and minerals, required by the body in relatively small amounts.

microorganism, any microscopic plant or animal, e.g. a bacterium, a protozoon, a fungus, a rickettsia, *Chlamydia* or a virus.

microphthalmos, *(mī-krof-thal-mos),* abnormally small eyes.

microscope, an instrument which magnifies objects which are normally invisible. They may be of the type which utilizes light or the very powerful electron microscope.

microscopic, an object which is invisible without the aid of a microscope.

Microsporum, a genus of fungi which causes disease of the skin and hair, e.g. ringworm.

microsurgery, surgery involving very small structures such as blood vessels and nerves, requiring the use of an operating microscope.

microtome, an instrument for cutting fine sections for microscopic examination.

microwaves, electromagnetic waves of high frequency and short wave length.

micturition, *(mik-tū-rish'-on),* the act of passing urine.

micturating urethrogram, *(mik-tū-rā ting ū-rē-thrō-gram), see* URETHROGRA PHY.

midbrain, part of the brain stem between the cerebrum and pons. *Se* MESENCEPHALON.

middle ear, *see* EAR.

midstream specimen of urin (MSSU), sample collected durin the middle part of the urine flow f microbiological examination. *S* CLEAN CATCH.

midwifery, the professional practi which involves the conduct ar supervision of a normal pregnanc labour and puerperium.

migraine, *(mī-grān),* a condition cha acterized by severe period headaches, nausea, visual distu bances and other neurological ma festations. It is caused by reduced cerebral blood flow and changes in the extracranial arteries that appear to be linked to the amount of 5-hydroxytryptamine in the blood. Attacks may be triggered by various factors such as bright lights, certain foods and stress etc.

milestones, the developmental norms against which an individual child's development may be measured.

milia (*sing.* **milium**), small white cysts of the epidermis of the face and neck. Result from obstruction of a sebaceous gland duct. *M. neonatorum*: those occurring in the newborn.

miliaria papulosa, (*mil-i-ar-i-a pa-pū-lō-za*), prickly heat. Caused when sweat ducts become obstructed.

miliary, like millet seed. Thus *m. tuberculosis* is an acute form of infection in which the tissues are studded with small tubercles so as to resemble a mass of millet seeds.

milieu, (*mil-yu*), the environment or setting. *M. intérieur*: the physical and chemical environment experienced by individual cells, e.g. the pH of the fluid surrounding the cells.

milk, the secretion of the mammary glands. Its production is stimulated by prolactin and its release or 'let down' is controlled by oxytocin. Human milk contains all the essential nutrients required by neonates in the correct proportions. The presence of IgA and lactoferrin increases the infant's resistance to infection. *M. sugar. see* LACTOSE. *M. teeth*: the first or deciduous teeth. *See* TEETH.

Miller-Abbott tube, a double-bore tube with a balloon at its distal end. Used to aspirate intestinal contents when the small bowel is obstructed.

milligram (mg), one thousandth part of a gram.

millilitre (ml), one thousandth part of a litre. Equal to a cubic centimetre.

millimetre (mm), one thousandth part of a metre.

millimole (mmol), a thousandth part of a mole.

millisecond (ms), a thousandth part of a second.

Milwaukee brace, an appliance used in the treatment of abnormal spinal curvatures, e.g. scoliosis.

mineralocorticoids, (*min-er-al-ō-kaw-ti-koyd*), steroid hormones secreted by the adrenal cortex, they regulate electrolyte levels by causing sodium reabsorption in the renal tubules, e.g. aldosterone.

minerals, inorganic elements. *See* NUTRITION APPENDIX.

minimally invasive surgery, minimal access surgery, a surgical technique which utilizes tiny incisions and endoscopic equipment to perform a variety of operations, e.g. cholecystectomy. Also known as **keyhole surgery.**

minute volume, *see* PULMONARY VENTILATION.

miosis, (*mī-ō-sis*), contraction of the pupil. *Syn.* **meiosis.**

miotic, (*mī-o-tik*), a drug which causes the pupil to contract. *Syn.* **meiotic.**

miscarriage, spontaneous abortion. *See* ABORTION.

Misuse of Drugs (Act 1971, Regulations 1985), in the UK. Controls the possession, supply, storage, prescription and administration of certain groups of habit-forming drugs that are liable to misuse. They are available to the public by medical prescription only; heavy penalties may follow any illegal possession or supply. The substances are known as controlled drugs and include the opioids, synthetic narcotics, cocaine, hallucinogens and barbiturates (with exceptions). They include: morphine, diamorphine, methadone, pethidine, etc.

mite, minute arthropod which is responsible for skin conditions such as scabies.

mitochondria, (mī-tō-kon-drē-a), cellular organelles responsible for the production of energy (ATP) from the oxidation of fuel molecules.

mitosis, (mī-tō-sis), a process of nuclear division (usually followed by cytokinesis) by which somatic (body) cells replicate themselves. It results in the production of two genetically identical 'daughter' cells with the diploid number of chromosomes.

mitral, (mī-tral), shaped like a mitre. *M. valve*: bicuspid. The left atrioventricular valve. *M. incompetence*: the valve fails to close properly with a resultant back-flow of blood. Usually treated surgically. *M. stenosis*: narrowing of the valve orifice. Usually treated surgically.

mittelschmerz, (mit-el-shmerts), middle pain. Abdominal pain occurring around ovulation.

MMR, abbreviation for the **measles, mumps and rubella vaccine**.

mnemonic, a memory aid which helps an individual remember through a variety of cues.

mobilization, to make mobile or movable, applied either to a specific part or to the person.

mode, the most common (frequent) value in a series of scores. *See* CENTRAL TENDENCY STATISTIC.

model, a conceptual framework or theory which can be used to explain situations or problems such as a nursing model, or a diagram.

modelling, in psychology, the way people learn from watching and copying the behaviour of others.

modem, acronym for MODulator/DEModulator. A peripheral device

able to transmit data from one computer to another via the telephone system.

moist wound healing, achieved by application of an occlusive, semipermeable dressing which permits the exudate to collect under the film to perform its bactericidal functions.

molality, the number of moles of substance (solute) per kilogram of solvent. The concentration of a solution.

molar, 1. large grinding teeth. *See* TEETH. **2.** a solution which contains one mole of the substance (solute) per litre of solution.

molarity, the concentration of a solution, expressed as a number of moles of the substance per litre of solution (mol/l).

mole (mol), 1. a measurement of amount of substance. One of the seven base units of the International System of Units (SI). One mole of any substance will contain the same number of particles (atoms or molecules): 6.02×10^{23} (also known as Avogadro's numbers). **2.** dark pigmented area on the skin. *See* CARNEOUS MOLE, HYDATIDIFORM MOLE.

molecular, pertaining to molecules. *M. biology*: the science of biological molecules and their role in living systems. *M. weight*: the total of the atomic weights of atoms in a molecule.

molecule, a particle consisting of two or more atoms from the same or different elements joined by a chemical bond.

molluscum, (mol-us-kum), skin conditions having soft tumours. *M. contagiosum*: a viral skin condition characterized by the development of white papules.

Monckeberg's medial sclerosis, (munk-bergz), sclerosis of the muscle layer and calcium deposition in medium-sized arteries resulting in the 'pipe-stem' arteries of old age.

Mongolian blue spot, blue-black discoloration seen on the sacral region of some neonates.

Monilia, (mo-ni-li-a), see CANDIDA, CANDIDIASIS.

monitoring, sequential recording. Term is also used to describe the automatic visual display of such measurements as temperature, pulse, respiration and blood pressure.

monoamine, (mon-ō-am-een), organic molecule containing one amine group, e.g. dopamine.

monoamine oxidase, (mon-ō-am-een oks-i-dāz), an enzyme which catalyses the breakdown of monoamines such as adrenaline (epinephrine) and 5-hydroxytryptamine (5-HT). *M. o. inhibitors (MAOIs)*: drugs which inhibit this enzyme activity are used as antidepressants. They have been largely superseded by other drugs with fewer side-effects and greater clinical efficacy. During their administration it is necessary to abstain from foods rich in tyramine (precursor of monoamines), e.g. cheese, yeast extract and red wine, and to avoid the use of certain drugs, e.g. pethidine. Selective MAOIs are used in the treatment of parkinsonism.

monochromatism, (mon-ō-krō-matizm), a rare type of colour blindness where all objects are seen as grey shades.

monoclonal, (mon-ō-klō-nal), derived from a single cell. *M. antibodies*: produced by a single cell, and on cell division its clones continue to make the single identical antibody. Widely used for the production of highly specific antibodies for research, diagnostic and therapeutic purposes.

monocular, (mon-ok'-ū-la), relating to one eye only.

monocyte, (mon-ō-sīt), large phagocytic white blood cell. Moves into the tissues where they differentiate into macrophages. Part of the monocyte-macrophage system (reticuloendothelial). *See* BLOOD, BLOOD COUNT, MACROPHAGE.

monocyte – macrophage system, a widely scattered system of specialized phagocytic cells in the liver, lymph nodes, spleen, bone marrow and other tissues. They break down blood cells and haemoglobin, dispose of cell breakdown products and have an important defensive role against infection. Also known as reticuloendothelial system.

monocytosis, (mon-ō-sī-tō-sis), abnormal increase in the number of monocytes in the peripheral blood.

monomania, (mon-ō-mā-nē-a), an obsession with a single idea or subject.

mononeuropathy, (mon-ō-nū-rop'-athi), disease of a single peripheral nerve.

mononuclear, with one nucleus.

mononucleosis, (mon-ō-nū-kle-ō'-sis), increase in monocytes in peripheral blood. *Infectious m.*: see INFECTIOUS MONONUCLEOSIS.

monoplegia, (mon-ō-plē'-ji-a), paralysis of one limb.

monorchid, monorchis, (mon-or'-kid), having only one testis.

monosaccharide, (mon-ō-sak-ar-īd), a simple sugar such as glucose, fructose or galactose. The basic unit from which other carbohydrates are formed.

monosomy, (mo-no-so-mi), a genetic abnormality where there is one chromosome missing (45 rather than 46). *See* TURNER'S SYNDROME.

monovular, (mon-ov-ū-la), see UNIOVULAR.

monozygotic, *(mon-ō-zī-got'-ik),* one zygote. Used to describe identical twins who develop from one zygote which splits into two embryos.

mons veneris, *(monz ven-ĕr-is),* the eminence lying over the symphysis pubis in the female.

Montgomery's glands, sebaceous glands of the breast areola. They enlarge during pregnancy and lactation.

mood, a person's emotional state or attitude, e.g. sad. *See* AFFECT.

moon face, a rounded face characteristic of Cushing's disease or syndrome.

Mooren's ulcer, a gutter-like excoriation of the peripheral cornea.

morbid, diseased, disordered, pathological.

morbidity, being diseased. *Standardized m. ratio:* the amount of self-reported limiting long-term illness indirectly standardized for variations in age and sex.

morbilli, *(mor-bil-ē),* measles.

moribund, dying.

morning after pill, *see* POST COITAL CONTRACEPTION.

morning dip, an early morning decline in respiratory function seen in some types of asthma.

morning sickness, *see* VOMITING OF PREGNANCY.

Moro reflex, the startle reflex, a normal reaction present in newborn babies (Figure 49).

morphine, morphia, an alkaloid obtained from opium. Its medicinal uses include the treatment of severe pain and acute pulmonary oedema. Controlled by the Misuse of Drugs Act and Regulations, it is addictive and subject to considerable criminal misuse.

morphoea, *(maw-fē-a),* scleroderma which affects the skin and subcutaneous connective tissues.

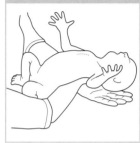

49 Moro or startle reflex

morphology, the science of form and structure of organisms.

mortality, 1. being mortal and subject to death. **2.** death rate. The annual death rate is expressed as the number of deaths x 1000 and divided by the mid-year population. Specialized death rates include: *Infant m.:* the number of infant deaths in the first year of life per 1000 related live births. *Maternal m.:* the number of women who die from causes associated with pregnancy and childbirth per 1000 total births. *Neonatal m.:* the number of deaths in the first four weeks of life per 1000 related live births. *Perinatal m.:* the number of stillbirths plus deaths in the first week of life per 1000 total births. *Postnatal m.:* the number of deaths in infants aged from 28 days to 1 year per 1000 live births. *Standardized m. rate:* number of deaths per 1000 population standardized for age.

morula, an early stage in the developing zygote.

mosaicism, *(mō-zā-ik-izm),* where an individual has cells of differing genetic composition.

motile, (mō-tīl), able to move independently.

motion, 1. movement. **2.** evacuation of the bowel. *M. sickness:* nausea and vomiting associated with the motion of a car, ship or plane.

motivation, the conscious or unconscious desire to achieve a specific goal. The incentive or reason for an action.

motor, pertaining to movement. *M. end plate:* communication between axon terminal and muscle fibre. *See* NEUROMUSCULAR JUNCTION. *M. neurones:* efferent nerves which convey impulses from the central nervous system to a muscle or gland where they cause activity. *See* EXTRAPYRAMIDAL, LOWER MOTOR NEURONE, PYRAMIDAL, UPPER MOTOR NEURONE. *M. neurone disease:* condition characterized by progressive degeneration of motor neurones in the cortex, brain stem and spinal cord. It is invariably fatal. *M. unit:* a group of muscle fibres innervated by a particular lower motor neurone axon.

mould, a fungus.

moulding, alteration in the shape and size of the fetal head as it is forced through the birth canal. The skull bones may overlap at the fibrous sutures.

mountain sickness, associated with the reduced partial pressure of oxygen at high altitudes. Prior to physiological acclimatization it causes rapid respiration, tachycardia, fatigue, vomiting and headache.

mourning, a response which assists the individual to adjust to a loss. *See* BEREAVEMENT.

mouth, a cavity bounded by the closed lips and facial muscles, the hard and soft palate, and lower jaw. It contains the teeth and the tongue and receives saliva. *M. care:* oral hygiene. The measures taken to keep the mouth clean and healthy. They include: assessment, adequate hydration, especially oral fluids, cleaning the teeth and oral surfaces, lip creams and mouth washes.

mouth-to-mouth/nose resuscitation, expired air artificial respiration where the first aider forces expired air from his or her lungs into the victim's mouth or mouth and nose simultaneously.

moving and handling, *see* MANUAL HANDLING.

movement, 1. motion. **2.** defaecation. *See* ACTIVE MOVEMENTS, PASSIVE MOVEMENTS.

movements (fetal), *see* QUICKENING.

MRI, abbreviation for **magnetic resonance imaging.**

MRSA, abbreviation for **methicillin-resistant *Staphylococcus aureus*.**

mucin, (mū-sin), a glycoprotein present in mucus.

mucocele, (mū´-kō-sēl), cyst distended with mucus, as of the gallbladder or lacrimal sac.

mucociliary, pertaining to the clearance of mucus and debris, by the ciliated mucosa, from the respiratory tract.

mucocutaneous, pertaining to mucous membranes and the skin.

mucoid, resembling mucus.

mucolytic, (mū-kō-lit-ik), a substance which reduces the viscosity of mucus, e.g. acetylcysteine, used in cystic fibrosis.

mucopolysaccharides, (mū-kō-pol-ē-sak´-a-rīdz), a group of complex connective tissue polysaccharides.

mucopolysaccharidoses, (mū-kō-pol-ē-sak´-a-rid-ō´-sis), *see* GARGOYLISM, HUNTER'S SYNDROME, HURLER'S SYNDROME.

mucoprotein, (mū-kō-prō-tēn), *see* GLYCOPROTEIN.

mucopurulent, (mū-kō-pū-roo-lent), with mucus and pus.

219

mucosa, *(mū-kō'-za)*, a mucous membrane.

mucositis, inflammation of a mucous membrane, such as the lining of the mouth and throat.

mucous membrane, *(mū-kus)*, mucus-secreting epithelium such as the varieties which line the gastrointestinal, respiratory and genitourinary tracts.

mucus, viscous secretion from the mucous glands.

müllerian ducts, primitive embryonic ducts which develop to form the internal genitalia in a genetically female embryo. *see* WOLFFIAN DUCTS.

multicellular, having many cells.

multigravida, *(mul-ti-gra'-vi-da)*, a pregnant woman who has previously had one or more pregnancies.

multinuclear, having several nuclei.

multipara, a woman who has had two or more pregnancies resulting in a live infant.

multiple myeloma, *(mī-el-ō-ma)*, myelomatosis. A malignant disease of plasma cells (derived from B lymphocytes) in which an abnormal immunoglobulin is produced. There is infiltration of bone marrow with plasma cells leading to anaemia, leucopenia and thrombocytopenia with bone pain and hypercalcaemia. *See* BENCE JONES PROTEIN.

multiple organ dysfunction syndrome (MODS), describes a situation where the functions of interdependent organ systems, such as kidneys, respiratory system, coagulation and gastrointestinal tract, are so compromised as to lead to metabolic derangement. It requires organ support, e.g. haemofiltration and mechanical ventilation.

multiple sclerosis, *(skle-rō-sis)*, a condition of unknown aetiology where there is demyelination within the CNS. Clinical features depend upon the site and extent of the lesions but include: weakness, ataxia, visual defects, and speech problems. A characteristic of the disease is its tendency to relapse and remit.

multivariate statistics, analysis of three or more variables at the same time. Used to elucidate the association of two variables after allowing for other variables.

mumps, infectious parotitis caused by a paramyxovirus. Spread by droplets, it has an incubation period of around 18 days. There is fever, swelling of the salivary glands and pain. Complications include: orchitis, oöphoritis, pancreatitis and meningitis. Immunization is available as part of the routine programme, in conjunction with protection against measles and rubella (MMR).

Munchausen's syndrome, *(mun-chow-zenz)*, a disorder where individuals attempt to obtain medical treatment or investigation for non-existent illnesses. *M.'s by proxy*: here a parent, usually the mother, or both parents, or other carers produce false stories for the child and falsify signs and symptoms.

mural, pertaining to the wall of an organ or structure.

murmur, abnormal sound heard on auscultation such as with valvular disease of the heart.

Murphy's sign, a physical sign which may be present when the gallbladder is acutely inflamed. Continuous pressure over the organ during a deep breath in will cause the individual to 'catch' his or her breath at the point of maximum inspiration.

muscae volitantes, *(mus-kē vol-i-tan-tēz)*, filaments, visible to the individual as black spots or floaters, floating in the vitreous humour.

muscarine, *(mus-ka-rīn)*, a poisonous alkaloid found in some fungal species.

muscarinic, describes a type of cholinergic receptor where muscarine would, if present, bind instead of the neurotransmitter acetylcholine. *See* NICOTINIC. *M. agonist*: drugs that stimulate or mimic the parasympathic nervous system, e.g. pilocarpine, used in glaucoma. *M. antagonist* (*antimuscarinic*): drugs that inhibit cholinergic nerve transmission, e.g. atropine, ipratropium bromide.

muscle, one of four basic body tissues. Specialized contractile tissue formed from excitable cells. There are three types: **1.** striated or voluntary (skeletal) m. **2.** smooth or involuntary m. **3.** cardiac m. which has features of both striated and smooth muscle (Figure 50).

muscular, pertaining to muscle. *M. dystrophy*: an inherited disease characterized by progressive muscle weakness and atrophy. *See* DUCHENNE-TYPE M.D.

musculoskeletal, relating to skeletal and muscular systems.

mutant, a cell (or individual) which carries a genetic change or mutation.

mutation, *(mū-tā-shon)*, a change in genetic material which alters the way a gene is expressed. It may be induced, e.g. exposure to radiation, or spontaneous.

mute, without the power of speech. Dumb.

myalgia, *(mī-al-ji-a)*, muscle pain. *Epidemic m.*: caused by the coxsackie virus. *See* BORNHOLM DISEASE.

myalgic encephalomyelitis (ME), *(mī-al-jik en-kef-a-lō-mī-el-ī-tis)*, post-viral syndrome or chronic fatigue syndrome. A condition with very variable presentation causing difficulties with diagnosis.

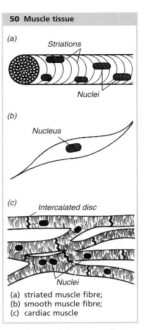

50 Muscle tissue

(a) striated muscle fibre;
(b) smooth muscle fibre;
(c) cardiac muscle

Its effects include: extreme fatigue, sore throat, anorexia, limb pains, headache, poor concentration, depression, enlarged liver and lymph nodes, etc.

myasthenia, *(mī-as-thēn-i-a)*, muscle weakness. *M. gravis*: a disease characterized by difficulty in sustaining muscle contraction and extreme fatigue. Autoantibodies block receptor sites and prevent the proper functioning of acetylcholine at the neuromuscular junction. In many cases there is some abnormality of the thymus gland.

myatonia, lack of muscle tone.

mycelium, (mī-sē´-li-um), the filaments of fungus forming an interwoven mass.

mycetoma, (mī-se-tō-ma), **Madura foot.** A fungal infection of the soft tissues and bones which commonly affects the limbs. It is caused by several species of actinomycetes and eumycetes.

Mycobacterium, (mī-kō-bak-teer-i-um), a genus of Gram-positive, acid-fast bacteria. M. tuberculosis causes tuberculosis, and M. leprae, leprosy.

mycology, study of fungi.

Mycoplasma, (mī-kō-plaz-ma), a genus of small microorganisms. M. pneumoniae is a cause of primary pneumonia.

mycosis, (mī-kō´-sis), disease caused by fungus.

mydriasis, (mi-drī-a-sis), pupil dilatation. Can relate to abnormal dilatation.

mydriatics, (mid-rē´-at-iks), drugs which dilate the pupil.

myelencephalon, (mi-el-en-kef´-al-on), part of the developing brain forming the medulla.

myelin, (mī-el-in), the white, fatty insulating material covering some nerves.

myelitis, (mī-e-lī´-tis), 1. inflammation of the spinal cord. 2. inflammation of the bone marrow.

myeloblast, (mī-el-ō-blast), a precursor cell of the polymorphonuclear series of granulocytes.

myelocele, (mī-el-ō-sīl), a spina bifida defect, commonly in the lumbar region, wherein development of the spinal cord itself has been arrested, and the central canal of the cord opens on to the skin surface, exposing the meninges and discharging cerebrospinal fluid.

myelocyte, (mī-e-lō-sīt), precursor cells of the polymorphonuclear series of granulocytes.

myelogram, (mī-el-ō-gram), an X-ray which demonstrates abnormalities of the spinal cord following injections of contrast into the subarachnoid space.

myelography, (mī-el-og-raf-i), a radiographic technique which visualizes the spinal cord following the introduction of contrast medium or gas into the subarachnoid space.

myeloid, (mī-el-oyd), pertaining to bone marrow, or the granulocyte precursor cells; myeloblasts and myelocytes in the bone marrow, or spinal cord.

myeloma, see MULTIPLE MYELOMA.

myelomatosis, see MULTIPLE MYELOMA.

myeloproliferative syndromes, (mī-el-ō-prō-lif-er-at-iv), any condition (premalignant or malignant) characterized by a proliferation of one or more of the cellular components of the marrow, they include: polycythaemia, myelosclerosis (myelofibrosis) and thrombocythaemia. See LEUKAEMIA.

myelosclerosis, (mī-el-ō-skle-rō-sis), replacement of haemopoietic marrow with cancellous bone or collagen.

myocardial, (mī-ō-kar´-di-al), pertaining to the myocardium. M. infarction: necrosis of the heart muscle following coronary artery occlusion, usually by thrombosis.

myocarditis, (mī-ō-kar-dī´-tis), inflammation of the myocardium such as that resulting from viral infections, or rheumatic fever.

myocardium, (mī-ō-kar´-di-um), the middle layer of the heart wall, it consists of highly specialized cardiac muscle tissue.

myoclonus, clonic spasmodic muscle contraction.

myofibril, bundles of fibres contained in a muscle fibre. They are formed from filaments of contractile proteins. *See* ACTIN, MYOSIN, TROPOMYOSIN, TROPONIN.

myofibroblasts, type of fibroblast that contains contractile protein filaments. They are responsible for the contraction that decreases wound size during healing.

myofibrosis, condition characterized by the replacement of muscle by fibrous tissue.

myogenic, *(mī-ō-jen-ik),* originating from muscular tissue.

myoglobin, *(mī-ō-glō-bin),* myohaemoglobin, the haem-containing protein molecule found in skeletal muscle. It facilitates oxygen transport. When massive muscle damage occurs such as in crush injuries, it is released into the blood causing renal damage.

myoglobinuria, *(mī-ō-glō-bin-ūr-i-a),* the presence of myoglobin in the urine.

myoma, *(mī-ō'-ma),* any tumour composed of muscular tissue.

myomectomy, *(mī-ō-mek'-to-mi),* removal of a myoma; usually referring to a fibroid from the uterus.

myometrium, *(mī-ō-mē'-tri-um),* the uterine muscle.

myopathy, *(mī-op'-path-i),* any disease of a muscle.

myope, *(mī'-ōp),* shortsighted person. *Myopic:* pertaining to shortsightedness.

myopia, *(mī-ō'-pi-a),* shortsightedness; corrected by use of a biconcave lens (Figure 51).

myosarcoma, *(mī-ō-sar-kō'-ma),* a malignant tumour of muscle.

myosin, *(mī-ō-sin),* a contractile protein, one of the component filaments of a muscle myofibril.

myosis, *(mī-ō'-sis),* contraction of the pupil of the eye. Also called miosis.

myositis, *(mī-ō-sī-tis),* inflammation of muscle. *M. ossificans:* a condition

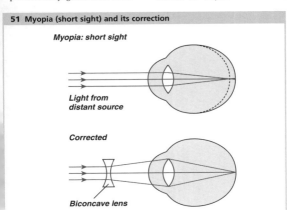

51 Myopia (short sight) and its correction

Myopia: short sight

Light from distant source

Corrected

Biconcave lens

where muscle is replaced by bone cells.

myotics, *(mī-ot-iks),* drugs which cause the pupil to contract. *Syn.* **meiotics, miotics.**

myotomy, *(mī-ot'-o-mi),* cutting through a muscle.

myotonia, *(mī-o-tō'-ni-a),* group of conditions characterized by tonic muscle spasm.

myringa, *(mir-in'-ga),* the tympanic membrane of the ear.

myringitis, *(mir-in-jī'-tis),* inflammation of the tympanic membrane of the ear.

myringoplasty, *(mi-ring-go-plas-ti),* plastic operation to repair the tympanic membrane.

myringotome, *(mir-in-go-tōm),* knife used in myringotomy.

myringotomy, *(mir-in-got-o-mi),* incision into the tympanic membrane. Used to drain fluid or pus from the middle ear. Middle ear ventilation is maintained by insertion of a grommet or Teflon tube.

myxoedema, *see* HYPOTHYROIDISM.

myxoma, *(miks-ō'-ma),* tumour of connective tissue containing mucoid material.

myxosarcoma, *(miks-ō-sar-kō-ma),* a malignant myxoma.

myxoviruses, *(miks-ō-vī-rus-es),* two families of RNA viruses (orthomyxoviruses and paramyxoviruses) that include the influenza viruses, respiratory syncytial virus, measles and mumps virus.

N

nabothian, also called **Naboth's.** *N. follicles or cysts*: small cysts arising in the uterine cervical glands due to duct obstruction. *N. glands*: mucous glands of the uterine cervix.

naevus, *(nē-vus)*, a birthmark. A congenital pigmented lesion usually consisting of dilated blood vessels. *See* HAEMANGIOMA.

Nägele's rule, a way of calculating the expected date of delivery – three months is subtracted from the date of the last menstrual period and seven days are added.

nanogram (ng), 10^{-9} of a gram. One thousandth part of a microgram (µg).

nanometre (nm), 10^{-9} of a metre. One thousandth part of a micrometre (µm). Used as a measurement of wavelength.

napkin rash, inflammation and soreness in the 'nappy area'. Causes include: contact with urine decomposition products, diarrhoea, detergents and infection.

narcissism, *(nar-sis'-izm)*, an abnormal love for oneself; named after Narcissus, a mythological character, who fell in love with the reflection of himself.

narcoanalysis, *(nar-kō-an-al-i-sis)*, a technique used in psychotherapy where individuals are encouraged to talk freely following the administration of narcotic drugs.

narcolepsy, *(nar-ko-lep-si)*, a condition characterized by sudden attacks of sleep occurring repeatedly during the day.

narcosis, *(nar-kōs-is)*, a state of altered consciousness produced by a narcotic drug.

narcotic, *(nar-kot-ik)*, a drug which produces narcosis or altered consciousness. Strong analgesic narcotics, e.g. opioids such as morphine, may cause respiratory depression.

nares, the nostrils. *Anterior n.*: openings into the nasal cavities from the outside. *Posterior n.*: openings from the nasal cavity into the nasopharynx.

nasal, pertaining to the nose. *N. cannula*: tube used to administer oxygen via the nares.

nascent, *(nās'-sent)*, at the moment of birth.

nasendoscope, an endoscope used for viewing the nasal passages and postnasal space and larynx.

nasoduodenal, *(nā-zō-dū-ō'-dē-nal)*, pertaining to the nose and duodenum. *N. tube*: a fine-bore tube passed via the nose into the duodenum for enteral feeding.

nasogastric, *(nā-zō-gas-trik)*, relating to the nose and stomach. *N. tube*: a tube passed into the stomach via the nose. Used to aspirate the gastric contents or for feeding.

nasojejunal, *(nā-zō-je-joon-al)*, pertaining to the nose and jejunum. *N. tube*: a weighted tube which is allowed to pass into the jejunum for feeding purposes.

nasolacrimal, *(nā-zō-lak'-ri-mal)*, relating to the nose and lacrimal apparatus.

225

nasopharyngeal, (nā-zō-far-in-jē-al), pertaining to the nasopharynx.

nasopharynx, (nā-zō-far-inks), the upper part of the pharynx, above the soft palate.

nates, (nā'-tēz), the buttocks.

National Framework for Assessing Performance, a framework that includes six areas for the assessment of NHS performance: effective delivery of appropriate healthcare; efficiency; fair access; health improvement; health outcomes and the patient/carer experience.

National Health Service (NHS), the system of preventive and therapeutic healthcare services and facilities available within the United Kingdom. It is financed by central government through money raised by taxation.

National Institute for Clinical Excellence (NICE), a Special Health Authority set up to generate and distribute clinical guidance based on evidence of clinical and cost-effectiveness. Functions include: identify health interventions for consideration; gather evidence via systematic approach, and produce protocols for practice (evidence: based). These protocols are disseminated by NICE to appropriate bodies.

National Service Frameworks (NSFs), evidence-based frameworks for major care areas and particular groups of disease, e.g. mental health and coronary heart disease, that state what patients/clients can presume to receive from the NHS.

National Vocational Qualifications (NVQ), Scottish Vocational Qualifications (SVQ), in the UK. Work-based qualifications available in many fields and areas of work, e.g. healthcare, catering, etc. NVQs are available at several levels of attainment and are recognized nationally.

natural childbirth, labour and delivery where medical input is minimal.

natural family planning, methods of family planning which use no drugs or appliances.

natural killer cell (NK), a type of lymphocyte which destroys, by lysis, virus-infected cells and some cells showing malignant changes. *See* INTERFERON.

naturopathy, (na-tūr-op-a-thi), a multidisciplinary approach to healthcare which includes all aspects of one's lifestyle, based upon the belief that the body has the power to 'heal itself'.

nausea, (naw'-sē-a), a feeling of sickness.

navel, the umbilicus.

navicular, (na-vi-kū-la), boat-shaped. One of the tarsal bones.

nebula, (neb'-ū-la), a cloud or mist. Term applied to filmy corneal opacities.

nebulizer, a device which produces a very fine spray. Used to administer drugs, especially those acting on the respiratory tract.

neck, 1. constricted area between head and body. **2.** narrow area of an organ or other structure, e.g. neck of femur. *Derbyshire n.*: *see* GOITRE. *Wry n.*: *see* TORTICOLLIS.

necrobiosis, (ne-krō-bī-ō-sis), death or degeneration of tissue.

necrophilia, (ne-krō-fil-i-a), **1.** a liking for dead bodies. **2.** a sexual perversion which involves sexual intercourse with a corpse or sexual gratification in the presence of a corpse.

necropsy, examination of a body after death.

necrosis, (ne-krō'-sis), death of tissue.

necrotic, (ne-krot'-ik), relating to necrosis.

necrotizing enterocolitis, *(ne-kro-tī-zing en-te-rō-ko-lī-tis),* a condition occurring primarily in preterm or low-birth-weight babies. Caused by hypoxia, leading to acute ischaemia of the bowel. The bowel becomes necrotic and there is obstruction, gangrene and peritonitis. Especially associated with respiratory distress syndrome and heart lesions in low-birth-weight babies.

necrotizing fasciitis, rare infection caused by some strains of group A *Streptococcus pyogenes.* There is severe infammation of the muscle sheath and massive soft tissue destruction. The mortality is high.

needlestick injury, occupational hazard of healthcare workers where accidental injury with contaminated needles or other items may infect them with various hepatitis viruses or, more rarely, HIV. All healthcare settings should have a risk assessment, staff training, and policies and procedures in place for protective clothing, proper disposal of equipment and action to be taken should injury occur.

needling, perforation with a needle, especially in cataract. See DISCISSION.

negative feedback, see FEEDBACK.

negativism, a state of mind in which the ideas and behaviour of an individual are in opposition to those of the majority and contrary to suggestion.

negligence, one form of professional malpractice which includes the omission of acts that a prudent professional nurse would have done or the commission of acts which a prudent professional nurse would not do. See MALPRACTICE.

Neisseria, *(ni-sē-ri-a),* a genus of bacteria. Gram-negative diplococci. *N. meningitidis* or *meningococcus* causes meningitis; *N. gonorrhoeae* or *gonococcus* causes gonorrhoea.

nematodes, *(nem-at-ōdes),* parasitic worms which include *Ascaris lumbricoides* (roundworms), *Enterobius vermicularis* (threadworms), *Loa loa* (filarial worms) and those from other species, such as *Toxocara canis.*

neoadjuvant therapy, chemotherapy given prior to surgery or radiation to reduce the size of a tumour.

neologism, *(nē-ol-o-jizm),* a specially coined word, often nonsensical; may express a thought disorder.

neonatal, *(nē-ō-nā-tal),* pertaining to the first four weeks of life. *N. mortality.* See MORTALITY. *N. respiratory distress syndrome (NRDS):* caused by a failure of the type II pneumocytes to secrete pulmonary surfactant (protein–lipid complex). It occurs most frequently in preterm infants and causes atelectasis and hypoxia that may be fatal. Management involves assisted ventilation and intratracheal administration of surfactant.

neonate, newborn. An infant during the first 28 days of life.

neonatology, *(nē-ō-nā-tol-o-ji),* branch of medicine dealing with the newborn.

neoplasm, a new growth or tumour. It may be benign or malignant. Neoplasia is the process of tumour formation.

nephrectomy, *(nef-rek'-tō-mi),* removal of a kidney.

nephritis, *(nef-rī'-tis),* inflammation of the kidney. A general term which covers a diverse group of disorders affecting the kidney. See GLOMERULONEPHRITIS, NEPHROTIC SYNDROME.

nephroblastoma, *(nef-rō-bla-stō-ma),* Wilm's tumour. A highly malignant tumour of the kidney arising from embryonic tissue. It occurs in early childhood.

nephrocalcinosis, *(nef-rō-kal-sin-ō-sis),* deposition of calcium within the renal tubules. It may occur in damaged tissue or as a result of hyperparathyroidism, malignancy and hypervitaminosis D, etc.

nephrocapsulectomy, *(nef-rō-kap-sū-lek'-to-mi),* operation to remove the kidney capsule.

nephrogram, *(nef-rō-gram),* radiograph of the kidney following administration of radiopaque contrast. *See* PYELOGRAPHY, UROGRAPHY.

nephrolith, *(nef-rō-lith),* kidney stone (calculus).

nephrolithiasis, *(nef-rō-lith-ī'-ā-sis),* stone (calculus) in the kidney.

nephrolithotomy, *(nef'-rō-lith-ot'-o-mi),* removal of a stone from the interior of the kidney. Now also accomplished by extracorporeal shock-wave lithotripsy. *Percutaneous n.:* removal of the stone via a small incision using a nephroscope.

nephrology, the study of the kidneys and the disorders that affect them.

nephroma, *(nef-rō'-ma),* tumour of the kidney.

nephron, the microscopic functional unit of the kidney consisting of the renal tubule (convoluted tubules, loop of Henle and collecting duct) and a knot of capillaries known as the glomerulus (Figure 52).

nephropathy, *(nef-ro'-path-i),* disease of the kidney.

nephropexy, *(nef-rō-pek'-si),* fixing a movable kidney.

nephroptosis, *(nef-rō-tō'-sis),* floating kidney. Downward displacement of a kidney.

nephropyelolithotomy, *(nef-rō-pi-el-ō-lith-ot'-o-mi),* removal of a stone from the renal pelvis.

nephropyeloplasty, *(nef-rō-pī-el-ō-plas-ti),* plastic surgery on the renal pelvis.

nephrosclerosis, *(nef-rō-skle-rō-sis),* kidney disease where there are changes in the renal vessels and ischaemia. Associated with hypertension or atheroma.

nephroscope, *(nef-rō-skōp),* a fibreoptic device used percutaneously to remove renal calculi.

nephrosis, *(nef-rō-sis),* degenerative changes in kidney.

nephrostomy, *(nef-ros'to-mi),* an operation to establish an opening into the renal pelvis for drainage.

nephrotic syndrome, *(nef-ro-tik),* characterized by heavy proteinuria, hypoproteinaemia and gross generalized oedema, it occurs in a variety of kidney diseases.

nephrotomy, *(nef-rot'-o-mi),* cutting into the kidney.

nephrotoxic, *(nef-rō-tok-sik),* a substance toxic to nephrons, e.g. the drug gentamicin.

nephroureterectomy, *(nef-rō-ū-rē-ter-ek'-to-mi),* surgical removal of the kidney and ureter.

nerve, bundles of conducting fibres which convey impulses between a nerve centre and muscles and glands. *See* ENDONEURIUM, EPINEURIUM, MOTOR, NEURONE, PERINEURIUM, SENSORY, VASOMOTOR. *N. block: see* ANAESTHESIA. *N. growth factor (NGF):* a protein important for growth of nervous tissue during embryonic development and its later maintenance. *N. impulse: see* IMPULSE. *N. root:* the dorsal and ventral roots of a spinal nerve which arise from the spinal cord.

nervous, 1. pertaining to nerves. **2.** anxious or excited. *N. system: see* AUTONOMIC NERVOUS SYSTEM, CENTRAL NERVOUS SYSTEM, PERIPHERAL NERVOUS SYSTEM.

nettle-rash, urticaria.

network, connecting computers together so they can share files and resources. *See* INTRANET, LAN, WAN.

52 A nephron

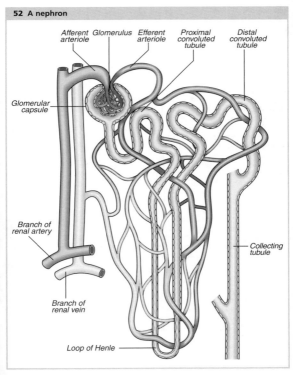

Afferent arteriole — Glomerulus — Efferent arteriole — Proximal convoluted tubule — Distal convoluted tubule

Glomerular capsule

Branch of renal artery

Branch of renal vein

Loop of Henle

Collecting tubule

neural, relating to nerves. *N. tube*: embryonic structure from which the central nervous system develops. *N. tube defects*: congenital developmental abnormalities affecting the nervous system, e.g. spina bifida. *See* FOLATES.

neuralgia, *(nū-ral-ji-a)*, pain in the distribution of a nerve, e.g. trigeminal.

neurapraxia, *(nū-ra-prak-si-a)*, temporary loss of nerve impulse conduction in a peripheral nerve; causes include nerve compression.

neurectomy, *(nū-rek'-to-mi),* excision of part of a nerve.

neurilemma, *(nū-ri-lem'-a),* outer sheath of a nerve fibre.

neurinoma, *(nū-ri-nō-ma),* a neuroma. Tumour of neurilemma, e.g. acoustic n.

neuritis, *(nū-rī'-tis),* inflammation of a nerve.

neuroblast, *(nū-rō-blast),* embryonic nerve cell.

neuroblastoma, *(nū-rō-blas-tō-ma),* a malignant tumour of embryonic nervous tissue, occurring in the adrenal medulla or sympathetic ganglia.

neurodermatitis, *(nū-rō-der-ma-tī-tis),* characteristic hyperkeratosis that is associated with habitual scratching.

neuroepithelium, *(nū-rō-ep-i-thē-li-um),* specialized epithelium containing receptors for external stimuli. Associated with the sense organs, e.g. olfactory epithelium in the nose.

neurofibrillary tangles, common pathological change occurring in the brain of people with Alzheimer's disease. Abnormal neurones, filled with filaments, form clusters of tangles.

neurofibroma, *(nū-rō-fī-brō'-ma),* tumour arising from connective tissue surrounding peripheral nerves.

neurofibromatosis, *(nū-rō-fī-brō-ma-tō-sis),* inherited condition where there are multiple neurofibromas on cranial and peripheral nerves. *See* VON RECKLINGHAUSEN'S DISEASE.

neurogenic, *(nū-rō-jen-ik),* caused or derived from nervous activity. *N. bladder:* functional disorder of the bladder caused by a disruption to its nerve supply, e.g. spinal cord injury, multiple sclerosis, diabetes mellitus and spina bifida. It causes either retention of urine, which presents as overflow incontinence, or continuous dribbling without retention. *N. shock: see* SHOCK.

neuroglia, *(nū-rō-gli-a),* glial cells. Nonexcitable supporting cells of the central nervous system. *See* ASTROCYTES, EPENDYMAL CELLS, MICROGLIAL CELLS, OLIGODENDROCYTES, SCHWANN CELLS.

neurohypophysis, *(nū-rō-hi-pof-i-sis),* the posterior lobe of the pituitary gland.

neurolemma, *(nū-rō-lem-ma), see* NEURILEMMA.

neuroleptics, *(nū-rō-lep-tik),* antipsychotics. Drugs that act on the nervous system. They are used in the management of schizophrenia, affective disorders, e.g. depression and organic psychoses. Basically they are all antagonists of dopamine receptors. They are classified as typical, e.g. fluphenazine and haloperidol, and atypical, e.g. sulpiride and clozapine. The typical neuroleptics may cause extrapyramidal side-effects, e.g. tremor, rigidity. *See* TARDIVE DYSKINESIA. The atypical drugs cause fewer side-effects.

neurological, pertaining to neurology. *N. assessment/observations:* used to assess neurological status, e.g. after head injury. They include: colour, respiration, blood pressure, pulse, temperature, level of consciousness, limb movement and pupil size and reaction. *See* GLASGOW COMA SCALE.

neurologist, *(nū-rol'-o-jist),* physician who specializes in neurology.

neurology, *(nū-rol'-o-ji),* medical science of diseases of the nervous system.

neuroma, *(nū-rō'-ma),* a tumour composed of nerve tissue.

neuromuscular, *(nū-rō-mus-kū-lar),* pertaining to nerves and muscles. *N. junction:* motor end plate. The communication between the axon and muscle fibre. *See* SYNAPSE.

neurone, a nerve cell. Highly differentiated excitable cells capable of transmitting an action potential. They have a nerve cell body with a nucleus, a long process called an axon and several short branching processes called dendrites (Figure 53). Types include: interneurone, motor and sensory.

neuropathy, *(nū-rop'-ath-i),* any disease of the nervous system, e.g. diabetic neuropathy.

neuropeptides, large group of neurotransmitters. They include: endorphins, somatostatin and enkephalins.

neuroplasticity, ability of nerve cells to regenerate.

neuroplasty, *(nū-rō-plas-ti),* operation to repair a nerve.

neurosis, *(nū-rō-sis),* a mental health problem where the person generally

---

53 Neurone (arrow shows the direction of impulse transmission)

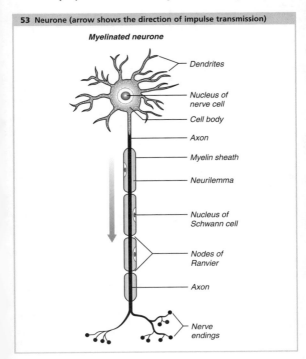

Myelinated neurone

- Dendrites
- Nucleus of nerve cell
- Cell body
- Axon
- Myelin sheath
- Neurilemma
- Nucleus of Schwann cell
- Nodes of Ranvier
- Axon
- Nerve endings

has some insight into his or her condition and may function as normal in some areas of his or her life. Associated with anxiety, stress and interpersonal problems, it is a functional disorder. Types include: anxiety, phobic, hysterical, obsessive-compulsive and depressive.

neurosurgery, surgery of peripheral and central nervous system.

neurosyphilis, (nū-rō-sif-il-is), involvement of the central nervous system by syphilis.

neurotic, 1. pertaining to a neurosis. **2.** a person with a neurosis. *N. disorder: see* NEUROSIS.

neurotmesis, (nū-rot-mē'-sis), severing or crushing of a peripheral nerve with loss of function.

neurotomy, (nū-rot-o-mi), division of a nerve.

neurotoxic, a substance which is toxic to nervous tissue.

neurotransmitter, a chemical released by nerve endings which allows the passage of the nerve impulse across a junction, e.g. acetylcholine, noradrenaline (norepinephrine), dopamine.

neurotripsy, (nū-rō-trip-si), the crushing of a nerve.

neurotropism, (nū-rō-trō-pizm), the predilection which some microorganisms have for nerve tissue, e.g. viruses of rabies and poliomyelitis.

neurula, (nū-ru-la), early embryonic stage when differentiation of nervous tissue commences.

neutral, 1. neither acid nor alkaline: pH 7.0. having no electrical charge.

neutron, subatomic particle without an electrical charge. *N. beam:* used for external beam therapy in radiotherapy.

neutropenia, (nū-trō-pē-ni-a), a reduction in the number of neutrophils in the peripheral blood.

neutrophil, (nū-trō-fil), a phagocytic leucocyte, forming the majority of

the polymorphonuclear series. *See* BLOOD, BLOOD COUNT, PHAGOCYTOSIS.

neutrophilia, (nū-trō-fi-li-a), an increase in the number of neutrophils in the peripheral blood.

neutrophilic, (nū-trō-fil-ik), having a predilection for neutral dyes/stains.

newton (N), SI unit of force, a derived unit.

NHS Trust, public accountable body that provides NHS healthcare to the population, either as a hospital or community trust.

niacin, (nī-a-sin), generic term which includes nicotinic acid and nicotinamide.

nicotinamide, (nik-o-tin-a-mīd), part of the vitamin B complex. It is obtained from food, formed from nicotinic acid or synthesized from the amino acid tryptophan. Required for the coenzymes NAD and NADP involved in glycolysis and oxidative phosphorylation. *See* PELLAGRA.

nicotine, poisonous alkaloid present in tobacco.

nicotinic, (ni-kō-tin'-ik), describes a type of cholinergic receptor where nicotine would, if present, bind instead of the neurotransmitter acetylcholine. *See* MUSCARINIC.

nicotinic acid, (ni-ko-tin-ik), part of vitamin B complex. *See* NIACIN, NICOTINAMIDE.

nictitation, (nik-ti-tā'-shon), involuntary blinking of the eyelids.

nidation, (ni-dā-shon), implantation, such as the ovum in the uterus.

NIDDM, abbreviation for **non-insulin-dependent diabetes mellitus.**

Niemann–Pick's disease, an inherited lipid storage disease where there is an accumulation of cholesterol and sphingomyelin in the liver, brain, spleen and bone marrow.

night-blindness, *see* NYCTALOPIA.

nipple, (nip'-pl), small eminence in the centre of each breast.

Nissl granules, *(nis-l)*, the rough endoplasmic reticulum present in the cytoplasm of a nerve cell body of a neurone.

nit, the egg of the louse.

nitrates, a salt of nitric acid. Some are used as coronary vasodilators for people with angina, e.g. glyceryl trinitrate.

nitric acid, a highly corrosive mineral acid.

nitric oxide (NO), naturally occurring neuromodulator. It is involved in areas such as learning, memory, nociception, etc. May be used therapeutically in acute respiratory distress syndrome.

nitrite, a salt of nitrous acid.

nitrogen (N), a colourless gaseous element which forms 78–79% of the atmosphere. Nitrogenous foods (protein) are required for the formation of proteins and nucleic acids. In health the body maintains a positive nitrogen balance.

nitrogenous, substances containing nitrogen such as amino acids.

nitrous oxide, an anaesthetic gas.

NMC, abbreviation for **Nursing and Midwifery Council.**

NMR, nuclear magnetic resonance, *see* MAGNETIC RESONANCE IMAGING.

nociceptors, *(no-si-sep-tors)*, sensory receptors which respond to stimuli which are harmful to tissues and cause pain, e.g. trauma, inflammatory chemicals.

nocturia, *(nok-tū-ri-a)*, passing urine at night.

nocturnal, at night. *N. enuresis:* bedwetting during sleep.

node, a swelling. *Atrioventricular n.:* see ATRIOVENTRICULAR (A-V). *Heberden's n.:* see HEBERDEN'S NODE. *Lymph n.:* see LYMPH. *N. of Ranvier:* constrictions in the neurilemma of a nerve fibre. *Sinoatrial n.:* see SINOATRIAL NODE.

nodule, a small node.

nominal data, categorical data where the classes have no particular order or value, such as colours. *See* ORDINAL DATA.

nomogram, a graph with several variables used to determine another related variable, e.g. body surface area from height and weight.

non-accidental injury (NAI), physical maltreatment of children by their parents, other adults or sometimes other children. It is characterized by injuries such as fractures and burns and the results of neglect, e.g. starvation. *See* CHILD ABUSE.

non-compliance, failure of an individual to adhere to a therapeutic regimen, such as medication, dietary modification or appointments, for a variety of reasons.

non compos mentis, not of sound mind.

non-insulindependent diabetes mellitus (NIDDM), *see* DIABETES MELLITUS.

non-maleficence, doing no harm. Cf. BENEFICENCE.

non-parametric test, statistical test that makes no assumption about the distribution of data.

non-rapid eye movement sleep (NREM), describes four stages of sleep (progressing from wakefulness to deep sleep without rapid eye movements) which occur in alternating cycles with rapid eye movement sleep.

non-starch polysaccharides (NSP), polysaccharides, other than starch, found in plant cell walls. They provide most of the dietary fibre in the diet.

non-steroidal anti-inflammatory drugs (NSAIDs), large group of drugs with variable anti-inflammatory, analgesic and antipyretic properties, e.g. naproxen.

non-union, failure of a fracture to heal.

noradrenaline (norepinephrine), (*nor-ad-ren-a-lin*), a catecholamine hormone produced by the adrenal medulla and a neurotransmitter functioning in the sympathetic division of the autonomic nervous system. Its physiological effects include: vasoconstriction and a rise in blood pressure.

norm, a standard against which values can be measured.

normal, the average or usual form. *N. distribution curve:* in statistics. When scores are plotted they form a bell-shaped curve which has the mean, mode and median in the centre. *N. flora:* the microorganisms which normally live in or on the body. *N. solution:* contains the equivalent weight of the substance in grams dissolved in a litre of solution.

normalization, the philosophy underpinning learning disability nursing and service delivery. Programmes of learning and individualized goal setting can help in acquiring the skills of daily living and maximum levels of independence.

normoblasts, immature nucleated red cells present in red bone marrow.

normocyte, (*nor'-mō-sīt*), a normally sized erythrocyte.

normotensive, having normal pressure. Usually applied to normal blood pressure for age and gender.

Norton scale, a scale devised by Norton, McLaren and Exton-Smith and used to identify those patients at risk of pressure ulcer development.

nose, the organ of smell. Also used for warming, filtering and moistening the air breathed in.

nosocomial infection, an infection acquired in hospital.

nostrils, the anterior apertures of the nose.

notifiable, diseases, incidents or occurrences that must by law be made known to the appropriate agency. Diseases such as food poisoning, diphtheria and measles must be reported to the relevant health authority.

NPF, abbreviation for **Nurse Prescribers' Formulary**.

nuclear, pertaining to a nucleus. *N. family: see* FAMILY. *N. magnetic resonance (NMR): See* MAGNETIC RESONANCE IMAGING. *N. medicine:* radionuclide techniques used for diagnosis, treatment and study of disease.

nucleated, (*nū'-klē-ā-ted*), with a nucleus.

nucleic acid, (*nū'-klā-ik*), long-chain organic molecule formed from many nucleotides. *See* DEOXYRIBONUCLEIC ACID, NUCLEOTIDE, RIBONUCLEIC ACID.

nucleolus, (*nū'-klē-ō-lus*), situated within the nuclear membrane, usually two in number, containing DNA and RNA and involved in nuclear division.

nucleoprotein, (*nū-klē-ō-prō-teen*), compound of protein and nucleic acid in nuclei.

nucleoside, (*nū'-klē-ō-sīd*), compound of a sugar and nitrogenous base (a purine or pyrimidine).

nucleotide, (*nū-klē-ō-tīd*), a compound of a sugar, a nitrogenous base (purine or pyrimidine) and phosphate groups. *See* NUCLEIC ACID.

nucleus, 1. of the cell, the structure containing the genetic material. *See* CELL. **2.** of the brain, an anatomically distinct area of cells within the brain. *N. pulposus:* a pulpy mass in the centre of the intervertebral discs. May become prolapsed into the spinal canal causing pressure on the cord and spinal nerves.

null hypothesis, a statement that declares there to be no relationship between dependent and independent variables.

nullipara, *(nul-lip'-a-ra),* a woman who has never had a child.

nurse, a person educated, skilled and qualified in the practice of nursing. A person whose name appears on the register of nurses administered by the United Kingdom Central Council for Nursing, Midwifery and Health Visiting (UKCC)/Nursing and Midwifery Council (NMC).

nurse consultant, new role for experienced clinical practitioners who have the necessary level of expertise in an area of practice; professional leadership and consultancy; education, training and development; and practice and service development, research and evaluation. Those appointed have considerable patient contact and work in diverse areas that include: critical care, mental health, continence care, dermatology, etc.

nurse practitioner, a nurse who has undergone specific role preparation to enable him or her to function at an advanced level within a particular working environment. This may be within primary healthcare, in an accident and emergency setting, or working with certain client groups, such as homeless people. Nurse practitioners can offer a nurse-led service and invariably have highly developed skills in client assessment.

nurse prescribing, in the UK limited drug prescribing by suitably registered health visitors and district nurses who have recorded their qualification with the UKCC. Individuals concerned have completed an appropriate course, demonstrated prescribing competence and are accountable for their prescribing from the Nurse Prescribers' Formulary.

nursing, the activities and interventions used by professional nurses to fulfil their role in preventing ill health, maintaining and restoring health and caring for people with ill health. *Barrier n.: see* BARRIER NURSING. *N. audit: see* AUDIT. *N. care plan: see* CARE PLAN. *N. diagnosis: see* DIAGNOSIS. *N. model:* the theoretical framework used by nurses to make sense of practice, identify their role and provide care which is consistent and of high quality. Particular nursing models may be widely used or developed for more local or specific use.

Nursing and Midwifery Council (NMC), a smaller council established in 2001, for the regulation of nursing, midwifery and health visiting in the UK. The new body replaces the UKCC and the four National Boards.

nursing process, the systematic, problem-solving approach to individualized nursing care within the framework of a particular nursing model. There are four overlapping stages: assessment, planning, implementation and evaluation.

nutation, *(nū-tā'-shon),* involuntary nodding of the head.

nutrient, nourishing. *N. foramen:* opening in a bone for the nourishing vessels.

nutrition, the science of food and its utilization by the body. Or the total process of receiving and utilizing the materials needed for survival, growth and repair. *See* ENTERAL NUTRITION, PARENTERAL.

nyctalopia, *(nik-tal-ō'-pi-a),* a state of the eyes which causes vision to be worse at night than during the day.

nyctophobia, *(nik-tō-fō'-bi-a),* abnormal fear of darkness.

nymphae, *(nim-fē),* labia minora.

nymphomania, excessive sexual desire in females.

nystagmus, *(nis-tag-mus)*, involuntary oscillations of the eyeball, may be caused by neurological disorders, vestibular apparatus problems or as a side-effect of some drugs.

O

oat cell carcinoma, a type of bronchial carcinoma characterized by ectopic hormone production, e.g. ACTH, ADH.

obesity, a common nutritional disorder characterized by excess body fat. Definitions vary but a body mass index in excess of 30 is accepted as obese by many authorities.

objective, 1. the lens nearest the object being viewed in a microscope. **2.** pertaining to matters external to oneself. **3.** an aim or purpose. *O. signs*: the observed signs of a disease, as distinct from the symptoms of which the patient complains.

obligate, mandatory or essential. *O. aerobe*: a microorganism which cannot grow or divide without oxygen. *O. anaerobe*: a microorganism which cannot grow or divide with oxygen in its environment.

oblique, inclined or slanted. *O. muscles*: **1.** two extrinsic muscles of the eyeball (superior and inferior). **2.** two large muscles of the abdominal wall (internal and external).

observation, using the senses to assess a situation and to collect data required to plan individualized care.

observational study, one where the researchers observe, listen and record the events of interest.

obsession, recurring thoughts. May be experienced by healthy individuals but often a feature of mental health problems.

obsessive-compulsive disorder (OCD) neurosis, a neurotic disorder where there may be obsessional thoughts which the patient tries to stop or a compulsion to repeat an act which the patient recognizes as being senseless and absurd. Attempts by the patient to control the behaviour lead to anxiety. *See* NEUROSIS.

obstetrician, *(ob-stet-rish-un),* doctor who practises obstetrics.

obstetrics, *(ob-stet-riks),* the medical science which deals with pregnancy, labour and the puerperium.

obstruction, 1. blockage of a hollow structure or passage such as the intestine or bile duct. **2.** whatever is causing the blockage, e.g. gallstone.

obturator, that which closes an aperture. *O. foramen*: a hole on either side of the pelvis, closed by ligaments and muscles.

obtusion, a blunting, as of sensitivity.

occipital, *(ok-sip′-i-tal),* relating to the back of the head. *O. bone*: bone forming the back of the cranium and part of the base of the skull.

occipito-anterior, *(ok-sip′-i-tō-an-tēr-ē-or),* a vertex presentation where the fetal occiput lies in the anterior part of the maternal pelvis.

occipito-posterior, *(ok-sip′-i-tō-pos-tēr-ē-or),* a vertex presentation where the fetal occiput lies in the posterior part of the maternal pelvis.

occiput, back of the head.

occlusion, *(ok-lū-zhon),* closure. *Coronary o.*: such as caused by a thrombosis in a coronary artery. *Dental o.*: the fit between the upper and lower teeth when they are in contact.

occlusive, *(ok-lū-siv),* something that covers or closes completely. *O. dressing*: one which completely seals a wound or ulcer.

occult, *(ok-ult),* hidden, not visible to the naked eye *O. blood*: term applied to minute quantities of blood passed in the faeces which can only be demonstrated chemically.

occupational, pertaining to an individual's work. *O. disease*: *see* INDUSTRIAL DISEASE. *O. health nurse*: a nurse with specialist skills and qualifications who provides professional services within a workplace location. *O. therapist*: health professional who practises occupational therapy. *O. therapy*: the treatment of physical and psychiatric conditions through specific activities in order to help people reach their maximum level of function and independence in all aspects of daily life.

oclophobia, *(ok'-lō-fō-bi-a),* abnormal fear of crowds.

ocular, *(ok'-ū-lar),* relating to the eye.

oculist, *(ok'-ū-list),* an eye specialist. An ophthalmologist.

oculogyric, *(o-kū-lō-ji-rik),* making the eyes roll.

oculomotor nerves, *(ok-ū-lō-mō-tor),* third pair of cranial nerves. They innervate four extrinsic muscles of the eyeball and alter pupil size and lens shape.

Oddi, sphincter of, a muscular sphincter at the opening of the common bile duct into the duodenum.

odontalgia, *(o-don-tal'-jia),* toothache.

odontoid, *(o-don'-toyd),* toothlike. *O. process*: peglike projection of second cervical vertebra.

odontolith, *(o-don'-to-lith),* calcareous matter deposited on teeth; tartar.

odontology, *(o-don-tol'-o-ji),* dentistry.

odontoma, *(o-don-tō'-ma),* tumour arising from a tooth or a developing tooth.

oedema, *(e-dē-ma),* swelling due to excess fluid in the tissue (interstitial) spaces and serous cavities. Causes include: (a) increased capillary permeability, e.g. release of inflammatory chemicals; (b) reduced osmotic pressure due to hypoproteinaemia, e.g. liver failure; (c) lymphatic obstruction, e.g. with malignancy and (d) increased venous hydrostatic pressure, e.g. heart failure. *Pulmonary o.*: fluid within the alveoli caused by acute left ventricular failure.

Oedipus complex, *(ē-di-pus),* an unconscious attachment of a son for his mother with jealousy of his father. This is suppressed with the production of guilt and conflict. Named after Oedipus who, according to mythology, unknowingly killed his father and married his mother.

oesophageal, *(ē-sof-a-jē-al),* pertaining to the oesophagus. *O. atresia*: developmental defect where the oesophagus ends in a blind pouch, often associated with a tracheal fistula. *O. reflux*: *see* GASTROOESOPHAGEAL. *O. varices*: varicosities at the gastrooesophageal junction. Associated with hepatic portal hypertension, they can cause massive haematemesis.

oesophagectasis, *(ē-sof-a-jek-tā-sis),* dilatation of the oesophagus.

oesophagectomy, *(ē-sof-a-jek-to-mi),* resection of part of the oesophagus.

oesophagitis, *(ē-sof-a-jī-tis),* inflammation of the oesophagus, especially that caused by the reflux of acid gastric contents due to hiatus hernia.

oesophagogastrectomy, *(ē-sof-a-go-gas-trek-to-mi),* removal of part of the oesophagus and the stomach.

oesophagogastroduodenoscopy (OGD), (ē-sof-a-go-gas-trō-dū-ō-dē-nō-skōp), endoscopic examination of the upper gastrointestinal tract.

oesophagoscope, (ē-sof-a-go-skōp), an endoscope used to view the interior of the oesophagus. Usually a flexible fibreoptic endoscope is used, but rigid metal instruments may be used occasionally.

oesophagostomy, (ē-sof-a-gos'-to-mi), operation where an artificial opening is made into the oesophagus.

oesophagus, (ē-sof-a-gus), the canal which runs from the pharynx into the stomach.

oestradiol (estradiol), (ē-stra-di-ol), principal oestrogen hormone produced by the corpus luteum during the second part of the menstrual cycle.

oestriol (estriol), (ē-strē-ol), an oestrogen produced by the placenta and the fetus. Oestriol levels in maternal blood or urine have been used as an indicator of placental function and fetal well-being.

oestrogenic, (ēs-trō-jen-ik), a substance having an oestrogen-like action.

oestrogens (estrogens), (ēs-trō-jens), a group of steroid hormones, oestriol, oestrone and oestradiol, which are responsible for the development and functioning of the female genital organs and the female secondary sexual characteristics. They are produced by the ovaries, the placenta and to a lesser extent in the adrenal cortex of both sexes.

oestrone (estrone), (ēs-trōn), an oestrogen produced by the ovary, important in menstrual cycle regulation.

ointment, an external application with a soft base impregnated with a drug.

old age mental illness, a term increasingly applied to mental health problems of older people, instead of elderly mentally ill.

olecranon, (o-lek-ra-non), a process on the upper end of the ulna forming part of the elbow. See ELBOW.

olfaction, the sense of smell.

olfactory, (ol-fak-tur-i), relating to the sense of smell. O. nerves: first pair of cranial nerves. They carry impulses from the olfactory epithelium to the olfactory cortex.

oligaemia, (ol-i-gē'-mi-a), lack of blood.

oligodendrocyte, (ol-i-gō-den'-drō-sīt), a type of neuroglial cell within the central nervous system.

oligohydramnios, (ol-i-gō-hī-dram'-ni-os), deficiency of amniotic fluid.

oligomenorrhoea, (ol-i-gō-me-no-rēa), infrequent or sparse menstruation.

oligospermia, (ol-i-gō-sper-mē-a), reduction in the number of spermatozoa in semen.

oliguria, (ol-ig-ūr-i-a), a decrease in the amount of urine produced by the kidneys.

ombudsman, a commissione (e.g. health) appointed by government to hear complaints in situations where it has not been possible to reach a satisfactory resolution at local level.

omentum, (ō-men-tum), a fold of the peritoneum. The greater o. is suspended from the greater curvature of the stomach and hangs in front of the gut. The lesser o. passes from the lesser curvature of the stomach to the transverse fissure of the liver.

omphalitis, (om-fal-ī-tis), inflammation of the umbilicus.

omphalocele, (om'-fal-ō-sēl), an umbilical hernia.

omphalus, (om-fal-us), the umbilicus.

Onchocerca, (on-kō-ser-ka), a genus of parasitic filarial nematodes.

onchocerciasis, (on-kō-ser-ki'-a-sis), river blindness. An infection of the skin, subcutaneous tissue and the eye by the filarial worm *Onchocerca volvulus*.

oncogene, a gene which has the potential to cause malignant changes.

oncogenic, *(on-kō-jen-ik)*, an agent or substance which causes tumour development, e.g. by viruses, chemicals. *See* CARCINOGENIC.

oncology, *(on-kol-o-ji)*, the study and treatment of tumours.

onychia, *(ōn-ik'-i-a)*, inflammation of the matrix of the nail.

onychogryphosis, *(on-ik-ō-gri-fō-sis)*, bizarre overgrowth of the nails, often the nail of the great toe.

onychomycosis, *(on-ik-ō-mī-kō-sis)*, fungal infection of the nails.

oöcyte, *(ō-o-sīt)*, an immature ovum. A female gamete prior to its penetration by a spermatozoon.

oögenesis, *(ō-o-jen'-e-sis)*, the production of oöcytes in the ovary.

oöphorectomy, *(ō-of-or-ek'-to-mi)*, removal of an ovary. *See* OVARIECTOMY.

oöphoritis, *(ō-of-or-ī'-tis)*, inflammation of an ovary.

oöphoron, *(ō-of-or-on)*, the ovary.

oöphorosalpingectomy, *(ō-of-or-ō-sal-pin-jek'-to-mi)*, removal of the ovary and its associated uterine tube.

opacity, *(ō-pas'-i-ti)*, want of transparency, cloudiness.

operant, *see* CONDITIONING.

operating system, a program that the computer must automatically load before it can run any other programs, e.g. MS-DOS, UNIX.

operculum, *(ō-per-kū-lum)*, plug of mucus which occludes the cervical canal during pregnancy.

ophthalmia, *(of-thal-mi-a)*, ophthalmitis. Inflammation of the eye. *O. neonatorum*: purulent inflammation of the eyes of the newborn. A notifiable condition which occurs as the infant passes through the vagina.

May be caused by chlamydial or gonococcal infections. *Sympathetic o.*: inflammation of the uveal tract which follows damage or disease in the other eye.

ophthalmic, *(of-thal'-mik)*, pertaining to the eye.

ophthalmitis, *(of-thal-mī-tis)*, inflammation of the eye.

ophthalmologist, *(of-thal-mol-o-jist)*, a doctor specializing in the treatment of eye diseases.

ophthalmology, the study of diseases of the eye.

ophthalmoplegia, *(of-thal-mō-plē'-ji-a)*, paralysis of the muscles of the eye.

ophthalmoscope, *(of-thal'-mō-skōp)*, a small instrument fitted with lenses and a light used to examine the interior of the eye.

opiate, *(ō-pē-āt)*, *see* OPIOIDS.

opioids, a group of morphine-like drugs that produce the same effects as morphine and can be reversed by antagonists such as naloxone. It includes: morphine analogues, e.g. morphine, diamorphine, codeine, naloxone; synthetic derivatives, e.g. pethidine, fentanyl, methadone, dextropropoxyphene, pentazocine, buprenorphine, etc.

opisthotonos, *(op-is-thot'-o-nōs)*, severe muscle spasm causing backward retraction of the head with arching of the back. Seen in tetanus and meningitis.

opium, obtained from poppy juice, it contains several alkaloids which include: morphine, codeine, papaverine. A narcotic and strong analgesic.

opponens, *(op-ō'-nens)*, opposing. Applied to muscles, e.g. o. pollicis brings the thumb towards the little finger.

opportunistic infection, a serious infection in an immunocompromised individual. Caused by organisms which normally have little or no pathogenic activity. *See* ACQUIRED IMMUNE DEFICIENCY SYNDROME.

opsins, the protein component of the visual pigments present in the rods and cones.

opsonic index, a measurement of the ability of phagocytes to destroy bacteria.

opsonins, substances such as antibodies or complement which make bacteria more susceptible to phagocytosis.

opsonization, the process by which bacteria are rendered more susceptible to phagocytosis.

optic, relating to sight. *O. atrophy*: degeneration of the optic nerve. *O. chiasma*: the point at the base of the brain where some optic nerve fibres cross over (Figure 54). *O. disc*: the point at which the optic nerve fibres

leave the eye. *See* BLIND SPOT. *O. nerves*: second pair of cranial nerves. They carry impulses from the photoreceptors of the retina to the visual cortex.

optical, pertaining to sight. *O. density*: the amount of light absorbed by a solution, used to determine the concentration of substances being measured.

optician, a person qualified to make or prescribe spectacles and contact lenses to correct refractive errors. *Ophthalmic o.*: a person who also tests eyes.

optics, the study of the properties of light.

optimum, the best possible in the particular circumstances.

optometry, measurement of visual acuity, performed by an optometrist.

oral, pertaining to the mouth, such as oral hygiene or contraceptive. *O.*

54 Optic chiasma

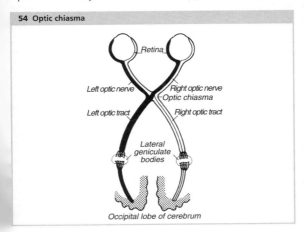

Retina

Left optic nerve

Right optic nerve

Optic chiasma

Left optic tract

Right optic tract

Lateral geniculate bodies

Occipital lobe of cerebrum

phase: a stage of development characterized by the infant's sensual interest in the mouth and activities such as sucking, biting and taking objects to the mouth. *O. rehydration solution (ORS)*: a solution of glucose and electrolytes used in oral rehydration.

orbicularis, *(or-bik-ū-la'-ris)*, a name given to the muscle which encircles an orifice, e.g. o. oris around the mouth.

orbit, bony cavity in the skull which holds and protects the eye.

orbital, pertaining to the orbit.

orchidalgia, *(or-kid-al-ji-a)*, pain in the testes.

orchidectomy, removal of one or both testes.

orchidopexy, *(or-kid-o-pek-si)*, operation to bring down an undescended testis and secure it within the scrotum.

orchiepididymitis, *(or-ki-ep-i-did-i-mī-tis)*, inflammation of the testis and epididymis.

orchis, *(or'-kis)*, testis.

orchitis, *(or-kī'-tis)*, inflammation of a testis.

ordinal data, categorical data that can be ordered or ranked, e.g. size in general terms, as in bigger than, or general condition – good, moderate or bad. *See* NOMINAL DATA.

orf, a virus transmitted from sheep and goats which may cause skin lesions in humans.

organ, a grouping together of tissues to form discrete functional units, they may be hollow or compact. *O. transplants*: *see* TRANSPLANTATION.

organelle, cellular structures with specific functions such as the mitochondria and ribosomes.

organic, pertaining to the organs. *O. compounds*: chemical compounds that contain carbon and hydrogen, e.g. glucose. Include the large biological molecules, such as proteins and carbohydrates. *O. disease*: one in which there is structural change in an organ.

organism, a living cell or cells.

organogenesis, *(or-gan-ō-jen'-i-sis)*, organ formation during embryonic and fetal development.

orgasm, the climax of sexual excitement.

oriental sore, Delhi boil. Cutaneous leishmaniasis seen in subtropical and tropical areas.

orientation, direction and position of acclimatization. 1. the location and knowledge of one's position and attitude in relation to the environment and time 2. dissemination of information prior to the commencement of a course etc.

orifice, an opening.

origin, anatomical term for the attachment of a muscle or the point at which a vessel or nerve branches from the main blood vessel or nerve.

ornithine, *(or-ni-thēn)*, an amino acid derived from arginine during the reactions of the urea cycle in the liver.

ornithosis, *(or-ni-thō-sis)*, a disease of birds, transmissible to humans, e.g. psittacosis.

orogenital, *(or-ō-jen-i-tal)*, pertaining to the mouth and external genitalia.

oropharynx, *(o-rō-fa-rinks)*, the part of the pharynx between the soft palate and the hyoid bone.

orthodontics, a branch of dentistry which deals with the prevention and correction of irregularities of the teeth.

orthopaedics, *(or-thō-pē-diks)*, the branch of surgery which deals with the correction of skeletal deformity and disease or injury of the locomotor system.

orthopnoea, *(or-thop'-nē-a)*, breathlessness where relief can be obtained only in an upright position.

orthoptics, (or-thop'-tiks), the practice of non-surgical correction of visual abnormalities such as strabismus by exercises, etc.

orthostatic, pertaining to or caused by standing upright. *O. albuminuria*: occurs in healthy people only when they stand upright.

Ortolani's test, (or-tō-la-nēz), used as one of the tests for developmental dysplasia of the hip in the newborn. *See* BARLOW'S TEST, DEVELOPMENTAL DYSPLASIA OF THE HIP.

os, 1. a mouth. *External os.*: opening of the cervix into the vagina. *Internal os.*: opening of the cervix into the uterine cavity. **2.** a bone. *O. calcis*: the heel bone.

oscheal, (os'-kē-al), pertaining to the scrotum.

oscillation, (os-si-la'-shon), a swinging movement.

oscilloscope, (os-sil-ō-skōp), a device which uses the fluorescent screen of a cathode ray tube to display various electrical waveforms such as that produced by the heart (ECG).

Osgood–Schlatter's disease, osteochondritis affecting the tibial tubercle.

Osler's nodes, painful tender swellings on the extremities, seen in subacute bacterial endocarditis.

osmolality, the osmotic pressure expressed as the number of osmoles (or milliosmoles) per kilogram of solution.

osmolarity, the osmotic pressure exerted by a given concentration of osmotically active solute in aqueous solution, defined in terms of the number of active particles per unit volume. The number of osmoles (or milliosmoles) per litre of solution.

osmole, standard unit of osmotic pressure which is equal to the molecular weight in grams of a solute divided by the number of

particles or ions into which it dissociates in solution. In low concentration solutions a smaller unit, the milliosmole, is used.

osmoreceptors, (oz-mō-rē-sep-terz), specialized cells in the hypothalamus which monitor the concentration (osmotic pressure) of the blood and extracellular fluid.

osmosis, (os-mō'-sis) the passage of water across a selectively permeable membrane under the influence of osmotic pressure. The movement of a dilute solution (lower solute concentration) to a more concentrated solution (higher solute concentration).

osmotic, (os-mo-tik), pertaining to osmosis. *O. pressure*: the pressure with which solvent molecules are drawn across a selectively permeable membrane separating two concentrations of the solute dissolved in the same solvent, when the membrane is impermeable to the solute but permeable to the solvent.

osseous, (os'-e-us), like bone, bony.

ossicle, (os'-sik-al), a small bone. Name applied to the tiny bones of the middle ear. *See* EAR.

ossification, process of bone formation. Also called **osteogenesis**.

ossify, to become bone.

osteitis, (os-tē-ī-tis), inflammation of bone. *O. deformans*: see PAGET'S DISEASE. *O. fibrosa cystica*: von Recklinghausen's disease of the bone. Where hyperparathyroidism causes calcium reabsorption from bone with cyst formation.

osteoarthritis, (os-tē-ō-ar-thrī-tis), osteoarthrosis (OA). A degenerative joint disease with loss of articular cartilage and underlying bone changes, e.g. osteophytes. It may be primary, where the aetiology is unknown, or secondary to joint injury or disease, usually affecting the hips, knees, spine and hands.

osteoarthropathy, *(os-tē-ō-ar-throp'-a-thi),* damage or disease affecting bones and joints.

osteoarthrotomy, *(os-tē-ō-ar-throt'-o-mi),* excision of joint and neighbouring bone.

osteoblasts, *(os-tē-ō-blasts),* bone-forming cells.

osteochondritis, *(os-tē-ō-kon-drī-tis),* inflammation of bone and cartilage. Usually applied to non-septic conditions, especially avascular necrosis involving the joint surfaces, e.g. o. dissecans, in which a portion of the joint surface may separate to form a loose body in the joint. *See* OSGOOD–SCHLATTER DISEASE, PERTHES' DISEASE.

osteochondroma, *(os-tē-ō-kon-drō'-ma),* benign tumour derived from bone and cartilage.

osteoclasia, *(os-tē-ō-klā-zi-a),* absorption of bone by osteoclasts during periods of growth, for remodelling and following injury.

osteoclasis, *(os-tē-ō-klā-sis),* intentional surgical fracture to correct a deformity.

osteoclastoma, *(os-tē-ō-klas-tō-ma),* tumour of osteoclasts.

osteoclasts, *(os-tē-ō-klasts),* cells involved in the absorption and removal of bone.

osteocyte, *(os-tē-ō-sīt),* a bone cell.

osteogenesis, *(os-tē-ō-jen-e-sis),* the process of bone formation. Also called **ossification**. *O. imperfecta*: congenital condition, affecting both sexes, where the bones are slender, brittle and easily fractured. Similar condition to fragilitas ossium.

osteogenic, *(os-tē-ō-jen-ik),* bone-producing or derived from such tissue. *O. sarcoma: see* OSTEOSARCOMA.

osteoid, organic matrix of bone containing collagen and other molecules.

osteology, *(os-tē-ol-o-ji),* the study of bones.

osteolytic, *(os-tē-ō-lit-ik),* bone destroying.

osteoma, *(os-tē-ō'-ma),* a bony tumour.

osteomalacia, *(os-tē-ō-ma-la-she-a),* softening of bone due to a failure to mineralize the osteoid. Caused by lack of vitamin D, it is sometimes known as **adult rickets**.

osteomyelitis, *(os-tē-ō-mī-e-lī-tis),* inflammation of bone tissue, usually due to acute or chronic bacterial infection.

osteon, *(os-tē-on),* a haversian system, the basic structural unit of bone.

osteopath, *(os-tē-ō-path),* one who practises osteopathy.

osteopathy, *(os-tē-op'-a-thi),* **1.** disease of the bone. **2.** a clinical discipline and established system of assessment, diagnosis and treatment. Osteopathy is concerned with the inter-relationship between structure and function of the body. It is known to be effective for the relief or improvement of a wide variety of conditions, such as 'glue ear' and some digestive disorders, as well as mechanical problems of the body. Osteopathy is one of only a few complementary therapies to have achieved statutory self-regulation on a par with medicine (Osteopaths Act 1993).

osteopetrosis, *(os-tē-ō-pe-trō'-sis),* inherited bone disease characterized by increasing bone density with loss of medullary space. The bones become extremely hard but brittle, which results in fractures. Loss of haemopoietic marrow leads to problems with blood cell formation. Also called **Albers–Schönberg's disease, marble bone disease**.

osteophony, *(os-tē-of'-o-ni),* conduction of sound by bone.

osteophyte, *(os-tē-ō-fīt),* a small bony outgrowth; occurs in osteoarthritis.

osteoplastic, *(os-tē-ō-plas-tik)*, pertaining to the repair of bones.

osteoporosis, *(os-tē-ō-po-rō-sis)*, loss of bone mass due to reabsorption without the usual balance of bone deposition. The bones, which retain their normal composition, are lighter and weaker. They deform and fracture more easily, and fractures of the wrist, neck of femur and vertebrae are especially common. Causes include: ageing in both sexes, nutritional deficiencies, immobility, hormonal, e.g. postmenopausal, Cushing's disease and corticosteroid therapy.

osteosarcoma, *(os-tē-ō-sar-kō'-ma)*, malignant tumour arising in osteoblasts.

osteosclerosis, *(os-tē-ō-skle-rō'-sis)*, increase in bone density.

osteotome, *(os-tē-ō-tōm)*, an instrument used for cutting bone.

osteotomy, *(os-tē-ot'-o-mi)*, the operation of cutting through a bone, usually performed for the relief or cure of bony deformities.

ostium, an opening. The orifice of any tubular passage.

otalgia, *(ō-tal'-ji-a)*, earache.

otic, pertaining to the ear.

otitis, *(ō-ti-tis)*, inflammation of the ear. *O. externa*: inflammation of the skin of the external ear. *O. interna*: inflammation of the internal ear vestibular structures. *O. media*: inflammation of the middle ear.

otoacoustic emission (OAE), a computer-linked hearing test used for screening infants soon after birth.

otolaryngology, *(ō-tō-la-rin-gol-o-ji)*, the study of the ear and larynx and the disorders affecting them.

otolith, *(ō-tō-lith)*, tiny calcium deposits associated with the saccule and utricle of the internal ear.

otologist, *(ō-tol-o-jist)*, ear specialist.

otology, *(ō-tol-o-ji)*, study of diseases of the ear.

otomycosis, *(ō-tō-mī-kō-sis)*, fungal infection of the external auditory canal.

otorhinolaryngology, *(ō-tō-rīn-ō-la-rin-gol-o-ji)*, the study of the disorders affecting the ear, nose and larynx.

otorrhoea, *(ō-tō-rēa)*, discharge of fluid from the ear especially pus.

otosclerosis, a hereditary condition causing hearing impairment. It affects the ossicles, especially the stapes, where bone changes alter their ability to conduct sound waves. Leads to progressive conductive hearing loss.

otoscope, an instrument, usually incorporating both illumination and magnification. It is used to examine the external ear, tympanic membrane and, through the tympanic membrane, the middle-ear ossicles. Also called an **auriscope**.

ototoxic, *(ō-tō-tok-sik)*, an agent toxic to the ear or vestibulocochlear nerves.

outcome criteria, in nursing the measurable and observable elements which result from nursing actions.

outlet, an opening or exit, such as that of the pelvis.

ovarian, *(ō-vair-i-an)*, pertaining to the ovary. *O. cycle*: the events occurring in the ovary during follicular development and oögenesis. There are two phases: follicular, including ovulation, and the luteal phase. *O. cyst*: fluid filled tumour which may be benign or malignant. *See* CHOCOLATE CYST, DERMOID, ENDOMETRIOSIS.

ovariectomy, *(ō-var-i-ek-to-mi)*, oöphorectomy. Excision of one or both ovaries.

ovaries, the female gonads. Two small structures situated either side of the uterus. Under the cyclical influence of pituitary hormones they produce oöcytes and ovarian hormones. *Polycystic o.: see* STEIN–LEVENTHAL SYNDROME.

ovariotomy, (ō-var-i-ot'-o-mi), incision into an ovary.

ovaritis, (ō-var-i-tis), *see* OÖPHORITIS.

ovary, *see* OVARIES.

overcompensation, a term used to describe exaggerated compensatory behaviour, e.g. aggressive in response to feelings of inadequacy.

overdosage, excessive blood levels of a drug causing toxic effects. May be due to a cumulative effect or from too high a dose.

overextension, extension beyond the normal limit, e.g. of a joint or muscle.

over-the-counter (OTC) drugs, drugs that can be sold to the public without a prescription. Countries vary as to which drugs are included in this category.

oviduct, (o'-vi-dukt), uterine or fallopian tube.

ovulation, the process by which a mature Graafian follicle ruptures to release the secondary oöcyte from the surface of an ovary.

ovum, (ō-vum), the female gamete. Strictly speaking it is known as a secondary oöcyte until penetration by a spermatozoon.

oxalic acid, (ok-sal-ik), poisonous organic acid found in rhubarb leaves and other plants.

oxaluria, (oks-al-ū-ri-a), the presence of oxalic acid and oxalates in the urine.

Oxford grading system, used to assess pelvic floor strength with genuine stress incontinence, prior to designing an individual pelvic floor exercise plan.

oxidation, the addition of oxygen to a substance such as in the formation of oxides. It is also the removal of hydrogen or the loss of electrons

from an atom or molecule. Fuel molecules in the body are oxidized to provide energy for metabolic processes. *See* REDUCTION.

oxidative phosphorylation, (oks-i-dā-tiv fos-for-il-ā'-shon), process occurring in the mitochondria which results in the synthesis of adenosine triphosphate (ATP).

oximeter, a device used to measure oxygen saturation of the haemoglobin.

oxygen (O), colourless gaseous element, forming some 20–21% of the atmosphere. It supports combustion and is essential to life. *O. administration*: used therapeutically to increase blood oxygenation by various means which include: mask, nasal catheters, endotracheal tube and, rarely, a tent. *O. concentrator*: device for removing nitrogen from air to provide a high concentration of oxygen. Used in the community for people requiring oxygen therapy for many hours per day. *O. debt* or *deficit*: occurs when the metabolic demand for oxygen exceeds supply such as with very strenuous exercise. The resultant anaerobic utilization of fuel molecules leads to the accumulation of metabolites, including lactic acid, which accounts for aching muscles after exercise.

oxygenation, to saturate with oxygen, the process which occurs when haemoglobin combines with oxygen to form oxyhaemoglobin.

oxygenator, a device used to oxygenate the blood, e.g. during open heart surgery. *See* BYPASS, CARDIOPULMONARY.

oxygen dissociation curve, each of the four haem groups of a haemoglobin molecule has a different affinity for oxygen, which is illustrated by the sigmoid-shaped dissociation curve. It indicates the ease with which the haem groups give up their oxygen to the tissues. This also depends on temperature, pH and carbon dioxide tension (Figure 55). *See* BOHR EFFECT.

55 Oxygen dissociation curve (at 37°C, pH 7.4, Hb 15g/dl)

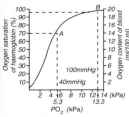

A = venous blood (at the tissues)
B = arterial blood (at the lungs)

oxyhaemoglobin, *(ok-si-hēm-o-glō-bin)*, the unstable compound formed by the combination of haemoglobin with oxygen.

oxyntic, *(ok-sin-tik)*, acid-producing. *O. cells:* gastric cells which produce hydrochloric acid. Also called **parietal cells.**

oxytocics, *(ok-si-tō-siks)*, agents that stimulate uterine contraction.

oxytocin, *(ok-si-tō-sin)*, hormone stored and secreted by the posterior pituitary gland. It causes uterine contraction during labour, and milk ejection during lactation.

oxyuriasis, *(ok-si-ū-rī-a-sis)*, infestation with threadworms (pinworms) of the genus *Enterobius* (*Oxyuris*).

Oxyuris vermicularis, *(ok-si-ūr-is ver-mik-ū-la-ris)*, *see* ENTEROBIUS VERMICULARIS, THREADWORM.

ozone (O₃), *(ō-zōn)*, a form of oxygen. Present as a layer in the earth's atmosphere. A powerful oxidizing agent.

P

pacemaker, the sinoatrial node which initiates the heart beat. *Artificial p.:* for arrhythmias such as heart block, electrical stimulation can be provided by means of wires placed in contact with the myocardium or in the oesophagus (temporary). The impulses are produced from an externally situated device on a temporary basis or permanently from a battery-powered device implanted subcutaneously, usually in the chest wall. They may be fixed-rate or demand-type which operate when the heart fails to maintain a specific rate.

pachydactyly, *(pak-i-dak-til-ē)*, thickening or enlargement of the digits.

pachydermia, *(pak-i-der'-mi-a)*, thickening of the skin.

pachymeningitis, *(pak-i-men-in-jī'-tis)*, inflammation of the dura mater, with thickening of the membrane.

pachyonychia, *(pak-i-ō-nik-i-a)*, thickening of the nails.

pack, 1. moistened material applied to a patient for various purposes, they may be: cold, ice, warm or hot. **2.** the material used to plug or fill an orifice or cavity, e.g. vaginal pack, abscess cavity. **3.** the dressing and/or instruments required for sterile procedures which are packed in paper bags prior to sterilization.

packed cells, plasma-reduced blood used for transfusion purposes when red cells rather than fluid volume are required. *P. cell volume (PCV):* **haematocrit.** The volume of red cells

expressed as a percentage of the total blood volume.

PaCO₂, abbreviation for the partial pressure or tension of carbon dioxide in arterial blood. The normal range is 4.4–6.1 kPa

PACO₂, abbreviation for the partial pressure of carbon dioxide in alveolar air.

paediatrician, *(pē-dē-a-tri-shon)*, specialist in diseases of children.

paediatric advanced life support, *see* ADVANCED LIFE SUPPORT, BROSELOW PAEDIATRIC RESUSCITATION SYSTEM.

paediatrics, *(pē-dē-at-riks)*, the science or study of diseases in children.

paedophilia, *(pē-dō-fil-i-a)*, a sexual attraction to children.

Paget's disease, 1. of bone. Osteitis deformans, a disease of unknown aetiology with irregular softening and thickening of various bones, e.g. skull. The effects include: pain, deformity, cardiac problems and malignant changes. **2.** of the nipple. Eczematous lesion associated with breast duct carcinoma.

pagophagia, *(pa-gō-fa-gi-a)*, eating ice, associated with iron deficiency anaemia.

pain, distressing sensation felt when certain nerve endings (nociceptors) are stimulated. It is a unique and subjective experience of physiological sensation and emotional response. It varies in intensity from mild to agonizing, but individual responses are influenced by factors which include: knowledge about cause, location, age, associated conditions, whether acute or chronic, culture and pain tolerance. *P. assessment*: the subjective nature of pain makes it difficult to measure, but various tools are available to help determine its intensity and the efficacy of pain relief. Usually the person with the pain is asked to describe it in terms of a set scale, e.g. 0–10 where 0 = no pain and 10 = worst pain possible. *P. control*: may be physical, e.g. basic comfort or ice packs; pharmacological, e.g. analgesic drugs or nerve blocks; psychological, e.g. distraction or reducing anxiety through explanation. Successful management requires a multidisciplinary approach. *P. threshold*: the lowest intensity at which a stimulus is felt as pain. There is little variation between people. *P. tolerance*: the greatest intensity of pain a person is prepared to endure. This varies considerably between people. *See* GATE CONTROL THEORY.

palate, roof of the mouth. *Hard p.*: anterior bony part. *Soft p.*: mobile posterior part formed from stratified epithelium and muscle, it tapers to become the uvula. *See* CLEFT PALATE.

palatine bones, bones of the face which form the hard palate, orbit and nasal cavity.

palatoplegia, *(pal-at-ō-plē-ji-a)*, paralysis of soft palate.

palliative, a treatment which relieves symptoms but does not cure.

palm, the hollow or flexor surface of the hand.

palmar, pertaining to the palm of the hand.

palpation, examination by the hand.

palpebra, *(pal-pe'-bra)*, the eyelid.

palpitation, an abnormal awareness of the heart beat. It may arise from anxiety, exercise or certain heart diseases.

palsy, paralysis. *See* BULBAR PALSY, ERB'S PALSY, CEREBRAL PALSY, PARALYSIS.

panacea, *(pan-a-sē'-a)*, a medicine which is claimed or advertised to cure all diseases.

panarthritis, *(pan-ar-thrī'-tis)*, inflammation of all joints or of all joint structures.

pancarditis, *(pan-kar-dī'-tis)*, generalized inflammation of the heart.

pancreas, *(pan-krē-as)*, a dual-purpose gland situated in the left upper abdomen (Figure 56). In its exocrine role it produces an alkaline secretion containing digestive enzymes which enter the duodenum via the pancreatic duct. The endocrine role is to produce hormones which regulate blood sugar levels. *See* AMYLASE, GLUCAGON, INSULIN, LANGERHAN'S ISLETS, LIPASES, PANCREOZYMIN, TRYPSIN.

pancreatectomy, *(pan-krē-a-tek'-to-mi)*, excision of the pancreas. *See* WHIPPLE'S OPERATION.

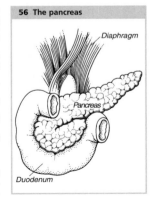

56 The pancreas

Diaphragm

Pancreas

Duodenum

pancreatitis, *(pan-krē-a-tī'-tis),* inflammation of the pancreas. It may be acute or chronic.

pancreozymin (PZ), *(pan-krē-ō-zī'-min),* an intestinal hormone identical to cholecystokinin (CCK), which is the name generally used. It stimulates pancreatic exocrine secretion.

pancytopenia, *(pan-sīt-ō-pē-ni-a),* a reduction in the number of all blood cells due to failure of the bone marrow.

pandemic, a widely spread epidemic.

panhypopituitarism, *(pan-hī-po-pi-tū-i-ta-rizm),* Simmond's disease. A deficient secretion of the hormones of the anterior pituitary. See HYPOPITUITARISM.

panhysterectomy, *(pan-his-te-rek'-to-mi),* total removal of the uterus.

panic, sudden overwhelming attacks of extreme fear and anxiety. Associated with anxiety states and other mental health problems.

panniculus, a layer of tissue or fascia.

pannus, corneal vascularization.

panophthalmia, panophthalmitis, *(pan-of-thal-mi-a, pan-of-thal-mī-tis),* generalized inflammation of the eyeball.

panproctocolectomy, *(pan-prok-tō-kol-ek'-to-mi),* complete excision of the rectum and colon with the formation of an ileostomy.

pantothenic acid, *(pan-tō-then-ik),* part of the vitamin B complex. Important in the formation of acetyl coenzyme A.

PaO₂, the partial pressure or tension of oxygen in arterial blood. The normal range is 12–15 kPa.

PAO₂, the partial pressure of oxygen in alveolar air.

Papanicolaou smear, Pap smear, *(pap-a-nik-ō-laow),* technique used in exfoliative cytology. Usually applied to cells obtained from the cervix by spatula or brush and examined for abnormal changes. See CERVICAL INTRAEPITHELIAL NEOPLASIA.

papilla *(pl.* **papillae),** a small nipple-shaped eminence. *Dermal p.:* projections of dermis into the epidermis. *Optic p.:* optic disc. *Tongue p.:* various types associated with the taste buds.

papillary, pertaining to a papilla. *P. muscle:* tiny muscles which, with the chordae tendinae, help to stabilize the atrioventricular valves of the heart.

papillitis, *(pap-pil-ī-tis),* inflammation of a papilla, e.g. optic disc.

papilloedema, *(pap-il-e-dē'-ma),* choked disc. Oedema of the optic disc indicative of raised intracranial pressure.

papilloma, *(pap-il-ō'-ma),* benign neoplasm of epithelial cells.

papillomavirus, *(pap-il-ō-ma-vī'-rus),* a virus responsible for the development of papilloma. See HUMAN PAPILLOMAVIRUS.

papovavirus, *(pap-ō-va-vī-rus),* a group of DNA viruses which includes the papillomavirus.

papule, *(pap'-ūl),* a small solid pimple.

papulopustular, *(pap-ū-lō-pus-tū-la),* a rash with both papules and pustules.

papulosquamous, *(pap-ū-lō-skwā-mus),* a papular and scaly skin condition.

para-aminobenzoic acid (PABA), *(par-a-a-mē-nō-ben-zō-ik),* an essential metabolite required for the growth of many microorganisms. Also used to filter ultraviolet rays, and in creams and lotions protects the skin from sunburn.

paracentesis, *(par-a-sen-tē-sis),* withdrawing fluid from a body cavity. Performed for diagnostic reasons or to relieve symptoms. See ASPIRATION.

paracrine, *(par-a-krēn),* hormone-like substances which have a local reglatory role, e.g. gastrin and gastric secretion.

paracusis, *(par-a-kū'-sis),* disordered hearing.

paradigm, an example, pattern, model or set of assumptions.

paradoxical, inconsistent or improbable. *P. breathing:* a feature of flail chest where part of the chest wall moves in during inspiration and vice versa. *P. sleep:* rapid eye movement (REM) sleep.

paraesthesia, *(par-es-thēz-i-a),* disorder of sensation, such as tingling and pins and needles.

paraffin, a hydrocarbon series obtained from petroleum. Uses include: ointment base, impregnated gauze dressings, wax baths, laxative and barrier for skin.

parafollicular cells, present in the thyroid gland, they secrete calcitonin.

paragonimiasis, *(par-a-gon-i-mī-ā-sis),* infection with flukes of the genus *Paragonimus.*

parainfluenza virus, types of myxovirus responsible for various respiratory diseases in children and sometimes adults.

paralysis, loss of movement and/or sensory function in a part of the body. Usually due to some disorder of the nervous system. *Flaccid p.:* mainly due to lower motor neurone lesions; there is loss of muscle tone and tendon reflexes are absent. *Spastic p.:* affected muscles are rigid and tendon reflexes are exaggerated, usually results from an upper motor neurone lesion. *See* PALSY, PARKINSONISM, POLIOMYELITIS.

paralytic, pertaining to paralysis. *P. ileus:* intestinal obstruction due to absent peristalsis. *See* ILEUS.

paramedian, close to the middle.

paramedical, allied to medicine.

parameter, 1. a statistical or mathematical measure of a population characteristic, e.g. mean or standard deviation. **2.** a numerically measurable property. **3.** a general term meaning limits.

parametric tests, statistical tests that assume the data are from a sample from a population that has a normal distribution curve.

parametritis, *(par-a-me-trī-tis),* inflammation of the parametrium. Pelvic cellulitis.

parametrium, *(par-a-mē-tri-um),* connective tissue surrounding the uterus.

paramnesia, *(par-am-nē'-si-a),* false memory; usually memory of events which did not occur in the connection related.

paramyxoviruses, *(par-a-mik-sō-vī-rus-ez),* a subgroup of myxoviruses which cause diseases such as mumps and measles.

paranasal, close to the nasal cavity. *P. sinuses: see* SINUS.

paranoia, *(par-a-noy-a),* a mental disorder characterized by the insidious onset of delusions of persecution.

paranoid, relating to paranoia. *P. schizophrenia: see* SCHIZOPHRENIA. *P. personality:* an individual who is mistrustful and abnormally sensitive to the reaction of others.

paranormal, something that cannot be explained by known scientific facts.

paraphasia, a speech disorder where similar words or sounds are substituted for the word intended.

paraphimosis, *(par-a-fi-mō'-sis),* retraction of the prepuce behind the glans penis with inability to restore it to the natural position.

paraphrenia, *(par-a-frē-ni-a),* a mental disorder of older people characterized by delusions, usually of a persecutory nature.

paraplegia, *(par-a-plē-ji-a),* paralysis of the lower limbs and trunk. Areas below the level of the spinal cord lesion are affected. It may include loss of bladder and bowel function.

paraprotein, an abnormal plasma protein.

parapsychology, involves areas, such as extrasensory perception, which cannot be explained by accepted scientific knowledge.

parasite, an organism which obtains food or shelter from another organism (the 'host').

parasiticide, (par-a-sīt-i-sīd) substance lethal to parasites.

parasomnias, a broad group of disturbances around sleep; it includes sleepwalking, bruxism and nightmares.

parasuicide, also known as deliberate self-harm (DSH). A suicidal gesture; an act, such as self-mutilation or drug overdose, which may or may not be motivated by a genuine desire to die. It is common in young people who are distressed but not mentally ill. It may be ASSOCIATED with low self-esteem. See SAMARITANS.

parasympathetic system, part of the autonomic nervous system, having craniosacral outflow. Opposing the action of the sympathetic system it tends to be involved with restful processes, e.g. digestion.

parasympatholytic, (par-a-sim-path-ō-lit'-ik), agent that blocks or opposes parasympathetic activity. Muscarinic antagonist.

parasympathomimetic, (par-a-sim-path-ō-mim-et'-ik), agent that produces the same effects as or causes parasympathetic activity. Muscarinic agonist.

parathormone, (par-a-thor-mōn), parathyroid hormone.

parathyroid, (par-a-thī-royd), four small endocrine glands normally situated on the posterior surface of the thyroid. *P. hormone (PTH)*: helps to maintain calcium and phosphorus homeostasis. See CALCITONIN.

parathyroidectomy, (par-a-thī-roy-dek-to-mi), excision of the parathyroid glands.

paratyphoid, (par-a-tī-foyd), an enteric fever caused by a bacterium *Salmonella paratyphi*.

paravertebral, (par-a-ver'-te-bral), to one side of the spinal column.

parenchyma, (par-en'-kī-ma), the functional part of an organ.

parenteral, (pa-ren'-ter-al), outside or apart from the alimentary tract. Therapy such as drugs, fluids and nutrition administered by a route other than the alimentary tract.

paresis, (par-ē-sis), partial or slight paralysis.

parietal, (pa-rī'-e-tal), pertaining to the outside wall of a cavity. *P. bones*: two bones forming the roof and sides of the skull. *P. lobe*: lobe of the cerebral hemisphere lying under the parietal bone. *P. pleura*: see PLEURA.

parity, (par-i-tē), the number of children a woman has borne.

parkinsonism, condition with features similar to those of Parkinson's disease (paralysis agitans). It is characterized by tremor, rigidity and impaired voluntary movement as the basal nuclei degenerate with loss of, or blockade of the neurotransmitter dopamine. Most cases of true Parkinson's disease are of unknown aetiology but parkinsonism may follow infection, trauma, tumours, phenothiazine drugs and Wilson's disease.

paronychia, (par-ō-nik'-i-a), whitlow. Inflammation and abscess around a fingernail.

parosmia, (par-oz-mi-a), disordered sense of smell.

parotid, near the ear. A pair of salivary glands, one in front of each ear.

parotitis, (par-ō-tī-tis), inflammation of the parotid gland. **1.** mumps (epidemic parotitis). **2.** spread of infection from oral sepsis.

parous, having borne a child or children.

parovarium, *(par-ō-va-rē-um)*, a vestigial structure in the broad ligament which occasionally becomes cystic.

paroxysm, *(par'-oks-izm)*, a sudden temporary attack.

paroxysmal, having the characteristics of a paroxysm. *P. atrial tachycardia*: a period of atrial tachycardia (150–200 beats/minute) that starts and stops suddenly. It is caused by an abnormal focus in the atrium. *P. nocturnal dyspnoea*: attacks of breathlessness occurring at night due to pulmonary oedema resulting from left ventricular failure. *P. ventricular tachycardia*: *see* SUPRAVENTRICULAR.

parrot disease, psittacosis.

partial pressure, the pressure exerted by an individual gas in a gas mixture or a liquid. This pressure is directly related to the concentration of the gas and the pressure exerted by the total mixture. *See* DALTON'S LAW.

partograph, a device used to record the progress of labour in a graphical format.

parturient, *(par-tū-rē-ent)*, relating to childbirth. Condition of giving birth.

parturition, *(par-tū-rish'-un)*, the act of giving birth to a child.

pascal (Pa), derived SI unit of pressure.

Pascal, a computer language.

passive, submissive. Not active or spontaneous. *P. immunity*: *see* IMMUNITY. *P. movements*: those performed by the therapist or nurse. The patient is relaxed. *P. smoking*: inhalation of tobacco smoke produced by another person.

Pasteurella, a genus of Gram-negative bacilli. *See* YERSINIA.

pasteurization, a method of destroying most pathogenic bacteria in milk and other fluids. Involves either

heating to 63–66°C for 30 minutes (holder process), or heating to 72°C for 15–20 seconds (high temperature short-time method), followed by rapid cooling. Pasteurization, using moist heat, is also used to disinfect medical equipment, such as instruments.

Patau's syndrome, an abnormality affecting chromosomes in group D (pairs numbered 13–15), the individual is trisomic for chromosome 13 with the result that he/she has 47 chromosomes. It is characterized by: central nervous system defects, learning disability, cataracts, and cleft lip and palate.

patch, a device for transdermal drug administration, e.g. nicotine, glyceryl trinitrate and hormone replacement.

patella, the kneecap. A sesamoid bone in front of the knee joint.

patellar, relating to the patella. *P. bursa*: the bursa around the patella which become inflamed with excessive kneeling (housemaid's knee). *P. reflex*: *see* KNEE JERK.

patellectomy, operation to excise the patella.

patent, open. *P. ductus arteriosus*: failure of the ductus arteriosus to close at birth. *P. foramen ovale*: failure of closure of the foramen ovale.

paternalism, restricting, over-protective, such as well-meaning rules and regulations which reduce individual autonomy.

pathogen, disease-producing, usually applied to a microorganism.

pathogenesis, *(path-ō-jen'-e-sis)*, the origin and progress of a disease.

pathogenic, *(path-ō-jen-ik)*, capable of causing disease.

pathogenicity, *(path-ō-jen-is-i-ti)*, the capacity to cause disease.

pathognomonic, *(path-og-no-mon'-ik)*, characteristic of, or peculiar to, a particular disease.

pathological, *(path-ō-loj'-i-kal),* relating to pathology. Morbid, abnormal.

pathology, *(path-ol'-o-ji),* the study of disease, particularly regarding the changes in the tissues resulting from disease.

patient, 1. an individual with a health deficiency who is receiving medical treatment and/or nursing care. **2.** a person whose name is on a list of a general practitioner, whether or not he or she is attending the surgery or clinic.

patient advocacy liaison service, provides an advocacy service to patients in NHS and primary care trusts by representing their concerns and complaints to the relevant department in the trust. Depending on the necessary legislation being in place it will replace some of the functions of the Community Health Council by 2002.

Patients' Charter, introduced by the UK government in 1991. It set out an individual's rights to treatment and national standards for care in the NHS. Now replaced by 'Your Guide to the NHS'.

patients' forum, a statutory and independent body comprising patients. It is planned that the body will exist in every trust to represent the views of patients about how their local NHS services are run. Depending on the necessary legislation being in place they will replace some of the functions of the Community Health Council by 2002.

patriarchy, *(pāt-rē-ar-kē),* a community or family where the male (father) dominates and is the highest authority.

Paul–Bunnell test, a serological test for infectious mononucleosis.

peak bone mass, the greatest density of bone, usually reached in the 30s.

peak expiratory flow rate (PEFR), respiratory function test. The flow of air during a forced expiration is measured using a peak-flow meter.

peau d'orange, *(pō-daw-rahnjh),* orange-skin appearance of skin overlying a carcinoma of the breast.

pectoral, relating to the chest. *P. muscles* are on the anterior surface of the chest.

pectus, the thorax, chest.

pedal, pertaining to the foot. *P. pulse:* palpation of the dorsalis pedis artery on the dorsum of the foot.

pedicle, the stalk of a tumour or organ. *P. graft:* a skin graft that is moved to the new site whilst still partially joined to the site of origin. This provides a blood supply until the graft is established.

pediculosis, *(pe-dik-ū-lō'-sis),* infestation with lice.

Pediculus, *(pe-dik'-ū-lus),* the louse. Genus of blood-sucking insects which act as vectors for disease (Figure 57). *P. capitis:* infests the head. *P. corporis:* infests the body. *P.* (more correctly, *Phthirius*) *pubis:* infests the pubic hair.

peduncle, a stalk. *Cerebral p.:* bulging structures on the midbrain which contain the descending voluntary motor tracts. *Cerebellar p.:* structures, also containing nerve tracts, which connect the cerebellum to the midbrain.

PEEP, abbreviation for **positive end-expiratory pressure.**

peer review, part of quality assurance where nurses of equal status review the practice and nursing actions of each other. *See* QUALITY ASSURANCE.

Pel–Ebstein fever, an intermittent fever which may occur in Hodgkin's lymphoma.

pellagra, a nutritional disorder caused by a deficiency of the B vitamin niacin and the amino acid trypto-

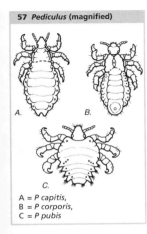

57 *Pediculus* (magnified)

A.

B.

C.

A = *P capitis*,
B = *P corporis*,
C = *P pubis*

phan. The effects include: stomatitis, glossitis, diarrhoea, dementia and dermatitis (initially resembling sunburn). Treatment is with oral nicotinamide.

pellet, a small pill, especially those used as implants.

pelvic, pertaining to the pelvis. *P. exenteration:* see EXENTERATION. *P. floor:* the muscles and ligaments supporting the pelvic organs. *P. inflammatory disease (PID):* inflammatory disease of the female internal genitalia. Usually due to bacterial infection. Can lead to infertility and chronic pain.

pelvimetry, measurement of pelvic dimensions.

pelvis, bony ring formed by the innominate bones and sacrum, encloses the bladder, rectum and reproductive structures. *Renal p.:* the funnel-shaped dilatation of the kid-

ney which receives urine from the calyces.

pemphigus, serious diseases characterized by bullae formation on the skin and mucous membranes. It has an autoimmune aetiology. *P. neonatorum:* a misnomer, it is in fact a very serious acute staphylococcal impetigo occurring in newborns.

pendulous, hanging down.

penicillinase, *(pen-i-sil-i-nāz),* See BETA LACTAMASE.

penicillins, large group of beta-lactam antibotics. Many have a wide spectrum of activity, but they produce hypersensitivity and some bacteria have developed resistance.

penile, pertaining to the penis.

penis, the male organ of urination and copulation.

pentose, a five-carbon sugar.

pepsin, proteolytic gastric enzyme. It converts protein into polypeptides.

pepsinogen, *(pep-sin'-ō-jen),* nonactive pepsin precursor secreted by the gastric zymogen cells. It is converted to active pepsin by gastric acid.

peptic, pertaining to digestion. *P. ulcer:* an ulcer occurring in any area exposed to pepsin/gastric juice: lower oesophagus, stomach, duodenum. Meckel's diverticulum and in the jejunum following surgical anastomosis to the stomach. *See* DUODENAL ULCER, GASTRIC ULCER.

peptidase, enzyme which splits peptides into amino acids, e.g. dipeptidase.

peptide, substance formed from two or more amino acids. *See* POLYPEPTIDE. *P. bond:* chemical bond formed in a dehydration synthesis reaction which holds amino acids together in a peptide.

peptone, the large fragment produced when a proteolytic enzyme (e.g. pepsin) or an acid acts upon a protein during the first stage of protein digestion.

perception, an awareness and understanding of impressions received through the senses.

percussion, a diagnostic method. The sound heard when the body is tapped; can be helpful in determining the condition of organs underneath.

percutaneous, *(per-kū-tā-nē-us),* through the skin – absorption of drugs or certain procedures. *P. endoscopic gastrostomy (PEG):* a gastroscope is used to aid the insertion of a feeding tube into the stomach which exits via the abdominal wall. *P. nephrolithotomy:* see NEPHROLITHOTOMY. *P. transhepatic cholangiography:* contrast medium is injected into a liver bile duct via the skin. *See* CHOLANGIOGRAPHY.

perforation, a hole in an organ caused by disease or injury. The act of perforating.

performance indicators (PIs), quantitative measures of activities and resources used in delivering healthcare.

perfusion, the flow of a fluid such as blood through an organ or tissue, e.g. lung.

perianal, *(per-i-ā-nal),* around the anus.

periarteritis, *(per-i-ar-ter-ī-tis),* inflammation of the outer coat of an artery.

periarthritis, *(per-i-ar-thrī'-tis),* inflammation of the tissues around a joint.

pericardial, *(per-i-kar-dē-al),* pertaining to the pericardium. *P. adhesions:* fibrosis following inflammation causing the two layers to adhere. *P. effusion:* collection of fluid between the two layers of the pericardium. *See* TAMPONADE.

pericardiocentesis, *(per-i-kar-dē-ō-sen-tē'-sis),* withdrawing fluid from the pericardial sac using a needle.

pericardiotomy, *(per-i-kar-dē-ot-o-mi),* an opening made into the pericardium.

pericarditis, *(per-i-kar-dī'-tis),* inflammation of the pericardium with or without effusion. Causes include: myocardial infarction, trauma, viral or bacterial infection, rheumatic fever, and uraemia. *See* DRESSLER'S SYNDROME, TAMPONADE.

pericardium, *(per-i-kar'-dē-um),* the serous membrane which encloses the heart. It consists of two layers, visceral (also called the epicardium) and parietal, between which is a small amount of serous fluid to prevent friction.

perichondritis, *(per-i-kon-drī'-tis),* inflammation of perichondrium.

perichondrium, *(per-i-kon'-dre-um),* the membranous covering of a cartilage.

pericolic, *(per-i-kōl-ik),* around the colon. *P. abscess:* local abscess formation, commonly associated with diverticulitis.

pericranium, *(per-i-krā'-ni-um),* the membrane covering the bones of the skull.

perilymph, fluid contained in the internal ear, between the bony and membranous labyrinth.

perimetritis, inflammation of the perimetrium.

perimetrium, *(per-i-me-trē-um),* peritoneum covering the uterus.

perimetry, measurement of a given field.

perimysium, *(per-i-mī-sē-um),* fibrous connective tissue which encloses bundles of muscle fibres.

perinatal, *(per-i-nā-tal),* relating to the time around birth. *P. mortality:* deaths in the first week of life plus stillbirths. *See* MORTALITY.

perineal, *(per-i-nē-al),* pertaining to the perineum.

perineoplasty, *(per-i-ne-ō-plas-ti),* perineorrhaphy.

perineorrhaphy, *(per-i-ne-or-raf-i),* operation to repair a torn or ruptured perineum.

perinephric, *(per-i-nef-rik),* round about the kidney. *P. abscess*: a collection of pus in the tissues round the kidney.

perineum or **perineal body,** *(per-i-nē-um),* wedge-shaped structure lying between the external genitalia and the rectum. Consists of muscle and connective tissue covered by skin.

perineurium, *(per-i-nū-rē-um),* connective tissue sheath around a bundle of nerve fibres.

periodic breathing, a period of apnoea in a newborn baby of 5–10 seconds followed by hyperventilation (50–60 breaths/minute), for a period of 10–15 seconds. Apnoea occurs quite frequently in very-low-birth-weight babies, often without definite cause. Attacks are only a problem if they are prolonged and do not respond to simple stimulation.

periodontal, *(per-i-ō´-don-tal),* pertaining to tissues around the teeth. *P. disease*: disease of the gums and supporting structures of the teeth. *P. membrane (ligament)*: structure attaching a tooth to its socket.

perioperative, the time around a surgical procedure; preoperative period, time in theatre and the immediate postoperative period.

periorbital, *(per-i-or´-bit-al),* area around the eye socket.

periosteal, *(per-i-os´-tē-al),* pertaining to periosteum.

periosteum, *(per-i-os-tē-um),* tough fibrous membrane covering a bone. It is protective and essential for regeneration.

periostitis, *(per-i-os-tī-tis),* inflammation of the periosteum.

peripheral, 1. relating to the circumference or outer surface. *P. nervous*

system (PNS): the general term for the part of the nervous system outside the brain and spinal cord. *P. neuritis*: inflammation of peripheral nerve. *P. resistance*: the resistance in the walls of the arterioles, vital in the control of blood pressure *P. vascular disease*: any abnormal condition arising in the blood vessels outside the heart, the main one being atherosclerosis, which can lead to thrombosis and occlusion of the vessel resulting in gangrene. **2.** in computing hardware devices which can be connected to the CPU, e.g. modem, printer.

periproctitis, *(per-i-prok-tī´-tis),* inflammation of tissue around the rectum or anus.

perisalpingitis, *(per-i-sal-pin-jī´-tis),* inflammation of the peritoneum covering the uterine tube.

peristalsis, *(per-i-stal-sis),* the rhythmic wave-like contraction and dilatation which occurs in a hollow tube, e.g. gastrointestinal tract where muscular action conveys food and waste through the tract.

peritoneal, *(per-i-to-nē-al),* pertaining to the peritoneum. *P. dialysis*: a method of removing waste products from the blood in renal failure. It uses the peritoneum as a selectively permeable membrane. Dialysing fluid is run into the peritoneal cavity; waste such as urea moves from the peritoneal blood vessels into the fluid which is then drained from the abdomen. May be intermittent or continuous. *See* CONTINUOUS AMBULATORY PERITONEAL DIALYSIS, DIALYSIS.

peritoneum, *(per-i-to-nē-um),* the serous membrane lining the abdominal cavity and covering many of the organs (Figure 58). The visceral layer covers the organs, and the parietal lines the cavity. *See* MESENTERY, OMENTUM.

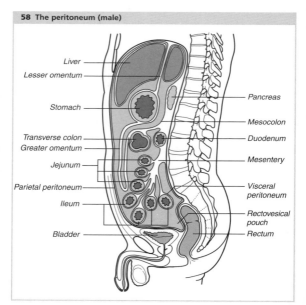

58 The peritoneum (male)

Liver
Lesser omentum
Stomach
Transverse colon
Greater omentum
Jejunum
Parietal peritoneum
Ileum
Bladder

Pancreas
Mesocolon
Duodenum
Mesentery
Visceral peritoneum
Rectovesical pouch
Rectum

peritonitis, *(per-i-ton-ī-tis),* inflammation of the peritoneum which may be bacterial or chemical. Results from: a perforated organ, intestinal obstruction, visceral inflammation, penetrating abdominal wounds, and blood-borne infections. It may be generalized or local with the formation of an abscess, e.g. pelvic or subphrenic.

peritonsillar, *(per-i-ton-si-la),* around a tonsil. *P. abscess*: an abscess forming in the tissues around a tonsil. Also known as **quinsy.** *See* TONSILLITIS.

perityphlitis, *(per-i-tif-lī-tis),* inflammation of the peritoneum around the caecum and appendix.

periurethral, *(per-i-ūr-ē′-thral),* around the urethra.

perlèche, *(per-lesh),* fissures and inflammation at the angles of the mouth. May be a sign of vitamin B deficiency, ill-fitting dentures or infection.

permeable, capable of being penetrated.

pernicious, tending to a fatal issue, highly destructive. *P. anaemia*: the megaloblastic anaemia caused by an inability to absorb vitamin B_{12} due to a failure of intrinsic factor (IF) secretion.

peroneal, *(per-ō-nē-al)*, pertaining to the fibula or the outer aspect of the leg. Applied to the muscles and nerve of the lower leg.

peroral, *(per-aw-ral)*, through the mouth.

perseveration, a recurring idea, feeling or way of action from which a person finds it difficult to escape.

persistent generalized lymphadenopathy (PGL), palpable lymph node enlargement (> 1 cm in diameter) at two distinct sites which persists for more than 3 months in the absence of an identifiable cause other than HIV infection.

persistent vegetative state (PVS), a totally dependent state occurring when the cerebral cortex is irreparably damaged, but the brainstem continues to function. The person, who appears awake, is unresponsive and unable to initiate any voluntary action.

personality, the make-up of a person with all his/her inherited characteristics, both inherited and acquired *P disorder*: an abnormality of personality where an individual does not conform to the norm, e.g. hysterical personality, sociopath.

perspiration, sweat excretion through the pores of the skin. *Insensible p.*: the fluid lost each day through the skin and respiratory tract of which we are unaware, usually around 500 ml/day. *Sensible p.*: fluid loss through visible sweating.

Perthes' disease, osteochondritis affecting the femoral head. There is avascular degeneration of the upper femoral epiphysis in children; revascularization occurs, but residual damage may lead to arthritic changes.

pertussis, *(per-tus-sis)*, whooping cough. A serious respiratory illness commonly occurring in young children. Caused by the bacteria *Bordetella pertussis*, it is spread by droplets and has an incubation period of 7–14 days. Its effects include: conjunctivitis and later bouts of paroxysmal coughing with a 'whoop' and vomiting. It may be complicated by pneumonia. Active immunization, as part of the DPTer triple vaccine (diphtheria, pertussis and tetanus), is available as part of the routine immunization programme in infancy.

pes, the foot. *P. cavus*: a greatly exaggerated longitudinal arch of the foot, with deformity of the toes. *P. planus*: flat foot.

pessary, 1. a supporting device placed in the vagina to correct uterine displacements. **2.** medicated suppository impregnated with drugs such as antimicrobials, hormones and prostaglandins for insertion into the vagina.

pesticide, an agent toxic to pests such as insects.

PET, *see* POSITRON EMISSION TOMOGRAPHY.

petechiae, *(pe-te'-chi-ē)*, small red or purple spots on the skin formed by an effusion of blood.

petit mal, *see* EPILEPSY.

petrous, stony; term applied to part of the temporal bone.

Peyer's patches, small areas of lymphoid tissue in the submucosa of the ileum.

pH, *see* HYDROGEN ION CONCENTRATION.

phaeochromocytoma, *(fe-ō-krō-mō-sī-tō'-ma)*, a rare tumour of the adrenal medulla and sympathetic chain. It secretes the catecholamines noradrenaline (norepinephrine) and adrenaline (epinephrine), causing hypertension which may be paroxysmal, palpitations and headache.

phage typing, *(fāj),* a method of identifying bacterial species according to their parasitic viruses. *See* BACTERIOPHAGE.

phagocytes, *(fag-ō-sītz),* white blood cells such as neutrophils and monocytes which are able to ingest and destroy bacteria and other foreign material. Other phagocytic cells include: the various types of macrophage and Kupffer cells.

phagocytosis, *(fag-ō-sī-tō-sis),* the process of enveloping and destroying bacteria and other particles by a phagocyte (Figure 59).

phalanges, the small bones of the fingers and toes.

phallic phase, the third stage of psychosexual development characterized by a child's sensual interest in the genitalia; the penis or clitoris, and attachment to the parent of the opposite sex.

phallus, the penis.

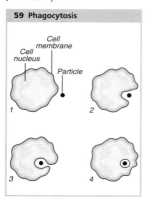

59 Phagocytosis

Cell nucleus

Cell membrane

Particle

1

2

3

4

phantasy, *(fan'-ta-si), see* FANTASY.

phantom limb, the sensation that an amputated limb still exists. Often involves the experience of pain and 'pins and needles'.

pharmaceutical, *(far-ma-sū-tik-al),* pertaining to drugs.

pharmacodynamics, *(far-ma-kō-dī-nam'-iks),* the study of drug action within living organisms and how it changes cellular processes to have an effect.

pharmacokinetics, *(far-ma-ko-kin-et'-iks),* the study of drug action within the body; absorption mechanism, distribution, metabolism and excretion. Each process occurs at a specific rate characteristic for that drug, and overall drug action (therapeutic and toxic) will be dependent on these processes.

pharmacology, *(far-ma-kol'-o-ji),* the science dealing with drugs.

pharmacopoeia, *(far-ma-kō-pē-a),* an authorized handbook of drugs available in a particular area. *See* BRITISH NATIONAL FORMULARY, *BRITISH PHARMACOPOEIA.*

pharmacy, 1. the science of preparing or mixing medicines or drugs. **2.** the place where medicines are prepared and distributed. *P. only medicines (P):* drugs that may be purchased by the public from a pharmacy, but only when a qualified pharmacist is present.

pharyngeal, *(fa-rin-jē-al),* pertaining to the pharynx. *P. pouch:* diverticulum occurring in a weak area of the inferior constrictor muscles.

pharyngectomy, *(fa-rin-jek'-to-mi),* excision of part of the pharynx.

pharyngismus, *(far-in-jiz-mus),* spasm of the pharynx.

pharyngitis, *(far-in-jī'-tis),* inflammation of the pharynx.

pharyngolaryngeal, *(far-in-go-lar-in-jē'-al),* relating to pharynx and larynx.

pharyngotympanic, *(far-in-gō-tim-pan-ik),* relating to pharynx and middle ear (tympanic cavity). *P. tube:* tube between the nasopharynx and the middle ear. Also called **auditory tube** and **eustachian tube.**

pharynx, funnel-shaped muscular structure lined with mucous membrane. Situated behind the mouth, it leads into the larynx and oesophagus. It is divided into three parts: *see* LARYNGOPHARYNX, NASOPHARYNX, OROPHARYNX.

phenol, a disinfectant. *See* CARBOLIC ACID.

phenomenology, *(fen-om-en-ol-o'-ji),* the study of occurrences as they form part of human experience.

phenothiazines, a group of typical neuroleptics, e.g. chlorpromazine, fluphenazine.

phenotype, *(fē-nō-tīp),* the physical characteristics of an individual which result from environmental factors and their genetic make-up. *Cf.* GENOTYPE.

phenylalanine, *(fē-nil-al-a-nēn),* essential (indispensable) amino acid.

phenylketonuria (PKU), *(fē-nil-kē-tō-nū-ri-a),* an inherited metabolic disorder where the enzyme phenylalanine hydroxylase which converts phenylalanine to tyrosine is absent or deficient. Toxic metabolites such as phenylpyruvic acid accumulate in the blood and are excreted in the urine. Untreated it leads to individuals with severe learning disabilities who have very fair hair and skin (lack of tyrosine needed for the pigment melanin). A routine screening blood test during the first few days of life ensures early diagnosis and a treatment regimen which includes reducing phenylalanine intake and monitoring for toxic metabolites. *See* GUTHRIE TEST.

pheromone, *(fer-o-mōn),* chemicals of specific odour secreted by an organism, e.g. in humans they are present in the sweat produced by the apocrine sweat glands. They may be involved in the communication between individuals and have an influence on sexual behaviour.

phial, *(fī-al),* a glass capsule or container for a drug.

Philadelphia chromosome (Ph), an anomaly affecting chromosome 22. Seen in the blood cells of individuals with chronic myeloid leukaemia.

phimosis, *(fi-mō-sis),* an abnormally tight prepuce which cannot be drawn back over the glans penis. Treatment is by circumcision. *See* PARAPHIMOSIS.

phlebectomy, *(fleb-ek'-to-mi),* excision of a vein.

phlebitis, *(fle-bī-tis),* inflammation of a vein. May be associated with thrombosis. *See* THROMBOPHLEBITIS.

phlebography, *(fleb-og-ra-fi),* *see* VENOGRAPHY.

phlebolith, *(fleb'-ō-lith),* concretion which forms in a vein.

phlebothrombosis, *(fleb-ō-throm-bō-sis),* thrombosis in veins, particularly the veins of the leg and pelvis. *See* DEEP VEIN THROMBOSIS, EMBOLISM.

Phlebotomus, (fleb-ot-o-mus), genus of sandfly which transmits leishmaniasis to humans. *P. alba dolens:* white leg; clotting and inflammation in a vein, may occur after childbirth. The leg is swollen, white, tense and very painful.

phlebotomy, *(fleb-ot-o-mi),* venesection.

phlegm, *(flem),* sputum. Abnormal mucus secretions from the respiratory tract.

phlegmasia, *(fleg-ma-zi-a),* inflammation. *P. alba dolens:* white leg; clotting and inflammation in a vein, may occur after childbirth. The leg is swollen, white, tense and very painful.

phlegmatic, *(fleg-mat'-ik),* describes an emotionally stable individual.

phlyctenule, *(flik-ten-ūl)*, small pink-yellow vesicles found on the conjunctiva or cornea. May be associated with tuberculosis.

phobia, a neurosis associated with irrational fears, e.g. agoraphobia (fear of open spaces). Causes the individual to experience anxiety and may seriously interfere with normal life if it is encountered frequently.

phocomelia, *(fō-kō-mē-li-a)*, an abnormality of limb development where the limb is incomplete or absent, e.g. such as those produced during the 1960s by the drug thalidomide taken during pregnancy.

phonation, *(fō-nā'-shon)*, the utterance of vocal sounds.

phonetic, relating to the voice.

phonocardiogram, *(fō-nō-kar-dē-ō-gram)*, a graphical record of heart sounds.

phonocardiography, *(fō-nō-kar-dē-og-ra-fi)*, a cardiac investigation where heart sounds and murmurs are recorded using a phonocardiograph.

phosphatases, *(fos-fa-tāz-ez)*, a group of enzymes concerned with reactions involving phosphate esters, e.g. carbohydrate metabolism, phospholipids and nucleotides. *Acid p.*: found in many tissue including red cells, bone, prostate and liver. High levels in the blood may indicate tumours of bone or prostate and blood diseases etc. *Alkaline p.*: found in liver, intestine and bone (osteoblasts), etc. Blood levels are commonly elevated in liver and bone disease.

phosphate, salt or ester of phosphoric acid.

phosphaturia, *(fos-fa-tū-ri-a)*, excess of phosphates in the urine.

phospholipid, *(fos-fō-li-pid)*, complex lipids which contain nitrogen and phosphorus. Especially important in the formation of cell membranes.

phosphonecrosis, *(fos-fō-ne-krō-sis)*, tissue destruction, usually affecting the jaw bone. An industrial disease associated with exposure to phosphorus.

phosphorus (P), poisonous nonmetallic element. Used in the body in the form of phosphates. The radioactive isotope ^{32}P is used in the treatment of primary proliferative polycythaemia and essential thrombocythaemia.

phosphorylases, *(fos-fo-ri-lāz-ez)*, enzymes concerned with carbohydrate metabolism.

photalgia, *(fō-tal-ji-a)*, pain in the eyes caused by exposure to bright light.

photochemotherapy, the effect of the administered drug is enhanced by exposing the patient to ultraviolet light.

photocoagulation, *(fō-tō-kō-ag-ū-lā-shon)*, see LASER.

photophobia, *(fō-tō-fō-bi-a)*, abnormal intolerance of light such as with inflammatory conditions of the eye or conditions of the nervous system, e.g. meningitis.

photoreceptor, see CONES, RODS.

photorefractive keratectomy, surgical reshaping of the cornea, using a laser, in order to correct a refractive error, usually myopia and/or astigmatism.

photosensitization, *(fō-tō-sen-si-tī-zā-shon)*, abnormal tissue reactions to light, usually resulting from the presence of chemicals in the tissues which increase the damaging effect of the radiation.

phototherapy, *(fō-tō-the-ra-pi)*, therapeutic use of light, such as the exposure to blue light used in the treatment of mild hyperbilirubinaemia in neonates.

phrenic, *(fren-ik)*, 1. relating to the mind. 2. relating to the diaphragm. *P. nerves*: a pair of nerves supplying the diaphragm.

phrenicotomy, *(fren-i-kot'-o-mi),* operation to divide the phrenic nerve on one side.

Phthirus pubis, *(thir-us pū-bis),* the public louse.

phylloquinone, *(fil-ō-kwin-ōn),* a plant substance that has vitamin K activity.

phylum, a major group in the classification of animals.

physical, relating to the body or the natural sciences. *P. activity level (PAL):* the ratio of energy used per day to the basal metabolic rate; varies between 1.4 and 1.9. *P. medicine:* a branch of medicine which makes use of physiotherapy and occupational therapy.

physician, a qualified medical practitioner. One who practises medicine rather than surgery.

physiological, *(fiz-ī-ō-loj-ik-al),* relating to physiology. Normal processes rather than pathological changes. *P. solution:* one having the same solute concentration and osmotic pressure as the plasma.

physiology, *(fiz-ī-ō-lo-ji),* science dealing with the functioning of living organisms.

physiotherapist, a health professional who practises physiotherapy.

physiotherapy, *(fiz-ē-ō-ther-a-pi),* traditionally, treatment to ameliorate, restore and sometimes cure, using electrotherapy, manipulation and exercise therapy and rehabilitation following injury or disease. Contemporarily, it also includes assessment and diagnosis, health education, health promotion and prevention of disabling conditions.

physique, *(fiz-ēk),* the form and constitution of the body.

phytates, phytic acid, *(fi-tik),* constituent of wholegrain cereals. In common with phosphates it inhibits the intestinal absorption of iron and calcium.

phyto-oestrogens, substances with oestrogenic properties found in plants, such as soya beans.

pia mater, *(pē-a mā-ter),* the fine membrane surrounding the brain and spinal cord. The inner layer of meninges.

pica, *(pī'-ka),* craving for unusual foods or non-food items.

Pick's disease, 1. a type of dementia occurring in mid-life due to brain atrophy. **2.** syndrome of ascites, hepatomegaly, oedema and pleural effusion occurring in constrictive pericarditis.

pickwickian syndrome, a disorder characterized by somnolence, obesity, polycythaemia and reduced pulmonary function.

picornavirus, *(pi-kor-na-vī-rus),* a group of RNA viruses which include the enteroviruses, e.g. hepatitis A virus and the rhinoviruses.

Pierre Robin syndrome, an inherited condition characterized by micrognathia, cleft palate, cleft lip and glaucoma.

pigeon chest, pectus carinatum. A deformity of the chest where the sternum is unusually prominent.

pigment, an organic colouring matter such as melanin, haemoglobin, bile pigments and those in the retina.

pigmentation, the coloration produced by pigment. *Abnormal p.:* such as may occur in Addison's disease or poisoning with metals, e.g. lead.

piles, *see* HAEMORRHOIDS.

pili, hair-like appendages of many bacteria. They transfer genetic material between different strains during conjugation.

pill, a small ball containing drugs, often sugar-coated. Taken orally.

pilonidal, *(pī-lō-nē-dal),* containing hair as in some cysts. *P. sinus:* sinus containing hairs which may form in anal cleft and become infected, resulting in an abscess.

pilosis, *(pī-lō-sis),* abnormal growth of hair.

pilot study, an initial smaller-scale trial used prior to the main research project to assess feasibility and to highlight deficiencies in methodology.

pineal body, *(pi-nē-al),* a structure situated close to the third ventricle of the brain. It secretes various substances which include: 5-hydroxytryptamine, histamine and melatonin. The release of melatonin is linked to the amount of light entering the eye. Melatonin appears to control the release of gonadotrophins, processes which follow diurnal rhythms such as sleep and influences mood. *See* SEASONAL AFFECTIVE DISORDER

pinguecula, *(pin-gwe-kū-la),* small yellow patch of connective tissue on conjunctiva occurring in old age.

pink-eye, infectious conjunctivitis.

pinna, the part of the external ear which projects from the head. The auricle.

pinocytosis, *(pī-nō-sī-tō-sis),* a process by which the plasma membrane surrounds a water droplet which is absorbed into the cell. *See* ENDOCYTOSIS, PHAGOCYTOSIS.

pinta, a treponemal disease of Central and South America caused by the spirochaete *Treponema carateum.* It affects the skin and spreads by contact within families.

pinworm, *see* THREADWORM.

pisiform, pea-shaped. One of the carpals or wrist bones.

pitting, pits are formed in the skin on pressure, as in oedema.

pituitary, *(pit-ū-it-a-ri),* hypophysis cerebri. An endocrine gland in the base of the skull connected by a stalk to the hypothalamus (Figure 60). It has two lobes: **1.** anterior lobe adenohypophysis) which produces adrenocorticotrophic hormone (ACTH), thyroid-stimulating hormone (TSH), the gonadotrophins – follicle-stimulating hormone (FSH) and luteinizing hormone (LH), growth hormone (GH), prolactin (PRL) and melanocyte-stimulating hormone (MSH). Anterior lobe activity is regulated by releasing and inhibitory hormones/factors released by the hypothalamus. **2.** posterior lobe (neurohypophysis) which stores and secretes oxytocin and antidiuretic hormone (ADH) which is also called vasopressin. Both these hormones are produced by the nerve fibres of two nuclei originating in the hypothalamus.

pityriasis, *(pit-i-rī-a-sis),* a group of skin diseases characterized by a scaly, erythematous macular eruption.

placebo, *(pla-sē-bo),* a harmless substance given as medicine. In a randomized placebo-controlled trial, an inert substance, identical in appearance with the material being tested, is used. When neither the researcher nor the patient knows which is which it is termed a double-blind trial. *P. effect*: a therapeutic effect that occurs following the administration of a placebo, or some non-drug intervention, e.g. information in advance of surgery may reduce the need for pain-relieving drugs.

placenta, *(pla-sen-ta),* afterbirth. The temporary hormone-secreting vascular structure which facilitates the exchange of substances: oxygen, nutrients, antibodies, carbon dioxide and nitrogenous waste between maternal and fetal blood (Figure 61). It is expelled from the uterus, along with the fetal membranes, during the

---

60 Pituitary gland with hormones

Hypothalamus

Special nuclei produce ADH and oxytocin

(travel in axons)

Stored in posterior pituitary

ADH and oxytocin released

Releasing and inhibiting hormones and factors made in hypothalamus (travel in portal system)

Anterior pituitary

Prolactin	GH	TSH	ACTH	MSH	FSH/LH
Breasts	Many tissues	Thyroid	Adrenal cortex	Skin pigment cells	Gonads

T_4 T_3

Glucocorticoids

Sex hormones

T_3 = Triiodothyronine
T_4 = Thyroxine

---

61 The placenta

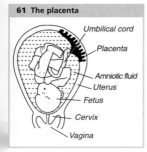

Umbilical cord
Placenta
Amniotic fluid
Uterus
Fetus
Cervix
Vagina

third stage of labour. *P. praevia*: a placenta situated partially or totally in the lower uterine segment. *See*

ANTEPARTUM HAEMORRHAGE, INEVITABLE HAEMORRHAGE.

placental, pertaining to the placenta. *P. hormones*: these include lactogen, oestrogens, progesterone, chorionic gonadotrophin and relaxin.

place of safety order, *see* EMERGENCY PROTECTION ORDER.

plague, an acute disease still endemic in Asia and areas of Africa with occasional cases in the United States, caused by the bacterium *Yersinia pestis*. It affects rats and is transmitted to humans by bites from rat fleas; human-to-human spread may occur by droplet infection. *See* BUBONIC PLAGUE, PNEUMONIC PLAGUE.

plane, in anatomy the imaginary lines drawn through the body: median (mid sagittal), coronal (frontal) and transverse.

planning, a stage in the nursing process where a care plan of nursing activities and interventions is developed that will achieve the goals and outcomes determined from the assessment.

plantar, relating to the sole of the foot *P. reflex* after infancy there is normally plantar flexion of the great toe when the outer aspect of sole is stroked. *Cf.* BABINSKI'S REFLEX.

plaque (*plahk*), **1.** small raised circular area. **2.** the layer of organic material and bacteria which forms on the surface of the teeth. A major cause of periodontal disease.

plasma, the fluid part of the blood in which the blood cells are suspended. *See* BLOOD. *P. cells:* immune cells derived from B lymphocytes. *See* LYMPHOCYTE. *P. thromboplastin antecedent (PTA):* factor XI in blood clotting.

plasma membrane, cell membrane.

plasmapheresis, (*plaz-ma-fe-rē-sis*), blood is withdrawn from an individual and the plasma is separated from the cells which are reinfused using a suitable isotonic solution. Uses include: the removal of autoantibodies in myasthenia gravis. *See* APHERESIS, MYASTHENIA GRAVIS.

plasmid, DNA present in the cytoplasm of some bacteria. During sexual reproduction, the genetic material in the plasmid is transferred between bacteria, thus allowing the genes for drug resistance to be exchanged.

plasmin, proteolytic enzyme which dissolves fibrin clots when healing is complete. Also called **fibrinolysin**.

plasminogen, (*plaz-min-ō-jen*), inactive precursor substance of plasmin.

Plasmodium, (*plas-mō-dē-um*), a genus of protozoa. Four species are responsible for causing malaria: *P. falciparum, P. malariae, P. ovale* and *P. vivax.*

plaster, *adhesive p.:* various types used to secure wound dressings, support or apply traction. *P. of Paris:* calcium sulphate which sets hard following the addition of water. Used in orthopaedics (casts for the immobilization of fractures) and in dentistry.

plastic, 1. capable of changing shape. **2.** forming tissue. *P. surgery:* restoration of tissue to its normal shape and appearance by operative means.

platelets, (*plāt-lets*), also called **thrombocytes**. Cellular fragments concerned with blood clotting. *See* BLOOD, BLOOD COUNT, BLOOD CLOTTING. Plateletpheresis is the removal of platelets from withdrawn blood prior to reinfusion of other blood components.

platelet plug, one of the four overlapping stages of haemostasis. Platelets adhere and aggregate at the site of blood vessel damage and form a temporary plug.

Platyhelminthes, (*plat-i-hel-min-thes*), flatworms. Includes flukes and tapeworms.

play, spontaneous or planned activities vital to normal social, physical, emotional and intellectual development during childhood. *P. group:* organized play and appropriate learning activities for a group of preschool children.

pleocytosis, (*plē-ō-sī-tō-sis*), increase of lymphocytes in cerebrospinal fluid.

pleomorphism, (*plē-ō-mor-fizm*), occurring in more than one form such as with microorganisms of the same species.

plethysmography, (*pleth-iz-mog-raf-i*), a technique for measuring changes in the volume and size of organs or extremities.

pleura, *(plū-ra)*, the serous membrane which covers the lungs (visceral layer) and lines the thoracic cavity (parietal layer). Between the layers is a small amount of serous fluid which reduces friction.

pleural, *(plū-ral)*, relating to the pleura. *P. effusion*: excess fluid between the layers of the pleura. *P. rub*: the sound produced by friction between the layers of the pleura.

pleurisy, *(plū-ri-si)*, inflammation of the pleura. It may be dry and fibrinous, associated with an effusion or purulent.

pleurodynia, *(plū-rō-din-i-a)*, pain in the intercostal muscles, such as in Bornholm disease.

pleurothotonos, *(plū-rō-thot-on-os)*, abnormal bending to one side due to muscle spasm on that side of the body.

plexor, small hammer used in testing deep reflexes, etc.

plexus, a network of nerves or blood vessels.

plicate, folded.

Plummer–Vinson syndrome, sideropenic dysphagia. Due to changes in the pharynx and oesophagus (post cricoid 'web'), it is associated with glossitis and iron deficiency anaemia.

pluripotent stem cells, *(plū-ri-pō-tent)*, uncommitted bone marrow cells which have the potential to differentiate into any one of several cell types including: erythrocytes, thrombocytes, granulocytes and lymphocytes.

pneumatocele, *(nū-mat-ō-sēl)*, **1.** a swelling containing air or gas. **2.** a lung hernia.

pneumaturia, *(nū-ma-tū-ri-a)*, the passage of air in the urine due to a fistula between the bladder and bowel.

pneumococcal, *(nū-mō-kok′-kal)*, pertaining to the pneumococcus.

pneumococcus, *(nū-mō-kok-us)*, *Streptococcus pneumoniae*. A Gram-positive diplococcus which causes pneumonia and meningitis.

pneumoconiosis, *(nū-mō-kō-nē-ō-sis)*, an occupational lung disease characterized by pulmonary fibrosis, caused by the inhalation of mineral dust, e.g. coal-workers' pneumoconiosis, asbestosis and silicosis.

Pneumocystis carinii, *(nū-mō-sis-tis)*, an opportunistic organism causing pneumonia in individuals who are immunologically compromised, e.g. with AIDS, after immunosuppression, in severely debilitated patients or infants.

pneumocyte, *(nū-mō-sīt)*, cells which line the alveoli (type 1) or secrete surfactant (type 2).

pneumoencephalography, *(nū-mō-en-kef-al-og′-raf-i)*, radiographic examination of cerebral ventricles after injection of air by means of a lumbar or cisternal puncture.

pneumomycosis, *(nū-mō-mī-kō′-sis)*, fungal disease of the lungs, e.g. aspergillosis, candidiasis.

pneumonectomy, *(nū-mō-nek′-to-mi)*, total or part excision of a lung.

pneumonia, an inflammation of lung tissue, usually due to bacterial or viral infection. It may be classified as: 1. primary, such as pneumococcal lobar pneumonia or viral which is commonly due to the influenza viruses. 2. secondary to existing respiratory infection, surgery, debility or immobilization; the 'non-specific' or aspiration pneumonias, *see* BRONCHOPNEUMONIA.

pneumonic plague, *(nū-mon-ik)*, a form of plague affecting the lungs. *See* PLAGUE.

pneumonitis, *(nū-mon-ī-tis)*, inflammation of the lung.

pneumoperitoneum, *(nū-mō-per-i-to-nē′-um)*, air in the peritoneal cavity.

Can be introduced for diagnostic or therapeutic purposes.

pneumotaxic centre, (*nū-mō-tak-sik*), a respiratory centre in the pons which ensures a smooth respiratory rhythm. *See* APNEUSTIC CENTRE.

pneumothorax, (*nū-mō-thor-aks*), air in the pleural cavity due to rupture of the visceral pleura or the perforation of the chest wall. Management involves the insertion of a cannula into the chest and connecting it either to a non-return valve or an underwater-seal drainage system. The underlying cause is treated. *Artificial p.*: air introduced into the pleural cavity for therapeutic purposes. *Spontaneous p.*: caused by the rupture of an air sac or bulla. *Tension p.*: large amounts of air become trapped in the chest, causing mediastinal shift and lung collapse requiring immediate emergency treatment.

pock, a pustule or the scar left by it.

podalic version, an obstetric manoeuvre which seeks to produce a breech presentation.

podiatrist, a person qualified in the diagnosis, care and treatment of disorders of the feet.

podiatry, the theory and practice relating to the maintenance of feet in a healthy condition and the treatment of disease and disability.

poikilocytosis, (*poy-kil-ō-sī-tō-sis*), variation in the form of the red blood cells.

poison, a substance which is deleterious to the body, causing injury or death.

polar, describes a molecule without electrical balance.

polar body, two small haploid bodies formed during the meiotic divisions of oögenesis.

polarized, describes the resting state of the plasma membrane of an excitable cell in which no impulse transmission is occurring. The inside of the membrane is electrically negative relative to the outside.

poliomyelitis, (*pō-lē-ō-mī-el-ī-tis*), inflammation of the anterior horn cells of the spinal cord. It is due to infection by the polioviruses and may lead to paralysis. Immunization, using an oral vaccine, is available as part of the routine programme during infancy with pre-school and school-leaving boosters. Cases of poliomyelitis have occurred following immunization and people are advised to wash their hands after defaecation or contact with recently vaccinated babies, especially after changing napkins. *See* SABIN VACCINE, SALK VACCINE.

polioviruses, (*pō-lē-ō-vī-rus-ez*), three related organisms which cause poliomyelitis. *See* ENTEROVIRUSES, PICORNAVIRUSES.

Politzer bag, device used to insufflate the middle ear and pharyngotympanic tubes.

pollenosis, (*pol-en-ō-sis*), hay fever. Allergy to grass pollen.

polyarteritis nodosa, (*pol-i-ar-ter-ī-tis*), a disease characterized by the formation of nodules on the smaller arteries with necrosis of the vessel wall leading to dilatation and thrombosis. The presentation depends upon the site and extent of the arterial changes.

polyarthritis, (*po-li-ar-thrī'-tis*), inflammation of many joints.

Polya's operation, *see* BILLROTH'S GASTRECTOMY.

polycystic, (*pol-i-sis-tik*), composed of many cysts. *P. kidneys*: a congenital abnormality leading to uraemia and renal failure. *P. ovaries*. *See* STEIN–LEVENTHAL SYNDROME.

polycythaemia, (*pol-i-sī-thē'-mi-a*), an increase in the number of red cells in the blood. It may be: **1.** primary proliferative polycythaemia, (p. vera), an idiopathic myeloproliferative disorder with an increase in red cells causing increased blood viscosity. **2.** secondary where the increase in red cells is in response to a low oxygen tension such as at high altitude or with chronic respiratory disease.

polydactyly, *(pol-i-dak'-ti-li)*, the presence of supernumerary fingers or toes.

polydipsia, *(pol-i-dip-si-a)*, excessive thirst.

polygene, a group of genes which act together to exert a cumulative influence on the same trait.

polymer, *(pol-i-mer)*, a substance formed from many smaller molecules, e.g. glycogen is a glucose polymer.

polymorphonuclear, *(pol-i-mor-fō-nū-kle-ar)*, having nuclei of various shapes. *P. white cells*: neutrophils, eosinophils and basophils. *See* BLOOD, BLOOD COUNT.

polymorphous, *(pol-i-mor-fus)*, having several forms.

polymyalgia rheumatica, *(pol-i-mī-al-ji-a rū-ma-ti-ka)*, a condition common in older people where there is acute pain and stiffness in the neck, back, shoulders, arms and thighs, especially in the morning.

polymyositis, *(pol-i-mī-ō-sī'-tis)*, weakness and wasting of muscles due to inflammation of unknown aetiology.

polyneuritis, *(pol-i-nū-rī'-tis)*, inflammation of several peripheral nerves at the same time.

polyneuropathy, *(pol-i-nū-ro-pa-thi)*, generalized diseases affecting the peripheral nerves. Varied aetiology, e.g. vitamin B deficiency.

polyopia, *(pol-i-ō'-pi-a)*, seeing multiple images of the same object.

polyp or **polypus,** *(pol-ip, pol-i-pus)*, a small tumour commonly occurring in the nose, cervix, endometrium and intestine.

polypectomy, *(pol-i-pek-to-mi)*, removal of a polyp.

polypeptide, *(pol-i-pep-tid)*, substance formed from amino acids joined in a chain by peptide bonds. Between a peptide and a protein in size.

polypharmacy, describes a situation where multiple drugs are prescribed for the same person, usually inappropriately. Substantially increases the risk of adverse effects.

polyploidy, *(pol-i-ploy-di)*, a chromosome number that is a multiple of the normal haploid number (other than the normal diploid of 46) such as 69; it is not compatible with life.

polypoid, *(pol-i-poyd)*, like a polyp or polypus.

polyposis, *(pol-i-pō-sis)*, the presence of many polyps. *Familial p.*: an inherited condition where multiple polyps form in the colon. These eventually become malignant. Affected individuals are monitored carefully by colonoscopy and polyps are removed, but proctocolectomy may eventually be required to prevent cancer.

polysaccharides, *(pol-i-sak-ar-īdz)*, complex carbohydrates formed from the combination of monosaccharide molecules. Important as energy storage or structural compounds. e.g. glycogen, cellulose. *See* CARBOHYDRATE.

polyserositis, *(pol-i-se-rō-sī-tis)*, inflammation of serous membranes with effusion of fluid.

polyunsaturated fats (PUFA), fats containing two or more double bonds in their structure. Usually liquid at room temperature, e.g. sunflower oil and fish oils. Required by the body for the synthesis of cell membranes and prostaglandins. Their inclusion in the diet tends to be associated with lower serum cholesterol levels. *See* FATTY ACIDS, LIPOPROTEINS, SATURATED FATS.

polyuria, *(pol-i-ūr-i-a)*, passing large volumes of urine such as with diabetes insipidus.

pompholyx, *(pom-fol-iks)*, vesicular skin lesion occurring on the hands and feet.

pons varolii, *(ponzva-ro-lī)*, part of the brain stem connecting the cerebrum and medulla.

Pontiac fever, *See* LEGIONNAIRES' DISEASE.

pontine, *(pon-tīn)*, pertaining to the pons.

popliteal, *(pop-li-tē'-al)*, pertaining to the popliteal space, the area behind the knee. Also refers to the artery and vein of that region.

population, 1. a group of individuals that share a feature or trait. **2.** in genetics a group of interbreeding organisms. **3.** a group of individuals within a defined geographical area, e.g. the prison population.

pore, a minute opening, such as those on the skin, which discharge sweat onto the surface.

porphyria, *(por-fi-ri-a)*, group of rare inherited or acquired disorders where defective haem synthesis leads to a build-up of intermediate porphyrins. Its effects depend upon the type of disorder but include: abdominal pain, urine which turns red on standing, photosensitivity, neuropathy and mental health problems. Certain drugs such as barbiturates and the oral contraceptive may precipitate an acute attack.

porphyrins, *(por-fi-rins)*, group of pyrrole substances formed during the synthesis of haem and cytochromes.

porphyrinuria, *(por-fir-in-ū-ri-a)*, presence of porphyrins in the urine.

port, in computing an interface or socket on the computer for plugging in other devices. *Parallel p.*: a socket used to connect the computer to other devices with a parallel port such as a printer. Parallel ports carry information by a faster method than that used by a serial port. Often called a **Centronics port**. *Serial p.*: a type of socket used to connect the computer to other devices with a serial port such as a modem or mouse. They carry information by a slower method than parallel ports. Also known as **RS232**.

portacaval, *(por-ta-kā-val)*, relating to the hepatic portal vein and the inferior vena cava. *P. anastomosis/shunt*: the hepatic portal vein is joined to the inferior vena cava so that some blood bypasses the liver, used in the treatment of hepatic portal hypertension.

Portage system, a method of behaviour modification used by family and friends to assist a child with physical or learning difficulties to develop social skills.

portal hypertension, more properly called hepatic portal hypertension. High pressure in the hepatic portal vein resulting from serious liver disease such as cirrhosis. *See* OESOPHAGEAL VARICES.

portal vein, more properly called the **hepatic portal vein**, it carries venous blood from the gastrointestinal tract, spleen and pancreas to the liver.

portfolio, a personal and private collection of evidence, which demonstrates the owner's continuing professional and personal development. It documents the acquisition of knowledge, skills, attitudes, understanding and achievements; in recording these events, it deals with the past. It contains reflections on current practice and progress, and in doing this it deals with the present. However, it also contains an action plan for future career and personal development, and in this it looks to the future. It does not simply record outcomes, but rather it documents the journey taken *en route* to the outcomes. As such, it is a valuable tool in continuing professional development. A portfolio should allow the practitioner to select profiles for a number of different purposes.

position, attitude or posture.

positive end-expiratory pressure (PEEP), during mechanical ventilation the pressure at the end of expiration is kept sufficiently high to prevent alveolar collapse by keeping the lungs partially inflated.

positive feedback, *see* FEEDBACK.

positive pressure ventilation, *see* INTERMITTENT POSITIVE PRESSURE VENTILATION.

positron emission tomography (PET), uses cyclotron-produced isotopes of extremely short half-life that emit positrons. PET scanning is used to evaluate physiological functions of organs, such as the brain.

positrons, positively charged particles that combine with negatively charged electrons, causing gamma-rays to be emitted.

posseting, the regurgitation of feed by an infant.

Possum (patient-operated selector mechanism), a device used by individuals with severe paralysis to operate other equipment, e.g. computers, telephone or other communications systems.

postabsorptive state, the fasted state. Metabolic state that exists between meals, such as late morning, late afternoon and during the night. Fuel molecules are in short supply and catabolic processes predominate as the body strives to maintain blood glucose by glycogenolysis, lipolysis and, later, the breakdown of body protein. *See* ABSORPTIVE STATE.

postcibal, occurring after eating. *See* DUMPING SYNDROME.

postcoital, (*pōst-kō-it-al*), after coitus. *P. bleeding*: may indicate disease of the cervix such as polyp. *P. contraception*: oestrogen and progesterone (or progesterone alone) hormones administered within 72 hours of unprotected intercourse, or the insertion of an intrauterine contraceptive device. *P. test*: in infertility specimens of cervical mucus are obtained within a few hours of intercourse to demonstate the presence of viable sperm.

posterior, situated at the back. *P. chamber of the eye*: space between the anterior surface of the lens and the posterior surface of the iris. It contains aqueous humour.

posteroanterior, from back to front.

postganglionic, (*pōst-gan-glī-ōn-ik*), relating to a nerve fibre distal to a ganglion.

posthumous, (*pos-tū-mus*), after death.

postmature, infant born after the expected date of delivery, the pregnancy lasting longer than 40 weeks (280 days).

postmenopausal, (*pōst-men-ō-paw-zal*), after the menopause. *P. bleeding (PMB)*: vaginal bleeding occurring after the menopause. It may indicate serious pathology such as endometrial cancer and should be investigated.

post-mortem, after death. *P. examination*: autopsy; an examination of the body after death to ascertain the cause of death.

postnatal, (*pōst nay-tal*), after birth or delivery. *P. (postpartum) blues*:

271

describes emotional lability and or a low mood experienced by some women for a few days following the birth of a baby; sometimes called 'fourth-day blues'. Less severe than P. depression: see PUERPERAL PSYCHOSIS. *P. depression: see* PUERPERAL PSYCHOSIS. *P. examination:* routine examination 6 weeks after delivery. Includes general physical and mental health, involution of the uterus, the pelvic floor and perineal healing. *P. period:* the time of at least 10 days and no more than 28 days, during which the attendance of a midwife on mother and infant is mandatory.

postoperative, after operation.

postpartum, after labour. *P. depression:* that occurring in the postpartum period. It may range from 'baby blues' to a serious psychotic depression. *P. haemorrhage:* excessive vaginal bleeding following the birth of the baby.

postprandial, after a meal.

post-transfusion syndrome, a disorder occurring some weeks after a blood transfusion. It is probably due to the presence of cytomegalovirus (CMV) and is characterized by rash, jaundice, fever and an abnormal blood count. Also known as postperfusion syndrome.

post-traumatic stress disorder, anxiety with nightmares, irritability, poor memory and concentration, headaches and depression which may occur after involvement in any traumatic situation such as a serious road accident, fire, explosion, crime or natural disaster.

postural, pertaining to posture or position. *P. treatment:* certain positions are used to relieve or treat, e.g. dyspnoea may be relieved by adopting an upright (orthopnoeic) posture. *P. drainage:* different areas of the lungs are drained by a careful positioning of the patient. *P.*

hypotension: very low blood pressure which occurs when suddenly standing upright. A side-effect of drugs used to treat high blood pressure.

potassium (K), a metallic element. It is a major intracellular cation and is required for normal neuromuscular activity. *See* HYPERKALAEMIA, HYPOKALAEMIA.

Pott's disease, tuberculous osteomyelitis affecting the spine.

Pott's fracture, ankle fracture with or without joint displacement.

pouch of Douglas, *see* DOUGLAS' POUCH.

poultice, fomentation. Local applications such as kaolin used to improve circulation and relieve pain.

Poupart's ligament, *(poo-parz'),* the inguinal ligament. Stretching from the anterior superior spine of the ilium to the pubis.

power calculation, a measure of statistical power. The likelihood of the study to produce statistically significant results.

powerlessness, a situation where an individual is unable to control or influence a situation such as a healthcare problem.

poxvirus, a group of DNA viruses which cause vaccinia, variola and orf.

PQRST complex, on an electrocardiogram the letters to denote the five deflection waves of the typical waveform produced during a cardiac cycle. The P wave represents atrial depolarization as the impulse is conducted across the atria. The next three waves are known collectively as the QRS complex and represent ventricular depolarization which immediately precedes contraction. The T wave represents ventricular repolarization (Figure 62). *See* ELECTROCARDIOGRAM.

62 PQRST complex

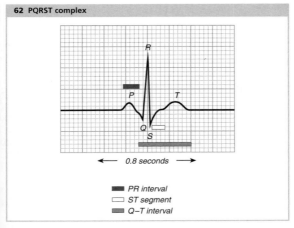

← 0.8 seconds →

- ▬ PR interval
- ☐ ST segment
- ▬ Q–T interval

practitioner, an individual qualified to practise a particular profession such as nursing.

Prader–Willi syndrome, inherited condition arising from mutations on the paternal chromosome 15 during gametogenesis. It is characterized by learning disability, hypotonia, short stature and obesity. *See* ANGLEMAN SYNDROME.

precancerous, obsolete term. *See* CAR-CINOMA-IN-SITU.

preceptorship, a system to help the newly qualified nurse achieve confidence in the early months of registered practice, under the guidance of a preceptor.

precipitate labour, a labour of very short duration in which very few contractions occur prior to the birth of the infant.

precipitins, *(pre-sip′-it-ins)*, antibodies present in the blood which destroy

soluble antigens by the formation of an immune complex which is then destroyed by precipitation. The principle can be used as the basis of diagnostic tests.

precognition, a knowledge of future events.

preconceptual, relating to the period prior to conception.

precordial, relating to the precordium. *P. thump*: a technique used in cardiopulmonary resuscitation (CPR).

precordium, *(pre-kor′-de-um),* the area of the chest over the heart.

precursor, a forerunner. Often describes an inactive enzyme or hormone.

prediabetes, having a predisposition to diabetes mellitus.

predigestion, partial digestion of foods prior to intake.

predisposed, susceptible.

pre-eclampsia, *(pre-e-klamp-si-a),* serious condition associated with

273

pregnancy. It is characterized by hypertension, proteinuria and oedema. *See* ECLAMPSIA.

prefrontal, lying in the anterior part of the frontal lobe of the brain. *P. leucotomy: see* LEUCOTOMY.

preganglionic, *(pre-gan-gli-on-ik),* relating to a nerve fibre proximal to a ganglion.

pregnancy, the state of being with child. Usually a period of some 280 days. *Ectopic p: see* ECTOPIC GESTATION. *P. test*: confirmation of pregnancy denoted by the presence of the hormone chorionic gonadotrophin in the urine or blood.

prejudice, a preconceived opinion or bias which can be negative or positive. It can be for or against members of particular groups and may lead to discrimination, racism, sexism or intolerance.

preload, the degree of stretch present in the myocardial muscle fibres at end diastole. It depends on the end diastolic volume (EDV). In situations where venous return is reduced, such as shock, there is a reduction in the degree of stretch or preload. *See* AFTERLOAD, STARLING'S LAW OF THE HEART.

premature, occurring before the correct time *P. baby: see* LOW BIRTH WEIGHT, PRETERM. *P. beat: see* EXTRASYSTOLE. *P. ejaculation*: emission of semen at the beginning of intercourse, often outside the vagina. *P. labour: See* PRETERM.

premedication, drugs given before another drug, such as those given before an anaesthetic. The use of premedication has decreased with the development of day case surgery. When they are given it may be to sedate and/or dry salivary and bronchial secretions.

premenstrual, before menstruation. *P. syndrome/tension (PMS/PMT)*: a col-

lection of signs and symptoms experienced by many women in the 7–10 days preceding the onset of menstruation. The aetiology is unknown but hormonal activity is one probable cause. Its effects include: mood change, fluid retention with weight gain, lethargy, food cravings, breast discomfort, bruising and joint pains.

premolar, the two bicuspid teeth in each jaw which lie between the canine and the molars. *See* TEETH.

prenatal, prior to birth, during the period of pregnancy.

preoperative, before surgery.

PREP, abbrev. for **Post-Registration Education and Practice.** Initiated by the UKCC; an ongoing system which will ensure that nurses, midwives and health visitors update their knowledge and skills as a requirement for continued registration. It became mandatory for all practitioners to comply by April 2001.

preprandial, before a meal.

prepubertal, relating to the period prior to puberty.

prepuce, loose skin covering the glans penis, foreskin.

presbycusis, *(pres-bi-koo-sis),* sensorineural deafness associated with increasing age.

presbyopia, *(pres-bi-o-pi-a),* longsightedness which develops as a result of the lens becoming less elastic with age. Near vision is affected.

prescription, a written formula signed by the prescriber, directing the pharmacist to supply the required drugs. *P. only medicine (POM)*: a drug that can be obtained only with a prescription, except in an emergency when it may be dispensed by a pharmacist, provided certain criteria are met.

presenility, *(pre-sen-il-i-ti),* premature ageing.

presentation, the part of the fetus which engages in the pelvis, it may be vertex, breech, foot, face, brow or shoulder.

pressor, substance causing blood pressure to rise.

pressure, exertion of force or compression by one object on another, e.g. blood on the arterial walls. *P. areas*: any area of the body subjected to pressure sufficient to compress the capillaries and disrupt the microcirculation. Usually occurs where tissues are compressed between a bone and a hard surface and where two surfaces are in contact, e.g. elbows, heels, buttocks and under breasts etc. *P. point*: the points at which pressure may be applied to arrest arterial haemorrhage (Figure 63). *P. ulcer*: previously known as pressure sore or decubitus ulcer. The European Pressure Ulcer Advisory Panel (EPUAP) defines a pressure ulcer as an area of localized damage to the skin and underlying tissue caused by pressure, shear, friction, or a combination of these factors. Pressure ulcers develop when any area of the body is subjected to unrelieved pressure that leads to tissue hypoxia, ischaemia and necrosis with inflammation and ulcer formation. Shearing forces also disrupt the microcirculation when they cause the skin layers to move against one another, such as a person slipping down the bed or being dragged instead of being moved correctly. Shearing injury damages the deeper tissues and can result in an extensive pressure ulcer. Friction from continual rubbing leads to blisters, abrasions and superficial pressure ulcers, and is exacerbated by the presence of moisture such as sweat or urine. Factors which predispose to pressure ulcer formation include: poor oxygenation, incontinence, age over 65–70, immobility, altered consciousness, dehydration and malnutrition. Assessment of the skin condition and the severity of existing pressure ulcers is an important part of the nursing assessment required for choosing the most appropriate interventions. There are several pressure ulcer grading scales, but the EPUAP recommends the use of a four-point grading scale. *See* BLOOD PRESSURE, CENTRAL VENOUS PRESSURE, INTRACRANIAL PRESSURE, PULMONARY ARTERY WEDGE PRESSURE.

pressure ulcer prevention, starts with assessment of skin condition and pressure areas using the most appropriate risk scale on a regular basis, e.g. Norton, Waterlow scale. Relief of pressure by moving or encouraging patients to change position, use of external aids, keeping skin clean and dry, ensuring that fluid and nutritional needs are met, and avoiding friction and shearing force.

presystole, (*prē-sis'-to-li*), period in the cardiac cycle before systole.

preterm, before term or premature. *P. baby/birth*: defined as the birth of a baby after 24 but before 37 weeks' gestation. The baby is likely to be of low birth weight and possibly small-for-dates or dysmature through placental insufficiency.

prevalence, the total number of cases of a disease existing in a population at a single point in time.

priapism, persistent erection of the penis without sexual stimulation, such as with spinal injuries and some types of leukaemia.

prickle cell, cells contained in the stratum spinosum in the germinative layer of the epidermis.

prickly heat, miliaria papulosa.

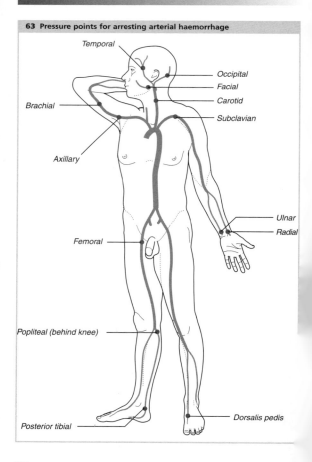

63 Pressure points for arresting arterial haemorrhage

Temporal

Occipital

Facial

Carotid

Brachial

Subclavian

Axillary

Ulnar

Radial

Femoral

Popliteal (behind knee)

Posterior tibial

Dorsalis pedis

primary, 1. first in terms of time, place or development. **2.** the most important in a series of events or features. *P. complex/focus:* first site of infection with tuberculosis. Usually heals spontaneously. Also known as Gnon's focus. *P. dentition: see* TEETH.

primary care group (PCG), in England, a grouping of primary health professionals and their services covering an area with a population of around 100 000. Working with the Health Authority, local authority and other relevant groups, they assess local health needs, plan and develop community and primary healthcare services and commission secondary services for the local population. In Scotland they are called local health co-operatives, and in Wales local health groups.

primary care trust (PCT), a freestanding body developed from a PCG which, having autonomy, can respond more flexibly to local need.

primary healthcare, the health care provided by health professionals who are community-based: community nurses, family doctors, health visitors, midwives and practice nurses, plus other health professionals such as physiotherapists. Based in health centres and doctors' surgeries the primary healthcare team are usually the person's first point of contact.

primary nursing, a professional model of practice, where one qualified nurse takes the main responsibility for assessing, planning, implementing and evaluating a patient's care. This is the primary nurse, who is supported by an associate nurse. Other nurses, including students, and healthcare assistants, may also provide care.

primary prevention, measures taken to prevent the occurrence of disease, e.g. immunization programmes.

primary sore, initial site of infection in syphilis.

prime mover, a muscle which has the main responsibility for a particular movement, e.g. biceps brachii in elbow flexion.

primigravida, *(prī-mi-gra-vid-a),* a woman pregnant for the first time.

primipara, *(prī-mip'-a-ra),* a woman who has borne one child.

primordial, *(prī-mor'-dē-al),* pertaining to the beginning, e.g. primitive cells formed during early embryonic development. *P. follicles:* follicles containing primary oöcytes, present in the ovary at birth.

prion, infectious agent consisting of protein, similar to viruses, but with no nucleic acids. Responsible for the transmission of diseases that include **Creutzfeldt–Jakob disease.**

proaccelerin, *(prō-ak-sel-er-in),* factor V in blood clotting. Also called the **labile factor.**

probe, a slender blunt-ended rod used for exploring wounds or cavities.

problem-oriented records, a multi-professional system of patient records in which each patient's problem has a numbered page and entries are made using the SOAP formula: S = subjective, O = objective, A = analysis of data, P = plan.

process, 1. in anatomy a projection or eminence of a part. **2.** a series of sequential steps such as the nursing process.

procidentia, *(pro-sid-en-she-a),* a falling down or prolapse. *Uterine p.:* when the uterine cervix is visible at the vaginal opening.

proconvertin, *(prō-kon-ver-tin),* factor VII in blood clotting. Also called **stable factor.**

proctalgia, *(prok-tal'-ji-a),* pain about the rectum.

proctectomy, *(prok-tek'-to-mi),* excision of rectum.

proctitis, *(prok-tī'-tis),* inflammation of the rectum.

proctocele, *(prok-tō-sēl),* prolapsed rectum.

proctoclysis, *(prok-tō-klī'-sis),* introduction into the rectum of fluid for absorption.

proctocolectomy, *(prok-tō-kol-ek-to-mi),* operation to remove the rectum and colon. *Restorative p.*: avoids a permanent stoma: an ileal reservoir is formed and ileoanal anastomosis carried out.

proctocolitis, *(prok-tō-kol-ī-tis),* inflammation of the rectum and colon.

proctology, *(prok-tol-o-ji),* a study of conditions of the rectum and anus.

proctorrhaphy, *(prok-tor-a-fi),* suturing of the rectum.

proctoscope, *(prok'-tō-skōp),* an instrument for viewing the interior of the rectum.

prodromal, *(prō-drō-mal),* relating to the period which elapses in an infectious disease between the first symptoms and the appearance of the rash. *P. rash*: one which precedes the true rash.

prodrug, a drug administered as an inactive form that is activated within the body, e.g. by liver enzymes. Used for a variety of reasons that include: overcoming gastrointestinal side-effects and damage such as with the cytotoxic drug cyclophosphamide that is activated in the liver.

proenzyme, *(prō-en-zīm),* zymogen. The inactive precursor of an enzyme, e.g. pepsinogen, trypsinogen.

progeria, *(prō-je-ri-a),* premature senility occurring during childhood.

progesterone, *(pro-jes-ter-ōn),* gestation hormone. A steroid hormone produced by the corpus luteum, placenta and to a limited extent the adrenal glands. It influences the endometrium, breasts, cervical mucus and myometrium and is important in preparing for and maintaining pregnancy.

progestogen, *(prō-jes-tō-jen),* substance having similar action to progesterone.

prognathism, *(prog-nath-izm),* protrusion of the jaw.

proglottis, *(prō-glo-tis),* segment of tapeworm.

prognosis, *(prog-nō-sis),* the expected course or outcome of a disease.

program, in computing a set of coded numeric instructions which let the CPU perform a specific task, e.g. word processing.

proinsulin, inactive precursor of the hormone insulin.

Project 2000, a system of preregistration nurse education, launched by the UKCC in the late 1980s. Nurses were educated to diploma level through a common foundation programme of 18 months, followed by a chosen branch of nursing: care of the adult, the child, people with mental illness and people with a learning disability. Curricula were rooted in health promotion and primary healthcare. Major changes to preregistration nurse education are planned, and new curricula are being piloted in several sites, based on the two documents: Commission for Education (1999) *Fitness for Practice*: London: UKCC and Department of Health (1999) *Making a Difference*: London: the Stationery Office.

projection, a mental defence mechanism where painful thoughts, feelings and motives are attributed to or transferred to another person.

prokaryote, a cell where the genetic material is scattered in the cytoplasm, such as in many microorganisms. There is no true nucleus. *See* EUKARYOTE.

prolactin (PRL), *(prō-lak-tin),* hormone produced by the anterior pituitary gland which stimulates milk production. Also called **lactogenic hormone**. *See* HYPERPROLACTINAEMIA.

prolapse, *(prō-laps),* sinking or falling down, e.g. uterus, rectum or umbilical cord. *See* PROCIDENTIA.

prolapsed intervertebral disc (PID), slipped disc due to prolapse of the central part of the cartilaginous intervertebral disc. *See* NUCLEUS PULPOSUS.

proliferation, reproduction. Rapid cell growth such as in tissue repair or cancer.

proliferative phase, 1. a stage of the menstrual cycle which commences after bleeding has ceased and lasts until ovulation. It is characterized by the regeneration of the endometrium and corresponds to the follicular phase of the ovarian cycle. **2.** phase of wound healing that includes: production of collagen network and granulation tissue, epithelialization and wound contraction.

proline, an amino acid.

promontory, a projecting part. An eminence.

promyelocyte, *(prō-mī-el-ō-sīt),* a precusor cell which eventually forms the white cells of the polymorphonuclear series.

pronation, downward turning of the palm of the hand.

pronator, muscle which pronates.

prone, lying with the face downwards.

pronephros, *(prō-nef-ros),* structure formed during the early embryonic development of the urinary tract.

prophase, *(prō-fāz),* first stage in mitosis and meiosis.

prophylactic, *(pro-fil-ak-tik),* pertaining to prophylaxis. An agent which tends to prevent disease, e.g. a drug or vaccine.

prophylaxis, *(pro-fil-ak-sis),* measures taken to prevent disease.

proprietary name, the brand name given to a drug by the company which produced it.

proprioception, *(pro-prē-ō-sep-shon),* a non-visual awareness of spatial orientation and the position of body parts.

proprioceptor, *(pro-prī-ō-sep-tor),* sensory end organ able to detect changes in body position. Situated in joints, muscles, tendons and the inner ear.

proptosis oculi, *(prop-tō'-sis ok'-ū-lē),* protrusion of eyeballs.

prosencephalon, *(pros-en-kef-al-on),* the forebrain. The part of the brain containing the telencephalon and diencephalon.

prospective study, research that collects data in the future, moving forward in time. *See* RETROSPECTIVE STUDY.

prostacyclin, *(pros-ta-sī-klin),* a prostaglandin derivative. It is produced in blood vessel walls and inhibits platelet aggregation and causes vasodilation. Important in preventing intravascular clotting.

prostaglandins, *(pros-ta-glan-dinz),* a large group of regulatory lipids derived from arachidonic acid (fatty acid). Very potent with a short duration of action, they modulate the action of several hormones. They are present in all tissues and affect a variety of physiological processes including: contraction of smooth muscle, gastric secretion, inflammation, blood flow, clotting and parturition. Used clinically to induce termination of pregnancy and labour, prevent platelet aggregation during haemodialysis, etc.

prostate, small structure consisting of several glands with a capsule surrounding the male urethra and bladder neck. It produces an alkaline fluid containing several enzymes which is added to semen prior to ejaculation.

prostate-specific antigen (PSA), an antigen which, if detected in the serum, acts as a tumour marker for prostate cancer. Levels may be raised in conditions other than cancer.

prostatectomy, *(pros-ta-tek'to-mi),* surgical removal of the prostate. Most commonly this is achieved by transurethral resection (TURP or TUR) but in some cases it may be necessary to remove the gland by opening the lower abdomen either by transvesical approach or by the retropubic operation (Millin's prostatectomy).

prostatic, *(pros-tak-ik),* pertaining to the prostate. *benign p. hyperplasia (BPH):* benign enlargement of the gland causing urinary problems such as retention in older men.

prostatitis, *(pros-ta-ti'-tis),* inflammation of the prostate gland.

prosthesis, *(pros-thē-sis),* the replacement of a structure or organ with an artificial part, e.g. heart valves, limbs, dentures, pacemaker, etc.

protamine sulphate, a naturally occurring heparin antagonist used in the treatment of heparin overdose.

protease, an enzyme which breaks down proteins.

protective isolation, reverse barrier nursing. Separation of patients who are immunocompromised to protect them from infection. This may include patients with AIDS, leukaemia, and during treatment with immunosuppressant drugs, chemotherapy or radiation or whenever the neutrophil count is low.

protein, complex nitrogenous organic compounds formed from amino acids linked in different combinations and sequences. Vital component of all living organisms, they are needed for cell division, growth and repair and to form functional proteins which include: enzymes, hormones and haemoglobin. *See* AMINO ACIDS. *P.energy malnutrition (PEM):* a form of malnutrition caused by an insufficient intake of protein and energy (kcal). May occur in hospitalized individuals who develop a negative nitrogen balance because protein is primarily being used to produce energy. A negative balance is associated with starvation or any severe physiological stress which increases protein catabolism, e.g. burns, sepsis, major surgery and multiple injuries. *See* KWASHIORKOR, MARASMUS.

proteinuria, *(prō-tin-ū-ri-a),* protein in the urine.

proteolysis, *(prō-tē-ol-i-sis),* process which breaks down proteins into less complex molecules by disrupting the peptide bonds.

proteolytic, *(prō-tē-ō-lit'-ik),* relating to proteolysis or substances such as p. enzymes which catalyse the breakdown of proteins.

Proteus, *(prō-tē-us),* a genus of Gram-negative bacteria normally found in the bowel, causes infection of the urinary tract and wounds.

prothrombin, *(prō-throm-bin),* factor II of blood clotting. A plasma protein which is the inactive precursor of thrombin. *P.time:* a test of blood clotting factor activity. *See* BLOOD CLOTTING.

proto-oncogene, a gene with the potential to become a cancer-causing oncogene if stimulated by mutagenic carcinogens.

proton, *(prō-ton),* subatomic particle with a positive charge.

protoplasm, *(prō-tō-plazm),* gel-like complex chemical mix of molecules which forms the main part of a cell

It is enclosed by the cell (plasma) membrane and contains the organelles.

prototype, (*prō'-tō-tīp*), the original form from which others are copied.

protozoa, (*prō-tō-zō-a*), microscopic unicellular animals. Diseases caused by protozoa include trichomoniasis (*Trichomonas vaginalis*), malaria, amoebiasis, leishmaniasis, etc.

proud flesh, excessive granulation tissue in a wound.

provitamin, (*prō-vi-ta-min*), substance that may be converted to a vitamin by the body, e.g. carotenes, tryptophan.

proxemics, (*proks-em-iks*), the study of how space and spatial relationships affect behaviour, e.g. population density.

proximal, (*proks'-i-mal*), in anatomy nearest to the centre. *Cf.* DISTAL.

prurigo, (*pru-rī'-gō*), a skin disease marked by irritating papules.

pruritus, (*pru-rī-tus*), itching. Severe skin irritation is a feature of some types of jaundice, allergy, malignant conditions, etc. *P. vulvae:* affecting the vulva, it is associated with vaginitis and glycosuria.

pseudoangina, (*sū-dō-an-jī-na*), chest pain in anxious individuals without evidence of heart disease.

pseudarthrosis, (*sū-dar-thrō'-sis*), a false joint.

pseudocyesis, (*sū-dō-sī-e-sis*), phantom pregnancy. The changes of pregnancy occur but without a fetus.

pseudohermaphrodite, (*sū-dō-her-ma-frō-dīt*), an individual whose external genitalia are of a different sexual type to the gonads.

pseudomembranous colitis, (*sū-dō-mem-brān-us*), a condition caused by superinfection with *Clostridium difficile* in patients whose normal bowel flora has been destroyed by broad

spectrum antibiotics. It is characterized by watery diarrhoea and can be life-threatening. Treatment is with antibiotics, e.g. metronidazole or vancomycin.

Pseudomonas, (*sū-dō-mo-nas*), a bacterial genus. Gram-negative motile bacilli. Found in water and decomposing vegetable matter. *Pseudomonas aeruginosa* causes wound, urinary and respiratory infection in humans. It can cause superinfection where the normal commensals have been destroyed by broad-spectrum antibiotics. Produces blue-green exudate or pus which has a characteristic musty odour.

pseudopodium, (*sū-dō-pō-di-um*), a temporary protrusion of a cell used for movement and to engulf material.

pseudosyncytium, a tissue where the boundaries between cells are poorly defined.

psittacosis, (*sit-a-kō-sis*), a chlamydial disease transmitted to humans from infected parrots or budgerigars. It causes an atypical pneumonia with headache and toxaemia.

psoas, (*sō-az*), *p. major* and *p. minor:* the large muscles of the back.

psoriasis, (*so-rī'-a-sis*), a chronic inflammatory skin disease characterized by an abnormality of keratinization producing lesions consisting of raised, red, scaly areas. It tends to be chronic with periods of acute exacerbation and remission and may be associated with a type of arthritis. Factors implicated in its aetiology include: genetic predisposition, immunological and biochemical factors.

psyche, (*sī'-ki*), the mind.

psychiatric, (*si-ki-at-rik*), pertaining to psychiatry.

psychiatrist, (*si-kī'-a-trist*), a doctor who specializes in the diagnosis,

281

treatment and management of mental health problems.

psychiatry, (sī-kī-at'-ri), the study and treatment of mental health problems.

psychoactive, drugs and other substances which may alter the processes of the mind.

psychoanalysis, (sī-kō-an-al-i-sis), a method of psychotherapy in which the relationship between patient and therapist is analysed back to the patient's earliest relationships.

psychodrama, a type of psychotherapy which utilizes spontaneous role play and drama. Group discussion aims at giving patients a greater awareness of the problems presented and possible methods of dealing with them.

psychodynamics, (sī-kō-dī-nam-iks), science of mental processes as a cause of mental activity.

psychogenic, (sī-kō-jen-ik), originating in the mind and having no physical cause.

psychogeriatrics, (sī-kō-je-rē-at-riks), old-fashioned term, pertaining to the mental health problems of older people. The term elderly mentally ill has also been used.

psychological, relating to psychology.

psychologist, (sī-kol-o-jist), an individual who specializes in psychology – development, processes of the mind and behaviour. *Clinical p.*: a suitably qualified person who provides professional services for people with emotional problems.

psychology, (sī-kol-o-ji), the study of behaviour, the mind and its processes.

psychometrics, (sī-kō-met-riks), the testing and measuring of mental processes, e.g. intelligence.

psychomotor, (sī-kō-mō-tor), pertaining to the motor effects of a mental process. *P. disorder*: mental conditions which affect muscular activity.

psychoneurosis, (sī-kō-nū-rō-sis), see NEUROSIS.

psychopathic personality, a persistent disorder or disability of mind which results in abnormally aggressive or seriously irresponsible conduct. The person lacks the ability to feel guilt for the consequences of his or her actions and often behaves in a destructive and antisocial manner.

psychopathology, (sī-kō-pa-thol-o-ji), study of the mechanism of mental disorders.

psychosexual, (sī-kō-seks-sū-al), pertaining to the mental aspects of sexuality. *P. development*. according to **Freud,** development occurs through five stages: oral, anal, phallic, latent and genital.

psychosis, (sī-kō-sis), a major mental health disorder in which individuals lack insight into their condition. It is usually characterized by loss of reality, hallucinations, delusions, impulses and disintegration of personality. Various classifications exist, but broadly it may be: **1** organic: acute as in delirium, e.g. electrolyte imbalance or alcohol etc. or chronic as in dementia which may be due to brain pathology, nutritional deficiencies, etc. **2.** functional: conditions occurring without brain disease or impairment, e.g. schizophrenia, major depression and manic-depressive illness, c.f. NEUROSIS.

psychosomatic, (sī-kō-so-mat-ik), relating to mind and body. *P. disorder*: physical condition caused by a psychological factor, e.g. some types of peptic ulcer.

psychotherapy, (sī-kō-ther-a-pi), a way of dealing with psychological and emotional problems by interaction between individuals or groups, usally by talking, but many different approaches exist.

psychotic, *(sī-kot-ik),* relating to a psychosis.

psychotropic, *(sī-kō-trop-ik),* drugs which affect the mind. They include: tranquillizers, sedatives and antidepressants, etc.

pterygium, *(te-rij-e-um),* a web of membrane growing inwards from the conjunctiva over the cornea.

ptosis, *(tō'-sis),* drooping of the upper eyelid.

ptyalin, *(ti-a-lin), see* AMYLASE.

puberty, the period during which the reproductive organs become functional, associated with the appearance of the secondary sexual characteristics.

pubes, *(pū-bēz),* the area over the pubic bones.

pubic, relating to the pubis.

pubiotomy, *(pū-bē-ot-o-mi),* cutting the symphysis pubis to enlarge the pelvis.

pubis, *(pū-bis),* the anterior part of the pelvis, the right and left pubic bones which meet at the symphysis pubis.

public health, area of medicine which deals with the health of a community or population. It includes: environmental aspects such as water and food safety, monitoring of disease patterns (especially communicable disease) and health promotion. *P. H. nursing*: health visitors, school nurses, practice nurses and other community nurses who promote public health and work to prevent ill health in a variety of settings, e.g. school, workplaces.

pudenda *(sing.* **pudendum),** *(pū-den'-da),* the external genitalia.

pudendal block, *(pū-den-dal),* anaesthesia of the external genitalia achieved by the transvaginal injection of local anaesthetic into the pudendal nerves during labour.

puerperal, *(pū-er-per-al),* relating to the puerperium. *P. psychosis*: severe mental health disorder occurring after childbirth. *P. sepsis* or *fever*: an infection of the genital tract as a result of childbirth.

puerperium, *(pū-er-per-i-um),* the period of about 6–8 weeks following childbirth in which the reproductive structures return to normal (involute).

Pulex irritans, *(pū-leksir-i-tans),* common flea. *See* FLEA.

pulmonary, *(pul-mon-a-ri)* relating to the lungs. *P. artery wedge pressure (PAWP)*: a method of measuring end diastolic left ventricular pressure by means of catheter, e.g. Swan-Gantz, passed into a small pulmonary artery via the right side of the heart. At intervals a small balloon in the catheter tip is inflated to wedge it and block off the pulmonary artery behind. Now the pressure being recorded in the p. capillaries will reflect that in the left atrium and ventricle. *P. circulation: see* CIRCULATION. *P. embolus: see* EMBOLISM. *P. function tests*: series of tests used to assess lung function, e.g. peak flow, blood gases. *P. hypertension*: increased pressure in the pulmonary vessels such as with congenital heart conditions or lung disease. *P. infarction*: necrosis of lung tissue resulting from an embolus. *P. oedema*: fluid within the alveoli. *P. stenosis*: narrowing of the pulmonary valve. *P. tuberculosis: see* TUBERCULOSIS. *P. valve*: semilunar valve situated between the pulmonary artery and right ventricle. *P. ventilation* or *minute volume*: the amount of air moved in and out of the lungs in one minute.

pulp, the interior, fleshy part of vegetable or animal tissue. *Digital p.*: the soft areas at the ends of the digits. *Splenic p.*: the interior of the spleen. *P. cavity*: the central part of a tooth.

pulsatile, (*pul-sa-tīl*), throbbing.

pulsation, (*pul-sā'-shon*), beating of the heart, or of the blood in the arteries.

pulse, the wave of expansion in an artery which corresponds to left ventricular contraction. It can be felt in a superficial artery, especially one that passes over a bone, e.g. radial artery at the wrist. The rate in a newborn is 120–130/min which decreases through infancy and childhood to reach the adult resting rate of 60–80/min. *P. deficit*: a difference in rate between the apical rate and the rate at the radial artery, due to some beats being too weak to reach the radial artery. *P. pressure*: the difference, in mm Hg, between the systolic and diastolic blood pressure readings.

pulse oximetry, a noninvasive method of measuring haemoglobin oxygen saturation using an oximeter. Sensors can be attached to the ear lobe, finger or the nose. It is used routinely in many situations including the perioperative period. Results of oxygen saturation can be misleading in some situations and must be interpreted carefully.

pulsus alternans, the pulse is alternately strong and weak, though regular in time.

punctate, dotted.

punctum (*pl.* **puncta**), a very small spot or point, e.g. the lacrimal puncta which are tiny openings through which tears enter the lacrimal ducts.

puncture, to make a hole with a sharp instrument. *See* CISTERNAL PUNCTURE, LUMBAR PUNCTURE, MARROW PUNCTURE.

pupil, variable size opening in the centre of the iris. *See* ARGYLL ROBERTSON PUPIL, EYE.

pupillary, (*pū-pil'-a-ri*), pertaining to the pupil. *P. reflex*: the reflex constriction and dilatation of the pupil in response to the amount of light entering the eye. It is controlled by the third cranial or oculomotor nerves.

purgative, (*per-gat-iv*), drug causing evacuation of fluid faeces. *see* APERIENT, LAXATIVE.

purines, (*pū-rēnz*), nitrogenous bases such as adenine and guanine, required in the formation of nucleosides, nucleotides and nucleic acids. Uric acid is a metabolite of purine breakdown.

Purkinje, (*per-kin-ji*), **1.** *P. cells*: nerve cells found in the cerebellum. **2.** *P. fibres*: the specialized conducting fibres of the heart.

purpura, red or purple spots (petechiae) or patches (ecchymoses) due to bleeding into the skin. Causes include: thrombocytopenia, meningococcal septicaemia, Cushing's syndrome, Henoch–Schönlein purpura, infections and old age.

purulent, (*pū'-rū-lent*), pus-like or containing pus.

pus, matter. Consists of dead leucocytes, dead bacteria, cell debris and tissue fluid.

pustule, (*pus'-tūl*), a pimple containing pus.

putrefaction, (*pū-tre-fak'-shon*), the rotting away of animal matter. Decomposition advanced to an offensive stage.

***P* value,** in inferential statistics there is a *P* value given. This is the probability that the results found have occurred by chance alone, e.g. $P = 0.05$ means 5% or 1 in 20 chance.

pyaemia, (*pī-ē-mi-a*), the circulation of septic emboli in the blood stream causing multiple abscesses.

pyarthrosis, (*pī-ar-thrō'-sis*), pus in a joint.

pyelogram, an X-ray of the kidney and ureter. *See* UROGRAM.

pyelography, (*pī-el-og-raf-i*), *see* URO-GRAPHY.

pyelolithotomy, (*pī-e-lō-lith-ot-o-mi*), operation to remove a stone from the renal pelvis.

pyelonephritis, (*pī-el-ō-nef-rī-tis*), inflammation of the renal pelvis and renal parenchyma. The causative organisms include: *Escherichia coli*, *Streptococcus faecalis* and *Pseudomonas aeruginosa* which usually spread upwards from a bladder infection but can spread to the kidney in the blood. It can lead to chronic renal disease and eventual failure.

pyeloplasty, (*pī-el-ō-plas-ti*), plastic surgery to relieve obstruction in the renal pelvis and for drainage in hydronephrosis.

pylorectomy, (*pī-lor-ek'-to-mi*), removal of the pyloric end of the stomach.

pyloric, (*pī-lor-ik*), pertaining to the pylorus. *P. stenosis*: narrowing of the pylorus. **1.** congenital hypertrophic p. s. occurs in the first few weeks of life and is characterized by projectile vomiting, dehydration, electrolyte imbalance, poor weight gain and palpable pylorus. Treatment is generally by pyloromyotomy (Ramstedt's operation). **2.** in adults it occurs secondary to tumours or peptic ulceration.

pyloromyotomy, (*pī-lor-ō-mī-ot-o-mi*), *see* RAMSTEDT'S OPERATION.

pyloroplasty, (*pī-lor-ō-plas-ti*), an operation which widens the pylorus and improves drainage from the stomach.

pylorus, (*pī-lor'-us*), region of the junction between the stomach and duodenum. A thickening of the circular muscle forms a sphincter which controls the rate at which chyme leaves the stomach.

pyocolpos, (*pī-o-kol'-pos*), pus retained in the vagina.

pyoderma, (*pī-ō-der-ma*), a skin condition associated with pus production.

pyogenic, (*pī-ō-jen'-ik*), producing or forming pus.

pyometra, (*pī-ō-mē'-tra*), pus retained in the uterus.

pyonephrosis, (*pī-ō-nef-rō'-sis*), pus in the kidney.

pyopericardium, (*pī-ō-per-i-kar'-di-um*), pus in the pericardium.

pyopneumothorax, (*pī-ō-nū'-mō-thor-aks*), pus and air in the pleural cavity.

pyorrhoea, a flow of pus. *P. alveolaris*: old term for periodontal disease characterized by pus formation.

pyosalpinx, (*pī-ō-sal-pinks*), pus in a uterine tube.

pyothorax, empyema. Pus in the pleural cavity.

pyramid, 1. a cone-shaped mass in the renal medulla. **2.** elevation on the medulla oblongata.

pyramidal, pyramid-shaped. *P. cells*: cells of the precentral motor cerebral cortex which stimulate voluntary muscles. Also called **Betz cells.** *P. tracts*: main motor pathways (tracts) in the brain and spinal cord carrying impulses from the p. cells. Most decussate in the medulla. *See* EXTRAPYRAMIDAL.

pyrexia, (*pī-rek-si-a*), fever. Elevation of the body temperature above normal. Usually applied to a temperature between 37.2 and 40–41°C, it may be intermittent or continuous. *P. of unknown origin (PUO)*: where no reason for the elevation in temperature is obvious. *See* HYPER-PYREXIA.

pyridoxine, (*pīr-i-dok-sēn*), vitamin B₆. A mixture of the phosphates of pyridoxine, pyridoxal and pyridoxamine, important as cofactors in amino acid and glycogen metabolism.

pyrimidines, *(pi-rim-id-ēnz),* nitrogenous bases such as cytosine, thymine and uracil required in the formation of nucleosides, nucleotides and nucleic acids.

pyrogen, *(pī-rŏ-jen),* a substance producing fever.

pyromania, *(pī-rŏ-mān-i-a),* strong impulses to start fires.

pyrosis, *(pī-rŏ-sis),* heartburn. Severe burning pain in the stomach.

pyrroles, substances forming part of the porphyrin which forms the organic portion of a haem molecule.

pyruvate, *(pī-rū-vāt),* salt of pyruvic acid.

pyruvic acid, *(pī-rū-vik),* an important product of glycolysis which is converted to acetyl coA which is utilized in the Krebs' cycle, or to lactic acid when glucose metabolism is anaerobic.

pyuria, *(pī-ū'-ri-a),* pus in the urine.

Q

QALYs, abbreviation for **quality-adjusted life years**. A method of evaluating healthcare outcomes by looking at quality of life, e.g. degree of dependence, pain, as well as life expectancy.

Q fever, caused by *Coxiella burnetii*, a rickettsia-like organism which is carried by cattle, sheep and many insects. Humans are infected by droplets or unpasteurized milk. It produces a fever, myalgia, headache and sweating; in some cases there is atypical pneumonia.

QRS complex, *see* PQRST COMPLEX.

quadriceps, *(kwod-ri-seps)*, having four heads. *Q. femoris*: large four-part extensor muscle of the anterior thigh (Figure 64).

quadriplegia, *(kwod-ri-plē-ji-a)*, paralysis of all four limbs. *See* TETRAPLEGIA.

quadrivalent, *(kwod-ri-va-lent)*, substance with a valence of four.

qualitative, relating to quality. *Q. research*: describes a research study based on observation and an interview to ascertain people's opinions, feelings or beliefs. *See* QUANTITATIVE.

quality assurance, systematic monitoring and evaluation of agreed levels of service provision which are followed by modifications in the light of the evaluation and/or audit. It has both clinical and management inputs, involves audit and usually applies to all aspects of a healthcare service. Some 'off the shelf' quality assurance tools such as Qualpacs

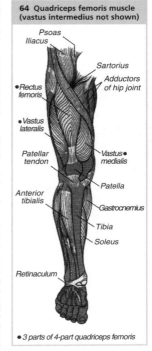

64 Quadriceps femoris muscle (vastus intermedius not shown)

Psoas
Iliacus
Sartorius
Adductors of hip joint
• Rectus femoris
• Vastus lateralis
Vastus • medialis
Patellar tendon
Patella
Anterior tibialis
Gastrocnemius
Tibia
Soleus
Retinaculum

• 3 parts of 4-part quadriceps femoris

and Monitor are available to assist staff. *See* AUDIT, BENCHMARKING, CLINICAL AUDIT, CLINICAL GOVERNANCE, PEER REVIEW, PERFORMANCE INDICATORS, QUALITY CIRCLES.

quality circles, group of staff who share a common interest and responsibility for care who meet on a regular basis to discuss quality issues as a means of improving standards of practice.

quality of life, the measure of the factors that allow individuals to cope successfully with every aspect of life and challenges encountered. Various scales are available; some are conceptual and others operational.

quantitative, relating to quantity. *Q. research*: describes a research study based on gained facts and statistics. *See* QUALITATIVE.

quarantine, the period of isolation required for infected or potentially infected people and animals, to prevent the spread of disease. For contacts it corresponds with the longest incubation period for the disease.

quartan, *(kwor-tan)*, recurring on the fourth day or every 72 hours. *Q. malaria*: a type caused by *Plasmodium malariae*, it is characterized by an intermittent fever occurring every 72 hours.

Queckenstedt's test, *(kwek-en-stetz)*, used to check the circulation of CSF. During a lumbar puncture, compression of the jugular veins will cause the fluid level in the manometer to rise. If there is some block to the free flow of CSF there will be little or no movement of the fluid level.

quickening, the first fetal movements felt by the mother. Usually around the 16th–18th week of gestation.

quiescent, *(kwē-es-sent)*, not active. Dormant.

quinism, *(kwin-izm)*, cinchonism. Toxic effects from overdose or prolonged use of quinine, including tinnitus, headache, nausea and visual disturbances.

quinsy, *(kwin'-zi)*, *see* PERITONSILLAR ABSCESS, TONSILLITIS.

quintan, *(kwin'-tan)*, recurring on the fifth day or every 96 hours.

quotient, result obtained by dividing one quantity by another. *See* ACHIEVEMENT QUOTIENT, INTELLIGENCE QUOTIENT, RESPIRATORY QUOTIENT.

R

rabid, having or pertaining to rabies.

rabies, hydrophobia. A viral disease of the central nervous system, transmitted to humans via the saliva of infected animals such as dogs, cats and foxes. It has a very variable incubation period and is characterized by severe muscle spasm, hydrophobia, hallucinations, delusions, paralysis and altered consciousness. Death usually occurs a week or so after the onset of symptoms. Vaccination is available for humans and susceptible animals.

race, often linked to ethnicity, but race only applies to biological features, e.g. skin colour, hair type, etc., that characterize a specific group.

racemose, *(ras'-e-mōs)*, resembling a bunch of grapes. *R. glands:* having the cells arranged in saccules with numerous ducts leading to a main duct, e.g. salivary glands.

rachitic, *(ra-kit'-ik)*, caused by or pertaining to rickets.

racism, a view of particular groups, based on race alone, that results in negative stereotyping, prejudice and discrimination. It may be overt or covert.

rad, old unit of absorbed dose of radiation, now replaced by the SI unit, the gray (Gy).

radial, in anatomy, relating to the radius. Describes the artery, pulse, vein and nerve.

radiation, emanation of radiant energy in the form of electromagnetic waves such as visible light, infrared, ultraviolet, X-rays and gamma rays. Subatomic particles such as electrons or neutrons may also be radiated. Radiation can be ionizing or non-ionizing and has numerous diagnostic and therapeutic uses. *R. sickness:* tissue damage from exposure to ionizing radiation results in diarrhoea, vomiting, anorexia and bone marrow failure. *See* IONIZING RADIATION.

radical, that which goes to the root; thus radical treatment aims to cure rather than palliate.

radiculography, *(rad-ik-ū-log-ra-fi)*, X-ray of the spinal nerve roots after rendering them radiopaque to locate the site and size of a prolapsed intervertebral disc.

radioactive, exhibiting radioactivity. Describes an unstable atomic nucleus which emits charged particles as it disintegrates. *See* ISOTOPE. *R. decay:* the spontaneous disintegration of radioactive atoms within a radioactive substance. *See* HALF-LIFE. *R. fallout:* release of radioactive particles into the atmosphere. Results from industrial processes or accidents and the testing or use of nuclear weapons.

radioactivity, the emission of radiant energy in the form of alpha, beta or gamma radiation from an element as it undergoes spontaneous disintegration.

radiobiology, science which studies the effects of radiation on living systems.

289

radiodermatitis, (rā-di-ō-der-ma-tī-tis), reddening of the skin occurring after exposure to ionizing radiation.

radiograph, a photographic image formed by exposure to X-rays.

radiographer, there are two types of radiographer, diagnostic and therapeutic. They are health professionals qualified in the use of ionizing radiation and other techniques, either in diagnostic imaging or radiotherapy.

radiography, the use of imaging techniques to create images of the body from which a medical diagnosis can be made (diagnostic radiography).

radioimmunoassay, (rā-di-ō-im-mū-nō-as-sā), a technique using radioactive substances to measure hormones, drugs and proteins in the blood.

radioisotope, (rā-di-ō-i-sō-tōp), an unstable isotope of an element that emits radioactivity. They may occur naturally or be produced artificially for various industrial and medical purposes. Also known as radionuclide.

radiologist, a doctor who has made a special study of radiology.

radiology, the science of radiation. Branch of medicine concerned with the use of radiation in diagnostic procedures.

radiolucent, substance which permits the passage of X-rays.

radionuclide, (rā-di-ō-nū-klīd), a radioisotope such as technetium (99m Tc). R. imaging/scanning: the use of radionuclides to scan and produce images of structures such as bone, liver, lung, thyroid and kidney. See GAMMA CAMERA, ISOTOPE, NUCLEAR MEDICINE.

radiopaque, (ra-di-ō-pāk), a substance which does not allow the passage of X-rays. Often used as contrast medium, e.g. barium sulphate.

radioresistance, (rā-di-ō-rē-zis'-tans), the ability of normal tissues and some tumours to withstand the effects of radiation.

radiosensitive, (rā-di-ō-sen-si-tiv), term applied to those normal tissues and tumours which are affected by radiation. In the case of tumours it can be enhanced by the use of radiosensitizing drugs.

radiotherapist, (rā-di-ō-ther-a-pist), a doctor specializing in radiotherapy. A radiation oncologist.

radiotherapy, (rā-di-ō-ther-a-pi), the treatment of proliferative disease, especially cancer, by X-rays and other forms of ionizing radiation.

radium (Ra), a radioactive element which results from the disintegration of uranium. It has a half-life of 1690 years and produces both alpha and gamma radiation. It has some uses in the treatment of malignant disease but has been largely replaced by other isotopes, e.g. caesium-137.

radius, the outer bone of the forearm, from the elbow to the wrist. See SKELETON.

radon, radioactive gas produced by the disintegration of radium.

raised intracranial pressure (RIP), a dangerous situation. Causes include: trauma, tumours, intracranial bleeding. The features depend on the cause, but may include: headache, vomiting, papilloedema, fits, bradycardia, arterial hypertension and altered consciousness.

râle, (rahl), an abnormal inspiratory sound heard on auscultation. It is a bubbling or gurgling associated with the presence of fluid in the airways or alveoli.

RAM, in computing an acronym for random access memory. That part of computer memory which holds data and programs whilst the CPU is working. Once the power supply is interrupted the RAM loses its contents.

Ramstedt's operation, pyloromyotomy. Operation to relieve congenital hypertrophic pyloric stenosis. The pyloric muscle layer is cut whilst leaving the mucosa intact. *See* PYLORIC STENOSIS.

ramus (*pl.* **rami**), **1.** a branch of a blood vessel or nerve. **2.** a thin projection from a bone.

random, completely by chance, aimless. *R. sampling*: selection process whereby every individual in the population has an equal chance of being selected.

randomized controlled trial (RCT), research using two or more randomly selected groups: experimental and control. Produces a high level of evidence for practice.

range, a measure of the span of values (lowest to highest) observed in a sample.

range of motion (ROM), the movements possible at a joint. *See* ACTIVE MOVEMENTS, PASSIVE MOVEMENTS.

ranula, cyst of mucous or salivary gland such as those under the tongue.

Ranvier nodes, *see* NODES.

rape, unlawful sexual intercourse without consent which is achieved by force or deception. Full penetration of the vagina (or other orifice) by the penis and ejaculation of semen are not necessary to constitute rape. Most rapes include force and violence, but acquiescence because of verbal threats should not be interpreted as consent. Incidents of rape are under-reported to the police because of the gruelling process of having to give evidence in court. If women are admitted to hospital, a police surgeon examines them and takes the necessary specimens in the presence of specially trained female police officers who then provide support throughout the interviews and subsequent investigation. Most police forces provide purpose-built facilities for dealing with the examination and interview of alleged rape victims. There are voluntary agencies to assist rape victims to regain confidence and rebuild their lives. Male rape, the rape of a man by another man, is increasingly recognized.

raphe, (*ra-fe*), a ridge, line, crease or seam forming a junction between two parts.

rapid eye movements (REM), rapid movements of the eyes associated with a stage of deep sleep with dreaming. REM sleep alternates with periods of non-rapid eye movement sleep (NREM).

rapport, a relationship of mutual understanding and respect between two people.

rarefaction, (*ra-re-fak'-shon*), the process of becoming less dense.

RAS, *see* RETICULAR ACTIVATING SYSTEM.

rat-bite fever, relapsing fever caused by the organisms *Spirillum minus* and *Streptobacillus moniliformis.* Usually transmitted by rat bites, they produce local inflammation, lymphadenitis and splenomegaly with rash and fever.

ratio data, measurement data with a numerical scale, e.g. height, that has an absolute zero. It is interval data with an absolute zero. *See* INTERVAL DATA.

rationalization, a justification of one's behaviour. A mental defence mechanism where the person seeks an acceptable explanation for a stressful or unacceptable event.

ray, a beam of radiant energy such as light moving from its source. *R.*

fungus: Actinomyces israeli. See ACTIN-OMYCOSIS.

Raynaud's disease/phenomenon, *(rā-nōz),* spasm of the digital arteries in response to cold, vibration, emotion and arterial disease. It produces numbness, colour changes in the digits with sensitivity to cold. Eventually it may lead to ischaemic changes, necrosis and gangrene.

RBC, abbreviation for **red blood cell**.

RCT, abbreviation for **randomized controlled trial**.

reaction, 1. response to a stimulus. **2.** chemical changes resulting in the formation of new molecules. *R. formation:* mental defence mechanism where the person exhibits behaviour which is opposite to stressful emotions, drives and impulses which are repressed.

reactive, 1. responding well to stimuli. **2.** in psychiatry a mental health problem which occurs in response to an outside event, e.g. depression associated with a bereavement.

reagent, an agent taking part in a reaction.

reality, real, existing, *R. orientation:* techniques used to help people regain or maintain awareness of person, place and time.

reasonable doubt, to secure a conviction in criminal proceedings, the prosecution must establish beyond reasonable doubt the guilt of the accused.

recalcitrant, resistant, especially of a disease to its treatment.

recall, bringing back a memory.

receptaculum chyli, *(re-sep-tak´-ū-lum ki-lē),* the lower expanded portion of the thoracic duct. The cisterna chyli.

receptor, 1. a sensory nerve ending. **2.** a protein molecule present on or in the cell membrane that reacts with hormones, other chemical mediators, or a specific antigen. Certain drugs work by combining with cell receptors.

recessive, tending to disappear. *R. gene:* a gene which produces its characteristic only if inherited from both parents, only in the homozygous state. The exception is for X-linked genes in males, in which the single recessive allele on the X chromosome will express itself so that the character is manifest. *Cf.* DOMINANT GENE.

recipient, individual receiving a blood transfusion or organ transplant.

Recklinghausen's disease, *(rek´-ling-how-sen), see* VON RECKLINGHAUSEN'S DISEASE.

recombinant DNA technology, genetic engineering. Fragments of DNA from one individual or species are introduced into the DNA molecule of another individual or species where they become part of their genetic makeup. There have been numerous applications, such as the production of human insulin by microorganisms, and there is research being done on the production of organs which can be transplanted from one species to another without the problems of rejection.

Recommended International Non-proprietiary Name (rINN), a new system by which drugs will have a recommended non-proprietary name that is used internationally.

recovery position, a first aid measure where an unconscious casualty is placed in such a position as to maintain the airway and prevent the aspiration of vomit and secretions.

recrudescence, *(re-krū-des-sens),* return of symptoms.

rectal, pertaining to the rectum. *R. examination:* digital examination of the rectum. *R. reflex:* defecation reflex. Urge to defecate as the rectum fills with faeces.

rectocele, *(rek'-tō-sēl),* prolapse of posterior vaginal wall. Strictly the term applies to any herniation of the rectum.

rectoperineorrhaphy, *(rek-tō-per-i-ne-or-a-fi),* operation to repair the rectal wall and perineum.

rectopexy, *(rek-tō-pek'-si),* surgical procedure to fix a prolapsed rectum.

rectoscope, *(rek'-tō-skōp),* proctoscope.

rectosigmoidectomy, *(rek-tō-sig-moy-dek'-to-mi),* operation to excise the rectum and the sigmoid colon.

rectouterine, *(rek-tō-ū-ter-īn),* pertaining to the rectum and uterus. *R. pouch:* see DOUGLAS' POUCH.

rectovaginal, *(rek-tō-va-jīn-al),* pertaining to the rectum and vagina. *R. fistula:* see FISTULA.

rectovesical, *(rek-tō-ves-ik-al),* pertaining to the rectum and bladder. *R. fistula:* abnormal opening between the rectum and bladder. *R. pouch:* peritoneal pouch between the rectum and bladder in the male.

rectum, lower part of the large bowel from the sigmoid colon to the anal canal. *See* BOWEL.

rectus, straight. Applied to various muscles. *R. abdominis:* two external abdominal muscles. *R. muscles of the eyeball:* four extrinsic muscles of the eyeball – lateral, medial, inferior and superior. *R. femoris:* part of the quadriceps muscle.

recumbent, lying down.

recuperate, to get better.

recurrent, returning after an interval. *R. laryngeal nerve:* supplies the vocal cords. May be damaged by tumour or during thyroid surgery, causing voice changes.

red blood cell (RBC), *see* BILE, BLOOD, BLOOD COUNT, ERYTHROCYTE, HAEMOGLOBIN.

reduction, 1. to replace in the normal position, e.g. after fracture, dislocation and hernia. 2. the division

occurring during meiosis when gametes are produced. 3. the removal of oxygen or the addition of hydrogen or electrons to a substance.

reference nutrient intake (RNI), the amount of protein, a vitamin or mineral which should be sufficient for around 97% of people within a population.

referred pain, pain felt at a point distant from the position of the affected part, e.g. pain from heart disease felt in the left arm.

reflective practice, where a health professional such as a nurse reflects upon an individual aspect of practice and evaluates the outcomes within the framework of available nursing theories so that practice and the practitioner can be developed and improved. This process may concentrate on an area of practice, perhaps ritualistic, or there may be analysis of a critical incident.

reflex, reflected. An instantaneous involuntary physiological response to a stimulus, which operates through a simple nerve pathway. Reflexes are postural or protective and include: tendon stretch, accommodation, corneal, plantar, abdominal, cough and swallowing. Various primitive reflexes are present in newborns and are used to assess their development, e.g. Moro, stepping, grasp and rooting. Reflexes may be inborn or conditioned (where a reflex develops by association with a repeated stimulus). *R. arc:* the sensory, connector and motor neurones through which some reflexes operate (Figure 65).

reflexology, *(rē-fleks-ol-o-ji),* a complementary therapy where the feet and/or hands are massaged. Each area of the foot and hands is thought

65 Reflex arc

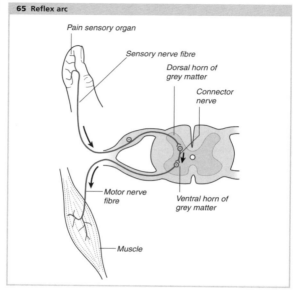

Pain sensory organ

Sensory nerve fibre

Dorsal horn of grey matter

Connector nerve

Motor nerve fibre

Ventral horn of grey matter

Muscle

to correspond to a specific part of the body.

reflux, flowing back. *Gastro-oesophageal r.*: where acid gastric contents flow into the oesophagus. *Vesicoureteric r.*: urine from the bladder flows back into the ureters, eventually causing kidney damage.

refraction, the bending of light waves as they pass from one medium to another. In the normal eye this occurs so that the image is focused on the retina.

refractory, stubborn; not amenable to treatment. *R. period*: the time during

which a nerve or muscle fibre is unable to respond to a stimulus. This may be relative where it can be overcome if the stimulus is sufficiently strong, or absolute when no response is possible.

regeneration, renewal of damaged tissue.

regimen, a prescribed course of treatment such as diet, drugs or exercise.

region, an anatomical term used to describe a specific area of the body, e.g. abdominal region.

Regional Cancer Centres, in the UK. Regional centres with facilities to support the site-specific treatment of common and rarer cancers.

regional ileitis, *(ĭ-lē-ī-tis), see* CROHN'S DISEASE.

registration, 1. the legal requirement officially to record all births, marriages and deaths. **2.** the process by which a list of qualified professionals such as nurses, midwives and health visitors is held and maintained by the United Kingdom Central Council (UKCC)/Nursing and Midwifery Council (NMC).

regression, 1. reverting to a more primitive state. **2.** in psychology, reverting to an earlier stage of development such as may occur in illness. **3.** when a disease process abates, such as a tumour decreasing in size. **4.** a tendency for genetically determined characteristics to move towards the norm for a population.

regression techniques, several analytical techniques used in multivariate statistics. Used to predict dependent variable(s) from independent variable(s).

regurgitation, *(re-ger-ji-tā-shon),* flowing back, e.g. food from the stomach into the mouth, or the back flow of blood through a defective heart valve.

rehabilitation, a planned programme in which the convalescent or disabled person progresses towards, or maintains, the maximum degree of physical and psychological independence of which he or she is capable.

rehydrate, to correct dehydration by the administration of oral or intravenous fluids.

reinforcement, in psychology the techniques used to enhance and strengthen a desired response, e.g. positive r. with a reward.

Reiter's complement fixation test, *(rī-terz),* a serological test previously used for syphilis.

Reiter's syndrome, *(rī-terz),* a syndrome characterized by arthritis, conjunctivitis and non-specific urethritis. It may follow exposure to a sexually transmitted infection or bacterial dysentery.

rejection, 1. immunological processes occurring in the recipient which destroy transplanted tissue. **2.** the act of excluding or denying affection to another person.

relapse, a deterioration in condition following an apparent improvement or recovery.

relapsing fever, a group of diseases caused by spirochaetes of the genus *Borrelia*: the organisms are tick- or louse-borne. Endemic in many areas of the world.

relaxant, any agent, drug or technique which leads to relaxation.

relaxation, a state of altered consciousness characterized by the release of muscle tension, anxiety and stress.

relaxin, hormone produced by the placenta which has a softening effect upon the cervix and pelvic tissues prior to labour.

releaser/releasing mechanism, describes a stimulus that initiates a cycle of instinctive behaviour.

releasing factor/hormone, substances produced by the hypothalamus that stimulate the secretion of anterior pituitary hormones.

reliability, in research consistency of results. The likelihood of producing the same findings using the same research conditions over a period of time or with different researchers.

REM, *see* RAPID EYE MOVEMENTS.

reminiscence therapy, a stimulation therapy used with older adults and others which involves their recall of important events assisted by articles, music, video, film and photographs etc. from that era. Sometimes

295

used as part of a reality orientation programme.

remission, period when a disease subsides and shows no symptoms.

remittent, returning at regular intervals, e.g. certain fevers.

renal, *(rē-nal),* relating to the kidney. *R. calculus:* kidney stone. *R. colic:* intense pain caused by the movement of a stone within the kidney or ureter. *R. cortex:* pale outer region of the kidney under the capsule. *R. erythropoietic factor (REF):* a substance released by the kidneys in response to renal hypoxia. It acts upon a plasma protein to form active erythropoietin prior to its release. *R. failure:* acute or chronic insufficiency of renal function for a variety of reasons. Treatment options include renal replacement therapy, such as dialysis and transplant. *See* HAEMODIALYSIS, PERITONEAL DIALYSIS. *R. function tests:* a variety of tests that include: routine urine testing, urine concentration/dilution tests, serum urea and electrolytes, serum creatinine and renal clearance. *R. medulla:* darker inner region of the kidney containing the renal pyramids. *R. threshold:* the level of a substance in the blood at which it is excreted in the urine, e.g. glucose. *R. transplant:* replacement of diseased kidneys with a single well-matched donor organ (living donor or cadaveric).

renin, *(rē-nin),* enzyme produced by the juxtaglomerular apparatus of the kidney in response to low serum sodium levels or low blood pressure. It initiates the angiotensin–aldosterone response causing increased reabsorption of sodium and water in the renal tubules and an increase in blood pressure. *See* JUXTAGLOMERULAR.

rennin, *(ren-in),* a milk-curdling enzyme present in the gastric juice.

reovirus, *(rē-ō-vī-rus),* a family of RNA viruses that includes the rotavirus which causes gastroenteritis.

repetitive strain injury (RSI), work-related upper limb disorder. The definition of this condition is controversial. It usually refers to pain and discomfort in the upper limbs as a result of repetitive movements or constrained posture. It encompasses a variety of symptoms, including tenderness, tingling and numbness, swelling, etc. Some clinicians include similar signs and symptoms in lower limbs.

replication, the duplication of genetic material during nuclear division.

repolarization, the stage of the action potential during which the membrane potential returns from the depolarized state to its polarized resting (negative) state.

repression, a mental defence mechanism where painful thoughts and memories are pushed back into the unconscious mind. The individual is unable consciously to recognize or accept these disturbing ideas.

reproduction, the processes by which organisms produce offspring.

reproductive, pertaining to reproduction. *R. system:* the male or female organs of reproduction, e.g. gonads (Figure 66).

research, systematic investigation of data, reports and observations to establish facts or principles. Research may be divided into two main types: qualitative or quantitative. Its stages may include: defining the problem, literature review, developing a hypothesis, preparing a research proposal, obtaining permission and considering ethical issues, designing the research,

66 Reproductive system (a) male (b) female

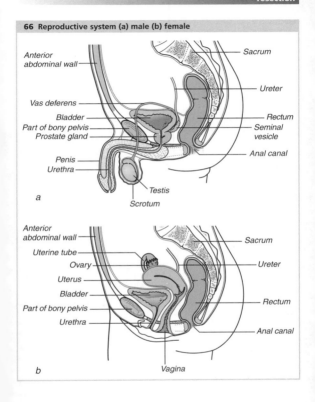

a

Anterior abdominal wall
Vas deferens
Bladder
Part of bony pelvis
Prostate gland
Penis
Urethra
Testis
Scrotum
Sacrum
Ureter
Rectum
Seminal vesicle
Anal canal

b

Anterior abdominal wall
Uterine tube
Ovary
Uterus
Bladder
Part of bony pelvis
Urethra
Vagina
Sacrum
Ureter
Rectum
Anal canal

and deciding on methods, collecting data, analysis and interpretation of data, conclusions and recommendations and dissemination of the results.

research methods, the varied methods used to collect data in a research study, e.g. survey.

resection, complete surgical removal of a part.

resectoscope, (rē-sek-to-skōp), instrument to view and remove pieces of tissue in transurethral prostatectomy.

reserve, used to describe something put by for later use. *Alkaline r.:* see ALKALI RESERVE. *Cardiac r.:* the ability of the heart to increase cardiac output during exercise.

residual, remaining. *R. urine:* the urine which remains in the bladder after apparent emptying has occurred. *R. volume:* amount of air left in the lungs after a maximal expiratory effort.

resistance, the degree of opposition to an action. See DRUG RESISTANCE, PERIPHERAL RESISTANCE.

resolution, 1. a resolve. **2.** return to normal with a regression of the inflammatory process.

resonance, increase of sound by reverberation, applied to voice sounds in auscultation.

resorption, absorption of secreted matter, e.g. callus following bone fracture.

respiration, the process which supplies atmospheric oxygen to the tissues for cellular metabolism and removes waste carbon dioxide. It consists of: 1. ventilation which involves inspiration and expiration. 2. external r.: gaseous exchange between alveolar air and pulmonary capillary blood. 3. internal r.: gaseous exchange between the blood and cells (via the tissue fluid). See ARTIFICIAL RESPIRATION, CHEYNE-STOKES BREATHING, KUSSMAUL RESPIRATION.

respirator, 1. appliance worn over the mouth and nose to prevent the inhalation of toxic substances. **2.** device used to maintain adequate respiration when the normal mechanisms are impaired. It may work on the principle of positive or negative pressure.

respiratory, pertaining to respiration. *R. acidosis:* a rise in arterial P_{CO_2} caused by hypoventilation associated with respiratory failure. *R. alkalosis:* a fall in arterial P_{CO_2} such as may be caused by the hyperventilation of severe anxiety. *R. centres:* specialized centres in the medulla and pons which control the rate, depth and rhythm of breathing. They receive inputs from chemoreceptors (which respond to carbon dioxide, pH and oxygen levels of the blood), stretch receptors, higher centres and the hypothalamus. See APNEUSTIC CENTRE, PNEUMOTAXIC CENTRE. *R. distress syndrome:* See PNEUMOCYTE, ACUTE RESPIRATORY DISTRESS SYNDROME, MULTIPLE ORGAN DYSFUNCTION SYNDROME, NEONATAL RESPIRATORY DISTRESS SYNDROME, SURFACTANT. *R. failure:* a situation where the respiratory efforts are insufficient to maintain the blood gases and pH at acceptable levels. It may be classified as either type I, where there is hypoxia, or type II (asphyxia), which is characterized by both hypoxia and hypercapnia. *R. function tests:* also known as lung or pulmonary function tests. They include: measuring lung volumes and capacities, e.g. vital capacity and peak expiratory flow. Other tests used include gas transfer tests and exercise tolerance tests. See ARTERIAL BLOOD GASES, PULSE OXIMETRY. *R. quotient:* the ratio between the volume of carbon dioxide given off to the volume of oxygen absorbed by the alveoli per unit of time. *R. syncytial virus (RSV):* responsible for bronchiolitis and pneumonia in infants and small children. *R. tract:* the organs and structures involved with breathing.

respite care, short-term or temporary care provided within a health or social care facility to allow relief for family and other home carers. May be provided on a daily or residential basis.

restitution, a movement to the right or left of the fetal head as it passes out of the birth canal.

restrictive respiratory disease, one characterized by a limited ability to expand the lungs or chest such as with the presence of fibrosis.

resuscitation, (re-sus-si-tā-shon), measures taken to maintain vital body functions. See ADVANCED LIFE SUPPORT, BASIC LIFE SUPPORT, CARDIOPULMONARY RESUSCITATION.

retardation, a slowing down of activity; backwardness.

retching, ineffectual efforts to vomit.

retention, a holding back. *Urinary r.*: an inability to void urine, e.g. with an enlarged prostate gland.

reticular, (re-tik´-ū-la), resembling a network. Applied to tissues. *R. activating system (RAS)*: functional area in the brain stem concerned with the state of cortical arousal, level of consciousness and the modification of sensory inputs to prevent sensory overload.

reticulocyte, (re-tik-ū-lō-sīt), an immature red cell forming up to 2% of those circulating in the blood.

reticulocytosis, (re-tik-ū-lō-sī-tō-sis), an increase in the number of reticulocytes in the blood which represents an overactivity of the marrow such as in severe anaemia.

reticuloendothelial system, (re-tik-ū-lō-en-dōthē-lē-al), see MONOCYTE–MACROPHAGE SYSTEM.

reticulum, (re-tik-ū-lum), a network of fibres.

retina, (ret-i-na), the inner coat of the eye. It is a multiple-layer complex of pigment cells, rods and cones (photoreceptors) and other neurones. The photoreceptors receive the light entering the eye and convert it chemically to nerve impulses which leave the eye via the optic nerve. *Detached r.*: a condition where the layers of the retina become torn. Lasers are often used to repair the tear before vision is permanently impaired. See EYE.

retinal, (ret-i-nal), pertaining to the retina.

retinene, (ret-in-een), see RETINOL.

retinitis, (ret-in-ī-tis), inflammation of the retina. *R. pigmentosa*: an inherited condition where there are degenerative changes in the retina resulting in night blindness, tunnel vision and blindness. The term retinopathy is becoming more widely used.

retinoblastoma, (re-ti-nō-bla-stō´-ma), tumour arising from germ cells in the retina.

retinol, (ret-in-ol), vitamin A. Required by the body for the functioning of the retina and epithelial cells. Essential for the formation of rhodopsin (visual pigment) needed for night vision. Also called retinene.

retinopathy, (ret-in-op´-a-thi), any non-inflammatory pathology affecting the retina, e.g. diabetic r., hypertensive r.

retinoscopy, (ret-in-os-ko-pi), an examination to determine the refractive errors of the eye.

retractile, (re-trak-til), that which can be drawn back.

retraction, shortening, drawing backward, such as the permanent shortening of the uterine muscle fibres during labour. *R. ring or Bandl's ring*: an abnormal area felt between the upper and lower uterine segments when labour is obstructed.

retractor, an instrument or muscle that retracts.

retrieval, to recover or restore such as with data.

retrobulbar, (ret-rō-bul'-ba), behind or at the back of the eyeball. *R. neuritis*: inflammation of the optic nerve.

retrocaecal, (ret-rō-sē'-kal), behind the caecum.

retroflexion, (ret-rō-flek-shon), a bending back, especially of the uterus which is bent back at the acute angle.

retrograde, going backwards. *R. amnesia*: memory loss which involves events prior to an illness or injury. *R. ejaculation*: discharge of semen into the urinary bladder. *R. urography/pyelography*: see UROGRAPHY.

retrogression, moving backwards.

retrolental, (ret-rō-len-tal), behind the lens of the eye. *R. fibroplasia*: fibrosis of the tissues behind the lens which leads to visual impairment. Associated with the administration of high-concentration oxygen to preterm or low-birth-weight infants.

retro-ocular, (ret-rō-ok-ū-lar), posterior to the eye.

retroperitoneal, (ret-rō-per-i-to-nē-al), behind the posterior layer of the peritoneum, e.g. kidneys and adrenal glands. *R. fibrosis*: fibrous tissue developing behind the peritoneum. May occur as a side-effect of some drugs.

retropharyngeal, (ret-rō-far-in-jē-al), behind the pharynx. *R. abscess*: collection of pus between the pharynx and the cervical vertebrae.

retropubic, (ret-rō-pū-bik), behind the pubis. *R. prostatectomy*: see PROSTATECTOMY.

retrospection, looking back into the past.

retrospective, relating to a past event. *R. audit*: a type of nursing audit where the nursing records are examined and the outcomes assessed after the care has been completed or the person discharged. *R. study*: research that collects data from the past, moving backwards in time. *See* PROSPECTIVE STUDY.

retrosternal, behind the sternum.

retroversion, (ret-rō-ver-shon), a turning backwards. *R. of uterus*: a backward displacement of the uterus. During pregnancy it may prevent the uterus from rising out of the pelvis.

retrovirus, (ret-rō-vī-rus), a group of RNA viruses that include the human immunodeficiency viruses (HIV-1 and 2) and the human T-cell lymphotrophic viruses (HTLV-1 and 2).

Rett's syndrome, a very rare genetic defect caused by a sporadic mutation of a gene on the X chromosome. It is almost always seen in girls and is characterized by normal development during the first year, followed by gradual deterioration in motor and intellectual ability. Affected children have severe learning and physical disability, and are prone to epilepsy and abnormal breathing patterns, breath-holding and hyperventilation.

reverse barrier nursing, see BARRIER NURSING, PROTECTIVE ISOLATION.

Reye's syndrome, (rāz), a rare condition characterized by encephalopathy and cerebral oedema with acute fatty degeneration of the liver occurring in children after a viral infection. Associated with the administration of salicylates in some cases, which has led to the recommendation that children under the age of 12 should not receive products containing aspirin.

rhabdomyoma, (rab-dō-mī-ō-ma), a benign tumour of voluntary and cardiac muscle.

rhabdomyosarcoma, (rab-dō-mī-ō-sar-kō-ma), a malignant tumour occurring in voluntary muscle, genitourinary tract and other tissues.

rhabdovirus, (*rab-dō-vī-rus*), a family of RNA viruses that include the rabies virus.

rhagades, (*rag-ad-ez*), a crack or fissure in the skin, especially those radiating from the angle of the mouth.

rhesus factor (Rh), (*rē-sus*), see ANTI D, BLOOD GROUPS.

rheumatic, (*rū-mat-ik*), pertaining to rheumatism. *R. fever*: an acute inflammatory process of connective tissue which affects joints, serous membranes, skin and the heart. It occurs mainly in children and may follow a throat infection with a beta-haemolytic streptococcus (Lancefield group A). It is characterized by migratory polyarthritis with swelling and pain, fever, tachycardia, rash and pancarditis of varying severity. It may have neurological manifestations. *See* CHOREA. *R. heart disease*: chronic cardiac disease with valvular damage resulting from rheumatic fever.

rheumatism, (*rū-ma-tizm*), a general non-specific term for the ill-defined aches and pains affecting the musculoskeletal system.

rheumatoid, (*rū-ma-toyd*), similar to rheumatism. *R. arthritis*: an inflammatory condition of connective tissue characterized by progressive joint destruction with pain, swelling, deformity and eventual loss of function. Its systemic effects include: general ill health, damage to heart valves, aortitis, anaemia and lung changes. There is a genetic predisposition to the condition which has an autoimmune aetiology. *See* JUVENILE CHRONIC ARTHRITIS, STILL'S DISEASE.

rheumatologist, (*rū-mat-ol-o-jist*), a doctor who specializes in the management of rheumatic conditions.

rheumatology, (*rū-mat-ol-o-ji*), study of rheumatic diseases.

rhinitis, (*rī-nī-tis*), inflammation of the nasal mucosa. The cause may be: allergic, infective, atrophic or vasomotor.

rhinopathy, (*rī-nop-ath-i*), a disease of the nose.

rhinoplasty, (*rī-nō-plas-ti*), plastic surgery on the nose, involving partial repair or the formation of a new nose.

rhinorrhoea, (*rī-no-rē'-a*), discharge of mucus, blood-stained fluid, pus or cerebrospinal fluid from the nose.

rhinoscope, (*rī'-no-skōp*), instrument used to examine the inside of the nasal passages. *See* NASENDOSCOPE.

rhinoscopy, (*rī'-nos-ko-pi*), examination of the nasal passages.

rhinotomy, (*rī'-not-o-mi*), operation of cutting into the nose.

rhinovirus, (*rī-nō-vī-rus*), a group of picornaviruses which cause the common cold.

rhizotomy, (*rī-zot-o-mi*), division of spinal nerve roots.

rhodopsin, (*ro-dop-sin*), visual purple. Light-sensitive pigment protein found in the rods of the retina. It is derived from vitamin A (retinol).

rhombencephalon, (*romb-en-kef-al-on*), the hindbrain. The part of the brain containing the metencephalon and myelencephalon.

rhonchus, (*rong'-kus*), a rattling bronchial sound heard on auscultation.

rhythm, movement or other feature following a definite pattern, e.g. the electrical activity of the brain or heart. *R. method*: natural family planning where knowledge of fertile times is used to avoid conception or plan a pregnancy. Ovulation timing is determined by menstrual calendar, temperature or cervical mucus.

See BIORHYTHMS, CIRCADIAN RHYTHMS, DIURNAL RHYTHMS.

rib, one of the twelve pairs of curved bones which form part of the thorax, they are all joined to the vertebra. *True r.*: the first seven pairs which are joined to the sternum by separate cartilages. *False r.*: the lower five pairs, of which the first three pairs are joined to the sternum by a common cartilage; the two bottom pairs are not attached to the sternum and are known as the floating ribs.

riboflavin, (*rī-bō-flā-vin*), part of the vitamin B complex. Required by the body for the formation of coenzymes (flavoproteins), important in all oxidative processes.

ribonuclease, (*rī-bō-nū-kle-āz*), enzyme which degrades RNA.

ribonucleic acid (RNA), (*rī-bō-nū-klā-ik*), a nucleic acid found in the nucleus, cytoplasm and the ribosomes. There are three types – messenger (mRNA), transfer (tRNA) and ribosomal (rRNA), which perform specific roles during protein synthesis. *See* TRANSCRIPTION, TRANSLATION.

ribose, a pentose sugar found as a constituent of nucleic acids.

ribosome, (*rī-bō-sōm*), cellular organelles either free in the cytoplasm or associated with rough endoplasmic reticulum. The site of protein synthesis.

RICE, acronym for rest, ice, compression and elevation. Treatment for strains and sprains.

rice-water stools, the watery stools which occur in cholera.

rickets, disease due to a lack of vitamin D during childhood which results from a low dietary intake or insufficient exposure to sunlight. This leads to abnormal calcium and phosphate metabolism with faulty ossification and poor bone growth. It is characterized by features which

include: muscle weakness, anaemia, respiratory infections, bone tenderness and pain and hypocalcaemia. There is delay in: motor development such as walking, eruption of teeth and closure of the fontanelles. Later there may be bony deformities such as skull bossing and bow legs. *Adult r.: see* OSTEOMALACIA.

Rickettsiae, (*ri-ket-sē-a*), a group of microorganisms having features of both bacteria and viruses; they cause diseases such as typhus and the spotted fevers. They are parasitic in ticks, fleas, lice and mites; transmission to humans is by bites from these arthropods.

rights, the recognition in law that certain inalienable rights, such as the right to life, should be respected, e.g. Human Rights Act 1998.

rigidity, a feature of conditions such as parkinsonism where there is resistance to the passive movement of a limb.

rigor, (*ri-gor*), an attack of shivering occurring when the heat-regulating centre malfunctions. This causes a rapid increase in body temperature which may remain elevated or fall as profuse sweating takes place. *R. mortis*: contraction of the muscle fibres due to chemical changes occurring after death. Causes stiffness of the body which lasts for a variable period.

rima, (*rī'-ma*), a fissure; thus *r. glottidis*: slit between vocal cords.

Ringer's solution, an isotonic intravenous solution containing sodium chloride with potassium and calcium salts. *Lactated R. s.*: one which contains lactate.

ringworm, tinea or dermatophytosis. A fungal disease affecting the skin, hair or nails.

Rinne's test, (*rin-nes*), a test which differentiates between conductive and sensorineural (perceptive) hearing loss. A tuning fork is used to test the conduction of sound through air and bone.

RIP, acronym for raised intracranial pressure.

risk, a potential hazard. *attributable r*: describes the disease rate in people exposed to the risk factor minus the occurrence in unexposed people. *relative r*: the ratio of disease rate in exposed people to those who have not been exposed. It is related to the odds ratio, which is the odds (as in betting) of disease occurring in an exposed person divided by the odds of the disease occurring in an unexposed person. *R. factor*: any factor which causes a person or group of people to be more vulnerable to disease, injury or complications. They include behavioural factors, e.g. smoking, lack of exercise, and social factors such as job control or environmental factors such as pollution. *R. management*: the responsibility of healthcare professionals to identify, assess and minimize the potential hazards inherent in a given situation.

risus sardonicus, *(rē-sus sar-don-i-kus)*, abnormal grin produced by prolonged facial muscle contraction, seen in tetanus.

rite of passage, a ceremony or event which marks a specific age or life event of some importance, such as reaching puberty.

ritual, an action which is performed or follows a set pattern without good reason, such as may be seen in some mental health problems.

river blindness, *see* ONCHOCERCIASIS.

RNA, *see* RIBONUCLEIC ACID.

RNI, abbreviation for **reference nutrient intake**.

Rocky Mountain spotted fever, a disease seen in the United States, caused by the organism *Rickettsia rickettsii* which is transmitted to humans by ticks.

rodent ulcer, a basal cell carcinoma of the skin. It occurs on exposed parts, especially those of the face, nose, eyelid, and cheek.

rods, photoreceptors in the retina which contain rhodopsin. They are responsible for vision in low-intensity light.

Rogerian counselling, humanistic client-centred approach to counselling and psychotherapy, introduced by Carl Rogers in the 1950s.

role, a specific pattern of behaviour expected of a person in a particular social situation such as the role of the nurse vis-à-vis that of the doctor. *R. conflict*: where a person is faced with a role which he or she perceives to have contradictory elements or expected patterns of behaviour. *R. model*: a person who acts as a model for another person's behaviour in a particular role. This is important for both childhood and professional development. *See* MENTOR. *R. play*: a technique used in education and in psychotherapy where people act out roles to experience the feelings of others, develop interpersonal skills, or to resolve conflicts.

ROM, in computing an acronym for read-only memory. That part of a computer's memory which stores the fixed contents installed at manufacture. It can be read by the CPU but not altered in any way. The information remains even after the power supply is switched off.

Romberg's sign, an inability to stand erect (without swaying) when the eyes are closed and the feet are together.

rooting reflex, primitive reflex seen in newborns – when the cheek is touched the infant will turn his or her head to that side.

rosacea, *(rō-zā'-se-a),* chronic disorder of the skin of the face with flushing and acne.

roseola, *(rō-zē-ō'-la),* a rose-coloured rash.

rotation, turning or twisting. Applied to the movements of the fetal head as it passes through the curvatures of the birth canal. *External* and *internal r.:* movements of a limb as its anterior surface moves outwards or inwards.

rotators, muscles which cause circular movement.

rotavirus, *(rō-ta-vī-rus),* a virus causing gastroenteritis in infants and children. Belongs to the reovirus group.

roughage, *see* FIBRE.

rouleau, *(rū-lō),* structure formed when several red blood cells become piled upon each other.

round ligaments, fibrous uterine supports which run from each uterine cornu through the inguinal canal to the labium majora.

roundworm, *see* ASCARIS.

Rovsing's sign, in acute appendicitis, pressure in the left iliac fossa will cause pain in the right iliac fossa.

rubefacients, *(rū-be-fā'-sē-ents),* mild irritants which cause reddening of the skin.

rubella, *(rū-bel-la),* German measles. A mild infectious disease caused by a virus which is spread by droplets. The incubation period is around 18 days. It is characterized by mild

fever, headache, cold-like symptoms, lymph node enlargement and a rash. If infection occurs in the first trimester of pregnancy there is a risk of fetal abnormalities which include: heart defects, cataract, impaired hearing and brain damage. Immunization is available as part of the routine programme in conjunction with protection against measles and mumps (MMR) during the second year of life, and subsequently to those individuals who did not receive MMR or any non-pregnant woman of childbearing age with insufficient immunity.

rubor, redness.

rugae, *(rū-je),* creases or folds such as those found in the mucosa of the stomach or vagina.

rugose, *(rū'-jōs),* wrinkled.

rule of nines, *see* WALLACE'S RULE OF NINES.

rumination, *(rū-min-ā-shon),* **1.** a feature of some obsessional neuroses where the person is preoccupied with the same idea or thought. **2.** the habit of regurgitating small amounts of food which are reswallowed.

rupture, popular term for a hernia. Bursting or tearing such as an ectopic (tubal) pregnancy, an aneurysm or the membranes during labour.

Russell traction, *see* TRACTION.

Ryle's tube, a narrow-bore plastic nasogastric tube used to aspirate stomach contents and occasionally for feeding.

S

Sabin vaccine, a type of live oral poliomyelitis vaccine.

sac, small pouch such as the conjunctival sac.

saccharide, *(sa-ka-rīd),* a series of carbohydrates. *See* MONOSACCHARIDE, DISACCHARIDE, POLYSACCHARIDE.

sacculated, *(sak'-ū-lā-ted),* having many small sacs.

saccule, *(sa-kū-l),* a fluid-filled membranous sac in the internal ear. Part of the vestibular apparatus concerned with static equilibrium, it responds to head position relative to gravity and to linear changes in speed and direction.

sacral, *(sā-kral),* relating to the sacrum.

sacroanterior, sacrolateral, sacroposterior, positions of breech presentation.

sacrococcygeal, *(sā-krō-kok-si-jē-al),* relating to the sacrum and coccyx.

sacroiliac, *(sā-krō-i-lē-ak),* relating to the sacrum and ilium or the joint between the two bones.

sacroilitis, *(sā-krō-i-lē-i-tis),* inflammation occurring in the sacroiliac joint.

sacrum, *(sā'-krum),* a triangular bone, consisting of five fused vertebrae, which forms the posterior part of the pelvis.

saddle joint, a type of synovial joint, e.g. the base of the thumb, where two bones with both concave and convex surfaces fit together. Movement in two planes is possible.

saddle nose, flattened bridge. Seen in congenital syphilis.

sadism, where pleasure is derived from inflicting cruelty, pain or humiliation upon another person, especially a sexual partner.

safe-handling or no-lifting policies, policies that provide risk assessment, staff training with regular updates, and equipment that includes: hoists, slings, sliding devices, transfer boards, belts, etc.

sagittal, *(saj'-it-tal),* in the median plane. *S. section:* section made by cutting through a specimen from top to bottom so that there are equal right and left halves. *S. suture:* the suture between parietal bones.

salicylates, *(sal-i-si-lāts),* salts of salicylic acid, e.g. aspirin. They have analgesic, anti-inflammatory and antipyretic properties.

salicylic acid, *(sal-i-si-lik),* used as a topical application in various hyperkeratotic dermatological conditions, e.g. psoriasis. Also used to remove corns and warts.

saline, containing sodium chloride. *Physiological s.:* a 0.9% solution which is isotonic with blood.

saliva, secretion from the salivary glands containing water, mucus and salivary amylase.

salivary, *(sal-i-va-ri),* pertaining to saliva. *S. glands:* three pairs of glands, parotid, sublingual and submandibular (Figure 67).

salivation, increased production of saliva.

Salk vaccine, an inactivated vaccine used to confer immunity against

67 Salivary glands

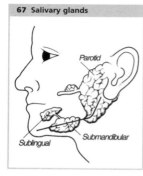

poliomyelitis in certain individuals. It is given by subcutaneous injection.

Salmonella, a genus of Gram-negative bacteria containing many hundreds of serotypes. The causative organism in the enteric fevers and in many cases of food poisoning.

salmonellosis, *(sal-mon-el-ō-sis)*, infection with salmonella.

salpingectomy, *(sal-pin-jek'-to-mi)*, surgical removal of one or both uterine tubes.

salpingitis, *(sal-pin-jī'-tis)*, inflammation of the uterine tubes, it may be acute or chronic.

salpingocyesis, *(sal-pin-gō-sī-ē'-sis)*, tubal pregnancy. *See* ECTOPIC GESTATION.

salpingography, *(sal-pin-gog'-ra-fi)*, a radiographic technique where the uterine tubes are visualized following the instillation of radiopaque contrast medium.

salpingo-oöphorectomy, *(sal-pin-gō-ō-of-o-rek'-to-mi)*, surgical removal of one or both uterine tubes and ovaries.

salpingostomy, *(sal-pin-gos'-to-mi)*, opening a uterine tube in an attempt to restore patency.

salpinx, a tube, pharyngotympanic or uterine.

salt, 1. a substance formed by the combination of an acid and base (alkali). **2.** popular term for sodium chloride (common table salt).

Samaritans, a voluntary befriending service, available 24 hours to suicidal or despairing people who phone in, visit local branches or make contact via e-mail.

sample, in research. The subset selected from a population.

sandfly, an insect (*Phlebotomus*) which transmits various tropical infections, e.g. leishmaniasis.

sanguineous, *(san-gwin'-e-us)*, pertaining to blood. Containing blood.

saphenous, apparent, manifest. The name given to two superficial veins in the leg, the long and short s. vein, and to the nerves accompanying them. The long s. vein is used for coronary artery vein grafts.

saprophytes, *(sap'-rō-fitz)*, organisms that exist only in dead matter.

sarcoidosis, *(sar-koy-dō-sis)*, a systemic granulomatous disease of unknown aetiology. It produces lesions similar to those which are produced by tuberculosis. The organs and structures affected include: skin, eyes, lungs, liver, spleen, lymph nodes, bone and salivary glands, etc. *See* KVEIM TEST.

sarcolemma, *(sar-kō-lem-ma)*, plasma membrane surrounding the sarcoplasm of a muscle fibre.

sarcoma, *(sar-kō-ma)*, a malignant tumour of connective tissue.

sarcomere, *(sar-kō-meer)*, segment of myofibril which forms the smallest contractile unit of skeletal muscle.

sarcoplasm, *(sar-kō-plazm)*, the cytoplasm of a muscle fibre.

Sarcoptes scabiei, *(sar-kop-tēz-skā-bē-ī),* the mite which causes scabies.

sartorius, *(sar-tor'-ē-us),* the long ribbon-shaped muscle of the front of the thigh.

satiety, *(sat-ī-et-ē),* feeling full and satisfied after eating.

saturated, a solution into which no more solute can be dissolved. *S. fatty acids:* fatty acids which have no double bonds in their structure. Usually solid at room temperature, e.g. lard, fat around meat. Mainly derived from animal sources but some are found in plants. High dietary intake is associated with elevated serum cholesterol levels and an unfavourable high density:low density lipoprotein ratio, both of which are linked with atherosclerosis. *See* FATTY ACIDS, LIPOPROTEINS, POLYUNSATURATED FATS, UNSATURATED FATS.

satyriasis, *(sat-i-rī-a-sis),* excessive sexual appetite in the male.

scabies, *(skā-bēz),* a contagious disease caused by *Sarcoptes scabiei.* There is severe itching as the mite burrows into the skin, especially between the fingers, on the genitalia and buttocks.

scala, *(ska-la),* fluid-filled chambers within the cochlea. *See* EAR.

scald, injury caused by hot liquids or vapours.

scale, 1. the layers of dead epidermis cells which are shed from the skin. **2.** to remove tartar deposits from the teeth. **3.** a device or graded system used for measurement.

scalenus syndrome, *(ska-lē-nus),* pain and tingling in arm and fingers, often with loss of power and muscle wasting, because of compression of the lower trunk of the brachial plexus behind scalenus anterior muscle at the thoracic outlet.

scaler, a metal instrument or ultrasonic device used for removing tartar from teeth.

scalp, the skin covering the cranium.

scalpel, a straight knife with convex edge, used in dissecting and surgery.

scan, a diagnostic procedure where detailed images of organs or tissues and sometimes their functions are produced. *See* COMPUTED AXIAL TOMOGRAPHY, IMAGING, MAGNETIC RESONANCE IMAGING, RADIONUCLIDE SCANNING, ULTRASOUND SCAN.

scanner, 1. the equipment used for scanning techniques, e.g. gamma camera. **2.** a device for converting pictures and text to computer files.

scanning, 1. visual examination. **2.** examination by scanner. *S. electron microscope:* a type of electron microscope. *S. speech:* staccato speech; a disorder of speech where there is hesitation between syllables which are equally stressed, characteristic of cerebellar disease.

scaphoid, *(skaf-oyd),* boat-shaped. One of the carpals or wrist bones.

scapula, *(skap'-ū-la),* triangular shoulder blade which articulates with the humerus and clavicle.

scar, the connective fibrous tissue found after any wound has healed.

scarification, *(skar-i-fi-kā'-shon),* shallow incisions just penetrating the epidermis. A technique used in vaccination.

scarlet fever, scarlatina. A disease which occurs with haemolytic streptococcal infections, usually of the throat. There is fever, sore throat, headache, red tongue and a widespread erythematous rash which is followed by desquamation.

SCAT, sheep cell agglutination test. A rheumatoid factor in the blood is detected by the sheep red cell agglutination titre.

Scheuermann's disease, *(shoy-er-manz),* osteochondritis of the spine affecting the ring epiphyses of the vertebral bodies. Occurs in adolescents and leads to kyphosis.

Schick test, a skin test for susceptibility to diphtheria.

Schiller test, the application of iodine to the cervix to demonstrate nonstaining abnormal cells for biopsy.

Schilling test, a test used to confirm the diagnosis of pernicious anaemia. The absorption of ingested radioactive vitamin B_{12} is assessed by measuring urinary excretion of the labelled vitamin.

Schirmer tear test, used to assess the functioning of the lacrimal apparatus.

Schistosoma, *(skis-to-sō-mah),* a genus of trematodes (flukes) which cause disease in humans. *See* SCHISTOSOMIASIS.

schistosomiasis, *(skis-tō-so-mī-a-sis),* bilharzia. A disease common in tropical areas caused by *Schistosoma haematobium, S. japonicum* and *S. mansoni.* The effects vary but may include involvement of: the urinary tract with haematuria, the liver with fibrosis and hepatic portal hypertension, the rectum with bleeding and the nervous system with paralysis and blindness.

schizoid, *(skit-zoyd),* resembling schizophrenia. *S. personality:* a personality disorder where the individual is solitary, detached, introverted and has difficulty forming relationships.

schizophrenia, *(skit-zo-frē-ni-a),* a psychosis. Major disorder characterized by withdrawal and disintegration of personality with a progressive loss of emotional stability, judgement and contact with reality. Commonly the person experiences hallucinations and delusions which may be of a paranoid nature. *See* SCHNEIDER'S FIRST RANK SYMPTOMS.

Schlatter's disease, *see* OSGOOD–SCHLATTER'S DISEASE.

Schlemm's canal, channel in the inner sclera, close to its junction with the cornea which drains excess aqueous humor to maintain normal intraocular pressure. Failure of this mechanism results in raised intraocular pressure and glaucoma.

Schneider's first rank symptoms, a list of 'first rank' symptoms used in the diagnosis and classification of schizophrenia. They include: certain types of delusions, hallucinatory voices and feelings of passivity.

school nurse, a registered nurse with a specialist qualification in the specific health needs of school-age children. Their expanding role includes: health surveillance and screening; monitoring growth and development; child protection; being accessible to pupils/students seeking advice; providing age-appropriate nurse-led clinics; advising and supporting the school management team on initiatives aimed at creating healthy schools, health and safety matters and the curriculum requirements of personal and social education and sex education. They are concerned with the provision for children with special educational needs, such as children with learning disability, behavioural problems and physical conditions that require extra care and support to enable them to benefit from inclusion in mainstream schools.

school refusal, a situation where a child or young person will not attend school. Reasons include: an irrational fear of school with anxiety, boredom or bullying.

Schwann cells, specialized neuroglial cells of the peripheral nervous system. They produce layers of neurilemma which form the myelin sheath enclosing some nerve fibres.

sciatic nerve, *(sī-at-ik),* largest nerve of the body. It arises from the sacral plexus and passes deep to the gluteus maximus muscle of the buttock and passes down the leg where it divides into the peroneal and tibial nerves at the knee.

sciatica, *(sī-at-i-ka),* pain in leg and buttock. Commonly caused by a prolapsed intervertebral disc.

scintillography, scintiscanning. Visual recording of radioactivity over selected areas after administration of suitable radioisotope.

scirrhous, *(ski'-rus),* hard and fibrous.

scirrhus, *(ski-rus),* a carcinoma containing connective tissue which makes it gritty and hard, such as in breast tissue.

scissor-leg deformity, deformity due to exaggerated tone in the adductor muscles usually resulting from cerebral lesions.

sclera, *(sklē'-ra),* outer fibrous coat which forms the 'white of the eye'. It covers the posterior five-sixths of the eyeball.

scleritis, *(skle-rī-tis),* inflammation of the sclera.

scleroderma, *(skler-ō-der-ma),* a group of connective tissue diseases leading to fibrosis and degenerative changes in many organs and the skin. Localized disease causes oedema of the skin, hardening, atrophy, deformity and ulceration. Diffuse fibrosis may occur in the myocardium, kidneys, lungs and gastrointestinal tract. *See* SCLEROSIS.

scleromalacia, *(skler-ō-ma-lā-sē-a),* thinning of the sclera.

sclerosis, *(skler-ō-sis),* hardening. *Amyotrophic lateral s.:* a presentation seen in motor neurone disease. There is muscle wasting, weakness and spasticity with abnormal reflexes. *See* ARTERIOSCLEROSIS, ATHEROSCLEROSIS, MULTIPLE SCLEROSIS.

sclerotherapy, *(skler-ō-ther-a-pi),* treatment of haemorrhoids, oesophageal varices or varicose veins by injecting them with a sclerosing chemical.

sclerotic, *(skle-ro-tik),* **1.** pertaining to the sclera. **2.** hard or indurated.

sclerotomy, *(skler-ot'-o-mi),* an operation on the sclerotic coat of the eye, for the relief of glaucoma.

scolex, *(skō'-leks),* head of a tapeworm.

scoliosis, *(skō-li-ō'-sis),* lateral curvature of the spine (Figure 68).

scotoma, *(sko-tō-ma),* a blind area in the visual field.

scratch test, a skin test for allergies where suspect allergens are applied to a scratched area. A wheal results if an allergy is present.

screening, 1. *see* FLUOROSCOPY. **2.** testing large numbers of people for a disease, e.g. cervical malignancy with exfoliative cervical cytology. *See* SENSITIVITY, SPECIFICITY.

scrotal, *(skrō-tal),* pertaining to the scrotum.

scrotocele, *(skrō'-tō-sēl),* hernia in the scrotum.

scrotum, *(skrō-tum),* bag of pigmented skin and fascia containing the testes.

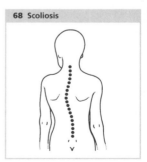

68 Scoliosis

scrub nurse, one who wears sterile gown and gloves to assist the surgeons during surgery. A role also undertaken by operating department assistant/technician.

scrub typhus, a mite-borne disease caused by the organism *Rickettsia tsutsugamushi.*

scurvy, a disease caused by the deficiency of vitamin C in the diet. In adults it causes spontaneous bruising, swollen and spongy gums that bleed, loose teeth, poor wound healing and anaemia. When it occurs in infants there may be swelling of the costochondral junctions and bleeding under the periosteum in long bones with severe pain.

scybala, *(sib′-a-la),* faeces passed as hard dry masses.

seasonal affective disorder (SAD), a disorder of mood where individuals experience depression and lethargy as the days shorten as winter approaches. It is linked to the amount of melatonin secreted by the pineal body/gland which is light-dependent. The treatment of choice is exposure to special lights during the autumn and winter, in addition to natural light, as spontaneous improvement occurs as the days lengthen in spring.

sebaceous, *(se-bā-shus),* fatty, secreting oily matter. *S. glands of the skin:* open into the hair follicles, secrete fatty material called sebum. *S. cyst:* sebum-filled cyst which develops if the opening of the gland becomes blocked.

seborrhoea, *(seb-o-rē′-a),* excessive secretion of the sebaceous glands.

sebum, fatty substance secreted by the sebaceous glands.

seclusion, a nursing intervention for mentally ill patients: they are isolated in a special room to decrease stimuli which might be causing or exacerbating their emotional distress. The use of seclusion is strictly controlled, monitored and audited.

second intention, type of wound healing. *See* GRANULATION.

second stage of labour, *see* LABOUR.

secondary, second in time or importance. *S. areola:* pigmented area appearing around the nipple during pregnancy. *See* AREOLA. *S. care:* care requiring admission to hospital. *S. cancer/deposits:* metastases or secondaries. *S. disease:* one that occurs as a result of some pre-existing disease. *S. haemorrhage: see* HAEMORRHAGE. *S. prevention:* detection of disease at an early stage, when serious effects may still be avoided. *S. sexual characteristics:* the physical changes occurring at puberty such as breast development, voice changes and growth of pubic hair.

secretin, *(se-krē-tin),* hormone produced by the duodenal mucosa which influences pancreatic secretion.

secretion, *(se-krē-shon),* **1.** the active production or extrusion of material, such as mucus or hormones, from a cell. **2.** the actual material produced by the cell.

secretory, relating to secretion. *S. phase:* a stage of the menstrual cycle which starts after ovulation and lasts until the next menstruation. It corresponds to the luteal phase of the ovarian cycle.

section, usually applied to the thin slices of tissue prepared for microscopic histological examination. *See* CAESAREAN SECTION.

secularization, *(sek-ūl-ar-i-zā-shon),* applied to society the increase in civil, state or non-religious influences and a decline in those of various religions.

sedation, a restful state of reduced activity.

sedative, an agent or drug which reduces excitement, anxiety, activity or tension.

sedentary, physically inactive.

sedimentation, a settling out of solids at the bottom of a fluid. *S. rate: see* ERYTHROCYTE SEDIMENTATION RATE.

segregation, a setting apart. In genetics, the separation from one another of two alleles, each carried on one pair of chromosomes; this happens during meiosis when the haploid gametes are produced. Isolation. *See* MENDEL'S LAWS.

selenium (Se), a trace element required by the body for important enzyme reactions which protect cells against oxidative damage. It is an antioxidant.

self, 1. in immunology the inherent cell antigens as opposed to those which constitute foreign non-self antigens. **2.** everything that makes the individual, the features of being a unique person.

self-actualization, reaching ones potential, fulfilment. *See* MASLOW'S HIERARCHY OF NEEDS.

self-advocacy, a process by which people are helped to acquire the skills and information required for them to speak out for themselves. See ADVOCACY.

self-care, 1. being able to meet one's own personal needs. **2.** meeting one's own medical or treatment needs after suitable instruction.

self-concept, a self-image that individuals have of their total characteristics, qualities and negative features.

self-esteem, the value or worth people place on themselves.

self-examination, a regular self-screening test where the person examines his or her own breasts or testes for changes which may indicate some pathology. *See* BREAST AWARENESS, TESTICULAR SELF-EXAMINATION.

self-harm, deliberate self-inflicted injuries. May be associated with low self-esteem.

self-help groups, groups of ordinary people with a common problem or goal who support and help each other through discussion and sharing, e.g. Alcoholics Anonymous.

self-image, the total concept of what one believes oneself to be vis-à-vis one's role in society.

self-medication, situation where the individual is responsible, following suitable education, for his or her own drug administration regimens.

self-poisoning, intentional consumption of potentially harmful substances such as drugs, often in combinations and with alcohol.

sella turcica, (*sel-a ter'-si-ka*), pituitary fossa of the sphenoid bone.

semantic, meaning of words.

semen, seminal fluid. It contains the spermatozoa and the secretions from the seminal vesicles, prostate gland and bulbourethral glands (Cowper's). The alkaline fluid discharged during ejaculation.

semicircular canals, three fluid-filled canals of the internal ear. Oriented in the three planes of space, they are part of the vestibular apparatus concerned with dynamic equilibrium and balance. *See* EAR.

semicoma, a state of altered consciousness from which the person can be roused by suitable stimuli.

semilunar, (*sem-i-lū-na*), shaped like a crescent or half moon. *S. cartilage*: menisci. Two cartilages in the knee joint between the femur and tibia. Very commonly injured and torn, especially during certain sports and other activities. *S. valve*: the valves at the entrance to the aorta and pulmonary artery which prevent the back flow of blood into the ventricles.

seminal, relating to semen. *S. fluid*: see SEMEN. *S. vesicles*: two accessory glands which contribute an alkaline fluid to semen. They are situated posterior to the male bladder.

seminiferous tubules, *(sem-in-if-er-us)*, coiled tubules within the testes which produce spermatozoa.

seminoma, *(sem-in-ō-ma)*, malignant testicular tumour.

semipermeable films, an adhesive polyurethane membrane designed to retain wound exudate, thereby creating a moist wound environment. Can be used on low-exudate wounds; as a secondary dressing with hydrogel dressings; and in the prevention of pressure ulcers.

semipermeable membrane, selectively permeable. One that allows the passage of molecules of a certain size, but not larger molecules.

semiprone, a position where the individual is partially prone with the face down and the knees flexed to one side. Useful in situations of altered consciousness.

senescence, *(se-ne'-sens)*, growing old.

Sengstaken–Blakemore tube, *(seng-sta-ken)*, oesophageal tube used to compress bleeding varices.

senile, relating to the changes occurring in old age. *S. dementia*: see DEMENTIA.

senility, mental and physical deterioration which occurs with old age.

sensation, feelings which result from the sensory information conveyed to the brain by the sensory neurones.

sense, faculties by which the environment can be perceived and interpreted, e.g. sight, hearing, taste, smell, proprioception and touch. *S. organ*: an organ which receives external sensory stimuli, such as the ears and eyes.

sensible, that which the senses perceive.

sensitive, 1. able to react to stimuli. **2.** being particularly perceptive in interpersonal skills. **3.** reacting adversely or being susceptible to a drug or antigen.

sensitivity, 1. being able to feel and respond. **2.** the position of being susceptible to a drug or antigen. *S. test*: in microbiology the tests performed to determine the sensitivity or resistance of a microorganism to a range of antimicrobial drugs. Used with other factors, such as toxicity, in making treatment choices. **3.** the ability of a test to identify accurately affected individuals, such as a screening test.

sensitization, production of an immunological state in which there is a disproportionate response to certain antigenic substances, such as with allergies. *See* ALLERGIC STATE, ANAPHYLAXIS, HYPERSENSITIVITY.

sensorimotor, having both sensory and motor components.

sensorineural hearing loss, *see* DEAFNESS.

sensorium, the consciousness; accurate memory and orientation for person, time and place.

sensory, pertaining to sensation. *S. cortex*: region of the cerebral cortex where sensory inputs are received. *S. nerves*: the afferent nerves which carry impulses from the peripheral receptors and sense organs to the central nervous system. *S. deprivation*: absence of usual sensory stimuli, e.g. patients in intensive care units. It may lead to mental changes, such as anxiety, depression and hallucinations. *S. loss*: reduced or total loss of function of any of the five senses. *S. overload*: a situation where the sense organs are excessively or inappropriately stimulated, which leads to an inability to sort the stimuli. May occur in intensive care units, e.g. bright lights, machine noise and people talking.

separation anxiety, a complication occurring in preschool children separated from their mothers for periods of time, such as due to hospital admission. It is characterized firstly by protest and then despair/depression, detachment and regression, such as loss of continence, clinging to parents or refusing to eat. The degree of distress is influenced by many factors, e.g. parental involvement/partnership in care, parenting styles, parent's response, the gender of the nurse, etc. The features of regression and emotional instability may continue long after discharge home but gradually resolve.

sepsis, the condition of being infected by pus-forming (pyogenic) bacteria.

septal, pertaining to a septum. *S. defect:* congenital abnormality where an opening exists between the two atria or the two ventricles of the heart.

septic, pertaining to or caused by sepsis. *S. shock:* shock occurring as a result of infection or an overwhelming inflammatory response. *See:* SYSTEMIC INFLAMMATORY RESPONSE SYNDROME.

septicaemia, *(sep-ti-sē-mi-a),* the circulation and multiplication of microorganisms in the blood.

septum, the division which separates two cavities, e.g. between the right and left side of the heart, and the nasal cavities.

sequelae, *(se-kwe'-lē),* morbid conditions remaining after, and consequent on, some former illness.

sequestrectomy, *(se-kwes-trek'-to-mi),* operation to remove a sequestrum.

sequestrum, *(se-kwes'-trum),* a fragment of dead bone.

serine, *(se-rēn),* an amino acid.

serological, *(se-rō-loj-i-kal),* pertaining to serology.

serology, *(se-rol-o-ji),* study of blood sera and its reactions, important in immunological diagnostic procedures.

serosa, *(se-rō-sa),* serous membrane. Includes the pleura, peritoneum and pericardium.

serosanguineous, *(se-rō-san-gwin'-e-us),* a discharge containing serum and blood.

serositis, *(se-rō-sī'-tis),* an inflamed serous membrane.

serotonin, *(ser-ō-tō-nin),* see 5-HYDROXYTRYPTAMINE.

serotyping, a classification of microorganisms based upon their antigenic features.

serous, pertaining to serum.

serpiginous, *(ser-pij'-in-us),* serpent-like in shape.

Serratia, (ser-ā-she-a), a genus of Gram-negative bacteria. *S. marcescens* causes infection in humans. It is an endemic hospital resident and causes nosocomial pneumonia and urinary tract infection.

serum, the fluid part of blood which remains after clotting. *S. sickness:* the allergic illness occurring 7–10 days following the injection of foreign serum for treatment or prophylaxis of infection. A rare event now that serum-containing antibodies from other species have been replaced by the use of human immunoglobulins.

sesamoid bones, *(ses-a-moyd),* small foci of bone formation in the tendons of muscles. The patella is the largest.

sessile, *(sis'-il),* having no stem (applied to tumours).

severe acute asthma (status asthmaticus), life-threatening asthma attack. There is respiratory distress, unproductive cough, central cyanosis, tachycardia, sweating, exhaustion and hypoxia. It is a medical emergency.

severe combined immunodeficiency (SCID), severe inherited disorder where there is a deficiency of T and B lymphocytes. The consequent lack of immunity will result in death from infection unless a compatible bone marrow transplant is performed.

sex, 1. coitus. **2.** being either male or female. *S. chromatin: see* BARR BODIES. *S. chromosomes*: the pair of chromosomes which determine genetic sex; females have XX and males have XY. *S. hormones*: the steroid hormones such as oestrogens, progesterone and testosterone which are produced by the gonads. They control secondary sexual characteristic development and reproductive function. *S.-linked*: an inherited characteristic which is carried by a gene on a sex chromosome, e.g. haemophilia is transmitted by the X chromosome.

sexism, a belief that members of one sex are superior to those of the other, and thereby have advantages. It leads to discrimination and can act as a limiting factor, e.g. in professional development.

sexual, pertaining to sex. *S. dysfunction*: lack of desire or the inability to achieve coitus in one or both partners.

sexuality, the sum of the structural, functional and psychological attributes as they are expressed by one's gender identity and sexual behaviour.

sexually transmitted infections (STI), also called diseases. The contagious conditions, including those defined legally as venereal, which are usually transmitted through sexual contact, but not exclusively so. They include: AIDS, candidiasis, chlamydial infection, genital herpes, genital warts, gonorrhoea, hepatitis, nonspecific urethritis, syphilis and trichomoniasis.

sharps, include used needles, razor blades, intravenous giving sets, central venous lines and cannulae. They should be put immediately into a rigid sharps' container of distinctive colour which is disposed of when three-quarters full. It is sealed in such a way that used needles cannot be recovered for misuse. Arrangements have to be made for safe disposal of those used by people in their own homes, district nurses, at health centres and doctors' surgeries.

shearing forces, a force which when applied will cause different layers, e.g. of tissues, to slide relative to one another. The deep blood vessels are stretched and angulated, thus deeper tissues become ischaemic with consequent necrosis. Responsible for the development of some types of pressure ulcers.

Sheehan's disease/syndrome, hypopituitarism due to infarction of the gland resulting from postpartum haemorrhage.

Shigella, (shi-gel-la), a genus of Gram-negative bacteria commonly found in the human gut. The following cause bacillary dysentery: *S. dysenteriae*, *S. flexneri* and *S. sonnei*.

shin-bone, the tibia. See SKELETON.

shingles, see HERPES ZOSTER.

Shirodkar suture, a purse-string suture used to close an incompetent cervix during pregnancy to prevent abortion. It is removed around the 38th week, or if labour commences or if loss of the pregnancy becomes inevitable.

shock, acute circulatory disturbance leading to cell hypoxia through inappropriate or inadequate tissue perfusion. There is a discrepancy between the circulating blood volume and the capacity of the vascular bed. It is characterized by tachycardia, shallow rapid respiration, pallor, sweating, hypotension, oliguria, restlessness and altered consciousness. Classifications of shock vary but may include: **1.** hypovolaemic, with loss of blood or other body fluids, e.g. severe haemorrhage, dehydration and surgery; or due to increased vessel permeability such as in septicaemia or anaphylaxis. **2.** cardiogenic or pump failure, e.g. after extensive myocardial infarction. **3.** neurogenic, which may be due to nervous system mechanisms, e.g. in response to spinal cord damage. *See* ANAPHYLACTIC SHOCK. *S. trousers*: 'pump up' garment used to improve venous return to the heart in hypovolaemia.

short circuit, anastomosis between gut or blood vessels which allows the contents to bypass a section of the normal pathway.

short-sightedness, *see* MYOPIA.

short-term memory, information which can only be recalled for a short time.

shoulder, joint formed by the humerus, scapula and clavicle. *See* FROZEN SHOULDER, SCAPULA. *S. presentation*: a variety of transverse lie which must be converted to a vertex or breech before vaginal delivery is possible.

show, popular term for the discharge of slightly bloodstained mucus common at the beginning of labour.

shunt, a diversion, especially of blood flow, due to congenital abnormality, acquired disease or surgery such as arteriovenous shunt.

SI, abbreviation for **Système International d'Unités,** *see* INTERNA-TIONAL SYSTEM OF UNITS, APPENDIX 4: UNITS OF MEASUREMENT.

sialoadenitis, (sī-al-ō-ad-en-ī´-tis), inflammation of a salivary gland.

sialogogue, (sī-al-ō-gog), any agent which increases the flow of saliva.

sialography, (sī-al-og-ra-fi), a radiographic examination of the salivary glands and ducts following the introduction of radiopaque contrast medium.

sialolith, (sī-al-ō-lith), a salivary calculus.

sibilus, (sib´-il-us), abnormal respiratory sound heard on auscultation. A hissing or whistling sound characteristic of airway narrowing such as in bronchitis.

sibling, one of two or more children of the same parents.

sick role, a sociological term which signifies the changes in role during illness. In acute illness, the person is relieved of usual activities and responsibilities, and can accept help from, and perhaps dependence on, others. In exchange, the person complies with treatment and relinquishes the sick role at an appropriate time. The concept is less useful in chronic illness.

sickle cell disease, an inherited condition which is due to an abnormal haemoglobin (HbS). Seen in individuals from areas where falciparum malaria is common (equatorial Africa, part of India and part of the Eastern Mediterranean) and their descendants in Europe, West Indies and the USA. The red cells become sickle-shaped, in hypoxia, dehydration or infection, which leads to reduced oxygen-carrying capacity, vessel blockage with pain and infarction and a chronic haemolytic anaemia as the abnormal red cells are destroyed in the spleen. When a sickle cell crisis occurs the person requires urgent rehydration and pain relief. At-risk populations should be screened for the abnormal HbS. *See* HAEMOGLOBINOPATHIES.

side-effect, any event occurring as a consequence of drug therapy or other treatment. Usually unwanted, but may have positive effects.

sideroblastic anaemias, (*si-der-ō-blas-tik*), rare anaemias due to abnormal iron metabolism, they may be inherited or acquired.

siderosis, (*sid-er-ō-sis*), **1.** inhalation of iron particles causing pneumoconiosis. May be combined with silica to produce silicosiderosis. **2.** excess iron in the blood or tissues which may be due to excessive intake.

sievert (Sv), the SI unit for radiation dose equivalent, it replaces the rem.

sigmoid, (*sig'-moyd*), like the Greek letter ς (sigma) applied especially to a bend in the pelvic colon just before it becomes the rectum. *S. sinus*: venous channel draining blood from the brain.

sigmoidoscopy, (*sig-moyd-os'-ko-pi*), an endoscopic examination of the rectum and sigmoid colon using a fibreoptic or rigid metal sigmoidoscope.

sigmoidostomy, (*sig-moyd-os'-to-mi*), opening into the sigmoid colon.

sign, an objective indication of disease which can be seen or elicited. *S. language*: various forms of signing (signs and gestures) used by hearing impaired people for communication. *See* BRITISH SIGN LANGUAGE, MAKATON. *Vital s.*: signs of life, such as blood pressure, pulse, respiration and temperature.

significance, *See* STATISTICAL SIGNIFICANCE.

silicones, water-repellent compounds with numerous medical uses, e.g. catheters and dressings.

silicosis, (*sil-i-kō-sis*), fibrotic lung disease due to the inhalation of silica particles. *See* PNEUMOCONIOSIS.

silver (Ag), metallic element. *S. nitrate*: a salt which is caustic, astringent and disinfectant.

Simmond's disease, *see* HYPOPITUITARISM, PANHYPOPITUITARISM.

simple fracture, *see* FRACTURE.

Sims', **1.** a position used for gynaecological examination and treatments (Figure 69). **2.** a type of vaginal speculum.

simulation, an educational technique where students are exposed to a set of circumstances (possibly computer-assisted) in the classroom, which are as close to reality as possible.

simulator, specialized equipment, often computer-linked, which is used to calculate exact treatment details prior to a course of radiotherapy.

sinciput, (*sin'-si-put*), the upper fore part of the head.

single-blind, a trial, usually for a drug, where either the researcher or the subjects know the identity of the controls and those taking the actual substance being tested.

sinistral, pertaining to the left.

sinoatrial (SA) node, (*si-nō-a-tri-al*), the pacemaker of the heart. An area of specialized autorhythmic cells in the wall of the right atrium near to the entrance of the superior vena cava. They regulate the cardiac

69 Sims' position

impulse and the muscular contraction which then spreads over the heart. *SA block*: *see* HEART BLOCK.

sinus, 1. a passage leading from an abscess or some inner structure, to an external opening. **2.** channels for venous blood, such as those draining the brain; cavernous, straight, sigmoid, transverse and sagittal sinuses. Or the heart. *Coronary s.*: *see* CORONARY. **3.** the paranasal (air) s. are air-filled cavities in the skull bones; frontal, maxillary, ethmoidal and sphenoidal. *Carotid s.*: *see* CAROTID.

sinus arrhythmia, (*sī-nus a-rith-mī-a*), *see* ARRHYTHMIA.

sinus rhythm, normal heart rhythm as demonstrated by a normal PQRST waveform.

sinusitis, (*sī-nu-sī-tis*), acute or chronic inflammation of a sinus, especially the mucous membrane lining a paranasal sinus.

sinusoid, (*sī-nū-soyd*), like a sinus. Channels for small blood vessels such as those in the liver and spleen.

siphonage, (*sī-fon-ij*), a method of transferring fluid from one vessel to another; the principle is utilized in gastric and rectal lavage.

sitz bath, a special shallow hip bath.

Sjögren's syndrome, (*sher-grens*), an autoimmune condition of unknown cause. It is characterized by keratoconjunctivitis with reduced secretions from salivary and lacrimal glands associated with connective tissue disease such as rheumatoid arthritis. Usually affects older women.

skeletal, relating to the skeleton. *S. muscle*: voluntary or striated muscle. *See* MUSCLE. *S. traction*: *see* TRACTION.

skeleton, the bony framework of the body (Figure 70). *Appendicular s.*: pectoral girdle, upper limb, pelvic girdle and lower limb. *Axial s.*: skull, spine, ribs, sternum and hyoid bone.

Skene's glands, two small glands which open into the female urethral meatus. Also known as **lesser vestibular glands.**

skewed distribution, in statistics. Any distribution of scores where there are more values one side of the mean than the other, i.e. not symmetrical. *See* NORMAL DISTRIBUTION CURVE.

skin, the outer covering of the body consisting of the dermis, epidermis and its appendages; hair, nails, glands. Its functions include: sensory, protective, storage, excretory, temperature regulation, absorption and synthesis. *S. fold thickness*: an anthropometric measurement used to assess nutritional status. *S. traction*: *see* TRACTION.

skin cancer, *see* BASAL CELL CARCINOMA, MELANOMA, RODENT ULCER, SQUAMOUS CELL CARCINOMA.

skin graft, *see* GRAFT.

skull, bony framework of the head; the bones of the cranium and face (Figure 71).

sleep, periods where the body and mind are at rest. There is an alteration in consciousness (which is easily reversed), suspension of volition and reduced activity. Typically sleep consists of alternating cycles of non-rapid eye movement sleep (NREM) which has four stages and rapid eye movement sleep (REM). *See* NON-RAPID EYE MOVEMENT SLEEP, RAPID EYE MOVEMENT SLEEP. *S. apnoea*: breathing pauses because of periodic upper airway closure during sleep. This results in a cycle of apnoea–wakening–apnoea, etc. throughout the night, disturbing sleeping and also daytime sleeping and risk of accidents. *S. terrors*: sudden wakening in a state of extreme fear, disorientation

70 The skeleton (a) front; (b) back view

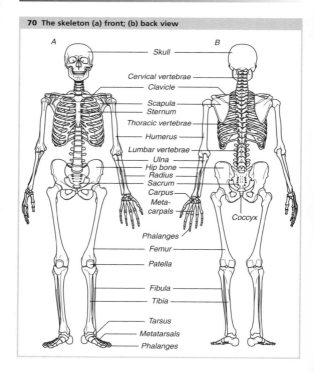

A

B

Skull

Cervical vertebrae

Clavicle

Scapula
Sternum

Thoracic vertebrae

Humerus

Lumbar vertebrae

Ulna
Hip bone
Radius
Sacrum
Carpus
Meta-
carpals

Coccyx

Phalanges

Femur

Patella

Fibula
Tibia

Tarsus
Metatarsals
Phalanges

and agitation. *S. walking*: see SOM-
NAMBULISM.

sleeping sickness, *see* TRYPANOSOMIASIS.

sliding board, device used to transfer
individuals unable to move independently or those with spinal
injuries.

sliding filament hypothesis, an
explanation of muscle contraction
which proposes that the filaments
slide against each other to cause
shortening.

slipped disc, *see* PROLAPSED INTERVERTE-
BRAL DISC.

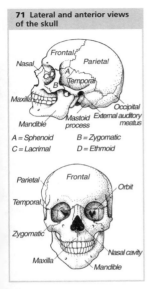

71 Lateral and anterior views of the skull

Nasal

Frontal

Parietal

Temporal

A

B

D

Maxilla

(slf)

Mandible

Occipital

Mastoid process

External auditory meatus

A = Sphenoid   B = Zygomatic
C = Lacrimal   D = Ethmoid

Parietal   Frontal

Temporal

Orbit

Zygomatic

Nasal cavity

Maxilla

Mandible

slit lamp, a device used for detailed examination of the eye.

slough, (sluf), **1.** necrotic tissue which separates from healthy tissue. **2.** to cast off.

slow virus, an infective agent known as a prion whose effects may take many years to become evident, e.g. Creutzfeldt-Jakob disease.

small for dates, *see* LOW BIRTH WEIGHT.

smallpox, variola. A virus disease now eradicated by the programme of disease control by the World Health Organization (WHO).

smear, material for examination or culture which is spread on to a slide or culture medium. *See* CIN,

EXFOLIATIVE CYTOLOGY, PAPANICO-LAOU SMEAR.

smegma, thick white sebaceous secretion which accumulates under the prepuce and around the clitoris.

Smith-Petersen nail, a nail used for the internal fixation of intracapsular fractures of the femoral neck.

smooth muscle, involuntary muscle. *See* MUSCLE.

Snellen's test types, a chart of different-sized letters used for testing visual acuity. The letters are arranged in lines that can be read by a normal (emmetropic) eye at 60, 36, 24, 18, 12, 9, 6 and 5 metres. Acuity is checked in each eye separately and expressed as 6 over the smallest line of letters that can be read, e.g. a person able to read the 6-metre line at 6 metres is said to have a visual acuity of 6/6 (Figure 72). Special E test-type charts (different orientations of the letter E) are used to test children and others unable to read the letters.

snow, *see* CARBON DIOXIDE. *S. blindness:* ophthalmia and photophobia caused by the glare of the sun from the snow.

snuffles, 1. partial breathing obstruction in babies with a 'cold'. **2.** snorting inspiration due to congestion of nasal mucosa. It is a sign of congenital syphilis, when the nasal discharge may be purulent or blood-stained.

social class, a socioeconomic classification based on the occupation of the householder. In the UK the Office of Population Censuses and Surveys has five categories: I professional II intermediate, III skilled (non-manual and manual), IV semiskilled and V unskilled. Other classifications are also in use. *See* CLASS.

social drift/mobility, the movement of individuals to other social class categories.

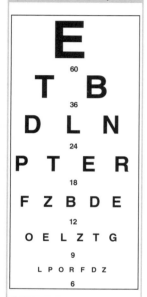

72 Snellen's type-test chart (5-metre line not shown)

E
60
T B
36
D L N
24
P T E R
18
F Z B D E
12
O E L Z T G
9
L P O R F D Z
6

social exclusion, refers to the multiple deprivation experienced by certain population groups who can become socially isolated and unable to participate in mainstream activities, such as education. Groups affected include: refugees, rough-sleepers, teenage mothers, young people, etc.

socialization, (so-shal-i-zā′-shon), in sociology, it describes the processes by which people learn the social norms and the value of adhering to them. Socialization occurs informally in the family and with friends, and more formally at school and in the workplace.

social network, the individuals who interact within a group, not necessarily related.

social norms, socially acceptable forms of behaviour. Norms may forbid certain behaviours and prescribe others.

social work, the professional practice of specially qualified social workers which involves helping people to adjust or cope with their social or environmental situation.

socially clean, describes articles required to be scrupulously clean, a condition achieved with disinfection. To prevent nosocomial infection, it must characterize all articles that patients use, e.g. baths, basins, etc.

sociobiological, (so-she-ō-bī-ō-loj-ik-al), pertaining to social and biological features.

sociocultural, pertaining to culture in its sociological setting.

socioeconomic, (so-she-ō-ek-on-om-ik), pertaining to social and economic features.

sociology, the scientific study of social organization, groups and relationships.

sodium (Na), white metallic element. Sodium is a major extracellular cation concerned with the integrity of fluid compartments and neuromuscular function. *S. hydrogen carbonate (bicarbonate)*: important buffer in the blood. Used intravenously to correct metabolic acidosis. *S. chloride*: used intravenously to replace fluids and electrolytes. *S. citrate*: an in vitro anticoagulant. *S. hypochlorite*: a powerful disinfectant solution which in suitable dilution will destroy HIV. *S. pump*: an active transport mechanism by which sodium ions pass through cell membranes.

soft sore, chancroid. A sexually transmitted condition caused by the bacteria *Haemophilus ducreyi*. It is characterized by the development of a necrotic ulcer, usually on the glans with inguinal lymphadenopathy which suppurates.

software, in computing a general term referring to data and programs.

solar plexus, a plexus of autonomic nerves and ganglia in the upper abdomen which supply the abdominal organs.

soleus, *(so'-le-us),* a muscle in the calf of the leg.

soluble, being dissolvable.

solute, a substance dissolved in a solvent.

solution, a liquid (solvent) containing a dissolved solid (solute). *Saturated s.: see* SATURATED.

solvent, a liquid able to dissolve another substance. *S. abuse:* 'glue sniffing' – inhalation of volatile substances such as those present in certain adhesives and fuels. It results in addiction and damage to nasal mucosa and the organs, e.g. brain. Death may occur due to asphyxia or toxicity.

somatic, *(so-mat-ik),* pertaining to the body. *S. cells:* body cells, not gametes.

somatostatin, *(so-ma-tō-stat-in),* growth hormone release-inhibiting hormone (GHRIH) produced by the hypothalamus. It is also secreted by cells in the pancreas and gastrointestinal tract where it influences both endocrine and exocrine functions.

somnambulism, *(som-nam'-bū-lizm),* walking and other activities during sleep.

Somogyi phenomenon, rebound hyperglycaemia following hypoglycaemia; seen in people with diabetes mellitus.

Sonne dysentery, *(son-ni),* bacillary dysentery caused by the organism *Shigella sonnei*.

sonography, *(son-og-ra-fi), see* ULTRASONOGRAPHY.

soporific, *(so-por-if-ik),* an agent that induces sleep.

sorbitol, *(saw-bi-tol),* a glucose derivative used as a sweetener in diabetic products and occasionally in total parenteral nutrition.

sordes, *(sor-dēz),* brown crusts forming on the lips and teeth in situations where normal oral hygiene mechanisms are impaired such as with dehydration and pyrexia.

souffle, *(soofl),* soft blowing sound heard on auscultation such as that heard over the pregnant uterus.

sound, a probe-like instrument used for exploring cavities such as the uterus, bladder, etc.

source isolation, required for patients who are sources of microorganisms which may spread from them to infect others. It may be strict for highly transmissible and dangerous diseases, or standard for other communicable diseases.

spasm, 1. sudden convulsive involuntary movement. **2.** sudden muscle contraction, the effects of which depend upon the structures involved. *Carpopedal s.:* spasm affecting the hands and feet. Seen where serum calcium is low. *See* TETANY. *Coronary artery s.:* a cause of angina pectoris and a cause of some cases of sudden death. *See* BRONCHOSPASM, CLONIC, TONIC.

spasmodic, 1. relating to a spasm. Occurring and recurring in spasms. **2.** agent causing spasms.

spasmolytic, *(spaz-mo-lit-ĭk),* substance which relieves spasm.

spastic, 1. pertaining to spasm. **2.** in a state of spasm with muscular rigidity. *S. colon:* see IRRITABLE BOWEL SYNDROME. *S. diplegia:* see LITTLE'S DISEASE. *S. paralysis.* see PARALYSIS.

spasticity, the condition of being spastic.

spatula, 1. a flat, flexible, blunt knife, used for spreading ointments and poultices. **2.** a tongue depressor.

spatulate, *(spat-ū-lāt),* shaped like a spatula.

species, a subdivision within a genus.

specific, 1. applied to a treatment which is curative for a particular disease. **2.** applied to a disease which is caused by a microorganism which causes that disease only. **3.** relating to a species. *S. gravity:* the density of a fluid compared with that of an equal volume of pure water. It depends on the quantity of solids dissolved in the fluid.

specificity, the ability of a test to identify accurately non-affected individuals, such as a screening test.

specimen, a sample used for diagnostic testing, e.g. tissue, blood or urine.

spectrophotometry, *(spek-trō-fo-tom-et-ri),* an analytical technique which uses a spectrophotometer to determine the amount of a substance present by measuring the light absorbed by its molecules.

spectroscopy, *(spek-tros'-ko-pi),* an analytical technique which detects and measures substances by using their individual absorption spectra.

spectrum, 1. a range of increasing or decreasing features or activity such as the types of electromagnetic waves arranged in terms of frequency or wavelength. **2.** the range of activity of an antimicrobial drug, e.g. broad-spectrum drugs act against several microorganisms.

speculum, *(spek'-ū-lum),* an instrument used to open a cavity so that the inside can be examined and/or treated, e.g. vagina, nose. Types of vaginal specula include: Cusco's and Sims'.

speech, the power of speaking; communicating a meaning by vocal sounds. *Oesophageal s.:* the use of air, regurgitated from the stomach, to produce sound following laryngectomy. *S. and language therapist:* the professional responsible for the assessment, diagnosis and treatment of speech and language disorders in children and adults. Disorders include: stammering, aphasia, dysarthria, and also problems with swallowing. *Telegraphic s.:* a type of speech seen in some organic brain disorders where answers contain only minimal information. *See* SCANNING SPEECH, STAMMERING.

sperm, spermatozoon. *S. bank:* storage of semen at very low temperatures prior to its use in artificial insemination. *S. count:* an investigation of male fertility levels where semen is examined for volume, chemical composition and sperm numbers, morphology and motility.

spermatic, pertaining to semen. *S. cord:* cord enclosing the artery, vein and vas deferens. It suspends the testis in the scrotum.

spermatocele, *(sper-mat-o-sēl),* cystic swelling containing semen.

spermatogenesis, *(sper-mat-o-jen-e-sis),* the formation of spermatozoa within the testes.

spermatorrhoea, *(sper-ma-to-rē-ă),* involuntary discharge of semen in the absence of an orgasm.

spermatozoon, *(sper-mat-o-zō'-on),* mature, male germ cell or gamete. It consists of a head containing the genetic material, a midpiece containing many mitochondria and a tail for motility. Each ejaculate of semen contains 50–150 million spermatozoa/ml (Figure 73).

spermicide, *(sper-mi-sīd)*, substance destroying spermatozoa.

sphenoid, *(sfe'-noyd)*, wedge-shaped. The name of one of the bones forming the base of the skull.

sphenoidal, *(sfen-oy'-dal)*, pertaining to the sphenoid bone.

spherocyte, *(sfe-rō-sīt)*, an abnormally shaped red cell, spherical instead of the normal biconcave disc.

spherocytosis, *(sfe-rō-sī-tō-sis)*, the presence in the blood of spherocytes. It may be hereditary due to defects in the red cell membrane or as a result of acquired haemolytic anaemias. Increased haemolysis of abnormal cells by the spleen results in anaemia, jaundice and splenomegaly.

sphincter, *(sfink-ter)*, a circular muscle which surrounds an orifice, e.g. anus, pylorus. Contraction of the muscle closes the opening.

sphincterectomy, *(sfink-ter-ek'-to-mi)*, excision of a sphincter.

sphincterotomy, *(sfink-ter-ot'-o-mi)*, division of sphincter muscles.

sphingolipid, *(sfin-gō-lip-id)*, sphingosine and a lipid. A component of biological membranes, especially in the brain and other nervous tissue.

sphingomyelin, *(sfin-gō-mī-el-in)*, a phospholipid formed from sphingosine found as a component of biological membranes. It is primarily found in the nervous system and in blood lipids.

sphingosine, *(sfin-gō-sīn)*, an amino alcohol with an unsaturated hydrocarbon chain. A constituent of sphingolipids and sphingomyelin.

sphygmocardiograph, *(sfin-gō-kar'-dē-ō-graf)*, apparatus recording both pulse and heart beats.

sphygmograph, *(sfig-mō-graf)*, an instrument which records the rate and characteristics of an arterial pulse.

sphygmomanometer, *(sfig-mo-man-om'-et-er)*, an instrument used for the noninvasive measurement of arterial blood pressure. *See* BLOOD PRESSURE.

spica, *(spi-ka)*, a bandage done in a series of 'figures of eight'. Used on the thumb, shoulder and hip, etc.

spicule, *(spi-kūl)*, fragment of bone.

spigot, plastic peg used to occlude the opening of a tube.

spina bifida, *(spī-na bif-i-da)*, a congenital neural tube defect where one or more neural arches fail to fuse in the midline. It may be accompanied by the protrusion of the meninges and nerve tissue. It is associated with a deficiency of folates in the diet and all women of child-bearing age are encouraged to have sufficient amounts; this is especially so around

73 Spermatozoon

Head containing nucleus

Body

Tail

Front view

Endpiece Side view

the time of conception and during early pregnancy. *See* MENINGOCELE, MENINGOMYELOCELE. *S. b. occulta:* a minor defect usually found by chance on X-ray.

spinal, relating to the spine. *S. anaesthetic: see* ANAESTHESIA. *S. canal:* canal formed by the vertebrae; contains the spinal cord and meninges. *S. column:* the backbone. Consists of 24 individual vertebrae – 7 cervical, 12 thoracic, 5 lumbar and 9 or 10 fused bones – 5 sacral, 4 or 5 coccygeal. *S. cord:* the part of the central nervous system within the s. canal, extending from the medulla oblongata to the level of the first or second lumbar vertebra in adults. *S. curves:* the normal curves are two primary (thoracic, sacral) and two secondary (cervical, lumbar). For abnormal curvatures *see* KYPHOSIS, LORDOSIS, SCOLIOSIS. *S. nerves:* 31 pairs of mixed nerves arising from the cord which form the peripheral nerves of the neck, trunk and limbs. *See* NERVE ROOT.

spinal cord compression (SCC), pressure on the spinal cord caused by tumour which, in most cases, is metastatic from breast, lung or gastrointestinal tract. Most cases present with pain, and prompt diagnosis is vital to prevent permanent paralysis.

spine, 1. backbone. **2.** a process on a bone.

spinhaler, a nebulizer (atomizer) that delivers a pre-set dose of the contained drug.

spinnbarkeit, (spin-bar-kīt), the slippery, elastic cervical mucus which can be drawn out on a glass slide. It is associated with ovulation and can be used to determine peak fertility. *See,* NATURAL FAMILY PLANNING.

spiral, a method of bandaging. *S. fracture: see* FRACTURE.

Spirillum, a genus of small spiral bacteria. *S. minus* causes one form of rat-bite fever.

spiritual beliefs, the system of religious or non-religious (secular) beliefs which an individual chooses as a personal guide to coping with moral issues and making sense of human existence and endeavour.

Spirochaetales, (spi-ro-kē-ta-les), the spirochaetes. An order of bacteria which includes the genera: *Treponema, Leptospira, Borrelia.* They are slender spiral structures capable of movement although they are non-flagellate. They cause diseases such as syphilis and Weil's disease.

spirograph, (spī-rō-graf), an instrument which records respiratory movements.

spirometer, (spi-rom′-e-ter), instrument for measuring the amount of air moved in and out of the lungs from which various capacities and changes in volumes can be calculated. Used as part of respiratory (pulmonary) function assessment.

Spitz–Holter valve, a device used in the treatment of hydrocephalus to drain cerebrospinal fluid from the ventricles of the brain into the venous circulation (superior vena cava or right atrium).

splanchnic, (splank′-nik), pertaining to the viscera. *S. nerves:* group of sympathetic nerve fibres which supply the viscera.

splanchnology, (splank-nol-o-ji), the study of the viscera.

spleen, a vascular lymphoid organ situated in the left upper abdomen. It forms part of the monocyte–macrophage system (reticuloendothelial), its functions include: destruction of old red cells and platelets, filtering blood for microorganisms, lymphocyte and antibody production, fetal red cell production and possibly serving as a reservoir for blood.

splenectomy, (*splen-ek´-to-mi*), removal of the spleen.

splenic, pertaining to the spleen. *S. flexure:* 90° bend of left colon near the spleen.

spleniculus, (*splen-ik-ū-lus*), an accessory spleen.

splenitis, (*splen-ī´-tis*), inflammation of the spleen.

splenocaval, relating to the spleen and inferior vena cava, usually referring to the anastomosis of the splenic vein to the vena cava to relieve hepatic portal hypertension.

splenomegaly, (*splen-ō-meg-a-li*), an enlarged spleen.

splenorenal, (*splē-no-rē-nal*), relating to the spleen and kidney. *S. anastomosis:* an operation to relieve hepatic portal hypertension where the splenic vein is joined to the renal vein.

splint, an appliance which supports or immobilises a part. Uses include: during healing, e.g. fractures, and the prevention and correction of deformity.

splinter haemorrhages, subungual haemorrhages. Characteristically occur in infective endocarditis.

spondyle, a vertebra.

spondylitis, (*spon-di-lī-tis*), inflammation of the vertebrae. *Ankylosing s.:* a rheumatic disease characterized by a rigid spine due to ossification of the ligaments and joints. It occurs mainly in young males and affects the spinal, sacroiliac and costovertebral joints. There is pain, loss of movement and deformity.

spondylolisthesis, (*spon-di-lō-lis-thē-sis*), defect occurring in the joints between the lower vertebral bodies. There is forward displacement and pressure on nerve roots.

spondylosis, (*spon-di-lō-sis*), ankylosis of the vertebral joints. The intervertebral disc is affected by

degenerative diseases that include osteoarthritis.

spontaneous, not forced or deliberate. Occurs without external aid. *S. abortion:* miscarriage. *See* ABORTION. *S. fracture: see* PATHOLOGICAL FRACTURE. *S. version:* unaided conversion of a transverse lie to a cephalic or podalic one.

sporadic, a disease occurring as a few isolated cases in a district. *Cf.* ENDEMIC, EPIDEMIC.

spore, 1. a reproductive body produced by certain plants, particularly fungi, and by protozoa. **2.** round or oval structures produced by some bacteria, e.g. the genus *Clostridium*. The spore has reduced metabolic activity and allows the organism to withstand unfavourable environmental conditions.

sporotrichosis, (*spo-rō-tri-kō-sis*), a subcutaneous infection caused by the fungus *Sporothrix schenckii*. It causes ulcers, abscess formation and lymphatic involvement.

spotted fever, 1. meningococcal meningitis. **2.** rickettsial diseases such as Rocky Mountain spotted fever.

sprain, joint injury due to sudden over-stretching of surrounding ligaments and tendons without dislocation or fracture. There is swelling due to effusion.

spreadsheet, a computer program which allows data manipulation in cells which are arranged in rows and columns.

sprue, chronic malabsorption associated with various conditions. It may be non-tropical or tropical and is characterized by: diarrhoea, abdominal pain, anaemia, sore tongue, weight loss and foul stools.

spur, a small projection of bone.

sputum, expectorated matter from the air passages. Different types

325

include: mucoid, mucopurulent, rusty (altered blood), frothy in pulmonary oedema and blood-stained.

squamous, (skwā-mus), scaly. *S. bone*: part of temporal bone. *S. cell carcinoma*: 1. common malignant tumour of the skin which responds well to treatment. 2. common malignant tumour of the bronchus is usually poorly differentiated. *S. epithelium*: the epithelium found covering body surfaces.

squint, see STRABISMUS.

St. Vitus' dance, Sydenham's chorea. May follow a streptococcal sore throat. See CHOREA.

stable factor, (proconvertin), factor VII in clotting.

staccato speech, (stak-ah-tō), see SCANNING SPEECH.

stages of labour, see LABOUR.

staging, a way of classifying malignant tumours according to type and extent. *TNM s.*: classification of malignancy on tumour size and infiltration (T), lymph node involvement (N) and metastatic spread (M). Important for assessing prognosis and choosing the most effective and appropriate treatment modality.

stain, dye used to colour tissue or microorganisms prior to microscopic examination, or to produce a reaction. See GRAM'S STAIN.

stammering, stuttering. A speech defect where there is hesitation and repetition of words or syllables.

standard deviation (SD), in statistics, a measure of dispersion of scores around the mean value.

standard error (SE), in statistics, a measure of variability of many mean values of different samples from a population. Used to calculate the chance of a sample mean being bigger or smaller than the mean for the population. Often used inappropriately instead of standard deviation, which should be used to measure variability of individuals in a sample.

stapedectomy, (stā-ped-ek-to-mi), removal of the stapes and insertion of a prosthesis and graft, which allows sound conduction. Used to treat otosclerosis.

stapediolysis, (sta-pe-de-ol'-i-sis), operation used in otosclerosis where the stapes is released.

stapes, (stā'-pēz), one of the three ossicles of the middle ear; stirrup-shaped. See EAR.

Staphylococcus, (staf-i-lo'-kok-us), a genus of Gram-positive bacteria which grow in clusters on culture plates. Some staphylococci are commensal on the skin and are found in the nasopharynx, axillae and perineum of some individuals. Staphylococcal infections include boils, wound infections, endocarditis, pneumonia, food poisoning, toxic shock syndrome and septicaemia. The genus includes the major pathogen *S. aureus* which produces the enzyme coagulase. Some strains produce a powerful exotoxin and others are methicillin-resistant. See METHICILLIN (MULTI)-RESISTANT STAPHYLOCOCCUS AUREUS. *S. epidermidis*: a skin commensal that does not produce coagulase. It causes wound infection and is increasingly responsible for infection involving prosthetic valves, intravascular devices and peritoneal dialysis catheters.

staphyloma, (staf-i-lō'-ma), any protrusion of the sclerotic or corneal coats of the eyeball due to inflammation.

starch, carbohydrate. A storage polysaccharide of plants, present in cereals and potato, etc.

Starling's law of the heart, the force of myocardial contraction is proportional to the length (stretching) of the ventricular muscle fibres (within physiological limits). As the heart fills during diastole the fibres stretch and the next contraction is more powerful. This relationship between length and tension is known as Starling's law.

startle reflex, also called **Moro reflex.** Normally present in newborns, who when startled throw out their limbs and then bring them together as if to embrace. *See* MORO REFLEX.

stasis, (stā-sis), standing still. Sluggish flow or stagnation. *Intestinal s.*: a holdup in the passage of the bowel contents. *Venous s.*: slowing of the circulation which results in congestion of blood in the organs and veins.

static, at rest; not moving. *S. electricity*: produced by friction. A hazard in places such as operating theatres where explosive gases are used.

statistical significance, in research an expression of how likely it is the results occurred by chance, e.g. 0.05, 0.01 and 0.001 levels. *See* P VALUE.

statistics, science of numerical data collection, analysis and evaluation.

status, condition. *S. asthmaticus*: *see* SEVERE ACUTE ASTHMA. *S. epilepticus*: a situation where epileptic fits occur in rapid succession without pause or recovery; it is an emergency and requires immediate treatment.

statute law, statutory. Law made by Acts of Parliament.

steatoma, (stē-at-ō-ma), **1.** a fatty tumour. **2.** a sebaceous cyst.

steatorrhoea, (stē-at-or-ē-a), passing undigested fat in the stools which are pale, bulky and offensive. Occurs when digestion or absorption of fat is defective.

steatosis, (stē-at-ō'-sis), fatty degeneration.

Stein–Leventhal syndrome, polycystic ovary syndrome. Increased ovarian and/or adrenal secretion of androgens causes hirsutism, obesity, menstrual irregularity, infertility and multiple follicular ovarian cysts.

Steinmann's pin, a pin inserted through a bone in order to apply extension in the case of fractures. *See* EXTENSION, TRACTION.

stellate, star-shaped. *S. ganglion*: sympathetic ganglion in the neck.

stem cell, *see* PLURIPOTENT STEM CELL.

stenosis, (ste-nō-sis), contraction of a canal or an orifice. *See* AORTIC STENOSIS, MITRAL VALVE, PULMONARY STENOSIS, PYLORIC STENOSIS, TRICUSPID STENOSIS.

stent, device used in a variety of situations to keep a tube or vessel open, or provide a shunt, e.g. stenting the ureters to overcome urinary obstruction.

Stensen's duct, the duct of the parotid gland. Opens into the cheek mucosa opposite the upper second molar.

stercobilin, (ster-ko-bi-lin), brown substance which colours faeces, formed from the action of intestinal bacteria on stercobilinogen.

stercobilinogen, (ster-ko-bi-lin-ō-jen), faecal urobilinogen. A substance formed by the action of intestinal bacteria on bilirubin, it is subsequently oxidized to stercobilin.

stercolith, (ster'-ko-lith), small hard mass of faeces. Faecolith.

stereognosis, (ster-ē-og-nō-sis), the ability to visualize the shape of objects by touch.

stereoscopic vision, (ster-ē-ō-skop-ik), the ability to perceive distance, depth and shape, resulting from binocular vision.

stereotactic surgery, (ster-ē-ō-tak-tik), stereotaxy. A method of operating on the brain after the exact position has been calculated using three-dimensional measurements.

stereotyping, making generalizations about particular groups in society.

sterile, 1. barren; unable to reproduce. **2.** free from microorganisms.

sterilization, 1. a surgical procedure which renders an individual sterile, e.g. division/occlusion of the uterine tubes, vasectomy. **2.** the destruction of microorganisms and spores by the use of heat, chemicals, filtration and radiation.

sternal, relating to the sternum. *S. puncture: see* MARROW PUNCTURE.

sternomastoid muscle, (*ster-nō-mas'-toyd*) muscle of neck, running from the inner end of clavicle and upper border of sternum to behind the ear. *See* TORTICOLLIS.

sternum, the breastbone.

steroids, group of organic compounds (lipids) having a common basic chemical configuration (three six-carbon rings and a five-carbon ring). They include: cholesterol, bile salts, vitamin D precursors in the skin and many hormones including the sex hormones and those from the adrenal cortex. *See* CORTICOSTEROIDS.

sterol, a compound with the basic steroid structure plus an alcohol group, e.g. ergosterol, cholesterol.

stertor, snoring type of respiration heard during sleep and in coma.

stertorous, pertaining to a snoring type of respiration.

stethoscope, instrument for listening to sounds, e.g. heart sounds, respiratory sounds.

Stevens–Johnson syndrome, a severe bullous form of erythema multiforme with ulceration of the mucous membranes and fever. It may follow infection or treatment with a sensitizing drug (allergic reaction).

stigma (*pl.* **stigmata**), mark on the skin. Also a defining characteristic

of a person or an action usually perceived negatively by others.

stilette, a probe.

stillbirth, a baby born after a period of gestation where it would be considered capable of a separate existence (viable), i.e. after 24 weeks, who shows no sign of life following complete expulsion from the uterus.

stillborn, born dead.

Still's disease, systemic-onset juvenile chronic arthritis. It is characterized by: swollen joints, arthralgia, myalgia, fever, rashes, lymphadenopathy, hepatosplenomegaly and cardiac involvement.

stimulant, an agent which causes increased activity in an organ.

stitch, 1. suture. *S. abscess:* infection around a stitch. **2.** pain in the side due to spasm of the diaphragm.

Stokes–Adams syndrome, syncope due to cerebral hypoxia resulting from intermittent complete heart block causing ventricular asystole. Also called **Adams–Stokes syndrome.**

stoma, 1. the mouth. **2.** an artificial opening of an internal organ on to the skin such as an ileostomy or colostomy. *S. nurse specialist:* a nurse specialist qualified in the support, care and management of individuals with stomas.

stomach, dilated portion of the digestive tract between the oesophagus and small bowel (duodenum) which produces gastric juice containing hydrochloric acid, enzymes and mucus (Figure 74). Its functions include: partial protein digestion, mechanical churning of food to produce chyme, destruction of some microorganisms and some absorption. *S. tube:* flexible tube used for gastric lavage. *See* HOURGLASS CONTRACTION.

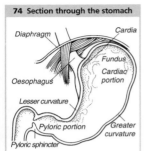

74 Section through the stomach

Diaphragm

Cardia

Oesophagus

Fundus

Cardiac portion

Lesser curvature

Pyloric portion

Greater curvature

Pyloric sphincter

stomatitis, *(stō-ma-tī'-tis)*, inflammation of the mouth. Causes include: fungal infection, bacterial infections and vitamin deficiency. *See* VINCENT'S ANGINA (UNDER ANGINA), APHTHOUS STOMATITIS.

stone, a calculus.

stools, faeces or motion discharged from the bowel. *See* MELAENA, RICE-WATER STOOLS, STEATORRHOEA.

strabismus, *(stra-biz-mus)*, squint. May be paralytic, which is due to a weakness in the muscles of the eyeball, or concomitant where there is failure to maintain the correct position of an eye which has defective vision.

strabotomy, *(stra-bot-o-mi)*, an operation to correct a squint.

strain, 1. to filter. **2.** condition due to stretching or unsuitable use of a part. **3.** a group of microorganisms within the same species.

strangulated, constricted, so that air or blood supply is cut off. *See* HERNIA.

strangury, *(stran-gu-ri)*, frequent painful desire to void small amounts of urine, due to muscle spasm associated with inflammation.

stratified, in layers. *See* EPITHELIUM.

stratum, *(stra'-tum)*, a layer.

Streptobacillus moniliformis, *(streptō-bas-il-us mon-il-ē-form-is)*, a bacteria causing a type of rat-bite fever.

Streptococcus, *(strep-tō-kok-us)*, a genus of Gram-positive bacteria which grow in pairs or chains on culture plates. They have varying haemolytic ability (beta, alpha and non-haemolytic) and some types produce a toxin. Some are commensals of the alimentary tract (*S. faecalis*) and respiratory tract (*S. viridans*). The commensal streptococci, along with the pathogens *S. pyogenes* and *S. pneumoniae*, cause serious infections that include scarlet fever, tonsillitis, otitis media, pneumonia, endocarditis, erysipelas, wound infections, meningitis, urinary tract infection and bacteraemia. Rheumatic fever and glomerulonephritis may follow haemolytic streptococcal infections. Group B streptococcus, a commensal of the vagina and gut, may cause serious infection in neonates infected by organisms present in the maternal genital tract. *See* GRIFFITHS TYPES, LANCEFIELD GROUPS.

streptodornase, *(strep-tō-dor-nāz)*, streptococcal enzyme used with streptokinase in liquefying pus and blood clots.

streptokinase, *(strep-tō-kin-āz)*, streptococcal enzyme. Plasminogen activator. Its fibrinolytic effect is used to treat various thromboembolic conditions. Used with streptodornase in wound management. *See* FIBRINOLYTIC THERAPY.

streptolysins, *(strep-to-li-sins)*, exotoxins produced by streptococci which cause red cell lysis.

Streptomyces, *(strep-tō-mī-sēz)*, a genus of branching bacteria which is an important source of antimicrobial agents such as streptomycin.

stress, the reaction to any of a variety of physical, psychological or social factors which affect physical and/or mental wellbeing. *See* GENERAL ADAPTATION SYNDROME, STRESSORS. *S. incontinence:* involuntary voiding of urine when intra-abdominal pressure rises such as with coughing. Commonly associated with cystocele and vaginal wall prolapse. *See* INCONTINENCE. *S. ulcer:* peptic ulcer associated with intense physiological stress. *See* CURLING'S ULCER.

stressors, factors which initiate stress responses. Examples include: pain, hunger, blood loss, overwork, a life crisis such as divorce, poor housing or low income. *See* GENERAL ADAPTATION SYNDROME.

striae, *(strī-ē),* scars on the thighs and abdomen caused by stretching of the dermis and rupture of elastic fibres when the abdomen enlarges, such as with pregnancy (s. gravidarum or stretch marks), tumours and ascites. Also seen with Cushing's disease and as a side-effect of glucocorticoid therapy.

striated muscle, *(strī-ā-ted),* striped voluntary muscle. *See* MUSCLE.

stricture, contraction or narrowing of a channel such as the oesophagus or urethra. It may be due to inflammation, malignancy, external pressure or spasm.

stridor, *(strī'-dor),* a harsh sound during breathing, caused by obstruction to the passage of air.

stroke, popular term for the sudden event (haemorrhage, embolus or thrombosis) affecting the cerebral blood supply. *See* CEREBROVASCULAR ACCIDENT. *Heat s.: see* HEAT STROKE.

stroke volume (SV), the difference between ventricular end diastolic volume and end systolic volume or,

put another way, the amount of blood pumped out of the heart by each ventricular contraction.

stroma, *(strō-ma),* connective or supporting tissue within an organ.

Strongyloides, *(stron-gi-loydz),* a small intestinal nematode worm.

strongyloidiasis, *(stron-gi-loy-dī-ā-sis),* a condition due to the parasitic nematode worm *Strongyloides stercoralis.* Common in the tropics, it causes diarrhoea, abdominal pain, malabsorption, anaemia, wheezing and urticaria where the larvae burrow into the skin. Systemic disease is an AIDS-defining condition.

strontium (Sr), a metallic element. Its radioactive isotope ^{90}strontium is used in radioisotope scanning.

structuralism, in psychology the study of consciousness, intellect, behaviour and feeling.

Stryker wedge frame, a special bed used to immobilize people with spinal injuries and in the management of extensive burns. It allows for turning to prone or supine by rotating the frame.

Stuart–Prower factor, factor X in blood clotting.

Student's paired test, a parametric test for statistical significance. Used to test differences in mean values for two related measurements, for example on the same individual.

Student's *t*-test for independent groups, a parametric test for statistical significance. Used to test differences in mean values of two groups.

Sturge–Weber syndrome, an inherited condition characterized by angioma of the face and underlying cerebrum, epilepsy and other neurological effects.

stuttering, *see* STAMMERING.

stye, hordeolum. Inflammation of sebaceous gland of eyelash.

stylet, *see* STILETTE.

styloid, (sti-loyd), a process of the temporal bone, ulna and radius.

styptic, agent applied to arrest bleeding; astringent, e.g. adrenaline (epinephrine).

subacute, a condition which progresses more quickly than a chronic disorder but does not become acute. *S. bacterial endocarditis: see* ENDOCARDITIS. *S. combined degeneration of the cord:* demyelination of the posterior columns and corticospinal tracts of the spinal cord due to a deficiency of vitamin B_{12}. Associated with pernicious anaemia.

subarachnoid, (sub-a-rak-noyd), below the arachnoid mater. *S. haemorrhage (SAH):* bleeding into the subarachnoid space. It may be due to the rupture of an aneurysm, extension of an intracerebral bleed or trauma. *S. space:* the space between the arachnoid and pia mater which contains cerebrospinal fluid.

subclavian, (sub-klā-vē-an), under the clavicle; the s. artery and s. vein pass under the clavicle.

subclinical, (sub-klin-ik-al), without any obvious signs of the disease.

subconscious, the part of the mind outside the range of clear consciousness, but capable of affecting conscious mental or physical reactions.

subcutaneous, (sub-kū-tā-nē-us), under the skin. *S. injection:* one given beneath the skin.

subdural, (sub-dū-ral), under the dura mater. *S. haematoma:* a collection of blood in the subdural space. It is associated with trauma and may be acute or chronic.

subinvolution, (sub-in-vo-lū-shon), a failure of the uterus to return to its normal size and position following childbirth.

subjacent, lying below.

subjective, not objective. Internal; pertaining to one's self.

sublimation, 1. the vaporization of a substance and condensation into a solid deposit. **2.** a mental defence mechanism where unacceptable motives, feelings or tendencies are transferred into an activity which is socially acceptable, e.g. aggression redirected into sport.

subliminal, (sub-lim-in-al), beneath the threshold of conscious perception.

sublingual, (sub-ling-gwal), under the tongue. *S. glands:* a pair of salivary glands.

subluxation, sprain and partial dislocation.

submandibular, below the mandible. *S. glands:* a pair of salivary glands.

submaxillary, (sub-mak-sil-a-ri), beneath the maxilla.

submucous, (sub-mū-kus), below a mucous membrane. *S. resection:* an operation to correct a deviated nasal septum.

subnormal, below normal, such as body temperature in hypothermia.

subphrenic, (sub-fren'-ik), under the diaphragm. *S. abscess:* a collection of pus beneath the diaphragm.

subpoena, an order of the court requiring a person to appear as a witness or to bring records/documents.

substance misuse, the overuse of a substance such as alcohol, tobacco or a drug to the point where health and/or social functioning is adversely affected.

substernal, under the sternum. *S. goitre:* one where part of the thyroid gland is under the sternum.

substrate, substance on which an enzyme works.

subungual, under a nail, such as a haematoma.

succussion, (su-kush-on), **1.** splashing sound produced by fluid in a hollow cavity when the patient moves. **2.** in homeopathy, the process by which natural diluted substances are shaken vigorously.

sucrase, *(sū-krāz)*, intestinal enzyme which splits sucrose into glucose and fructose.

sucrose, *(sū-krōz)*, a disaccharide present in beet and cane sugar. Consists of a glucose and fructose molecule.

suction, sucking. The use of reduced pressure to remove fluid and other material from cavities and wounds. Uses include: clearing the air passages, clearing blood from an operation site, wound drainage and evacuation of the uterine contents to terminate a pregnancy.

sudamina, *(sū-dam-i-na)*, a sweat rash.

sudden infant death syndrome (SIDS), cot death. Unexpected death of an apparently healthy infant. Aetiology is unknown but its occurrence is linked with: prone sleeping position, environmental temperature, exposure to tobacco smoke, respiratory illness and infection. Parents and others caring for infants are advised to place the baby on its back for sleeping, not to overheat, place the baby at the foot of the cot to prevent it wriggling under the bedclothes, not to smoke in the same room and to seek advice from a health professional if the baby seems unwell.

sudorific, *(sū-dor-if'-ik)*, an agent causing perspiration.

suffocation, cessation of breathing due to occlusion of air passages such as in drowning, resulting in coma and death. Asphyxia.

suffused, congested.

sugars, monosaccharide and disaccharide carbohydrates such as glucose, fructose, lactose, maltose and sucrose.

suggestibility, a state when the patient readily accepts other people's ideas and influences.

suicide, the act of deliberate self-destruction.

sulcus, *(sul'-kus)*, a furrow.

sulphaemoglobin, *(sulf-hē-mo-glō-bin)*, an abnormal haemoglobin pigment formed following the administration of some drugs. It cannot transport oxygen or carbon dioxide, and as it is not reversible in the body, it is an indirect poison. Also known as sulphmethaemoglobin.

sulphate, a salt of sulphuric acid, e.g. magnesium sulphate.

sulphuric acid, a strong inorganic acid. Highly corrosive.

summation, the accumulation of effects such as those concerned with sensory stimuli, transmission of nerve impulses or muscle contraction. It may be spatial or temporal.

summative evaluation, an assessment or judgement about performance done after the event, e.g. a nursing action evaluated on all the relevant features including the outcomes.

sunstroke, *see* HEAT STROKE.

superciliary, *(sū-per-sil-i-a-ri)*, relating to the eyebrow.

supercilium, *(sū-per-sil'-i-um)*, the eyebrow.

superego, *(sū-per-ē-go)*, according to Freud, one of the three main aspects of the personality (the other two being the id and ego); the part of the mind concerned with morality and self-criticism, it operates at a partly conscious, but mostly unconscious, level and corresponds roughly to what is called 'conscience'.

superfecundation, *(sū-per-fe-kun-dā-shon)*, the fertilization of two oöcytes, released during the same cycle, by spermatozoa from separate acts of insemination.

superfetation, *(sū-per-fet-ā'-shon)* the presence of two fetuses of different maturity. Resulting from oöcytes released and fertilized during different cycles.

superficial, near the surface, e.g. superficial veins of the leg.

superinfection, an infection that follows destruction of the normal flora with broad-spectrum antibiotics. This allows other microorganisms, such as *Clostridiuim difficile,* to flourish in the bowel without competition. *See* PSEUDOMEMBRANOUS COLITIS.

superior, above. The upper of two organs.

supernumerary, extra, not counted as part of normal numbers.

superoxide, *see* FREE RADICAL.

supervision, direction, surveillance and control. *Clinical s.*: process where a clinical supervisor assists another practitioner to develop his or her practice and knowledge. A continous process aimed at maintaining and enhancing standards of clinical practice in many disciplines, e.g. psychotherapy, nursing.

supination, turning the palm of the hand upwards.

supine, lying face upwards; in the case of the forearm, having the palm uppermost.

supplemental air, air which remains in the lung following normal expiration.

suppository, a cone of material which melts at body temperature, to which drugs may be added. It is inserted rectally (blunt end first to aid retention) as an evacuant or to administer a drug such as an antibiotic.

suppression, 1. failure to secrete. *S. of urine*: when no urine is produced in renal failure. 2. preventing an activity. 3. a mental defence mechanism, whereby individuals voluntarily force painful thoughts out of the mind.

suppuration, the formation of pus.

supracondylar, (*sū-pra-kon-dĭ-lar*), above the condyles. *S. fracture*: a

fracture above the lower end of the humerus or femur.

supraorbital, (*sū-pra-or'-bĭ-tal*), above the orbit such as the s. ridge of the frontal bone.

suprapubic, (*sū-pra-pū-bĭk*), above the pubic arch such as s. catheterization.

suprarenal, (*sū-pra-rē-nal*), above the kidney. *See* ADRENAL GLANDS.

supraventricular, (*sū-pra-ven-trik-ū-lar*), above the ventricles. *S. ectopic heart rhythms*: cardiac arrhythmias which arise from structures in the atria or AV node; they include: s. tachycardia, extrasystoles, atrial flutter and atrial fibrillation.

surfactants, (*sur-fak-tantz*), agents that reduce surface tension. In the lungs, pulmonary surfactant, a phospholipid which prevents alveolar collapse, is produced by type II pneumocytes. *See* NEONATAL RESPIRATORY DISTRESS SYNDROME.

surgery, the branch of medical science concerned with conditions requiring operative treatment.

surgical, pertaining to surgery. *S. neck*: narrow part of the humerus, below the tuberosities. *See* EMPHYSEMA.

surrogate, a substitute for a person or object.

survey, a data collection method. It may be postal, telephone, interview or via the internet.

susceptible, liable to, e.g. infection.

suspension, 1. hanging. 2. temporary stoppage of a function. 3. undissolved particles in water. *See* VENTROSUSPENSION.

suspensory, describes a structure that holds another in position such as the s. ligament of the eye. *S. bandage*: one used to give support to the testes and scrotum.

sutures, 1. ligatures or stitches of silk, catgut, nylon, dexon, and wire, etc. used internally and to close wounds. **2.** the union of flat bones by their margins, e.g. bones of the skull.

SVGA, abbrev. for **super video graphics array**. A type of screen display which supports high-resolution colour images.

swab, pieces of material used for a variety of purposes which include: cleaning wounds, absorbing exudate from wounds, and removing blood during surgery. Also describes a small piece of material, e.g. sterile cotton wool, on a shaft of wood, plastic or metal. It is used to collect material for microbiological examination.

Swan–Ganz catheter, used to monitor pulmonary artery wedge pressure. Useful in the management of cardiogenic and hypovolaemic shock. *See* PULMONARY ARTERY WEDGE PRESSURE.

sweat, perspiration. Secretion of the sweat glands containing water, electrolytes (sodium, chloride) and nitrogenous and other waste. Concerned mainly with temperature regulation. *S. glands*: *see* APOCRINE, ECCRINE. *S. test*: *see* CYSTIC FIBROSIS.

sycosis, (*si-kō-sis*), inflammation of the hair follicles, especially of the beard.

Sydenham's chorea, *see* CHOREA.

symbiosis, (*sim-b ī-ō ′-sis*), a close relationship between two organisms, whose mutual association is necessary to each, although neither is parasitic.

symblepharon, (*sim-blef′-a-ron*), adhesion of the eyelids to the eyeball.

symmetrical, equal. Both sides the same.

sympathectomy, (*sim-path-ek-to-mi*), surgical division of sympathetic nerves.

sympathetic, having sympathy. *S. nervous system*: part of the autonomic nervous system having thoracolumbar outflow. Its actions are usually concerned with stimulation; the flight or fight response which includes dilation of pupil and bronchi, increased heart rate and cessation of digestion. Adrenal medulla hormones augment the effects of the s. system which oppose those of the parasympathetic system. *S. ophthalmitis*: inflammation leading to blindness in the uninjured eye following a penetrating wound in the other eye.

sympatholytic, (*sim-path-ō-lit-ik*), agent that blocks or opposes sympathetic activity. An antagonist, e.g. propranolol. *See* ALPHA-ADRENOCEPTOR ANTAGONIST, BETA-ADRENOCEPTOR ANTAGONIST.

sympathomimetic, (*sim-path-ō-mi-met-ik*), agent whose action is similar to those of sympathetic nerves. An agonist, e.g. salbutamol. *See* ALPHA-ADRENOCEPTOR AGONIST, BETA-ADRENOCEPTOR AGONIST.

symphysiotomy, (*sim-fiz-ē-ot-o-mi*), operation to divide the symphysis pubis. May be required to facilitate delivery if the pelvis is contracted.

symphysis, (*sim-fi-sis*), a type of slightly movable cartilaginous joint where a pad of fibrocartilage separates the two bones. *S. pubis*: the joint formed by the two public bones.

symptom, a noticeable change in the body and its functions; evidence of disease. Usually refers to those perceived by the patient which are subjective, but those apparent to others are termed objective.

symptomatology, (*simp′-tō-ma-tol-o-ji*), a study of the symptoms of disease.

synapse, (*sī-naps*), the gap between the axon of one neurone and the dendrites of another, or the gap between an axon and an effector cell. Transmission of the nerve impulse across the gap depends upon the release of a chemical neurotransmitter such as acetylcholine.

synapsis, *(sin-ap-sis),* pairing of homologous chromosomes to form a bivalent during meiosis I.

synarthrosis, *(sin-ar-thrō-sis),* fibrous immovable joint such as the skull sutures.

synchondrosis, *(sin-kon-drō'-sis),* a cartilaginous joint formed by the epiphyseal plates prior to their ossification.

synchysis, *(sin'-ki-sis)* softening of the vitreous humor of the eye. *S. scintillans*: bright particles found in the vitreous humour.

synclitism, *(sin'-klit-izm),* descent of the fetal head through the pelvis with its planes parallel to those of the pelvis.

syncope, *(sin-ko-pe),* fainting. Due to a temporary interruption in cerebral blood flow.

syncytium, *(sin-sit-ē-um),* a mass of cytoplasm, containing many nuclei. A tissue where boundaries between individual cells do not exist or are poorly defined (pseudosyncytium). This facilitates the rapid passage of impulses, contraction waves, etc. across the tissue, such as in myocardial contraction.

syndactyly, webbed fingers or toes.

syndesmosis, *(sin-des-mō'-sis),* a type of synarthrosis where a membrane connects the bones to allow some 'give', e.g. inferior tibiofibular joint.

syndrome, collection of symptoms and signs which form a recognizable pattern of disease.

synechia, *(sin-ek'-i-a)* adhesion of the iris to the cornea, or to the crystalline lens.

synergist, *(sin-er-jist),* an agent cooperating with another. One partner in a synergic action, e.g. drug or muscle.

synergy, *(sin-er-ji),* the working together of two or more agents.

synovectomy, *(sī-nō-vek'-to-mi),* operation to remove synovial membrane.

synovial, *(sī-nō-vi-al),* pertaining to special membrane, fluid and the joints containing them. *S. fluid*: viscous lubricating fluid secreted by s. membranes. *S. joint*: diarthroses. Freely movable joints whose cavity is lined with specialized membrane. *S. membrane*: fluid-secreting membrane lining the cavity of a freely movable joint, it does not extend to the articulating surfaces.

synovitis, *(sī-nō-vī'-tis),* inflammation of the synovial membrane of a joint.

synthesis, building up complex substances from the combination of simpler units.

syphilide, a skin rash associated with secondary syphilis.

syphilis, a sexually transmitted infection which is classified legally as venereal. It is caused by the spirochaete *Treponema pallidum* and may be congenital or acquired. *Congenital s.*: transmitted from mother to fetus via the placenta. The affected infant may exhibit certain characteristic features which include: rash, abnormal teeth and keratitis. *Acquired s.*: contracted during sexual contact with an infected person. There are four stages: 1. primary with chancre development and lymphadenopathy. 2. secondary with rash, fever, condylomata lata, mucosal ulcers and lymphadenopathy. 3. tertiary occurs after many years with skin lesions such as gumma. 4. quarternary with cardiovascular and nervous system involvement. Syphilis is diagnosed by various serological tests which include: Venereal Disease Research Laboratory (VDRL) test and *T. pallidum* haemagglutination assay.

syringe, instrument for injecting fluids or for irrigating or aspirating cavities. *S. driver*: device used to administer a preset drug dose via a syringe over a given period of time.

syringomyelia, *(si-rin-gō-mī-el-i-a)*, a rare condition with cavity formation in the spinal cord and brainstem. The effects include: loss of pain and temperature sensation in the hands with muscle weakness and wasting.

syringomyelocele, *(si-rin-gō-mī-el-ō-sēl)*, a severe type of spina bifida. The central canal is dilated and the thinned-out posterior part of the spinal cord is in the hernia.

systematic review, a systematic approach to literature reviews (published and unpublished) that reduces random errors and bias.

Système International d'Unités, *see* APPENDIX 4.

systemic, affecting the whole body. *S. inflammatory response syndrome (SIRS)*: systemic inflammatory response syndrome (SIRS): and multiple organ dysfunction syndrome (MODS) frequently coexist in critically ill patients. Previously, septic shock, sepsis or septicaemia were terms used to describe the clinical scenario of pyrexia, tachycardia, tachypnoea and deranged white cell count. It was then discovered that a number of other factors, i.e. in the complete absence of infection, could also precipitate the same clinical features, including trauma, reduced perfusion, major burns and pancreatitis. This resulted in the adoption of the term SIRS. Regardless of the cause, SIRS results in a response of the inflammatory system which is unnatural, in that it is exaggerated and not localized, causing widespread physiological derangement and damage. *S. lupus erythematosus (SLE)*: a connective tissue disease with antibodies and immune complexes affecting many systems. The aetiology is multifactorial with genetic, immunological, environmental and possible infective elements. It affects joints, kidneys, heart, skin, lungs and blood vessels.

systole, contraction phase of the cardiac cycle when the heart contracts. *See* DIASTOLE, EXTRASYSTOLES.

systolic, pertaining to systole. *S. murmur*: heart murmur heard during systole. *S. blood pressure*: *see* BLOOD PRESSURE.

T₃, *see* TRIIODOTHYRONINE.

T₄, *see* THYROXINE.

T lymphocyte, *see* LYMPHOCYTES.

T tube, a tube inserted into the common bile duct to drain bile until the duct becomes patent again following surgery.

tabes, (*tā-bēz*), wasting. *T. dorsalis*: locomotor ataxia. Degeneration of the posterior columns in the spinal cord with sensory loss, occurs in quarternary syphilis. Results in 'lightning pains', loss of proprioception, staggering gait and Charcot's joints.

tablet, a solid form of a drug dosage. It may be swallowed whole, dissolved in water or in the buccal cavity or sublingually, or enteric-coated to ensure no absorption occurs until it reaches the small bowel.

taboos, behaviours banned by individual societies, such as incest.

tabular, data arranged in a table.

tachycardia, (*tak-ē-kar-di-a*), rapid heart rate (in excess of 100 beats/min in adults).

tachyphrenia, (*tak-ē-fren-i-a*), overactivity of mental processes.

tachypnoea, (*tak-ip-nē-a*), rapid respiratory rate (in excess of 20 breaths/min in adults).

tactile, relating to touch. *T. corpuscles*: cutaneous end organs of the tactile nerves.

taenia, (*tē-ni-a*), flat strip. *T. coli*: three bands of longitudinal muscle of the colon; shorter than the colon, they produce puckering or haustrations.

Taenia, (*tē-ni-a*), a genus of cestodes. Tapeworm. *T. saginata*: the beef tapeworm; *T. solium*: the pork tapeworm. *See* CYSTICERCOSIS, ECHINOCOCCUS, HYDATID CYSTS, TAPEWORM.

tail of Spence, a tail of breast tissue extending into the axilla.

talipes, (*tal'-i-pēz*), clubfoot (Figure 75). A foot deformity, often congenital. *T. calcaneus*: heel projected downwards. *T. equinus*: heel lifted from the ground. *T. valgus*: eversion: the foot is turned outwards. *T. varus*: inversion: the foot is turned inwards. Combinations of these four basic types also exist, e.g. t. equinovarus (Figure 76).

talus, (*tāl-us*), large bone of the ankle. One of the seven tarsal bones.

tampon, a plug used in the vagina or other orifice to absorb blood or secretions.

tamponade, compression. *Cardiac t.*: the presence of blood or fluid in the pericardium inhibits heart action. It may be due to trauma, surgery or effusion.

tantalum (Ta), (*tan'-ta-lum*), a relatively inert metallic element used in bone surgery as plates or wires.

tapeworm, cestodes. Humans are infected by eating contaminated undercooked meat (beef or pork). Or from undercooked fish contaminated by *Diphyllobothrium latum* (fish tapeworm). Treatment is with anthelmintic drugs. Cats and dogs are the definitive host for the tapeworm *Dipylidium caninum* which occasionally infects humans. *See* TAENIA.

337

75 Talipes

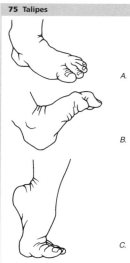

A = talipes valgus,
B = talipes calcaneus with some cavus deformity,
C = talipes equinus

76 Talipes equinovarus

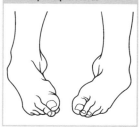

GLANDS. *T. plate*: connective tissue forming the eyelids.

tarsalgia, *(tar-sal'-ji-a)*, ankle pain.

tarsoplasty, *(tar-sō-plas'-ti)*, plastic surgery of the eyelid.

tarsorrhaphy, *(tar-sōr-a-fi)*, stitching the eyelids together to protect the cornea or to allow an abrasion to heal.

tarsus, 1. the seven bones of the ankle. **2.** the connective tissue framework of the eyelid.

tartar, calculus. Hard deposit which forms on the teeth.

taste, the chemical sense of gustation. It is closely linked with smell. *T. buds*: specialized sensory end organs on the tongue, epiglottis and pharynx. They are sensitive to four basic tastes: sweet, sour, bitter and salt.

taurocholic acid, *(taw-rō-kō-lik)*, one of the bile acids.

taxis, hand manipulation for restoring a part to its natural position, such as reducing a hernia.

taxonomy, a classification.

Tay–Sachs disease, an inherited lipid storage disease with accumulation of ganglioside (carbohydrate-rich sphingolipid) within the nervous system, resulting in mental deterioration, blindness and death. The

tapping, *see* ASPIRATION.

tardive dyskinesia, *(tar-div dis-kin-ē-zi-a)*, a disorder characterized by repeated involuntary movements of limbs, trunk and face. May be seen as a side-effect of treatment with typical neuroleptics, especially the phenothiazines.

target cells, abnormal red cells seen in certain liver diseases and haemoglobinopathies.

tarsal, 1. relating to the seven bones of the ankle or tarsus. **2.** relating to the eyelids. *T. glands: see* MEIBOMIAN recessive gene is most commonly carried by people of Ashkenazic Jewish origins.

team nursing, a method of care delivery designed to provide maximum continuity of patient-centred care. A small team of nurses, working together but led by one registered nurse, is responsible and accountable for the assessment, planning and implementation of the care of a particular group of patients for the length of time they require care in a particular setting. It differs from patient allocation or primary nursing in that it is based on the belief that a small group of nurses working together can give better care than if working individually, using the skills of all the team members to the benefit of each patient, but retaining continuity of care. Effective verbal and written communication between the team members is vital.

tears, secretion of the lacrimal gland.

technetium (Tc), (tek-ne-she-um), a radioactive element. The isotope ^{99m}Tc produced from molybdenum is widely used in radionuclide imaging.

teeth, 1. first dentition. *Deciduous t. (milk teeth):* 20 teeth which erupt between 5–6 months and $2\frac{1}{2}$ years (Figure 77a). **2.** second dentition: 32 teeth which start to replace the deciduous teeth at about 6 years. The process is nearly complete at 12 years; the third molars (wisdom teeth), if they erupt, will appear between 18 and 25 years (Figure 77b). *See* TOOTH.

teething, eruption of teeth, especially the first dentition.

tegument, the skin.

tela, tissue formed like a web.

telangiectasis, (te-lan-ji-ek′-tā-sis), a group of dilated capillaries. *Hereditary haemorrhagic t.:* lesions occur in the skin, mucosa and intestine.

telencephalon, part of the developing brain above the diencephalon, it forms the cerebrum.

teletherapy, (tel-ē-ther-a-pi), radiotherapy using rays produced by a source some distance from the tumour, e.g. linear accelerator, ^{60}Co (cobalt) machine.

telomeres, protective covering present on the ends of chromosomes. They normally prevent chromosomal

77a First dentition

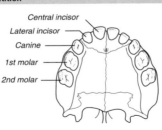

Central incisor
Lateral incisor
Canine
1st molar
2nd molar

77b Second dentition

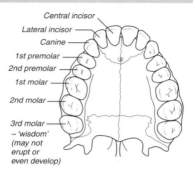

- Central incisor
- Lateral incisor
- Canine
- 1st premolar
- 2nd premolar
- 1st molar
- 2nd molar
- 3rd molar – 'wisdom' (may not erupt or even develop)

damage during cell division, but after 50 or so divisions the telomeres no longer function properly. This eventually leads to genetic disruption and cell death. *See* APOPTOSIS.

telophase, *(te-lo-fāz),* last stage in mitosis and meiosis.

temperament, a person's mental outlook.

temperature, measurement of the degree of heat. Average normal body temperature in humans is 37°C (98.6°F) with a diurnal variation of between 0.5 and 1.0°C over the 24-hour period. *T. method*: a type of natural family planning where the fertile period is determined by the slight increase in temperature occurring at ovulation which persists until the next menstruation.

temporal, 1. pertaining to time. *T. summation*: see SUMMATION. **2.** pertaining to the temple. *T. arteritis*: giant cell arteritis. Inflammation of the temporal, carotid and cerebral

arteries with severe headache, fever and thickened vessels. *T. artery*: vessel supplying the scalp. *T. bone*: one of the bones of the skull. *T. lobe*: cerebral lobe containing the auditory and olfactory cortex. *T. lobe epilepsy*: see EPILEPSY.

temporomandibular, *(tem-por-ō-man dib'-ū-lar),* pertaining to the temporal bone and mandible, such as the synovial joint of the lower jaw. *T. joint syndrome*: pain in the region of the joint, frequently caused by the malocclusion of the teeth, resulting in joint malposition and abnormal muscle activity and bruxism. There may be clicking and impaired jaw movement.

tenacious, thick and sticky such as sputum or mucus.

tenaculum, *(te-nak-ū-lum),* an instrument for grasping tissue.

tendinitis, *(ten-din-ī'-tis),* inflammation of a tendon.

tendon, band of fibrous tissue that attaches muscle to bone. *Achilles t*: the large tendon joining the gastronemius to the calcaneum. *T. reflex*: see REFLEX.

tendovaginitis, *(ten-dō-vaj-in-ī-tis)*, see TENOSYNOVITIS.

tenesmus, *(te-nes-mus)*, painful and ineffectual straining to defecate or micturate.

tennis elbow, pain near the insertion of the extensor muscles at the lateral epicondyle. Due to prolonged or unusual use.

tenoplasty, *(te-nō-plas'-ti)*, plastic surgery to a tendon.

tenorrhaphy, *(ten-or-a-fi)*, operation to suture a tendon.

tenosynovectomy, *(ten-ō-sin-ō-vek'-to-mi)*, operation to remove a tendon sheath.

tenosynovitis, *(ten-ō-sīn-ō-vī'-tis)*, inflammation of the tendon sheath.

tenotomy, *(ten-ot'-ō-mi)*, cutting a tendon.

tension, stretching. A state of stress or unrest.

tent, plastic cover such as an oxygen or isolation tent.

tentorial, pertaining to the tentorium. *T. herniation*: a bulging of brain tissue into the tentorium resulting from raised intracranial pressure.

tentorium cerebelli, *(ten-tor-i-um se-ri-bel-li)*, a fold of dura between the cerebrum and cerebellum. Damage during birth may result in haemorrhage.

teratogen, *(ter-at-o-jen)*, any agent such as drug, radiation or microorganism that may cause serious embryonic or fetal malformation.

teratoma, *(ter-at-ō-ma)*, a benign or more usually a malignant tumour which arises from residual embryonic cells. Sites include: ovary, testes and retroperitoneal structures.

teres, *(tēr-ēz)*, round and smooth. *Ligamentum t.*: ligament holding the femur in the acetabulum, or the fibrous remnant of the fetal umbilical vein within the falciform liga-

ment of the liver. *T. minor* and *major*: two muscles of the shoulder.

term, see FULL TERM.

terminal care, the management and care of the dying. The aims are pain relief, symptom control and the provision of emotional support for the individual, his/her family and friends.

termination of pregnancy (TOP), an induced therapeutic abortion which fulfils the criteria of the Abortion Act 1967 (amended 1990). The methods employed depend upon the stage of gestation and include: an oral progesterone agonist (mifepristone) with vaginal prostaglandin as an alternative to surgical termination (within 49 days of the last menstrual period), suction evacuation, dilatation and curettage and prostaglandins or other substances administered transcervically, abdominally in the amniotic sac or intravenously.

tertian, *(ter-shan)*, a form of malaria which recurs every 48 hours.

tertiary, *(ter-shē-er-ē)*, third. *T. care*: hospital care in a specialized regional centre, e.g. specializing in cardiac surgery. *T. prevention*: measures taken to minimize the effects of an established disease. *T. syphilis*: see SYPHILIS.

test, 1. a trial or examination. **2.** a reaction distinguishing one substance from another.

testicles, see TESTIS.

testicular, *(tes-tik'-ū-lar)*, pertaining to the testes. *T. self-examination*: a means of detecting changes, such as cancers, at a stage where curative treatment is possible.

testis *(pl. testes)*, male gonad. One of two glandular structures contained within the scrotum, which produce spermatozoa (spermatogenesis) and male hormones. *Undescended t.*: a testis which fails to migrate from the abdominal cavity to the scrotum.

testosterone, *(tes-tos'-ter-ōn),* the major androgen, a steroid hormone derived from cholesterol. Secreted by the testes, it is responsible for the development of the male secondary sexual characteristics and proper reproductive functioning.

tetanus, *(tet-a-nus),* **1. lockjaw.** Disease caused by *Clostridium tetani.* An anaerobic spore-forming bacteria which is commensal in the gut of humans and domestic animals, found in soil and dust. The organism enters through penetrating wounds contaminated with soil. Its powerful exotoxin affects motor nerves causing muscle spasm, convulsions and rigidity. Active immunization with t. toxoid and passive immunization with t. immunoglobulin is available as part of the routine programme; in conjunction with diphtheria and pertussis, as regular booster doses and at times of increased risk. *See* OPISTHOTONOS, RISUS SARDONICUS, TRISMUS. **2.** In muscle contraction the summation which increases force by increasing the frequency of stimulation to the maximum to produce a sustained contraction.

tetany, *(tet-a-ni),* a condition of muscular hyperexcitability. It is marked by cramps and spasm in the hands and feet (carpopedal spasm) due to a low serum calcium or to alkalosis where the amount of available calcium is reduced. Causes include: hypoparathyroidism, rickets, hyperventilation, and excessive intake of alkalis. *See* CHVOSTEK'S SIGN, TROUSSEAU'S TEST.

tetralogy of Fallot, *see* FALLOT'S TETRALOGY.

tetraplegia, *(tet-ra-plē'-ji-a),* paralysis of all four limbs. *Syn.* quadriplegia.

tetravalent, *(tet-ra-va-lent),* having a valence of four, such as carbon.

tetrogenesis, *(tet-rō-jen-e-sis),* defective embryonic development resulting in serious fetal malformation.

thalamic, *(thal-am-ik),* pertaining to the thalamus.

thalamus *(pl.* **thalami),** *(thal-am-us),* two areas of grey matter situated in the cerebral hemispheres. Acts as a relay station for most incoming sensory impulses.

thalassaemia, *(thal-a-sē-mi-a),* a group of inherited haemoglobinopathies resulting from reduced or absent synthesis of globin chains producing haemolytic anaemia. They are inherited in an autosomal recessive pattern. They are seen most commonly in populations around the Mediterranean and in South-East Asia. There are three main types: (a) Beta-thalassaemia major (Cooley's anaemia). A severe form where individuals are unable to synthesize beta-chains of adult haemoglobin (HbA). It is caused by inheriting two abnormal genes (homozygous). There is severe anaemia, jaundice and hepatomegaly and splenomegaly. Treatment includes bone marrow transplant, blood transfusion, folic acid and chelating agents, such as desferrioxamine for iron overload. (b) Beta-thalassaemia minor denotes the carrier state where the individual has only one abnormal gene (heterozygous). The individual may be asymptomatic or have mild microcytic, hypochromic anaemia with target cells and punctate basophilia. (c) Alpha-thalassaemia, a form where individuals are unable to synthesize alpha chains because the genes (4) have been deleted. The effects depend on the number of genes deleted; i.e. one gene has no effects, two genes deleted cause mild anaemia, if three genes are deleted the person ha haemoglobin H disease requiring treatment with folic acid, and still-birth occurs where all four are deleted. *See*: ANAEMIA.

thallium (Tl), a metallic element. Many of its compounds are highly toxic. ^{201}Tl, a radionuclide used in the localization of a myocardial infarction.

theca, *(thē'-ka),* a covering such as the dura mater of the spinal cord or a tendon sheath. *T. folliculi*: the hormone-secreting covering of a developing ovarian follicle.

thenar, *(thē'-nar),* relating to the palm of the hand or base of thumb.

therapeutic, of benefit. Pertaining to treatment. *T. abortion*: *see* TERMINATION OF PREGNANCY. *T. community*: one where the total environment supports the treatment of those with mental health problems. *T. index*: an indicator of the difference between the drug dose that produces a therapeutic effect and the dose which causes toxic effects. It alerts the prescriber to the safety margins for a particular drug, but the t. index will vary between people, who all process drugs in an individual way.

therapeutics, *(ther-a-pū'-tiks),* the branch of medicine which deals with treatment.

therapist, a person skilled and qualified in a particular area of treatment, e.g. psychotherapist.

therapy, treatment of disease such as physiotherapy, occupational t., and speech and language t.

thermal, pertaining to heat. T. dilution: a method of determining cardiac output.

thermistor, *(ther-mis-tor),* device able to detect minute changes in temperature.

thermogenesis, *(ther-mō-jen-e-sis),* heat production.

thermography, the detection of minute differences in temperature

over regions of the body using an infrared device (thermograph) sensitive to radiant heat. It can be used to study blood flow disorders, and in the detection of some cancers, e.g. breast cancer, that show as 'hot spots'.

thermolabile, *(ther-mō-lā-bīl),* substance which undergoes change with temperature.

thermometer, device for recording temperature. Types include: clinical, electronic, oral, rectal, room, subnormal, tympanic membrane.

thermophilic, *(ther-mō-fil-ik),* applied to an organism which flourishes at high temperatures.

thermoreceptor, heat-sensitive nerve ending.

thermoregulation, homeostatic mechanisms that maintain body temperature within a normal range.

thermostable, a substance unaffected by high temperatures.

thermostat, a device or structure which automatically regulates temperature.

thermotherapy, any therapeutic measure involving heat, e.g. warm compress.

thesis, dissertation offered for the award of a higher degree.

theta wave (rhythm), irregular brain waves with a frequency of 4–7 Hz. Common in childhood and in adults during the initial stages of sleep, but considered to be abnormal in awake adults.

thiamine or **thiamin,** vitamin B$_1$, an essential coenzyme required during the metabolism of carbohydrates, alcohol and fats. *See* BERIBERI, KORSAKOFF'S SYNDROME, WERNICKE'S ENCEPHALOPATHY.

Thiersch graft, *(tersh),* a partial-thickness skin graft.

thigh, the portion of the lower limb above the knee.

343

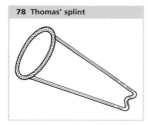

78 Thomas' splint

third stage of labour, *see* LABOUR.

Thomas' splint, used to immobilize fractures of the lower limb during transportation and to facilitate skeletal traction (Figure 78).

thoracic, *(thor-as-ik),* pertaining to the thorax. *T. cage:* bony framework which protects the thoracic organs and provides attachment for muscles. *T. cavity:* the chest. Body cavity superior to the diaphragm which contains the heart, lungs and great vessels. *T. duct:* large lymphatic vessel commencing in the abdomen which collects lymph draining from the legs, abdomen, left side of chest and head and left arm.

thoracocentesis, *(thor-a-kō-sen-tē'-sis),* puncture of the thorax, e.g. aspiration of pleural effusion.

thoracolumbar, pertaining to the thoracic and lumbar regions.

thoracoscopy, *(thor-a-kos-ko'-pi),* endoscopic examination of the pleural cavity. Also used for treatment, e.g. sympathectomy for excess sweating.

thoracostomy, *(thor-a-kos'-to-mi),* opening made in the chest for drainage of fluid.

thoracotomy, *(thor-a-kot'-o-mi),* surgical opening into the chest.

thorax, the chest. Cavity containing the lungs, heart and great vessels.

thorium (Th), a radioactive element with diagnostic and therapeutic uses.

threadworm, *Enterobius (oxyuris) vermicularis.* Pinworm. A common parasitic worm in children.

threonine, *(thrē-ō-nēn),* an essential (indispensable) amino acid.

threshold, the point at which a stimulus will produce a response. *Pain t.:* see PAIN. *Renal t.:* see RENAL THRESHOLD.

thrill, a vibratory impulse perceived by palpation.

thrombectomy, *(throm-bek'-to-mi),* removal of a thrombus from a vessel.

thrombin, enzyme formed from prothrombin. It converts fibrinogen to fibrin during the process of blood clotting.

thromboangiitis, *(throm-bō-an-ji-ī-tis),* inflammation of a blood vessel with clot formation. *T. obliterans:* **Buerger's disease.** Condition which affects young males who smoke heavily. The blood supply to the limbs is diminished with intermittent claudication and gangrene development.

thromboarteritis, *(throm-bō-ar-ter-ī-tis),* arteritis with thrombosis.

thrombocytes, *(throm-bō-sītz),* cell fragments concerned with blood clotting. Usually known as **platelets.** *See* BLOOD, BLOOD CLOTTING, BLOOD COUNT, PLATELETS.

thrombocythaemia, *(throm-bō-sī-thē-mi-a),* an increase in the number of platelets in the blood.

thrombocytopenia, *(throm-bō-sī-tō-pē-ni-ah),* deficiency of platelets in the blood. Causes include: drugs, infections, radiation, malignancy affecting the marrow and idiopathic.

thrombocytosis, *(throm-bō-sī-tā-sis),* an increase in the number of platelets in the blood. It can arise as a reaction to malignancy, chronic inflammation and chronic blood loss, or as part of thrombocythaemia and other myeloproliferative disorders.

thromboembolic, *(throm-bō-em-bol-ik),* a condition where a thrombus becomes detached and travels in the circulation, eventually occluding a vessel. *T. deterrents (TEDs): see* ANTIEMBOLIC HOSE.

thromboendarterectomy, *(throm-bō-end-ar-ter-ek-to-mi),* see ENDARTERECTOMY.

thrombokinase, *(throm-bō-kī-nāz),* see THROMBOPLASTIN.

thrombolysis, *(throm-bō-lī-sis),* see FIBRINOLYSIS.

thrombolytic, *(throm-bō-lit-ik),* pertaining to the disintegration of blood clot. *See* FIBRINOLYTIC.

thrombophlebitis, *(throm-bō-fle-bī′-tis),* inflammation of a vein with thrombosis.

thromboplastin, *(throm-bō-plas-tin),* also called thrombokinase. A lipoprotein released from damaged tissue which initiates the extrinsic coagulation pathway. *Activated partial t. time (APTT):* a test of blood coagulation function. *Intrinsic t.:* produced by the interaction of several factors during the clotting of blood. Much more active than tissue thromboplastin. *Tissue t.:* factor III of blood coagulation, it joins with other factors to activate factor X, needed for the formation of a fibrin clot. *See:* BLOOD CLOTTING.

thrombosis, *(throm-bō-sis),* intravascular clotting. Formation of a thrombus in the heart or vessels. *See* CAVERNOUS SINUS THROMBOSIS, CEREBRAL THROMBOSIS, CORONARY THROMBOSIS, DEEP VEIN THROMBOSIS.

thrombosthenin, *(throm-bos-then-in),* contractile protein present in platelets, important in the process of clot retraction.

thromboxanes, *(throm-bok-sān),* part of a group of regulatory lipids derived from arachidonic acid. Released from platelets, they cause vasospasm and platelet aggregation during platelet plug formation. *See* LEUKOTRIENES, PROSTAGLANDINS.

thrombus, a blood clot in the heart or vessels, at its site of formation.

thrush, fungal infection. *See* CANDIDIASIS.

thymectomy, *(thī-mek-to-mi),* operation to remove the thymus gland.

thymic, pertaining to the thymus gland.

thymine *(thī-mēn),* a nitrogenous base derived from pyrimidine, with other bases, a sugar and one or more phosphate groups it forms the nucleic acid DNA. *See* NUCLEIC ACIDS, DNA.

thymol, *(thī-mol),* an antiseptic often used for mouthwashes and gargles.

thymoma, *(thī-mō-ma),* a tumour of the thymus gland.

thymopoietin, thymic peptide hormone. *See* THYMUS.

thymosin, thymic peptide hormone. *See* THYMUS.

thymus, *(thī-mus),* a two-lobed gland situated in the mediastinum. It is important in fetal life, infancy and childhood, where it grows to reach a maximum at puberty, after which it becomes smaller. It consists of lymphoid tissue with many lymphocytes. The thymic hormones, thymosin and thymopoietin, stimulate the proper development of the T lymphocytes concerned with cell-mediated immunity. Various autoimmune conditions, such as myasthenia gravis, result from pathological activity of the thymus.

thyrocalcitonin, *(thī-rō-kal-sit′-ō-nin),* see CALCITONIN.

thyroglobulin, *(thī-rō-glob′-ū-lin),* a glycoprotein produced by the follicles of the thyroid gland. With iodine molecules it forms a colloid from which the thyroid hormones are produced.

thyroglossal cyst, *(thī-rō-glos-al),* a congenital cyst around the hyoid bone associated with the persistence of an embryonic structure.

thyroid, *(thī-royd)*, relating to the thyroid gland. *T. cartilage*: largest cartilage of the larynx. The Adam's apple. *T. crisis (thyrotoxic crisis)*: a sudden increase in metabolic rate characterized by tachycardia, pyrexia and dehydration. It is a very uncommon event seen after thyroidectomy in a person inadequately prepared with antithyroid drugs or infection in a person with hyperthyroidism. *T. gland* (Figure 79): an endocrine gland consisting of two lobes, one either side of the trachea. It secretes three hormones: triiodothyronine (T₃), thyroxine (T₄) under pituitary control which stimulate metabolism, and calcitonin which regulates calcium and phosphate homeostasis. *See* HYPERTHYROIDISM, HYPOTHYROIDISM. *T. hormones: see* TRIIODOTHYRONINE, THYROXINE. *T. stimulating hormone (TSH)*: thyrotrophin. Hormone produced by the pituitary gland which stimulates the secretion of thyroid hormones.

thyroidectomy, *(thī-royd-ek-to-mi)*, operation to remove part or all of the thyroid gland.

thyroiditis, *(thī-royd-ī-tis)*, inflammation of the thyroid gland. *See* HASHIMOTO'S THYROIDITIS.

thyrotoxicosis, *(thī-rō-tok-si-kō-sis)*, *see* HYPERTHYROIDISM.

thyrotrophic, *(thī-rō-trō-fik)*, stimulating the thyroid gland. *See* THYROID-STIMULATING HORMONE.

thyrotrophin-releasing hormone (TRH), hypothalamic hormone that stimulates TSH secretion by the anterior pituitary.

thyroxine (T₄), *(thī-rok-sēn)*, thyroid hormone required for metabolism and growth. It contains four atoms of iodine and is derived from the amino acid tyrosine.

tibia, the shin bone; the larger bone of the leg below the knee. *See* SKELETON.

tic, spasmodic twitching of muscles; usually of face and neck. *T. douloureux: see* TRIGEMINAL NEURALGIA.

tick, blood-sucking parasitic arthropod. Transmits diseases which include: relapsing fever, Rocky Mountain spotted fever and typhus.

tidal volume, the amount of air moved in and out of the lungs during one breath.

tincture, an alcoholic solution of a drug.

tine test, a skin test for tuberculosis. A device with several tines is used to inject tuberculin into the skin. *See* HEAF TEST.

Tinea, *(ti-nē-a)*, ringworm. A fungal infection of the skin. *T. barbae*: of the beard area. *T. capitis*: the scalp. *T. corporis*: of the body. *T. cruris*: of the groin area. *T. pedis*: of the feet (athlete's foot).

tinnitus, *(tin-ī-tus)*, ringing, roaring or buzzing noises in the ear.

tissue, a collection of specialized cells which perform a similar function, e.g.

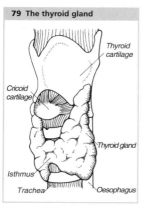

79 The thyroid gland

Thyroid cartilage

Cricoid cartilage

Thyroid gland

Isthmus

Trachea

Oesophagus

muscle, connective, epithelium and nervous. *T. culture:* cells and tissues grown under artificial conditions after their removal from the parent organism. *T. plasminogen activator (t-PA):* chemical required to activate plasminogen. Produced by endothelium lining the blood vessels.

titration, *(tī-trā-shon),* quantitative analysis using standard solutions.

titre, *(tē-ter),* a standard of strength. Measurement of antibody levels in the blood.

TNM, abbreviation for **tumour**, **node** and **metastasis**. *see* STAGING.

tocography, *(to-kog'ra-fi),* method of recording uterine contractions (pressure changes) during labour.

tocolytics, agents that relax uterine muscle. They have limited value in the inhibition of preterm labour.

tocopherols, *(to-kof'-er-ols),* a group of compounds with vitamin E activity which includes the important alpha-tocopherol. They act as antioxidants in biological membranes.

tocotrienols, *(to-ko'-trī-nols),* a group of compounds with vitamin E activity. They act as antioxidants in biological membranes but are less potent than tocopherols.

togaviruses, *(tō-ga-vī-rus-ez),* a family of RNA viruses that include the rubella virus and several spread by insects, e.g. yellow fever.

tolerance, reduction in the normal reaction. *Drug t.:* see DRUG TOLERANCE. *Immunological t.:* the immune system fails to initiate a response to a previously encountered antigen which can be harmful. With self-antigens this tolerance is normal. *Pain t.:* See PAIN. See GLUCOSE TOLERANCE TEST.

tomography, *(tom-og-ra-fi),* a radiographic technique used to produce images of specific areas of the body at different depths. *See* COMPUTED AXIAL TOMOGRAPHY, POSITRON EMISSION TOMOGRAPHY.

tone, 1. normal state of tension as found in muscles. **2.** quality of sound.

tongue, muscular organ in the floor of the mouth, concerned with mastication, swallowing, taste and speech. Its mucous membrane is arranged in papillae (tiny projections) and contains taste buds.

tonic, 1. popular term for a medicine which increases general wellbeing. **2.** sustained or continuous muscle contraction. *T. spasm:* prolonged muscle spasm. *Cf.* CLONIC.

tonicity, *(ton-is-i-ti),* **1.** normal muscle tone or tension. **2.** the effective osmotic pressure of a solution.

tonography, *(ton-og-ra-fi),* recording pressure, especially the intraocular pressure, by electrical tonometer.

tonometer, *(ton-om-et-er),* instrument for measuring tensions such as that used to measure intraocular pressure.

tonometry, *(ton-om-et-ri),* the measurement of tension or pressure.

tonsil, a body of lymphoid tissue found in the nasopharynx (pharyngeal t.), at the base of the tongue (lingual t.) and in folds formed by the soft palate and oropharynx (palatine t.). See ADENOID, WALDEYER'S RING.

tonsillectomy, *(ton-sil-ek'-to-mi),* operation to remove the palatine tonsils.

tonsillitis, *(ton-sil-ī-tis),* inflammation of tonsils.

tonsillotome, *(ton-sil'-o-tōm),* an instrument for cutting off a tonsil.

tonus, *(tō-nus),* the normal state of slight muscular contraction.

tooth, one of the structures in the mouth used to cut, tear and chew food. The types are: incisor, canine, premolar and molar. Each tooth consists of a root embedded in the jaw and an exposed crown. The bulk of the tooth is made of dentine surrounding a pulp cavity, the exposed portion is covered with enamel (Figure 80). *See* TEETH.

tophus, (*pl.* **tophi**) a gritty deposit due to gout, found in tendon sheaths and cartilage, especially that in the auricle of the ear.

topical, a substance applied locally to the surface of the body.

topography, a description of the various regions of the body.

torsion, twisting.

tort, a civil wrong, excluding breach of contract. It includes: negligence, trespass (to person, goods or land), nuisance, breach of statutory duty and defamation.

torticollis, (*tor-ti-kol-lis*), wry neck. The head is flexed and drawn to one side. It may be due to damage to one of the sternomastoid muscles during birth or spasmodic contractions of the muscles.

total lung capacity (TLC), volume of air in the lungs following greatest inspiratory effort.

total parenteral nutrition (TPN), provision of the entire nutritional requirements by the intravenous route using a central vein catheter.

Tourette's syndrome, Gilles de la Tourette syndrome. It is characterized by rude gestures and obscene speech. *See* COPROLALIA, COPROPRAXIA.

tourniquet, (*tor'-nē-kā*), device used to exert pressure on an artery to occlude flow or stop haemorrhage. Used in certain diagnostic, surgical and therapeutic procedures but no longer recommended for first aid.

toxaemia, (*tok-sē-mi-a*), circulation of toxins, usually bacterial, in the blood.

toxic, poisonous, caused by a poison. *T. epidermal necrolysis*: a serious condition characterized by severe skin rash, hyperpigmentation and extensive skin shedding. It can occur in response to serious drug reactions, staphylococcal infection, systemic illness, and it can be idiopathic. *T. shock syndrome (TSS)*: a potential complication of tampon use, but it does also occur in men and non-menstruating women. It is a rare occurrence caused by the toxins produced by the bacterium *Staphylococcus aureus* found at various sites, including the perineal area in healthy people. Bacterial contamination of the tampon occurs and the bacteria multiply within the vagina. The toxins enter the blood, causing pyrexia, vomiting and diarrhoea, a rash, and sometimes life-threatening hypovolaemic shock. Prevention involves: hand hygiene, use of lowest-absorbency tampons appropriate for the loss, changing tampons every 4 hours, using a sanitary pad rather than a tampon at night, remembering to remove the tampon at the end of menstruation and

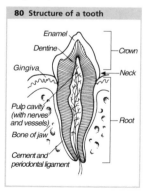

80 Structure of a tooth

Enamel — Dentine — Crown

Gingiva — Neck

Pulp cavity (with nerves and vessels) — Root

Bone of jaw

Cement and periodontal ligament

reporting illness occurring during menstruation. Women with a history of TSS are advised to use sanitary pads rather than tampons.

toxicity, the degree to which a substance is toxic.

toxicology, *(tok-si-kol'-o-ji),* science of poisons.

toxicosis, *(tok-si-kō'-sis),* any disease due to poisoning.

toxin, a poison, usually of bacterial origin. *See* ENDOTOXIN, EXOTOXIN.

Toxocara, (tok-sō-kar-a), a genus of nematode roundworm of dogs and cats, particularly *T. canis.* Humans may become infected by contact with affected animals and faeces, especially children. The worms affect the lungs, spleen and eyes.

toxocariasis, *(tok-sō-kar-ī-a-sis),* infestation with *Toxocara.* Characterized by fever, hepatomegaly and the possibility of blindness.

toxoid, *(tok-soyd),* a bacterial toxin treated to remove its pathogenicity while retaining its antigenicity. Used to produce active immunity to diseases such as diphtheria and tetanus.

Toxoplasma, (tok-sō-plaz-ma), a genus of protozoon, e.g. *T. gondii.* The definitive host is the domestic cat and other felines, and rodents are the intermediate host.

toxoplasmosis, *(tok-sō-plaz-mō-sis),* infection with the protozoa *Toxoplasma gondii.* It is transmitted by eating undercooked meat, contact with the faeces of infected cats, and from infected mothers to the fetus. The congenital form causes serious neurological defects such as hydrocephaly or microcephaly; the liver and the eyes are affected. Most infants, if they survive, are severely disabled and blind. Acquired infections may be asymptomatic but respiratory illness, rash, enlarged lymph nodes and eye problems may

occur. It also causes serious disease in immunocompromised individuals, e.g. AIDS patients, who develop encephalitis and eye problems.

trabecula, *(tra-bek'-ū-la),* a septum extending into the organ from its capsule or wall.

trabeculectomy, *(trab-ek-ū-lek'-to-mi),* operation for glaucoma.

trace elements, elements required by the body in minute quantities for metabolic processes and homeostasis, e.g. copper, cobalt manganese and selenium.

tracer, an instrument or substance used to gain information about metabolic processes. Radioactive tracers can be used to investigate thyroid disease or possible brain tumours.

trachea, *(tra-kē-a),* the windpipe; air passage from the larynx to the bronchi. It consists of incomplete rings of cartilage and is lined with ciliated mucous membrane.

tracheal, *(tra-kē-al),* pertaining to the trachea. *T. intubation:* insertion of an endotracheal tube into the trachea to provide a patent airway.

tracheitis, *(tra-kē-ī-tis),* inflammation of the trachea.

trachelorrhaphy, *(trak-el-or-a-fi),* the operation of suturing a torn cervix uteri.

tracheobronchitis, *(trak-ē-ō-bron-kī'-tis),* inflammation of the trachea and bronchi.

tracheo-oesophageal, *(trak-ē-ō-ē-sof-a-jē-al),* relating to the trachea and oesophagus. *See* FISTULA.

tracheostomy, *(tra-kē-os-to-mi),* an opening in the trachea, for establishment of a safe airway with the insertion of a plastic or metal tube. The tube may be inserted directly through an incision made between the tracheal cartilages, percutaneously or as a minitracheostomy. It may be performed to facilitate mechanical ventilation, where there is a respiratory obstruction, for the removal of secretions and following laryngectomy. May be temporary or permanent.

tracheotomy, (trak-ē-ot-o-mi), incision of the trachea. See TRACHEOSTOMY.

trachoma, (tra-kō-ma), a contagious chlamydial keratoconjunctivitis caused by *Chlamydia trachomatis*: a common cause of blindness in hot dry areas of the world. Infection may occur by contact; during birth an infant may become infected from vaginal discharge and unhygienic use of fomites. Also called trachoma inclusion conjunctivitis (TRIC).

traction, the act of pulling or dragging. It may be applied to the skeleton or the skin and uses a series of pulleys, cords and weights in conjunction with frames and splints. *Skeletal t.*: traction on a bone by means of a pin or wire passed through a lower fragment. This keeps the fractured bone in the correct position and overcomes muscle contraction. Tongs are used to apply skull traction in cervical spine injuries. *Skin t.*: extension – the traction is achieved by applying weights to foam or extension plaster attached to the skin. This type of straight pull traction is used prior to internal fixation of fractures of the femoral neck. *Hamilton–Russel t.*: a form of skin traction on the femoral shaft with the knee flexed. See EXTENSION.

tragus, (trā-gus), small eminence in front of the external auditory meatus.

trait, 1. a physical or personality characteristic special to an individual. **2.** a genetically determined characteristic or condition.

trance, used to describe hypnotic sleep and for certain self-induced stuporous states.

tranquillizer, a drug which relieves tension, agitation and anxiety.

transactional analysis, a type of psychotherapy founded on the theory that all individuals have three ego states, child, adult and parent, which are concurrent. The goal is to give the adult ego decision-making power over the child and parent egos.

transaminases, (trans-am-i-nāz-ez), now known as **aminotransferases.** See AMINOTRANSFERASES, CARDIAC ENZYMES, LIVER FUNCTION TESTS.

transcoelemic, (trans-se-lō'-mik), across a body cavity, such as the spread of malignant cells across the abdomen via the peritoneum.

transcription, process by which genetic information is transferred from DNA to mRNA, the first stage in protein synthesis.

transcultural, across cultures. *T. nursing*: the provision of professional nursing to different cultural groups which takes account of their customs, health beliefs, values and behaviours.

transcutaneous, (trans-kū-tā-nē-us), through the skin, such as the absorption of some drugs, or the monitoring by pulse oximetry. *T. electrical nerve stimulation (TENS)*: a non-invasive method of pain control where electrical impulses are used to prevent the transmission of pain sensation to the brain.

transdermal, through the skin, such as the absorption of drugs, many of which are administered via an impregnated patch applied to the intact skin or gels and creams. Drugs administered in this way include nitrates and hormone replacement.

transducer, a device which transforms one form of energy into another so that it may be transmitted electrically.

transfer RNA (tRNA), a type of ribonucleic acid involved in the translation stage of protein synthesis. It translates the base sequence in the mRNA codon into the amino acids required to build the protein and transfers them from the cytoplasm to the ribosome.

transference, in psychotherapy or psychoanalysis the transfer of a patient's emotions regarding a significant person in his or her life to the therapist.

transferrin, a protein to which iron is bound whilst in transit around the body.

transfusion, see BLOOD TRANSFUSION.

transient, of short duration. *T. ischaemic attack (TIA):* sudden attack of cerebral ischaemia usually followed by complete recovery within hours. However, it may precede a more severe stroke.

transillumination, *(trans-i-lū-min-ā-shon),* a bright light is used to illuminate a translucent structure such as a paranasal sinus.

translation, the second stage of protein synthesis. It involves tRNA and rRNA translating the base sequence required to make a new protein from amino acids within the ribosomes.

translocation, the transfer of segments from one chromosome to another. A cause of congenital abnormalities such as some types of Down's syndrome.

translucent, neither opaque nor transparent. Allows the passage of some diffused light.

transperitoneal, *(trans-per-i-to-ne′-al),* through the peritoneum.

transplacental, across the placenta, such as the exchange of substances between fetal and maternal blood.

transplantation, the transfer of a portion of tissue from one part of the body to another, as in skin grafts; or from one person to another, as in organ transplants, tissue from a compatible donor being used to replace a diseased structure, e.g. heart, lungs, liver, kidney, pancreas, bone marrow, etc. See HISTOCOMPATABILITY ANTIGENS.

transposition, 1. an embryonic abnormality where a structure is moved from one side of the body to the other. **2.** in genetics the movement of genetic material between chromosomes. *T. of the great vessels:* a developmental anomaly where the pulmonary artery arises from the left ventricle and the aorta from the right ventricle.

transsexualism, the condition where people feel that they are of the opposite gender to their biological gender. This can cause conflict, with severe psychological and emotional problems. Surgical and hormonal modification may eventually be undertaken to change the individual's gender to conform with his or her wishes.

transudation, oozing of fluid (transudate) through a membrane or from a tissue, e.g. ascites in the peritoneal cavity.

transurethral, *(trans-ū-rē′-thral),* via the urethra. See PROSTATECTOMY, TURP.

transverse, across. *T. colon:* see BOWEL. *T. lie:* where the fetus lies across the uterus, it must be converted to a longitudinal lie before a vaginal delivery is possible.

transvesical, *(trans-ves-i-kal),* through the bladder. See PROSTATECTOMY.

transvestism, *(trans-ves-tizm),* dressing in the clothes of the opposite gender.

trapezium, *(tra-pē-zē-um),* one of the carpals or wrist bones.

trapezius, *(tra-pē-zē-us),* large triangular muscle of the neck and thorax.

trapezoid, *(tra-pē-zoyd),* one of the carpals or wrist bones.

trauma, 1. a physical wound or other injury. **2.** a psychological injury caused by a severe emotional upset.

treatment, methods of curing disease or controlling its effects. *Conservative t.*: treatment with drugs, rest or diet rather than surgery or other drastic means. *Curative t.*: measures aimed at cure. *Palliative t.*: measures taken to control symptoms such as pain, without hope of cure. *Prophylactic t.*: preventive. Measures taken to prevent disease such as immunization.

Trematoda, *(trem-a-tōd-a)*, class of flukes which infect humans causing diseases such as schistosomiasis (bilharzia).

tremor, involuntary trembling associated with emotion, extreme fatigue or disease. *Intention t.*: occurs when the individual attempts to touch an object.

trench foot, occurs in frostbite and other conditions of exposure where there is deprivation of local blood supply and secondary bacterial infection.

Trendelenburg, *T.'s operation*: performed for varicosed veins; the long saphenous vein is ligated in the groin. *T. position*: used during certain operations; the head is lower than the pelvis and the legs are raised. *T.'s sign*: seen where there is inefficient functioning of the hip abductor muscles, e.g. developmental dysplasia of the hip. When the person stands only on the affected leg, the pelvis tilts down on the other side.

trephine, *(tre-fīn)*, an instrument for removing a disc of tissue such as a bone or cornea. Used to gain access to enclosed areas, e.g. trephining the skull.

Treponema, *(trep-ō-nē-ma)*, a genus of spirochaetes. *T. pallidum*: the organism that causes syphilis; other dis-

ease due to *Treponema* include yaws (*T. pertenue*) and pinta (*T. carateum*).

triacylglycerol, *see* TRIGLYCERIDES.

triage, *(tri-arjh)*, a system of classification of patients in any emergency situation. *T. nurse*: the nurse given this specific responsibility in an accident and emergency department.

triangular bandage, useful for making arm slings and securing dressings.

tricarboxylic acid cycle (TCA), *see* KREBS' CYCLE.

triceps, certain muscles with three heads. *T. brachii*: muscle of the upper arm which extends the elbow. *T. skinfold*: a measurement of the midarm subcutaneous fat layer, used as part of a nutritional assessment.

trichiasis, *(tri-kī-a-sis)*, inversion of eyelashes causing corneal friction and irritation.

Trichinella, a genus of parasitic nematode worms. *T. spiralis*: nematode worm which is a parasite of pigs and rats.

trichiniasis, *(trik-in-ī-a-sis)*, trichinosis. Infestation with the worm *T. spiralis* caused by eating raw or undercooked pork. It is characterized by diarrhoea, fever, oedema, pain at sites of larval invasion and the formation of skeletal muscle cysts.

trichloroacetic acid, *(tri-klor-ō-a-sē-tik)*, a caustic used to remove warts.

Trichomonas, *(trik-ō-mōn-as)*, a genus of protozoa which infects humans. *T. vaginalis*: a cause of vaginitis in females and genitourinary infection in males.

trichomoniasis, *(trik-ō-mōn-ī-a-sis)*, disease caused by *T. vaginalis*. In females there is a foul-smelling, green/yellow, frothy, vaginal discharge with intense itching, but in males the infection is usually asymptomatic. It is commonly, but not exclusively, sexually transmitted.

trichomycosis, (trik-ō-kī-kō'-sis), a fungal disease of hair.

trichonosis, (trik-on-ō'-sis), **trichopathy,** any disease of hair.

trichophagy, (trik-ō-fa-ji), hair biting or eating.

trichophytosis, (trik-ō-fī-tō-sis), fungal infection of the hair caused by an organism of the genus *Trichophyton*. See TINEA.

trichuriasis, (trik-ūr-ī-a-sis), infection with the worm *Trichuris trichiura* caused by ingesting contaminated soil or food. There are few symptoms but a heavy infection may cause diarrhoea.

Trichuris, (trik-ūr-is), a genus of parasitic nematode worms. T. trichiura: whipworm. An intestinal parasite in humans.

tricuspid, (tri-kus-pid), having three points, flaps or cusps. T. incompetence: failure of the t. valve to close properly which allows regurgitation of blood. T. stenosis: a narrowing of the t. valve impeding blood flow. T. tooth: a tooth with three points. T. valve: the right atrioventricular valve preventing backflow of blood into the right atrium during ventricular systole.

tricyclics, (tri-sīk-liks), an important group of organic compounds, some of which are used as antidepressant drugs.

trigeminal, (tri-jem-in-al), triple. T. nerves: the fifth and largest pair of cranial nerves which divide into three divisions: ophthalmic, maxillary and mandibular; they are sensory to the face and scalp and contain motor fibres which innervate the muscles of mastication. T. neuralgia: tic douloureux. Agonizing facial pain of unknown aetiology. The pain may be precipitated by simple stimuli, such as cold air or chewing.

trigger finger, a finger that can be bent but not straightened without

help. Caused by thickening of the tendon sheath at the metacarpophalangeal joint.

triglycerides, (trī-gli-se-rīdz), neutral fat. A lipid which consists of three fatty acids and a glycerol molecule. It forms the fat deposits of the body and provides the major source of stored energy. Also called triacylglycerols.

trigone, (tri-gōn), a triangle. T. of the bladder: the area in the bladder between the openings of the ureters and the urethra.

triiodothyronine (T_3), (trī-ī-ō-dō-thī-ro-nēn), thyroid hormone required for metabolism and growth. It contains three atoms of iodine and is formed by the conversion of thyroxine.

trimester, a three-month period. Pregnancy can be divided into three trimesters.

triphasic, having three phases. See GENERAL ADAPTATION SYNDROME.

triple test, blood test offered to pregnant women. It measures alpha-fetoprotein, unconjugated oestriol and total human chorionic gonadotrophin (hCG) in maternal serum and is used early in pregnancy to predict the estimated risk of conditions such as Down's syndrome. For example, a reduced alpha-fetoprotein and oestriol with an elevated hCG would indicate an increased risk for Down's syndrome. This test is a fairly crude screening of risk which is calculated in conjunction with age, gestation and weight. The test for Down's syndrome does produce false positives and negatives. Where the risk prediction is 1 in 250, the couple are offered more specific tests. See AMNIOCENTESIS, CHORIONIC VILLUS SAMPLING.

triple vaccine, contains diphtheria, tetanus and pertussis (whooping cough) antigens.

triplet, the three sequential bases in a DNA molecule which code for a specific amino acid in protein synthesis.

triploid (3n), having three sets of chromosomes; in the case of humans having 69 instead of 46 chromosomes is 3n (where n = 23). *See* POLYPLOIDY.

trismus, lockjaw. Spasm in the muscles of the jaw, such as that seen in tetanus.

trisomy, *(trī-so-mi),* an anomaly where there are three chromosomes instead of the normal two in one of the 23 pairs which constitute the normal diploid number. It results in an individual with 47 chromosomes rather than 46. *See* DOWN'S SYNDROME, EDWARD'S SYNDROME, PATAU'S SYNDROME.

trivalent, in chemistry, a substance with a valence of three.

trocar, *(trō-kar),* the perforating instrument used, with a cannula, to access a body cavity or other structure prior to the instillation or drainage of fluids.

trochanter, *(tro-kan'-ter),* two processes (the greater and the lesser), at the juncture of the neck and shaft of femur.

trochlear, *(trok-lē-ar),* relating to a pulley. *T. nerves:* the fourth pair of cranial nerves. They innervate the superior oblique muscle which moves the eyeball out and downwards.

trophic, relating to nutrition. *T. ulcer:* one occurring in tissue which lacks nourishment, due to either an impaired blood supply or a systemic nutritional deficiency.

trophoblast, *(trō-fō-blast),* outer cell layer surrounding the blastocyst. It secretes enzymes involved in implantation and nourishment, produces hormones and will eventually form the placenta.

tropomyosin, *(tro-pō-mī-ō-sin),* one of the proteins in the thin filaments of a muscle myofibril.

Trousseau's sign, a sign of latent tetany: forearm muscle spasm is seen within 3 to 4 minutes of inflating a cuff on the upper arm to a pressure greater than systolic blood pressure. *See* CARPOPEDAL SPASM, HYPOCALCAEMIA, TETANY.

truncus arteriosus, embryonic structure which becomes the aorta and pulmonary artery.

truss, an apparatus for retaining a hernia in place.

Trypanosoma, *(tri-pan-ō-sō-ma),* a genus of protozoa responsible for several human diseases.

trypanosomiasis, *(tri-pan-ō-sō-mī-a-sis),* sleeping sickness. Infection with *Trypanosoma brucei gambiense* and *T. rhodesiense* which are transmitted to humans by the bites of an infected tsetse fly. In South America the disease is also known as Chagas' disease, the organism being the *T. cruzi* which is transmitted via the faeces of bugs.

trypsin, a proteolytic enzyme produced by the pancreas in its precursor form. *See* TRYPSINOGEN.

trypsinogen, *(trip-sin'-o-jen),* the inactive precursor of trypsin. Activated by the enzyme enterokinase produced in the small bowel.

tryptophan, *(trip-to-fan),* an essential (indispensable) amino acid.

tsetse, *(tet-sē),* a type of fly responsible for the transmission of trypanosomiasis in Africa.

TSH, *see* THYROID-STIMULATING HORMONE.

tsutsugamushi disease, *(tut-sū-ga-mū-shē),* scrub typhus.

tubal, relating to a tube, especially the uterine tubes. *T. gestation or preg-*

nancy: see ECTOPIC GESTATION. *T. ligation:* female sterilization where the uterine tubes are ligated.

tube feeding, the administration of nutrients and fluid via a tube inserted into the gastrointestinal tract, e.g. via gastrostomy, nasoduodenal or nasogastric tubes. *See* ENTERAL NUTRITION.

tubercle, *(tū'-ber-kl),* **1.** a small bony eminence. **2.** the specific lesion of *Mycobacterium tuberculosis. See* GHON'S FOCUS.

tuberculide, *(tū-ber'-kū-līd),* any skin rash due to tuberculous infection.

tuberculin, *(tū-ber-kū-lin),* old tuberculin or PPD (purified protein derivative) products prepared from *Mycobacterium tuberculosis.* Used in skin testing for the diagnosis of tuberculosis or prior to BCG immunization. *See* HEAF, MANTOUX, TINE TESTS.

tuberculoma, *(tū-ber-kū-lō'-ma),* walled-off region of caseating tuberculosis.

tuberculosis (TB), *(tū-ber-kū-lō-sis),* a chronic granulomatous infection caused by an acid-fast bacillus, *Mycobacterium tuberculosis* (human type), *M. bovis* (cattle) and atypical mycobacteria, e.g. avian. *Primary t.:* occurring in childhood, there is lung involvement, fever and skin rash. *Miliary t.:* widespread disease which spreads via the blood to all areas of the body. *Multidrug-resistant t. (MDR-TB):* a serious event where the *M. tuberculosis* is resistant to antituberculous drugs. It is a particular problem in patients with AIDS and in certain countries, e.g. Russia. *Post primary t.:* the most common form which affects the lung but other sites may be affected. Tuberculosis is characterized by systemic effects such as fever, night sweats and weight loss plus those dependent upon the site, e.g. cough in pul-

monary disease, haematuria in renal TB and infertility if the uterine tubes are affected. Diagnosis is made on: clinical signs, X-rays, skin tests and the presence of acid-fast bacilli in sputum, urine, etc. Treatment is based on antituberculosis drugs in combination. Immunization with BCG is used to protect vulnerable individuals usually detected by skin testing.

tuberculous, *(tū-ber-kū-lus),* relating to tuberculosis.

tuberosity, *(tū-ber-os'-i-ti),* rough bony prominence.

tuberous sclerosis, *(tū-be-rus skle-rō-sis),* see EPILOIA.

tubo-ovarian, *(tū-bo-ō-vā-ri-an),* relating to both the uterine tube and ovary, such as a cyst.

tubular, relating to a tube. *T. necrosis:* affecting the kidneys, it is caused by bacterial toxins, toxic agents such as metals and ischaemia as in shock. A cause of acute renal failure.

tubule, *(tū-būl),* a small tube. *Renal t.:* the tubular part of the nephron.

tularaemia, *(tū-la-rē-mi-a),* a bacterial disease caused by *Francisella tularensis* which is transmitted to humans from rabbits by ticks or by handling the infected animals.

tumefaction, *(tū-me-fak-shon),* becoming swollen.

tumour, **1.** a swelling; an abnormal enlargement. **2.** an abnormal uncontrolled proliferation of cells, it may be benign or malignant. *T. marker:* a substance detected in the serum that may be associated with the presence of a specific cancer or sometimes a non-malignant disease. They include: alpha-fetoprotein, prostate-specific antigen, etc.

tunica, term applied to a coat, lining or covering. *T. adventitia/externa:* outer covering of blood vessels. *T. intima:* smooth endothelial lining of blood vessels. *T. media*: muscle and elastic tissue coat forming the middle layer of the vessel wall. *T. vaginalis*: outer covering of the testes.

tuning fork, an instrument used to test hearing (*see* RINNE'S TEST, WEBER'S TEST), or sense of vibration.

turbid, not clear, cloudy.

turbinate bones, *(ter-bin-āt)*, nasal conchae. Three thin convoluted plates of bone situated on the lateral walls of each nasal cavity.

turbinectomy, *(ter-bi-nek-to-mi)*, operation to excise a turbinate bone.

turgescence, swelling due to blood or other fluid in the tissues.

turgid, swollen, distended.

turgor, the firmness and resilience of the skin derived from the cells and tissue fluid.

Turner's syndrome, ovarian dysgenesis. An anomaly of female sex chromosomes, usually there is only one X chromosome (XO with a total number of 45). It is characterized by underdevelopment of the genital tract and secondary sexual characteristics, short stature, neck webbing and other abnormalities.

TURP, abbrev. for **transurethral resection of the prostate gland.** *See* PROSTATECTOMY.

tussis, a cough.

twin, one of two infants resulting from a single pregnancy. *Conjoined t.*: one joined, to some degree, to its fellow twin. A failure of early separation when uniovular twins are forming from one ovum. Siamese twins. *See* BINOVULAR, DIZYGOTIC, MONOZYGOTIC, UNIOVULAR.

tylosis, *(tī-lō-sis)*, *see* KERATOSIS.

tympanic, *(tim-pan-ik)*, pertaining to the tympanum or ear drum. *T. cavity*: middle ear. *T. membrane*: the ear drum. Membrane between the external auditory canal and the middle

ear. *T. thermometer*: electronic probe introduced into the external auditory canal to record body temperature. *See* EAR.

tympanites, *(tim-pan-ī-tēz)*, distension of the abdomen caused by gas in the intestine.

tympanitis, *(tim-pa-nī-tis)*, inflammation of tympanic membrane, otitis media.

tympanoplasty, *(tim-pa-no-plas-ti)*, operation to reconstruct the ear drum or middle ear ossicles to improve sound conduction.

tympanum, *(tim-pan-um)*, 1. tympanic cavity. The cavity of the middle ear. 2. tympanic membrane or ear drum.

type A behaviours, characterized by high competitiveness resulting in compulsive working schedules, believed by some to be associated with an increased risk of coronary heart disease.

type B behaviours, behaviours which display minimal hostility and aggression; not highly competitive and believed to have a lower risk of heart disease.

type I and type II errors, in research, a type I error (alpha error) is rejecting a null hypothesis that is true, and a type II error (beta error) is not rejecting a null hypothesis that is false.

typhlitis, *(tif-lī-tis)*, inflammation of the caecum.

typhoid fever, an infectious enteric fever caused by *Salmonella typhi* transmitted by contaminated food, milk or water. It is commonly associated with a lack of clean water and poor sanitation, but outbreaks may occur in other areas, usually by contamination of food by carriers of the bacteria (especially food handlers). There is bacteraemia and inflammation of small bowel lymphoid tissue (Peyer's patches) which ulcerates and may perforate or bleed. The onset is characterized by a 'stepladder' rise in temperature, slow pulse, headache, drowsiness and cough. Later there is a rose red spot rash on the abdomen, splenomegaly and typical pea-soup diarrhoea with abdominal tenderness, delirium and bronchitis.

typhus fevers, a group of rickettsial diseases transmitted by lice, ticks, fleas and mites. Associated with overcrowding and poor hygiene they include: epidemic typhus (*Rickettsia prowazekii*), endemic typhus (*R. mooseri*), scrub typhus (*R. tsutsugamushi*) and Rocky Mountain spotted fever (*R. rickettsii*). Presentation varies between types but all include high temperature and a rash which is usually petechial.

typing, identifying and classifying blood groups, tissue and microorganisms.

tyramine *(tī-ra-mēn)*, an amine present in some foods, e.g. mature cheese, yeast extract, broad beans, bananas and some red wines, etc. All of these should be avoided by people taking monoamine oxidase inhibitors (MAOI) antidepressants to minimize the risk of hypertensive crisis.

tyrosine, *(tī-rō-sēn)*, an amino acid.

tyrosinosis, *(tī-rō-sin-ō-sis)*, an inborn error of metabolism where large quantities of tyrosine and intermediates are excreted in the urine. Leads to severe hepatic disease.

U

UKCC, abbreviation for **United Kingdom Central Council for Nursing, Midwifery and Health Visiting.**

ulcer, a break in the continuity of the skin or mucous membranes; suppuration may be present. Types include: arterial, Curling's, peptic, pressure ulcer, rodent, venous.

ulcerative, *(ul-ser-a-tiv)*, pertaining to ulceration. *U. colitis:* an inflammatory bowel disease which affects the colon and rectum. It causes diarrhoea with blood and mucus, pain, anaemia, weight loss and serious complications which include: toxic dilatation, perforation, dehydration, electrolyte disturbances, malignant changes and liver damage.

ulna, the inner bone of the forearm. *See* SKELETON.

ulnar, relating to the ulna. The artery, vein and nerve which run beside the ulna.

ultrafiltration, *(ul-tra-fil-trā-shon)*, filtration under pressure. The use of very fine filters to remove minute particles from a solution, such as the technique used in haemofiltration where the blood is filtered under pressure.

ultramicroscopic, *(ul-tra-mī-krō-skop-ik)*, particles too small to be seen with a light microscope.

ultrasonic, *(ul-tra-son-ik)*, pertaining to sound waves of very high frequency.

ultrasonography, *(ul-tra-son-og-ra-fi)*, sonography. A technique which uses ultrasound to produce images of organs and structures which aid diagnosis. *See* ECHOCARDIOGRAPHY, ECHOENCEPHALOGRAPHY.

ultrasound, ultrasonic waves of a frequency over 20 000 Hz that are inaudible to the human ear used in ultrasonography to scan soft tissues and produce images and in fetal monitoring. *U. scan:* abbreviated to USS.

ultraviolet (UV) rays, electromagnetic rays of short wavelength. Not in the visible spectrum of light. Vitamin D is produced by the action of UV rays on substances in the skin.

umbilical, *(um-bil-i-kal)*, pertaining to the umbilicus. *U. cord:* the funis. The cord which connects the fetus with the placenta. It contains two arteries and one vein and gelatinous embryonic connective tissue called Wharton's jelly. *U. hernia: see* HERNIA.

umbilicated, *(um-bil-i-kāt-ed)*, having a navel-like depression.

umbilicus, *(um-bil-i-kus)*, small depressed scar on the anterior abdominal wall remaining from separation of the umbilical cord. The navel.

unciform, *(un'-si-form)*, hook-shaped. *See* HAMATE.

unconditioned reflex, an innate reaction or response which occurs spontaneously without training. *See* CONDITIONED REFLEX.

unconscious, insensible to stimuli. *U. mind:* that part of the mind which contains feelings, instincts and experiences of which the individual is not normally aware, although they influence behaviour.

unconsciousness, the state of being unconscious, not responding to stimuli, e.g. after a stroke, during a general anaesthetic. The depth of unconsciousness varies from deeply unconscious and not responding to painful stimuli to easily rousable and able to respond to simple questions. *See* GLASGOW COMA SCALE.

underclass, describes a group in society who are deprived, disenfranchised and marginalized in society, such as the homeless. *See* SOCIAL EXCLUSION.

underwater seal drain, a closed system of drainage used to drain the pleural space following surgery or trauma and to allow lung expansion after a spontaneous pneumothorax. A chest tube with its other end under water allows the drainage of air or fluids but prevents air entering the chest (Figure 81), as long as the drainage bottle is lower than the cavity and the integrity of the closed system is maintained.

undifferentiated, a primitive cell without any development (differentiation) to a more specialized type. A characteristic of certain tumour cells.

undine, *(un'-dēn),* a thin glass flask with two spouts. Used for irrigation of the eye.

undulant *(un-dū-lant),* wave-like. *U. fever. See* BRUCELLA.

ungual, *(un-gwal),* pertaining to a finger or toenail.

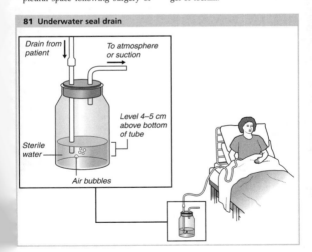

81 Underwater seal drain

Drain from patient

To atmosphere or suction

Level 4–5 cm above bottom of tube

Sterile water

Air bubbles

unguentum (*un-gū-en'-tum*), an ointment; abbreviation, **ung.**

unguis, (*un'-gwis*), a finger or toenail.

unicellular, (*ū-ni-sel-ū-la*), organisms which consist of one cell, e.g. protozoa.

unilateral, (*ū-ni-lat-er-al*), on one side.

uniocular, (*ū-ni-ok'-ū-la*), relating to one eye.

union, healing, such as that occurring after a fracture. *Delayed u.*: where healing is slower than normal.

uniovular, (*ū-ni-ov-ū-la*), one ovum. *U. twins*: develop from a single fertilized ovum. They are identical.

uniparous, (*ū-nip'-a-rus*), having borne only one child.

unipolar, *see* DEPRESSION.

United Kingdom Central Council for Nursing, Midwifery and Health Visiting (UKCC), the Council was established by an act of Parliament in 1979, and resulted in the formation of the UKCC and the four national boards for England, Northern Ireland, Scotland and Wales. These statutory bodies had certain functions, including the establishment and maintenance of a professional register for all nurses and midwives, the power to remove individuals from the register in cases of misconduct, and the establishment and maintenance of education and training regulations and standards. The UKCC consisted of 60 members from across the relevant professions and with lay membership, some members being elected to post and others being nominated by the Secretary of State for Health. Following a review of the UKCC in 1999, the UK government recommended that a new and smaller council be established with the end of the four national boards. *See* NURSING AND MIDWIFERY COUNCIL.

See APPENDIX: CODE OF PROFESSIONAL CONDUCT, PREP.

univalent, having a valance of one.

univariate statistics, descriptive statistics that analyse a single variable, such as the mean.

universal precautions, the routine precautions taken during contact, or the possibility of contact, with blood and body fluids, e.g. wearing plastic aprons and gloves.

unsaturated, a solution into which more solute can be dissolved. *U. fats*: *see* POLYUNSATURATED FATS. *See* FATTY ACIDS, LIPOPROTEINS, SATURATED FATS.

unstable bladder, instability of the detrusor muscle leads to powerful bladder contractions which cannot be controlled. A common cause of female incontinence with frequency, urgency and urge incontinence.

upper motor neurone, that part of the descending pyramidal motor tracts from the Betz or pyramidal cell in the motor cortex to the anterior horn of the spinal cord. *U. m. n. disease*: any disease affecting upper motor fibres, e.g. stroke. Characterized by spastic paralysis and no muscle wastage.

urachus, (*ū-ra-kus*), a canal which connects the bladder and umbilicus in the fetus. It becomes a fibrous remnant known as the median umbilical ligament. It may persist, giving rise to a vesico-umbilical fistula with infection or cyst formation.

uracil, (*ū-ra-sil*), nitrogenous base derived from pyrimidine; with other bases, a sugar and one or more phosphate groups it forms the nucleic acid RNA. *See* NUCLEIC ACIDS, RNA.

uraemia, (*ū-rē-mi-a*), azotaemia. A syndrome characterized by high levels of urea and other toxic nitrogenous substances in the blood, with disturbance of electrolytes and acid–base balance.

It occurs when renal function is impaired, either from kidney disease or by events occurring elsewhere in the body, e.g. hypotension associated with hypovolaemia. The clinical effects include: lethargy, headache, nausea, vomiting, visual problems, cardiac arrhythmias, hiccups, pruritus, altered consciousness and fits.

uranium (U), a heavy metallic radioactive element which is a source of energy and other substances such as radium.

urate, (ū-rāt), a salt of uric acid. A constituent of some calculi and concretions.

urea, (ū-rē-a), nitrogenous waste product formed in the liver and excreted by the kidneys. *U. cycle*: the biochemical cycle occurring in the liver whereby ammonia derived from amino acids is combined with carbon dioxide to form urea.

urease, (ū-rē-āz), bacterial enzyme which catalyses the breakdown of urea.

uresis, (ū-rē-sis), urination.

ureter, (ū-rē-ter), the tube which conveys urine from the renal pelvis to the bladder.

ureteral, (ū-rē'-ter-al), pertaining to the ureter.

ureterectomy, (ū-rē-ter-ek'-to-mi), excision of a ureter.

ureteric, (ū-rē-ter-ik), pertaining to the ureter. *U. catheter*: very fine tube used to introduce contrast medium for a retrograde urogram (pyelogram) or for drainage. *U. colic*: see RENAL COLIC. *U. transplantation*: the ureters are implanted into an isolated loop of ileum (ileal conduit) or into the sigmoid colon.

ureteritis, (ū-rē-ter-ī-tis), inflammation of a ureter.

ureterocele, (ū-rē-ter-ō-sēl), prolapse and dilatation of the part of the ureter within the bladder wall.

ureterocolostomy, (ū-rē-ter-ō-ko-los'-to-mi), implanatation of the ureters into the colon.

ureteroileostomy, (ū-rē-ter-ō-il-ē-os-to-mi), also known as ileoureterostomy. *see* ILEAL CONDUIT.

ureterolith, (ū-rē'-ter-o-lith), stone in the ureter.

ureterolithotomy, (ū-rē-ter-ō-lith-ot-o-mi), removal of a stone from the ureter.

ureteronephrectomy, (ū-rē-ter-ō-nef-rek-to-mi), removal of the ureter and kidney.

ureterosigmoidostomy, (ū-rē-ter-ō-sig-moyd-os-to-mi), implantation of the ureters into the sigmoid colon. Ureterocolostomy.

ureterostomy, (ū-rē-ter-os'-to-mi), the creation of a fistula/opening which drains urine. *Cutaneous u.*: the ureters are brought out on to the skin surface from where they drain urine into a suitable appliance.

ureterovaginal, (ū-rē-ter-ō-va-jī-nal), pertaining to the ureter and the vagina. *U. fistula*: abnormal communication between ureter and vagina which results in the leakage of urine via the vagina. It may be congenital or the result of disease such as cancer of the cervix.

ureterovesical, (ū-rē-ter-ō-ve-si-kal), pertaining to a ureter and the bladder.

urethra, (ū-rē'-thra), the canal between the bladder and the exterior through which the urine is discharged.

urethral, (ū-rē'-thral), pertaining to the urethra. *U. caruncle*: a prolapse of mucosa from the urethra in the female. *U. dilatation*: instrumental treatment for stricture. *U. stricture*: a narrowing of the urethra which usually follows infection or trauma.

urethritis, (ū-rē-thr ī-tis), inflammation of the urethra.

urethrocele, *(ū-rē-thrō-sēl)*, prolapse of the urethral wall into the vagina, as a result of damage during childbirth. May be accompanied by descent of the bladder neck and bladder, causing stress incontinence.

urethrography, *(ū-rē-throg-ra-fi)*, radiographic examination of the urethra following the instillation of radiopaque contrast medium via a catheter. May be combined with radiographic examination of the bladder (cystourethrography), cystometry and uroflometry. *Micturating* or *voiding u.: see* CYSTOGRAPHY.

urethroplasty, *(ū-rē-thrō-plas-ti)*, plastic repair to the urethra.

urethroscope, *(ū-rē-thrō-skop)*, an instrument for viewing the interior of the urethra.

urethrostomy, *(ū-rē-thros-to-mi)*, an artifical opening into the urethra to overcome a stricture.

urethrotomy, *(ū-rē-throt'-o-mi)*, incision of the urethra to overcome a stricture.

urge incontinence, *see* INCONTINENCE, UNSTABLE BLADDER.

urgency, an immediate need to void urine, such as that which occurs with detrusor muscle instability.

uric acid, *(ū-rik)*, a derivative of purine metabolism, which is a constituent of nucleic acids and some foods and beverages. It is excreted by the kidneys and can form renal calculi. Blood levels may rise when purine intake is high, when excretion is decreased or in the abnormal breakdown of cells, e.g. leukaemia. *See* GOUT.

uridrosis, *(ū-rid-rō-sis)*, excessive amounts of nitrogenous waste such as urea in the perspiration.

urinalysis, *(ū-rin-al-i-sis)*, analysis of urine. Physical, chemical or microbiological examination.

urinary, *(ū-rin-a-ri)*, pertaining to urine. *U. tract*: the kidneys, ureters, bladder and urethra (Figure 82).

urination, *(ū-ri-nā'-shon)*, micturition. The act of discharging urine.

urine, clear straw-yellow to amber fluid secreted by the kidneys. Normal daily volume varies according to age, fluid intake and other conditions, but in adults is around 1.5 litres. The normal constituents are water, electrolytes and nitrogenous waste. The pH is around 6.0 but a range of 4.5–8.0 is possible and the specific gravity is usually in the range 1.005–1.030. In health the pH and specific gravity vary according to homeostatic needs.

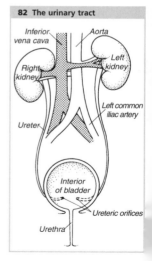

82 The urinary tract

Inferior vena cava
Aorta
Right kidney
Left kidney
Left common iliac artery
Ureter
Interior of bladder
Ureteric orifices
Urethra

urinometer, *(ū-rin-om-ēt-er),* an instrument (hydrometer) used for measuring the specific gravity of urine.

URL, abbreviation for **uniform resource locator**. Used to identify specific web site locations, such as http://www.doh.gov.uk/dhhome.htm.

urobilin, *(ū-rō-bi-lin),* a pigment derived from the oxidation of urobilinogen and excreted in the faeces. Sometimes found in urine left standing in contact with air.

urobilinogen, *(ū-rō-bi-lin'-o-jen),* microbial action in the bowel converts bilirubin to the pigment stercobilinogen. Some of this is excreted in the faeces, but some is reabsorbed into the circulation and passes through the liver and is excreted as urobilinogen by the kidney. Levels in the urine are decreased in obstructive jaundice and increased in liver disease and haemolysis.

urochrome, *(ū-rō-krōm),* pigment colouring urine.

urodynamics, the use of sophisticated equipment to measure bladder function. Particularly useful in diagnosing the cause of urinary incontinence.

uroflometry, *(ū-rō-flō-met-ri),* non-invasive method of assessing urinary flow rates by voiding into a receptacle incorporating a transducer which records rates electronically.

urogenital, *(ū-rō-jen-it-al),* relating to the urinary and genital organs.

urogram, radiographic image of the urinary tract.

urography, *(ū-rog-ra-fi),* also called pyelography, but urography is more correct as it involves more than the kidney. Radiographic examination of the urinary tract; kidney and ureter, following the administration of radiopaque contrast medium by various methods: 1. *antegrade u.:* where contrast is injected into the kidney via a catheter inserted percutaneously. 2. *intravenous u. (IVU):* where contrast is administered intravenously. 3. *retrograde u.:* the contrast is introduced into the renal pelvis via a cystoscope and ureteric catheters.

urokinase, *(ū-rō-ki-nāz),* a thrombolytic enzyme. A plasminogen activator produced by the kidney. Used therapeutically in vitreous haemorrhage, thrombosed arteriovenous shunts and other thromboembolic conditions.

urolith, a stone in the urinary tract.

urolithiasis, *(ū-rō-lith-i-a-sis),* urinary calculi.

urologist, *(ū-rol-o-jist),* a specialist in urology.

urology, *(ū-rol-o-ji),* the study of diseases of the urinary tract in females and the genitourinary tract in males.

urostomy, *(ū-ros-to-mi),* an opening or stoma which drains urine. *See* ILEAL CONDUIT, URETEROSTOMY.

urticaria, *(er-ti-ka-ri-a),* nettlerash; hives. Often due to allergic reaction to certain foods, e.g. shellfish, or drugs such as penicillin. Characterized by wheals, erythema and intense itching.

uterine, *(ū-ter-īn),* pertaining to the uterus. *U. prolapse: see* PROCIDENTIA. *U. tubes:* paired tubes extending laterally from the uterus which open into the peritoneal cavity close to the ovaries. The site of fertilization. Previously called fallopian tubes.

uterography, *(ū-ter-og-ra-fi), see* HYSTEROSALPINGOGRAPHY.

uterosacral, *(ū-ter-ō-sa'-kral),* pertaining to the uterus and sacrum. *U. ligament:* uterine support extending from the cervix backwards to the sacrum.

uterovesical, *(ū-ter-ō-ve-si-kal),* relating to the uterus and the bladder.

uterus, womb. Hollow pear-shaped muscular organ situated in the pelvis. It has three parts: the top or fundus, the body and the cervix. *See* CERVIX. It connects bilaterally with the uterine tubes and opens inferiorly into the vagina (Figure 83). Its three layers are: 1. perimetrium, an outer serous coat. 2. myometrium, a thick layer of interlocking smooth muscle fibres. 3. endometrium, a mucosal lining of highly vascular epithelium containing many glands which is influenced by the cyclical secretion of hormones. *See* MENSTRUAL CYCLE, MENSTRUATION. The uterus receives the fertilized ovum and provides the environment for implantation and fetal development, and expels the fetus through the vagina. When the ovum is not fertilized, the endometrial living is shed, resulting in menstrual flow.

utilitarianism, *(ū-til-i-tair-ē-an-izm)*, ethical theory that supports the view that an action should always produce more benefits than harm. It aims to provide the greatest good for the majority of people. *See* DEONTOLOGY.

utricle, *(ū-trikl)*, fluid-filled membranous sac in the internal ear. Part of the vestibular apparatus, it contains

83 Uterus, left tube and ovary

the receptors for static equilibrium, hair cells and otoliths, which respond to head position relative to gravity and changes in linear speed and direction.

uvea, *(ū-vē-a)*, uveal tract. The middle pigmented coat of the eyeball. The choroid, ciliary body and iris as a whole.

uveitis, *(ū-vi-ī′-tis)*, inflammation of the uvea.

uvula, *(ū′-vū-la)*, a small fleshy body hanging down at the back of the soft palate.

uvulectomy, *(ū-vū-lek′-to-mi)*, excision of uvula.

uvulitis, *(ū-vū-lī′-tis)*, inflammation of the uvula.

V

vaccination, protective inoculation. The use of vaccines to produce artificial active immunity to specific diseases. *See* IMMUNITY, IMMUNIZATION.

vaccine, an extract prepared from: attenuated organisms, e.g. BCG, rubella; bacterial toxins, e.g. tetanus and inactivated virus or bacterial preparations, e.g. typhoid. The antigenicity of the organism is retained but the pathogenicity is reduced. *See* BCG, HIB VACCINE, MMR SABIN, SALK.

vaccinia, a poxvirus causing disease in cattle. It is used to confer immunity against smallpox in people whose work puts them at risk of contact with poxviruses, such as laboratory staff.

vaccum, a space from which the air or gas has been extracted. *V. aspiration*: a method of terminating a pregnancy up to the 14th week. *V. drainage system*: a closed system of suction drainage used for surgical wounds. The amount and type of wound drainage or exudate is visible in the drainage container. *V. extraction (Ventouse)*: a method of delivery where a vacuum is used to fix a cap to the fetal head and exert traction.

vagal, (*vā'-gul*), pertaining to the vagus nerve.

vagina, (*va-jī-na*), the passage leading from the cervix to the vulva. Lined with mucous membrane arranged in folds or rugae which allows considerable distension.

vaginal, (*va-jī-nal*), pertaining to the vagina. *V. hysterectomy*: removal of the uterus via the vagina. *See* HYSTERECTOMY. *V. prolapse*: vaginal wall prolapse. *See* CYSTOCELE, RECTOCELE, URETHROCELE. *V. repair*. *see* COLPORRHAPHY. *V. speculum*: *see* SPECULUM.

vaginismus, (*vaj-in-iz-mus*), involuntary spasm of the muscles around the vagina whenever the vulva is touched, such as during examination or sexual contact. It results in dyspareunia and makes sexual intercourse difficult or impossible.

vaginitis, (*vaj-in-ī-tis*), inflammation of the vagina. *Atrophic v.*: occurs as a result of the oestrogen lack associated with the hormonal changes of the climacteric. Thinning of the vaginal mucosa and loss of acidic secretions make the vagina more prone to infection. Candidiasis is particularly common in older women. *Infective v.*: may be caused by *Trichomonas vaginalis*, *Chlamydia trachomatis*, *Gardnerella vaginalis*, *Neisseria gonorrhoeae* and yeasts, especially *Candida albicans*.

vaginosis, bacterial infection of the vagina. *See* GARDNERELLA VAGINALIS.

vagotomy, (*va-got'-o-mi*), surgical division of the vagus nerve. An operation used to reduce gastric acid secretion in peptic ulceration.

vagus, (*vā-gus*), tenth pair of cranial nerves. They are parasympathetic and innervate the pharynx, larynx, trachea, lungs, heart, oesophagus and abdominal organs which

365

include: stomach, liver, spleen, intestine and kidney. They are sensory or motor depending on the structure supplied.

valence, **1.** in chemistry the combining ability of an element. **2.** in immunology the number of binding sites for either an antibody or an antigen molecule.

valgus, *(val'-gus),* turned outward (bowlegged). *Talipes v.: see* TALIPES.

validity, a term in research which indicates the degree to which a method or test measures what it intends to measure.

valine, *(va-lēn),* an essential (indispensable) amino acid.

Valsalva's manoeuvre, a forced expiration against a closed glottis. it increases pressure in the thorax and abdomen, and reduces venous return to the heart. Occurs naturally when straining to lift, change position or defaecate.

values, an individual and personal view of the worth of an idea or way of behaving.

value systems, an accepted set of values, conduct and way of behaving in a particular social group.

valve, a fold of membrane across a channel allowing flow in one direction, e.g. heart valves, ileocaecal valve. *V. replacement*: operation to replace a heart valve.

valvotomy, incision into a valve, especially heart valve. The purpose of the operation is to widen the orifice of a stenosed valve.

valvular, pertaining to a valve. *V. heart disease*: disease affecting the heart valves which may become stenosed (narrowed) or incompetent (leaky). The mitral and aortic valves are most commonly affected and the tricuspid less often. The pulmonary valve is rarely affected. *See* FALLOT'S TETRALOGY.

valvulitis, *(val-vū-lī'-tis),* inflammation of a valve.

valvulotomy, *(val-vū-lot'-o-mi), see* VALVOTOMY.

vancomycin-resistant enterococci (VRE), enterococci that have developed resistance to the antibiotic vancomycin, such as *Enterococcus faecium.*

van den Bergh's test, a test which measures bilirubin in serum; both the conjugated and unconjugated bilirubin are estimated.

vanillylmandelic acid (VMA), *(van-il-ĕl-man-del-ik),* a metabolite of adrenaline (epinephrine) which is excreted in the urine. Levels of VMA detected in a 24-hour urine collection can be used to assess the function of the adrenal medulla.

vapour, a liquid or solid in its gaseous form, e.g. steam.

variables, in research any factor or circumstance which is part of a research study. *Confounding v.*: a variable that affects the conditions of the independent variables unequally. *Dependent v.*: depends upon the experimental conditions. The factor being studied. *Independent v.*: the variable conditions of an experimental situation, e.g. experimental or control. *Random v.*: background factors, e.g. noise, which may affect any conditions of the independent variable conditions equally.

variance, a mathematical term used in statistics. The distribution range of a set of results around the mean. Standard deviation is the square root of variance.

varicella, *(var-i-sel'-la),* chickenpox.

varicella/zoster immunoglobulin (VZIG), a blood product which when injected, gives immunity to varicella and zoster. Used for neonates exposed to infection and immunocompromised individuals.

varicella-zoster virus (VZV), the herpesviruses that cause chickenpox (varicella) and shingles (herpes zoster).

varices (*sing.* **varix**), dilated twisted veins. *Oesophagogastric v.*: dilated veins at the lower end of the oesophagus and in the proximal stomach. Associated with hepatic portal hypertension they may give rise to massive haematemesis.

varicocele, *(var-i-kō-sēl),* a varix present in the veins of the spermatic cord.

varicose, *(var-i-kōs),* dilated or swollen. *V. veins*: tortuous, dilated veins. Commonly affect the superficial veins of the leg in which the valves have become incompetent. Other examples are the oesophagogastric varices and haemorrhoids.

variola, *(var-i-ō-la), see* SMALLPOX.

varus, *(vā'-rus),* turned inwards (knock-kneed). *Talipes v.: see* TALIPES.

vas, a vessel or duct. *V. deferens*: ductus deferens. Duct continuous with the epididymis of the testis, conveys spermatozoa to the ejaculatory ducts.

vasa vasorum, *(va-zah va-zor-um),* network of tiny blood vessels which supplies blood to the outer layer of larger arteries and veins.

vascular, *(vas-kū-lar),* relating to or possessing many blood vessels. *V. system*: the system of blood vessels.

vascularization, *(vas-kū-lar-ī-zā-shon),* growth of new blood vessels within an organ or structure. Occurs during the healing process.

vasculitis, inflammation of blood vessels.

vasectomy, *(vas-ek-to-mi),* resection and ligation of the vas deferens. Bilateral operation renders the individual sterile and is used as male sterilization.

vasoactive intestinal peptide (VIP), regulatory peptide hormone which inhibits gastric motility.

vasoconstriction, *(vā-zō-kon-strik'-shon),* contraction or narrowing of the lumen of a blood vessel.

vasoconstrictor, *(vā-zō-kon-strik'-tor),* a drug or nerve that causes the narrowing of blood vessels with a decrease in flow and an increase in blood pressure. Also called vasopressor.

vasodilatation, *(vā-zō-di-la-tā'-shon),* dilatation of blood vessels.

vasodilator, *(vā-zō-dī-lā'-tor),* a drug or nerve that causes the widening of blood vessels with an increase in flow and a decrease in blood pressure.

vasomotor, *(vā-zō-mō-tor),* pertaining to the nerves and muscles concerned with vessel lumen size. *V. centre*: part of the cardiovascular centre, situated in the medulla oblongata, which controls the lumen size of peripheral arterioles. It operates through sympathetic activity in response to signals from baroreceptors. The size of vessels controls peripheral resistance which is a factor contributing to arterial blood pressure.

vasopressin, *(vā-zō-pres-in), see* ANTIDIURETIC HORMONE. A synthetic preparation, desmopressin, is available, which is used in the treatment of diabetes insipidus.

vasospasm, *(vā'-zō-spazm),* spasm of the blood vessels.

vasovagal attack, *(vā-zō-vā-gul),* syncope due to bradycardia and peripheral vasodilatation due to vagal activity. Causes include: fluid loss, prolonged standing, unpleasant or frightening experiences and pain.

Vater's ampulla, duodenal papilla. The point where the bile and pancreatic ducts enter the duodenum.

VDRL (Venereal Disease Research Laboratory) test, a serological test for syphilis.

VDU, in computing the abbreviation for **visual display unit**. The computer monitor screen.

vector, 1. a carrier. Animal that conveys an organism from one host to another, e.g. mosquito, tick. **2.** a quantity which has both direction and magnitude.

vegan, a vegetarian who excludes all animal products from his or her diet. Nutritional deficiencies can occur without careful selection of food, with particular attention to obtaining the essential amino acids, minerals and vitamins, such as vitamin B_{12}.

vegetal pole (vegetative), situated at the opposite end of the ovum to the animal pole, it is relatively inactive.

vegetarian, an individual whose diet is selected from foods derived from plants and vegetables. However, some people choose to include eggs, milk and milk products in their diet. See LACTOVEGETARIAN, LACTO-OVOVEGETARIAN, VEGAN.

vegetations, concretions of organic debris on diseased heart valves in infective endocarditis.

vegetative, 1. pertaining to growth. **2.** a resting stage, not active. **3.** functions occurring involuntarily. **4.** in psychiatry a state of lethargy and passivity.

vehicle, a substance in which a drug is administered.

vein, vessel carrying blood to the heart (Figure 84). The lining coat of veins in the limbs is modified to form valves that allow flow in one direction and prevent pooling of blood in the limbs.

vellus, soft, fine fluffy hair that forms the body hair of children and women. Also appears on the scalp when the hair thins. See LANUGO.

84 Structure of a vein

Tunica intima
Tunica media
Tunica adventitia
Lumen

vena cava, (vē-na kā-va), superior and inferior, the two large veins which empty venous blood into the right atrium.

venepuncture, (vē-ne-punk'-tūr), inserting a needle into a vein to withdraw blood or introduce fluids or drugs.

venereal, (ven-eer-ē-al), pertaining to sexual intercourse. *V. diseases (VD)*: in Britain these are still defined legally as syphilis, gonorrhoea and chancroid, but they are now classified and included in a larger and more comprehensive group of sexually transmitted infections. See SEXUALLY TRANSMITTED INFECTIONS.

venereology, (ven-eer-ē-ol'-o-ji), the study of venereal disease.

venesection, (ve-ne-sek-shon), phlebotomy. Opening a vein to drain off a quantity of blood via a wide-bore needle. Used to collect blood for transfusion and as a treatment in polycythaemia.

venogram, (ven-ō-gram), an X-ray of veins.

venography, (ve-nog'-ra-fi), radiographic examination of veins following the administration of radiopaque contrast medium.

venom, poisonous substance produced by snakes, insects and other animals.

venotomy, (ven-ot-o-mi), incision of a vein. See VENESECTION.

venous, (vē-nus), pertaining to veins. *V. pressure*: pressure within the veins. *See* CENTRAL VENOUS PRESSURE. *V. sinuses*: channels which carry venous blood, such as those in the brain or heart. *V. thrombosis*: thrombus formation in a vein. *See* DEEP VEIN THROMBOSIS. *V. ulcer*: also called gravitational ulcer. An indolent ulcer with a venous aetiology. They are usually near the ankle or between the ankle or knee. The surrounding skin is often pigmented (brown-staining) and there may be varicose (gravitational stasis) eczema and contact dermatitis; ulcers tend to be large and shallow with copious amounts of exudate. Patients often have a history of varicose veins and deep vein thrombosis, and complain of local tenderness and aching legs. *See* DERMATITIS, ECZEMA.

ventilation, 1. supply of fresh air. 2. the mechanical process of breathing. *See* ALVEOLAR VENTILATION RATE, PULMONARY VENTILATION. *V. perfusion imaging*: used to detect pulmonary emboli. It involves imaging of the lungs following the inhalation of a radioactive gas and an intravenous injection of radioactive albumen. *V. perfusion ratio (V/Q)*: the ratio between the gases in the alveoli (alveolar ventilation) and blood flow in the pulmonary capillaries (pulmonary perfusion). The ratio is subject to homeostatic controls that ensure that gas exchange is efficient. Healthy subjects may have a small mismatch between ventilation and perfusion in some parts of the lung, but the V/Q is 1.

ventilator, respirator. Device which maintains the flow of gases in and out of the lungs, used in assisted ventilation. *See* INTERMITTENT POSITIVE PRESSURE VENTILATION.

ventral, relating to the abdomen or front (anterior) surface. *V. nerve root*: anterior or motor nerve root.

ventricles, (ven-tri-kls), 1. the two thick-walled lower chambers of the heart which pump blood into the circulation. 2. four cavities within the brain containing cerebrospinal fluid.

ventricular, (ven-trik-ū-la), relating to a ventricle. *V. arrhythmias*: abnormalities of cardiac rhythm which arise in the ventricle. They include: *V. ectopics*: ventricular contractions occurring without atrial activity. *V. fibrillation*: commonest cause of sudden death. There is an uncoordinated rhythm in the ventricles which is ineffective in pumping blood around the body. *See* CARDIAC ARREST, FIBRILLATION. *V. tachycardia*: rapid ventricular rate of between 140 and 200 beats/min, a serious arrhythmia which may progress to fibrillation or 'pulseless' ventricular tachycardia. *V. septal defect (VSD)*: a congenital heart defect where there is a communication between the right and the left ventricles.

ventriculoatrial shunt, (ven-trik-ū-lō-a-tri-al), a surgical procedure where excess cerebrospinal fluid from a cerebral ventricle is diverted to the right atrium via a plastic shunt. Used in the treatment of hydrocephalus.

ventriculography, (ven-trik-ū-log-ra-fi), 1. a radiographic examination of the heart ventricles following the instillation of radiopaque contrast medium or a technique using radionuclide imaging. 2. rarely performed radiographic examination of the ventricular system of the brain. *See* ENCEPHALOGRAPHY.

ventriculoperitoneal shunt, (ven-trik-ū-lō-peri-tō-nē-al), a surgical procedure where excess cerebrospinal fluid from a cerebral ventricle is diverted to the peritoneal cavity via a plastic shunt. Used in the treatment of hydrocephalus.

ventrosuspension, *(ven-trō-sus-pen-shon),* operation to correct uterine retroversion.

Venturi effect, a principle of gas behaviour utilized in certain medical equipment for the mixing and delivery of gases, such as Venturi oxygen masks.

Venturi mask, an oxygen therapy mask designed to mix atmospheric air to a given flow of oxygen which allows the administration of different concentrations of oxygen, e.g. 24% or 28%.

venule, *(ve'-nūl),* small vein.

verbigeration, *(ver-bij-er-a-shon),* repetition of words and phrases which are meaningless.

vermiform, *(ver'-mi-form),* wormlike. *V. appendix: see* APPENDIX VERMIFORMIS.

verminous, infested with animal parasites.

vermis, 1. a worm. **2.** worm-like structure which connects the hemispheres of the cerebellum.

vernix caseosa, *(ver'-niks kā-sē-ō'-sah),* fatty sebaceous substance which covers and protects the fetal skin. Its production commences around the 30th week of gestation.

verruca, *(ver-ū'-ka),* a wart. *See* CONDYLOMA.

version, alteration of fetal presentation in the uterus to facilitate delivery. It may be achieved internally or externally. *Bipolar v.:* the version is performed by acting on both fetal poles. *See* CEPHALIC VERSION, PODALIC VERSION, SPONTANEOUS VERSION.

vertebra, one of the 33/34 bones forming the spinal column. There are 24 individual bones and 9 or 10 fused bones. *See* SPINAL COLUMN.

vertebral, relating to the vertebra. *V. arteries:* two arteries which form the basilar artery which is part of the circle of Willis at the base of the brain. *V. column: see* SPINAL COLUMN.

vertex, the crown of the head. *V. presentation:* presentation of the vertex of the fetus.

vertical transmission, disease passing from mother to fetus, via the placenta, at delivery or through breast milk, e.g. HIV.

vertigo, giddiness; a sensation of whirling and rotation.

vesical, *(ves-i-kal),* relating to the bladder.

vesicant, *(ves-i-kant),* a blistering agent.

vesicle, *(ves-i-kl),* **1.** a small blister containing serum. **2.** a small fluid-filled bladder, e.g. seminal vesicles.

vesicoenteric, *(ves-i-kō-en-ter-ik),* vesicointestinal, relating to the bladder and intestine. *See* FISTULA.

vesicoureteric, *(ves-i-kō-ū-rē-ter-ik),* relating to the bladder and the ureter. *V. reflux:* back flow of urine into the ureter. A cause of pyelonephritis.

vesicovaginal, *(ves-i-kō-va-jī-nal),* relating to the bladder and the vagina. *See* FISTULA.

vesicular, *(ves-ik-ū-la),* pertaining to or having vesicles. *V. breathing:* sounds heard on auscultation in normal quiet respiration. *V. mole: see* HYDATIDIFORM MOLE.

vesiculitis, *(ves-ik-ū-lī-tis),* inflammation of seminal vesicles.

vesiculopapular, *(ves-ik-ū-lō-pap-ū-la),* a rash with both vesicles and papules.

vesiculopustular, *(ves-ik-ū-lō-pus-tū-la),* a rash with both vesicles and pustules.

vessel, a tube or channel which conveys body fluids, e.g. blood or lymph.

vestibular, *(ves-tib-ū-la),* relating to a vestibule. *V. apparatus:* structures in the internal ear concerned with balance and position: semicircular canals, and the saccule and utricle in the vestibule. *V. glands*: four mucus-secreting glands which open into the vestibule of the female genitalia. Two greater v. glands, *see* BARTHOLIN'S GLANDS, and two lesser v. glands, *see* SKENE'S GLANDS. *V. nerve*: the vestibular branch of the vestibulocochlear (VIIIth cranial) nerve. Damage may cause tinnitus, vertigo, dizziness and nausea.

vestibule, (*ves-ti-būl*), **1.** area bounded by the labia minora. **2.** part of the bony labyrinth of the internal ear, situated between the semicircular canals and the cochlea. **3.** part of the mouth between the lips and gums/teeth.

vestibulocochlear, (*ves-tib-ū-lō-kok-lē-a*), relating to the vestibule and the cochlea of the ear. *V. nerve*. the eighth pair of cranial nerves. Also known as the auditory nerve.

vestigial, (*ves-tij'-i-al*), rudimentary. Bearing a trace of something now vanished or degenerate.

VGA, in computing the abbreviation for **video graphics array**. A type of screen display which supports high-resolution (but less so than SVGA) colour images.

viable, capable of living or surviving independently. Usually applied to a fetus of 24 weeks' gestation or more.

Vibrio, (*vib-ri-ō*), a genus of curved comma-shaped Gram-negative bacteria. *V. cholerae* is the causative organism of cholera.

vicarious liability, the liability of an employer for the wrongful acts of an employee committed whilst in the course of employment.

vicarious, (*vi-kār-i-us*), when one organ performs the work of another.

villi (*sing.* **villus**), (*vil-lī*), minute finger-like processes that project from some cells. *Intestinal v.*: in the small bowel, each contains a central lacteal surrounded by a plexus of capillar-

ies. They greatly increase the surface area available for absorption (Figure 85). *See* CHORIONIC VILLI.

vinca alkaloids, cytotoxic drugs extracted from the periwinkle plant, e.g. vincristine.

Vincent's angina, *see* ANGINA (VINCENT'S ANGINA), STOMATITIS.

viraemia, (*vī-rē-mi-a*), viruses present in the blood stream.

viral, relating to or caused by viruses, such as v. hepatitis. *See* HEPATITIS. *V. haemorrhagic fevers*: occurring mainly in the tropics; they may be transmitted by mosquitoes and ticks. Examples include: Ebola, Lassa fever, Marburg disease and yellow fever.

virilization, (*vir-il-ī-zā-shon*), the development of masculine characteristics in the female.

virology, (*vī-rol-o-ji*), the study of viruses and the diseases caused by them.

virulence, (*vir-ū-lens*), the pathogenicity of a microorganism (its ability to produce disease). It depends upon several factors, e.g. the level of host resistance and the strain of organism involved.

virulent, (*vir-ū-lent*), violent. *V. disease*: one causing severe and serious illness.

virus, 1. any of a diverse group of microorganisms which are only visible using an electron microscope. They contain either DNA or RNA and can only replicate within the host cell. Viruses infect animals, plants and other microorganisms. *See* BACTERIOPHAGE. Diseases caused by viruses in humans include: colds, rubella, influenza, measles, rabies, hepatitis, poliomyelitis and AIDS. There is increasing evidence to support the view that some viruses are carcinogenic. *See* EPSTEIN–BARR VIRUS,

85 A villus (intestinal)

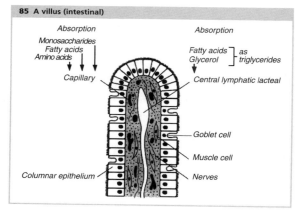

Absorption

Monosaccharides
Fatty acids
Amino acids

Capillary

Absorption

Fatty acids
Glycerol } as triglycerides

Central lymphatic lacteal

Goblet cell

Muscle cell

Columnar epithelium

Nerves

HUMAN PAPILLOMAVIRUS, HUMAN T-CELL LYMPHOTROPHIC VIRUSES. **2.** in computing a program which is generally installed maliciously and without the user's knowledge. Such programs copy automatically (replicating like viruses in living cells) and usually disrupt or destroy data, but some have no ill effects.

viscera *(sing.* **viscus***), (vis-er-ah),* the internal organs of the body cavities, especially those in the abdomen.

visceral, *(vis-er-al),* pertaining to viscera (organs).

viscid, viscous, *(vis'-kid, vis'-kus),* sticky, thick, adhesive.

viscosity, *(vis-kos-i-ti),* quality of being sticky and adhesive. As the viscosity of a liquid increases it flows with more difficulty.

vision, the faculty of seeing. *Binocular vision*: using both eyes without seeing two images. *Double v.: see* DIPLOP-IA. May be due to a defect in the eye,

the muscles of the eye or to nervous system disease. *See* STEREOSCOPIC VISION.

visual, pertaining to vision. *V. acuity*: sharpness of vision, ability to see the difference between two points of light. *See* ACUITY, SNELLEN'S TEST TYPES. *V. fields*: the area in which objects can be seen while looking straight ahead. *V. purple: see* RHODOPSIN.

vital, pertaining to life. *V. capacity (VC)*: maximum volume expired after greatest respiratory effort. *See* ACUITY. *V. signs*: signs indicating life; temperature, pulse and respiration. Blood pressure is also usually included. *V. statistics*: statistical information relating to populations; births, marriages, deaths and morbidity.

vitallium, *(vi-ta'-li-um),* an alloy used in bone surgery for nails, screws, plates, etc.

vitamins, a group of organic substances required in small amounts by the body. They are vital for many metabolic processes in which they often function as coenzymes. Most are obtained from the diet but some are synthesized by the body, e.g. vitamin D. They include: **1.** fat-soluble group – vitamins A, D, E and K. **2.** water-soluble group – vitamin C and the vitamin B complex which consists of thiamine, niacin, riboflavin, pyridoxine, biotin, folates, cobalamins and pantothenic acid. *See* APPENDIX 8: NUTRITION.

vitiligo, *(vit-il-i-go),* leucoderma. Patchy areas of depigmentation occurring in the skin.

vitreous, *(vit-rē-us),* glass-like. *V. chamber of the eye*: posterior cavity of the eyeball behind the lens. *V. humor*: clear gel filling the v. chamber where it contributes to intra-ocular pressure. A closed system formed during embryonic development, it lasts for life.

vocal, relating to the voice or its production. *V. cords*: vocal folds. Two membranous folds running antero-posteriorly in the larynx. Sound is produced as expired air is forced through the larynx to vibrate the v. cords. Pitch or frequency of the voice changes with the length (tension) of the v. cords.

void, to empty, such as passing urine from the bladder during micturition.

volatile, 1. having violent, changeable or explosive characteristics. **2.** a liquid which evaporates quickly.

volition, act or power of willing. Conscious exercise of will.

Volkmann's ischaemic contracture, *see* CONTRACTURE, SUPRACONDYLAR FRACTURE.

volt (V), a derived SI unit used to measure electrical potential, potential difference or electromotive force.

volume, the space taken up by a substance, e.g. a fluid, or an object. *See*

PACKED CELL VOLUME, STROKE VOLUME, TIDAL VOLUME.

voluntary, free. Regulated by will and choice. *V. muscle*: striated skeletal muscle under voluntary control. *V. organization*: one that is run and controlled by volunteers, e.g. Samaritans, MIND. Many have charitable status, some have grants from local and central government, and some employ professionals and other paid staff to assist in their activities.

volvulus, *(vol-vū-lus),* twisting of a loop of small bowel or sigmoid colon with its mesentery. Causes gangrene and intestinal obstruction (Figure 86).

vomer, *(vō'-mer),* a bone of the septum of the nose.

vomit, 1. ejection of the stomach contents through the mouth. **2.** the material ejected from the stomach. Types include: bile-stained, faeculant and 'coffee ground' in appearance due to partially digested blood.

vomiting, the disagreeable experience that occurs when stomach contents are reflexly expelled through the

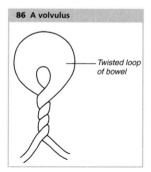

86 A volvulus

Twisted loop of bowel

373

mouth. It is often accompanied by feelings of nausea. It may be effortless, associated with abdominal pain, or projectile, such as with pyloric stenosis. A person who is vomiting generally needs: privacy and support, a suitable receptacle and a denture container if appropriate, facilities for teeth cleaning, a mouthwash and a wash and bedding/clothing change as appropriate. Postoperatively, people should be encouraged to support wounds with their hands. The vomit and type of vomiting, e.g. projectile, should be observed and accurate records of fluid balance kept. Apart from these simple measures, nurses should ensure that the most appropriate antiemetic drugs, e.g. metoclopramide, are administered as prescribed. Antiemetics should always be given in anticipation of expected vomiting, such as with cancer chemotherapy with cytotoxic drugs. *V. of pregnancy*: occurs commonly during the first trimester. Excessive or prolonged vomiting is abnormal and may lead to dehydration, electrolyte imbalance and ketosis. *See* HYPEREMESIS GRAVIDARUM.

von Gierke's disease, *(von-ger-kes)*, a glycogen storage disease. An inherited condition where the enzyme glucose-6-phosphatase (G6P) nor-

mally found in the liver and kidney is absent.

von Kupffer's cells, *see* KUPFFER'S CELLS.

von Recklinghausen's disease, 1. neurofibromatosis. An inherited condition characterized by multiple tumours of cranial and peripheral nerves with areas of skin pigmentation. **2.** of bone. *See* OSTEITIS FIBROSA.

von Willebrand's disease, a condition where there is excessive bleeding from injuries, bruising and mucous membrane bleeding. It is inherited as an autosomal dominant deficiency of factor VIII which affects either sex. *Cf.* HAEMOPHILIA.

voyeurism, *(voy-er-izm)*, a psychosexual disorder where the individual derives sexual gratification from watching the sexual behaviour of others.

VRE, abbreviation for **vancomycin-resistant enterococci.**

vulva, the external genitalia in the female.

vulvectomy, *(vul-vek'-to-mi)*, excision of vulva.

vulvitis, *(vul-vi'-tis)*, inflammation of the vulva.

vulvovaginal, *(vul-vō-va-ji-nal)*, pertaining to the vulva and the vagina.

vulvovaginitis, *(vul-vō-vaj-in-i-tis)*, inflammation of both the vulva and the vagina.

Waldenström's disease, macroglobulinaemia. A condition characterized by the presence of high molecular weight immunoglobulins in the plasma.

Waldeyer's ring, *(vul-dā´-yers)*, a ring of lymphoid tissue around the pharynx formed by the lingual, palatine and pharyngeal tonsils.

walking aids, sticks, crutches, tripods and various metal frames that allow people to regain or retain independence for walking.

Wallace's rule of nine, a chart for calculating the percentage of body surface area affected by a burn in adults (Figure 87). *See* LUND AND BROWDER'S CHART.

Wallerian degeneration, *(va-lār-i-an)*, degeneration of a nerve after it has been isolated from its nerve cell body.

WAN, in computing an acronym for wide area network. A multiple site network where local area networks (LANs) are linked by various methods to LANs in other locations to share files and resources.

wart, small horny tumour of the skin induced by viruses, may also affect mucous membranes. *See* CONDYLOMA, HUMAN PAPILLOMAVIRUS.

wasting, loss of weight and or muscle mass. Emaciation.

Wasserman reaction (WR), *(vas-er-man)*, obsolete complement fixation test for syphilis. *See* SYPHILIS.

water (H₂O), colourless fluid compound. Its molecules contain two

87 Wallace's rule of nine (adult)

9% (head)

18% front and back 18% of trunk

9% (arm)

9% (arm)

1% (perineum)

18% (leg)

18% (leg)

atoms of hydrogen and one of oxygen. The body consists of 50–70% water depending upon age and build. *W. bed*: water-filled mattress used in the prophylaxis of pressure ulcer.

water-hammer pulse, *see* CORRIGAN'S PULSE.

Waterhouse–Friderichsen syndrome, *(fri-de-rik'-sen),* syndrome resulting from bilateral adrenal haemorrhage accompanying the purpura of acute septicaemia, usually meningococcal.

Waterlow scale, a scale devised by Waterlow in the 1980s and used to identify those patients at risk of pressure ulcer development. It is more comprehensive than earlier scales and includes six main criteria: build/weight for height, continence, skin type/visual risk areas, mobility, age/sex and appetite, and a number of special risks: tissue malnutrition, neurological deficit, major surgery/trauma and medication.

Waterston's operation, palliative surgical procedure for Fallot's tetralogy, where the right pulmonary artery is anastomosed to the aorta.

watt (W), a derived SI unit used to measure electrical power.

wavelength, the distance between two adjacent crests of any wave motion.

weal, wheal, a white or pinkish elevation on the skin, as in urticaria.

weaning, describes the process that involves the gradual addition of solid food to the milk-only diet of babies. It should not start before the baby is 4 months old, but should start before 6 months, because it is not possible to provide the full nutritional needs after this age, and it becomes more difficult to teach the baby to accept and/or chew lumpy solid foods. The word 'weaning' is also used in the sense of helping to withdraw a person from something on which he or she is dependent, e.g. assisted ventilation.

web site, a collection of one or more pages that can be accessed via the internet or an intranet by using the specific URL. *See* INTERNET, INTRANET.

Weber's test, a tuning fork test which may be helpful in the diagnosis of conductive hearing loss. Especially useful when only one ear is affected.

wedge pressure, *see* PULMONARY ARTERY WEDGE PRESSURE, SWAN–GANZ CATHETER.

Weil's disease, *(vīlz),* serious disease caused by bacteria of the genus *Leptospira*, e.g. *L. icterohaemorrhagiae,* carried by rats and other animal hosts. Causes fever, jaundice, purpura, haemorrhage and renal failure. *See* LEPTOSPIRA.

Weil–Felix reaction, *(vīl-fē-liks),* a non-specific agglutination reaction for rickettsial disease, such as typhus.

Welch's bacillus, *Clostridium perfringens,* a spore-forming organism found in gas gangrene.

well baby clinic, mothers are encouraged to bring their new babies during the early years for monitoring by health visitors. General advice and information, and immunization are available.

well-man clinic, a primary health initiative where screening checks are undertaken on men who are apparently well, e.g. weight, blood pressure, urine testing, blood tests. It is an opportunity to discuss life-style influences on health and to promote health, e.g. diet, exercise, smoking, alcohol safe limits and testicular self-examination.

well-woman clinic, a primary health initiative where screening checks are undertaken on women who are apparently well, e.g. weight, blood pressure, urine testing, blood tests, cervical smear and breast awareness education. It is an opportunity to discuss life-style influences on health and to promote health, e.g.

diet, smoking, alcohol use and exercise.

wen, *see* SEBACEOUS CYST.

Wenckebach phenomenon, a type of second-degree heart block where the PR interval becomes progressively longer until a beat is dropped.

Wernicke's encephalopathy, a syndrome occurring in association with the polyneuritis of long-term alcohol misuse. It is characterized by vertigo, nystagmus, ataxia and stupor. A manifestation of thiamine deficiency. *See* KORSAKOFF'S SYNDROME.

Wertheim's hysterectomy, *(vār'-tīms)*, a radical operation for uterine cancer, whereby the uterus, tubes, ovaries, upper vagina and pelvic fascia and lymph nodes are entirely removed.

West nomogram, used to calculate body surface area in children.

Western blot, method of testing for HIV infection. Usually carried out after two positive results from the less specific ELISA test.

Wharton's jelly, *(wor-tonz)*, gelatinous embryonic connective tissue within the umbilical cord.

wheeze, difficult breathing with a characteristic whistling sound, associated with the bronchospasm of asthma and other conditions.

whiplash injury, injury to the structures of the cervical region following sudden, violent, jerking movements of the head and neck. Seen commonly in road traffic accidents where there is sudden deceleration or acceleration.

Whipple's operation, radical surgery for carcinoma of the head of pancreas. It involves: partial pancreatectomy, excision of the bile duct, duodenum and pylorus, a gastrojejunostomy with the pancreas and gallbladder joined to the jejunum (Figure 88).

88 Whipple's operation

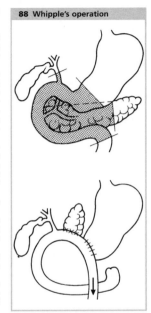

whipworm, *see* TRICHURIS TRICHIURA.

white cell, *see* BLOOD, LEUCOCYTE.

white matter, white nerve tissue of the central nervous system, the myelinated nerve fibres. *See* GREY MATTER.

whiteleg, *see* PHLEGMASIA ALBA DOLENS.

whitlow, *see* PARONYCHIA.

WHO, abbreviation for **World Health Organization**.

whooping cough, pertussis.

Widal reaction, *(vē'-dal)*, an agglutination blood test for typhoid fever.

377

Wilcoxon test, in statistics, a non-parametric alternative to Student's paired *t*-test.

will, voluntary effort. Conscious choice of action.

Wilm's tumour, see NEPHROBLASTOMA.

Wilson's disease, hepatolenticular degeneration. A rare inherited autosomal recessive condition where copper metabolism and excretion are abnormal. Copper accumulates in the liver, eye, basal nuclei, kidneys and bone.

windpipe, the trachea.

wisdom teeth, third molars (four in number). The last teeth to erupt, usually during late teens and early twenties.

withdrawal, the physical or psychological retreat from a frightening or stressful situation. *W. method*: see COITUS INTERRUPTUS. *W. symptoms*: the symptoms occurring when a substance, to which a person has physical dependence, is withheld or is unavailable.

wolffian duct, pair of embryonic ducts which develop to form the genitourinary tract in the male fetus under the influence of androgens secreted by the fetal testes.

Wolff–Parkinson–White (WPW) syndrome, a supraventricular ectopic rhythm caused by the presence of an abnormal portion of atrioventricular conducting fibres. It is characterized by a shortening of the PR interval, a change in the QRS complex, tachycardia and the risk of life-threatening ventricular arrhythmias.

Wood's light, special ultraviolet light used for the detection of fungal infections, e.g. ringworm.

woolsorter's disease, see ANTHRAX.

word blindness, see DYSLEXIA.

word processor, in computing a program which allows text to be entered, edited, corrected and printed prior to storage. Most word processing packages contain facilities for spell checking, cut and paste blocks of text and the production of contents and index pages. Advanced programs support printers which can produce graphics, varied fonts and even full 'desk-top publishing' facilities.

word salad, a jumble of disconnected words characteristic of the speech of psychotic patients, such as those with schizophrenia.

World Health Organization, an agency of the United Nations which is concerned with health promotion, epidemiology, environmental conditions and access to health facilities on a regional and global scale.

worm, invertebrate animal. See ASCARIS, OXYURIS, SCHISTOSOMA, STRONGYLOIDES, TAENIA, TRICHURIS, etc.

wound, a break in the continuity of tissue, it may be due to injury or surgery. Types include: abrased, contused, incised, infected, lacerated, penetrating, puncture and fungating. They may be acute or chronic and are classified as: clean, clean contaminated, contaminated or dirty. *W. dressings*: proprietary materials applied to medical or surgical wounds. Modern dressings aim to be permeable to water vapour and gases but not to bacteria or liquids; this retains serous exudate which is actively bactericidal. They do not adhere to the wound surface and, on removal, do not damage new tissue.

wound healing, normally consists of four overlapping phases: haemostasis, inflammation, proliferative and maturation. See ANGIOGENESIS, EPITHELIALIZATION, FIRST INTENTION, GRANULATION.

wrist, the joint between the hand and the forearm. The carpus.

wryneck, *see* TORTICOLLIS.

wuchereriasis, *(voo-ker-e-rī´-a-sis)*, infestation with filarial worms such as *Wuchereria bancrofti* which causes elephantiasis.

www, abbreviation for **worldwide web**.

X

X chromosome, sex chromosome which is paired in the homogametic sex (female). It carries many major genes. Present in every female gamete and in half the male gametes. *Cf.* Y CHROMOSOME.

X-linked inheritance, the inheritance of traits carried by genes on the X chromosome, e.g. haemophilia is inherited by males in this way.

X-rays, short rays of electromagnetic spectrum. The word is popularly used for radiograph.

xanthelasma, *(zan-the-las'-ma),* a condition in which yellow patches or nodules occur on the skin, especially in the eyelids.

xanthine, *(zan-thīn),* an intermediate metabolite in the degradation of nucleotides to uric acid. Large amounts are excreted in the urine in the inherited condition, xanthinuria, a disorder where renal calculi may develop.

xanthochromia, *(zan-thō-krō-mi-a),* yellow discoloration of the cerebrospinal fluid; may be due to the presence of degraded haemoglobin following a subarachnoid haemorrhage.

xanthoderma, *(zan-thō-der'-ma),* yellowness of the skin.

xanthoma, *(zan-thō'-mah),* see XANTHELASMA.

xanthomatosis, *(zan-thō-mat-ō'-sis),* yellow discoloration of tissues seen in various inherited lipid storage disorders. *See* GAUCHER'S DISEASE, NIEMANN–PICK DISEASE.

xanthopsia, *(zan-thop-sē-ah),* visual disorder where all objects appear to be yellow.

xanthosis, *(zan-thō-sis),* yellow discoloration of the skin associated with a high intake of some foods, e.g. carrots, or malignant disease.

xenograft, *(zen-ō-grahft),* heterograft. Graft with material obtained from a donor of different species.

xenon (Xe), an inert gas.

Xenopsylla, *(zen-op-sil-a),* a genus of fleas. *Xenopsylla cheopis* is the rat flea that transmits typhus and bubonic plague.

xeroderma, *(ze-rō-der'-ma),* dry skin. *X. pigmentosum (Kaposi's disease):* rare inherited condition where an excessive photosensitivity results in skin changes which include tumour formation.

xerophthalmia, *(zer-of-thal-mi-a),* ulceration of the cornea occurring in vitamin A deficiency.

xerosis, *(zer-ō'-sis),* abnormal dryness, e.g. of the conjunctiva or the skin.

xerostomia, *(ze-rō-stō'-mi-a),* dryness of the mouth.

xiphoid process, *(zif'-oyd),* a sword-shaped cartilage attached to the breastbone. Also called the **ensiform cartilage.**

XO, an anomaly where there is only one sex chromosome. *See* TURNER'S SYNDROME.

XX, sex chromosomes of a normal female.

XXX syndrome, multiple X syndrome occurring in females where the cells have an extra X chromosome, bringing the total to 47, or occasionally two extra (XXXX). Affected individuals may have underdeveloped secondary sexual characteristics and may have mild learning disability.

XXY syndrome, *see* KLINEFELTER'S SYNDROME.

XY, sex chromosomes of a normal male.

xylose, *(zī-lōz)*, a pentose sugar. *X. absorption test*: used in the diagnosis of intestinal malabsorption.

XYY syndrome, a condition in males where the cells have an extra Y chromosome, bringing the total to 47, or occasionally two extra (XYYY). Affected individuals tend to be tall with mild learning disability and behavioural problems such as aggression.

Y

Y chromosome, sex chromosome found only in the heterogametic sex (male). It is shorter than the X chromosome and carries fewer major genes.

yaws, framboesia. Tropical granulomatous disease. It resembles syphilis, but is not sexually transmitted. Lesions affect skin and bone caused by the spirochaete *Treponema pertenue.*

yeast, unicellular fungus. Some are pathogenic, e.g. *Candida albicans, Cryptococcus neoformans.*

yellow card reporting system, in the UK, a system by which prescribers report suspected adverse drug reactions to the Committee on Safety of Medicines (CSM), the body responsible for monitoring drug safety and advising on the licensing of new drugs.

yellow fever, viral disease transmitted by mosquitoes. Occurs in the tropics and is characterized by fever, jaundice, anuria and gastrointestinal haemorrhage.

Yersinia, *(yer-sin-i-a),* a genus of Gram-negative bacteria, *Y. pestis* is the causative organism of plague.

yoga, a discipline which utilizes breathing techniques, exercises and postures to relax, reduce stress and generally enhance physical and mental well being.

yolk sac, an embryonic structure which forms from endodermal cells. Important as a site of early blood cell production and as a source of primordial germ cells in humans (Figure 89).

yttrium-90 (⁹⁰Y), *(it-ri-um),* the radioactive isotope of yttrium is used in the treatment of malignant disease.

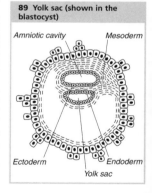

89 Yolk sac (shown in the blastocyst)

Amniotic cavity

Mesoderm

Ectoderm

Endoderm

Yolk sac

Z

Z-plasty, a plastic surgery technique for relieving scar tissue.

Z-track, an intramuscular injection technique used to prevent leakage and staining such as with iron preparations (Figure 90).

Ziehl–Neelsen stain, (*zēl-nēl-sens*), an acid-fast staining technique used in the microscopic identification of *Mycobacterium tuberculosis.*

zinc (Zn), a metallic element required in trace amounts, it is a cofactor in certain enzyme reactions, needed for insulin storage and promotes wound healing. Its salts are used in ointments and as disinfectants and caustic agents.

Zollinger–Ellison syndrome, ectopic source of gastrin production, usually a pancreatic neoplasm. Gastric acid secretion increases in response to the hormone release, resulting in peptic ulceration and inactivation of intestinal enzymes.

zona, 1. literally, a girdle. **2.** may be applied to shingles; Z. facialis. *See* HERPES ZOSTER. *Z. fasiculata, glomerulosa* and *reticularis:* three layers of the adrenal cortex. *Z. pellucida:* membrane around the oöcyte.

zonula ciliaris, (*zon-ū-la sil-i-ar-is*), suspensory ligament of lens of the eye.

zonulolysis, (*zon-ū-lŏ-lī-sis*), use of enzymes to break down the zonula ciliaris, used sometimes prior to intracapsular lens extraction.

zoology, that part of biology which deals with the study of animal life.

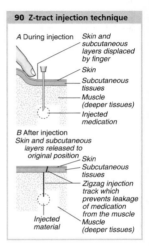

90 Z-tract injection technique

A During injection — Skin and subcutaneous layers displaced by finger
— Skin
— Subcutaneous tissues
— Muscle (deeper tissues)
— Injected medication

B After injection
Skin and subcutaneous layers released to original position
— Skin
— Subcutaneous tissues
— Zigzag injection track which prevents leakage of medication from the muscle
— Injected material
— Muscle (deeper tissues)

zoonosis, (*zō-o-nō-sis*), a disease transmitted from animals to humans, e.g. rabies, anthrax, psittacosis.

zoophilia, (*zō-o-fil-i-a*), abnormal liking for animals. Including a psychosexual disorder in which the individual derives sexual gratification from fantasy involving animals, sexual or other close contact with animals.

zoophobia, (*zō-o-fŏ-bi-a*), excessive and irrational fear of animals.

zoster, shingles. *See* HERPES.

zwitterion, *(tsvit-er-i-on)*, a dipolar ion having both positive and negative regions, such as an amino acid in a neutral solution.

zygoma, *(zig-ō-ma)*, the cheekbone.

zygote, *(zī-gōt)*, the fertilized ovum. The diploid cell produced by the fusion of the female (ovum) and male (spermatozoon) nuclei. *Z. intrafallopian transfer (ZIFT)*: an assisted conception technique where mature oocytes are retrieved, mixed with sperm and after fertilization the resultant zygote is placed in the the ulterine (fallopian) tube.

zymogen, *(zī-mō-jen)*, a proenzyme. An inactive proteolytic enzyme, e.g. clotting factors and proteolytic enzymes produced by the stomach and pancreas. *Z. (chief) cells*: gastric cells which secrete the proteolytic enzyme precursor pepsinogen.

Appendix 1
Code of professional conduct for the nurse, midwife and health visitor

Each registered nurse, midwife and health visitor shall act, at all times, in such a manner as to: safeguard and promote the interests of individual patients and clients; serve the interests of society; justify public trust and confidence; and uphold and enhance the good standing and reputation of the professions.

As a registered nurse, midwife or health visitor, you are personally accountable for your practice and, in the exercise of your professional accountability, must:

1. act always in such a manner as to promote and safeguard the interests and well-being of patients and clients;
2. ensure that no action or omission on your part, or within your sphere of responsibility, is detrimental to the interests, condition or safety of patients or clients;
3. maintain and improve your professional knowledge and competence;
4. acknowledge any limitations in your knowledge and competence and decline any duties or responsibilities unless able to perform them in a safe and skilled manner;
5. work in an open and co-operative manner with patients, clients and their families, foster their independence and recognise and respect their involvement in the planning and delivery of care;
6. work in a collaborative and co-operative manner with health care professionals and others involved in providing care, and recognise and respect their particular contributions within the care team;
7. recognise and respect the uniqueness and dignity of each patient and client, and respond to their need for care, irrespective of their ethnic origin, religious beliefs, personal attributes, the nature of their health problems or any other factor;
8. report to an appropriate person or authority, at the earliest possible time, any conscientious objection which may be relevant to your professional practice;

9. avoid any abuse of your privileged relationship with patients and clients and of the privileged access allowed to their person, property, residence or work-place;

10. protect all confidential information concerning patients and clients obtained in the course of professional practice and make disclosures only with consent, where required by the order of a court or where you can justify disclosure in the wider public interest;

11. report to an appropriate person or authority, having regard to the physical, psychological and social effects on patients and clients, any circumstances in the environment of care which could jeopardise standards of practice;

12. report to an appropriate person or authority any circumstances in which safe and appropriate care for patients and clients cannot be provided;

13. report to an appropriate person or authority where it appears that the health or safety of colleagues is at risk, as such circumstances may compromise standards of practice and care;

14. assist professional colleagues, in the context of your own knowledge, experience and sphere of responsibility, to develop their professional competence, and assist others in the care team, including informal carers, to contribute safely and to a degree appropriate to their roles;

15. refuse any gift, favour or hospitality from patients or clients currently in your care which might be interpreted as seeking to exert influence to obtain preferential consideration and

16. ensure that your registration status is not used in the promotion of commercial products or services, declare any financial or other interests in relevant organisations providing such goods or services and ensure that your professional judgement is not influenced by any commercial considerations.

N.B.: the Code of Professional Conduct is currently (2001) being reviewed and a new version which includes key points from other documents (*Guidelines for Professional Practice* and *The Scope of Professional Practice*) is being prepared.

Appendix 2
Prefixes and suffixes

Prefixes

A

a/an- without, not
ab- away from
abdo- abdominal
acro- extremity
ad- towards
adeno- glandular
adip- fat
aer- air
ambi- both
amyl- starch
ana- up
andro- male
angio- blood vessel
aniso- unequal
ante/antero- before, in front
anti- against
apo- away, from
arthro- joint
auto- self

B

bi/bis- two
bili- bile
bio- life
blast- germ, bud
blenno- mucus
bleph- eyelid

brachi- arm
brachy- short
brady- slow
broncho- bronchi
bucc- cheek

C

calc- chalk
carcino- cancer
cardio- heart
carpo- wrist
cata- down
cent- hundred
cephal- head
cerebro- brain
cervic- cervix/neck
cheil/cheilo- lip
cheir- hand
chemo- chemical
chol/chole- bile
cholecysto- gallbladder
choledocho- bile ducts
chondro- cartilage
chrom- colour
cine- motion
circum- around
co/col/con- together, with
coli- bowel
colpo- vagina
contra- against

cost- rib
cox- hip
crani- skull
cryo- cold
crypt- hidden
cyan- blue
cysto- bladder
cyto- cell

D

dacry- tear
dactyl- finger
de- away
deci- tenth
demi- half
dent- tooth
derma- skin
dextro- right
di/diplo- twos, double
dia- through
dis- separation, against
dors- back
dys- difficult, painful

E

ec- out from
ecto- outside
electro- electrical
em- in
en/end/endo- in, into, within

ent- within
entero- intestine
epi- above, on, upon
erythr- red
eu- well, normal
ex/exo- away from, out of
extra- outside

F

faci- face
ferri/ferro- iron
feto- fetus
fibro- fibrous, fibre
flav/flavo- yellow
fore- before, in front of

G

galacto- milk
gastr/gastro- stomach
genito- genitals
ger- old age
gloss/glosso- tongue
glyco- sugar
gnatho- jaw
gynae- female

H

haem/haemo/haemato- blood
hemi- half
hepat/hepato- liver
hetero- different
hexa- six
hist- tissue
homeo- like

homo- same
hydro- water
hygro- moisture
hyper- above
hypno- sleep
hypo- below
hyster/hystero- uterus

I

iatro- physician
idio- peculiar to an individual, self
ileo- ileum
ilio- ilium
im/in- not, in, within
immuno- immunity
infra- below
inter- between
intra- within
intro- inwards
ischio- ischium
iso- same, equal

K

karyo- nucleus
kerato- keratin, horn, cornea
kin- movement, motion
kypho- rounded

L

lacri- tears
lact- milk
laparo- abdomen, flank
laryngo- larynx

later- side
lepto- soft, thin
leuco/leuko- white
lip/lipo- fat
litho- stones
lympho- lymphatics

M

macro- large
macul- spot
mal- bad
mamm/mast- breast
medi/meso- middle
mega/megalo- large
melano- black
meta- after, between
metro- uterus
micro- small
milli- thousand
mio- smaller
mono- single, one
morph/morpho- shape
muco- mucus
multi- many
myc- fungal
myel- marrow, spinal cord
myo- muscle

N

nacro- stupor
naso- nose
necr- dead
neo- new
nephr/nephro- kidney
neuro- nerves, nervous system
noct/nyct- night

normo- normal
nucleo- nucleus
null/nulli- none

O

oculo- eye
odonto- tooth
oligo- diminished
onc/onco- mass, tumour
onycho- nail
oö- egg
oöphor- ovary
ophthalmo- eye
opisth- backwards
orchido- testis
oro- mouth
orth- normal, straight
os- mouth, bone
oss/osteo- bone
oto- ear
ovari- ovary
ovi- egg, ovum
oxy- oxygen

P

pachy- thick
paed- child
pan- all
para- beside, near
part- birth
path- disease
pent- five
peps- digest
per- through
peri- around
perineo- perineum

phag- ingest, swallow
pharmac- drug
pharyngo- pharynx
phil/philo/phillic- affinity for
phlebo- vein
phono- voice, sound
photo- light
phren- diaphragm, mind
physi- nature, form
pilo- hair
plas- form, grow
pleur/pleuro- pleura
pneumo- air, lung
podo- foot
poly- many
post- after
pre/pro- in front, before
proct- anus, rectum
proto- first
pseudo- false
psycho- mind
pulmon- lung
pyelo- renal pelvis
pyloro- pylorus
pyo- pus
pyr- fever, fire

Q

quadri- four
quint- five

R

radio- radiation
re- back, again

ren- kidney
retro- backward
rhin- nose
rub- red

S

sacchar- sugar
sacro- sacrum
salpingo- uterine tube (fallopian)
sapro- decaying, dead
sarco- flesh
sclero- hard
semi- half
sept- seven
sero- serum
socio- sociology
somat- body
somni- sleep
sphygm- pulse
splen/spleno- spleen
spondyl/spondylo- vertebra
steato- fat
steno- narrow
sterno- sternum
sub- below
supra/super- above
sym/syn- together, union, with

T

tachy- fast
tars/tarso- foot, eyelid
teno- tendon
tetra- four

thermo- heat
thorac/thoraco- chest
throm/thrombo- clot
thyro- thyroid
tox- poison
trache/tracheo- trachea
trans- across, through
tri- three
trich- hair
troph- growth, nourishment

U

ultra- beyond, extreme
uni- one
uretero- ureter
urethr/urethro- urethra
uri/uro- urine
uter/utero- uterus

V

vas/vaso- vessel, duct
vene- vein
vesico- bladder
viscer- organs

X

xanth- yellow
xero- dry

Z

zoo- animal

Suffixes

A

-able capable of
-aemia blood
-aesthesia sensation
-algia pain
-asis/esis state of
-ase enzyme

B

-blast germ, bud

C

-caval pertaining to the vena cava
-cele swelling
-centesis to puncture
-cide killing
-cle/cule small
-cyte cell

D

-derm skin
-desis bind or fix together
-dynia pain

E

-ectasis dilation
-ectomy removal
-emesis vomiting

F

-facient making
-ferent carry

-form having the form of
-fuge expelling

G

-genesis/genetic formation, origin
-genic capable of causing
-gogue increasing flow
-gram a tracing or drawing
-graph instrument for recording

I

-ia/iasis state of, condition
-iatric(s)/iatry healing, medical specialty
-ician person skilled in a particular field
-ism condition, state
-itis inflammation

K

-kin/kinesis/kinetic movement, motion

L

-lith stones
-lithiasis presence of stones

-logy science or
study of
-lysis breakdown

M

-malacia softening
-megaly enlargement
-meter measure
-morph shape

O

-ogen precursor
-oid likeness
-ology science or
study of
-oma tumour
-opia eye
-opsy looking
-ose sugar
-osis condition
-ostomy/stomy
opening
-otomy/tomy incision
-ous like

P

-pathy disease
-penia lack of

-pexy fixation
-phage ingest,
swallow
-phagia swallowing
-phasia speech
-phil/philia affinity for
-phobe/phobia fear of
-phylaxis protection
-plas form, grow
-plasty reconstruct
-plegia paralysis
-pnoea breathing
-poiesis making

R

-rhythmia rhythm
-rrhage/rrhagia to
burst, pour,
excessive flow
-rrhaphy to repair
-rrhoea flow,
discharge

S

-saccharide
carbohydrate
-scope instrument for
examining

-scopy to examine,
looking
-soma/somatic body
-somy pertaining to
chromosomes
-sonic sound
-stasis lack of
movement, stand
still

T

-taxia/taxis/taxy
order,
arrangement
-tome instrument for
cutting
-trophy growth,
nourishment
-trophic changing,
influencing

U

-uria urine

Appendix 3
Chemical symbols and formulae commonly encountered in nursing

Aluminium	Al	Lithium	Li
Ammonia	NH_3	Magnesium	Mg
Ammonium	NH_4	Manganese	Mn
Barium	Ba	Mercury	Hg
Calcium	Ca	Molybdenum	Mo
Carbon	C	Nitrogen	N
Caesium	Cs	Nitrate	NO_3
Carbon dioxide	CO_2	Oxygen	O
Chlorine	Cl	Phosphate	PO_4
Chromium	Cr	Phosphorus	P
Cobalt	Co	Potassium	K
Copper	Cu	Radium	Ra
Fluorine	F	Selenium	Se
Gold	Au	Silicon	Si
Helium	He	Silver	Ag
Hydrogen	H	Sodium	Na
Hydrogen carbonate		Strontium	Sr
(bicarbonate)	HCO_3	Sulphate	SO_4
Hydrogen phosphate	HPO_4	Sulphur	S
Hydroxide	OH	Technetium	Tc
Iodine	I	Vanadium	V
Iridium	Ir	Water	H_2O
Iron	Fe	Yttrium	Y
Lead	Pb	Zinc	Zn

Appendix 4
Units of measurement

International System of Units (SI)

The International System of Units or *Système International d'Unités* is the measurement system used for scientific, technical and medical purposes in most countries. SI units have replaced those of the Imperial System, e.g. the kilogram is the unit of mass rather than the pound in the United Kingdom.

The International System has seven base units and several derived units. Units of measurement have their own symbols and can be expressed as a decimal multiple or submultiple of the base unit by using the appropriate prefix, e.g. a milligram is one thousandth of a gram.

Rules for Using SI Units and Writing Decimals and Large Numbers

- Only the singular form of the unit symbol is used, plurals are not in use:

    10 kg not 10 kgs

- Large numbers are written in three-digit groups (working from right to left) with spaces, but not commas (which are used as a decimal point in some countries):

    twenty thousand is written as   20 000

    two hundred thousand is written as   200 000

- Numbers with four digits are written without the space, e.g.

    five thousand is written as   5000

- Decimals should always have a zero (0) before the decimal point, which is written as a full stop positioned near the line, e.g. 0.75 or 0.005. Decimals with more than four digits are also written in three-digit groups with spaces, but this time working from left to right, e.g. 0.000 25.

- 'Squared' and 'cubed' are expressed as numerical powers and not by abbreviation: square centimetre is cm^2, not sq.cm.

Base Units and Symbols

Measurement	Base Unit and Symbol
Length	metre (m)
Mass	kilogram (kg)
Temperature	kelvin (K)
Time	second (s)
Amount of substance	mole (mol)
Electric current	ampere (A)
Luminous intensity	candela (cd)

Derived units for measuring different quantities are reached by multiplying or dividing two or more base units.

Derived Units (Some Commonly Encountered Examples)

Measurement	SI-Derived Unit and Symbol
Frequency	hertz (Hz)
Power	watt (W)
Electrical potential ⎫	
Potential difference ⎬	volt (v)
Electromotive force ⎭	
Force	newton (N)
Pressure	pascal (Pa)
Energy/quantity of heat/work	joule (J)
Absorbed dose of radiation	gray (Gy)
Radioactivity (radionuclide)	becquerel (Bq)
Dose equivalent	sievert (Sv)

Factors, Prefixes and Symbols for Decimal Multiples and Submultiples of SI Units

Factor	Prefix	Symbol	Factor	Prefix	Symbol
10^{12}	tera	T	10^{-2}	centi	c
10^{9}	giga	G	10^{-3}	milli	m
10^{6}	mega	M	10^{-6}	micro	μ
10^{3}	kilo	k	10^{-9}	nano	n
10^{2}	hecto	h	10^{-12}	pico	p
10^{1}	deca	da	10^{-15}	femto	f
10^{-1}	deci	d	10^{-18}	atto	a

Units Requiring Further Explanation

Temperature – although the SI base unit for temperature is the kelvin (K), by international convention temperature is measured in degrees Celsius (°C).

Volume – volume is calculated by multiplying length, width and depth. Using the SI unit for length we end up with a cubic metre (m³), which is huge volume. For clinical purposes the litre (l or L) is used. A litre is based on the volume of a cube which measures 10 cm × 10 cm × 10 cm. Smaller units, e.g. millilitre (ml) or one thousandth part of a litre are commonly used in clinical practice.

Time – the SI base unit for time is the second, but it is perfectly acceptable to use minute (min), hour (h) or day (d). In clinical practice it is usual to use 'per 24 hours' for the excretion of substances in urine and faeces.

Energy – the energy composition of food or energy requirements is measured in kilojoules (kJ); the SI base unit for energy is the joule (J). However, in practice many people still use an old non-SI unit in the kilocalorie (kcal) for these purposes.

Pressure – the SI unit for pressure is the pascal (Pa), and the kilopascal (kPa) should replace the old non-SI unit of millimetres of mercury pressure (mmHg) for blood pressure and blood gases, but mmHg is still widely used for blood pressure. Other pressure measurement anomalies include: central venous pressure (CVP) which is measured in centimetres of water pressure (cm/H_2O) and cerebrospinal fluid (CSF) pressure which is still measured in millimetres of water pressure (mm/H_2O).

Amount of Substance – the mole (mol) is the SI base unit for amount of substance. The concentration of many substances is expressed in moles per litre (mol/l) or millimoles per litre (mmol/l) which replaces milliequivalents per litre (mEq/l). Exceptions to this include: plasma proteins which are measured in grams per litre (g/l), haemoglobin measured in grams per decilitre (g/dl) and enzyme activity in International Units (IU, U or i.u.).

Measurements, Equivalents and Conversions (SI or metric and imperial)

Weight or mass

1 kilogram (kg)	=	1000 grams (g)
1 gram (g)	=	1000 milligrams (mg)
1 milligram (mg)	=	1000 micrograms (µg)
1 microgram (µg)	=	1000 nanograms (ng)

N.B. To avoid any confusion with milligram (mg) the word microgram should be written in full on prescriptions.

Conversions

1 kilogram (kg)	=	2.204 pounds (lb)
1 gram (g)	=	0.0353 ounce (oz)
453.59 grams (g)	=	1 pound (lb)
28.34 grams (g)	=	1 ounce (oz)

Volume

1 litre (l)	=	1000 millilitres (ml)
1 millilitre (ml)	=	1000 microlitres (µl)

N.B. The millilitre (ml) and the cubic centimetre (cm^3) are usually treated as identical.

Conversions

1 litre (l)	=	1.76 pints (pt)
568.25 millilitres (ml)	=	1 pint (pt)
28.4 millilitres (ml)	=	1 fluid ounce (fl oz)

Length

1 kilometre (km)	=	1000 metres (m)
1 metre (m)	=	100 centimetres (cm) or 1000 millimetres (mm)
1 centimetre (cm)	=	10 millimetres (mm)
1 millimetre (mm)	=	1000 micrometres (µm)
1 micrometre (µm)	=	1000 nanometres (nm)

Conversions

1 metre (m)	=	39.370 inches (in)
1 centimetre (cm)	=	0.3937 inches (in)
30.48 centimetres (cm) =		1 foot (ft)
2.54 centimetres (cm) =		1 inch (in)

Appendix 5
Normal values

Commonly performed investigations: blood, urine and cerebrospinal fluid (CSF)

The figures given below represent an 'average' range of reference values, in adults, for blood, urine and CSF. However, individual laboratories set local reference value ranges and readers should consult their own laboratory for those used locally. This is especially important in the case of enzyme assays where reference values depend upon the analytical equipment and temperatures used.

M = male   F = female

Blood Tests

Haematological values	SI units	Other units
Activated partial thromboplastin time	30–40 s	
Bleeding time (Ivy method)	up to 8 min	
Erythrocyte sedimentation rate (ESR)	less than 20 mm in 1 h (depending on age)	
Folate (serum)	2.2–18 μg/l	
Haemoglobin	M 130–180 g/l	M 13–18 g/dl
	F 115–165 g/l	F 11.5–16.5 g/dl

By convention haemoglobin concentration is expressed in g/dl instead of g/l.

Mean cell haemoglobin (MCH)	27–32 pg	
Mean cell haemoglobin concentration (MCHC)	30–35 g/dl	30–35%
Mean cell volume (MCV)	78–95 fl	
Packed cell volume (PCV or haematocrit)	M 0.4–0.54	M 40–54%
	F 0.35–0.47	F 35–47%
Platelets (thrombocytes)	150–400 × 10^9/l	

Blood Tests (*cont.*)

Haematological values	SI units	Other units
Prothrombin time	12–15 s	
Red cells (erythrocytes)	M 4.5–6.5 × 10^{12}/l F 3.8–5.8 × 10^{12}/l	
Reticulocytes (newly formed red cells)	10–100 × 10^9/l	0.2–2%
Total white cells (leucocytes)	4.0–11.0 × 10^9/l	
Differential count (white cells)		
Neutrophils	2.5–7.5 × 10^9/l	40–75%
Lymphocytes	1.0–3.5 × 10^9/l	20–45%
Monocytes	0.2–0.8 × 10^9/l	2–10%
Eosinophils	0.04–0.4 × 10^9/l	1–6%
Basophils	0.01–0.1 × 10^9/l	0–1%

Biochemistry	SI units	Other units
Alanine aminotransferase (ALT)		10–40 U/l
Alkaline phosphatase		40–125 U/l
Amylase		50–300 U/l
Ascorbic acid (serum)	23–57 µmol/l	
Aspartate aminotransferase (AST)		10–35 U/l
Bicarbonate	22–28 mmol/l	
Bilirubin (total)	2–17 µmol/l	
Caeruloplasmin	150–600 mg/l	
Calcium (total)	2.1–2.6 mmol/l	
Chloride	95–105 mmol/l	
Cholesterol	< 5.2 mmol/l (ideally)	
P_{CO_2} (arterial)	4.4–6.1 kPa	
Copper	13–24 µmol/l	
Creatine kinase (total) (CK)		M 30–200 U/l F 30–150 U/l
Creatinine	53–150 µmol/l	

Blood Tests (*cont.*)

Biochemistry	SI units	Other units
γ-Glutamyl transferase (γ-GT)		M 10–55 U/l F 5–35 U/l
Glucose (fasting)	3.9–5.8 mmol/l	
Glycosylated haemoglobin (HbA$_1$)	4.5–7.5%	
Hydrogen ion concentration [H$^+$]	36–44 nmol/l	
NB: pH 7.4 is equivalent to 40 nmol		
Iron	M 14–32 μmol/l F 10–28 μmol/l	
Iron-binding capacity total (TIBC)	45–72 μmol/l	
Lactate dehydrogenase (LD/LDH)		100–300 Ul
Lead	< 1.7 μmol/l (adult)	
Magnesium	0.7–1.0 mmol/l	
Osmolality	285–295 mmol/kg	
Po_2 (arterial)	12–15 kPa	
pH (arterial)		7.35–7.45
Phosphate (fasting)	0.8–1.46 mmol/l	
Plasma proteins (total)	60–80 g/l	
Albumin	35–47 g/l	
Globulins	24–37 g/l	
Fibrinogen	1.5–4.0 g/l	
Potassium	3.3–5.0 mmol/l	
Sodium	135–145 mmol/l	
Triglyceride (fasting)	0.6–1.7 mmol/l	
Urates	M 0.12–0.42 mmol/l F 0.12–0.36 mmol/l	
Urea	2.5–6.5 mmol/l	
Vitamin B$_{12}$ (as cyanocobalamin)	160–1600 ng/l	
Zinc	11–22 μmol/l	

N.B. The SI unit for enzyme activity is the *katal* but this is not widely used. Instead the International Unit (IU, U or i.u.) is generally used in clinical situations.

N.B. The amount of proteins and other complex molecules are usually expressed in g/l.

Urine

	SI units	Other units
Calcium	< 12 mmol/24 h (on normal diet)	
Copper	0.2–0.8 µmol/24 h	
Creatinine	9–17 mmol/24 h	
5-Hydroxyindole-3 acetic acid (5HIAA)	10–45 µmol/24 h	
Osmolality (random)	50–1400 mmol/kgH$_2$O	
Oxalates	M 80–480 mmol/24 h	
	F 40–320 mmol/24 h	
Phosphates	15–50 mmol/24 h	
Porphyrins (total)	90–370 nmol/24 h	
Potassium	25–100 mmol/24 h	
Protein	< 0.3 g/l	
Sodium	100–200 mmol/24 h	
Urates	1.2–3.0 mmol/24 h	

Cerebrospinal fluid (CSF)

	SI units	Other units
Cells		0–5/mm^3
Chloride	120–170 mmol/l	
Glucose	2.5–4.0 mmol/l	
Protein (total)	100–400 mg/l	

Appendix 6
Observing and testing urine

The routine observation and testing of urine for abnormalities is important for the early identification of potential problems, the diagnosis of disease and in monitoring existing diseases. Normally urine consists of:

- 96% water
- 4% solids (salts, nitrogenous waste, organic acids, hormones and drug metabolites)

The volume of urine passed and its colour, clarity and odour are important and all should be noted using a freshly voided specimen prior to measuring specific gravity, pH and testing with one of the commercially produced reagent strips/sticks which may include tests for specific gravity and pH.

Volume

During 24 h the normal output of urine is between 1 l and 1.5 l in an adult. The actual amount will depend upon factors which include: fluid intake, diet, activity, climate and health.

An increase in volume is known as *polyuria* and causes include:
- overhydration
- inability to form concentrated urine such as in chronic renal disease
- lack of ADH in diabetes insipidus
- presence of glucose in the urine in diabetes mellitus

A decrease in volume is known as *oliguria* and causes include:
- dehydration
- reduced renal function in shock
- acute renal failure, e.g. after an incompatible blood transfusion

Colour

Normal urine is straw-yellow to amber in colour due to the presence of urochrome, a substance derived from the breakdown of haemoglobin.

a. *Pale colour.* Is usually dilute and contains fewer solids than normal and has a low specific gravity. Causes include:
   - excess fluid intake
   - cold weather where sweating is decreased and most water is excreted via the urine
   - diabetes insipidus
   - chronic renal disease
   - diabetes mellitus (here the specific gravity is high because the urine contains glucose)

b. *Dark colour.* Is usually concentrated with more solids than normal and has a high specific gravity. Causes include:
   - reduced fluid intake
   - pyrexia such as with an acute infection
   - dehydration due to fluid loss from excess sweating, vomiting or diarrhoea

c. *Other colours.*
   - blood in the urine may be bright red or smoky depending on the amount and site of bleeding
   - dyes in certain foods may colour the urine, e.g. beetroot (red beet) colours urine red
   - certain drugs, e.g. rifampicin (anti-tuberculosis) colours urine (and other body secretions) red-orange
   - bile pigments in the urine cause brown-green frothy urine
   - dark red urine (after standing) occurs in porphyria

Clarity – Deposits

Urine is normally clear with possibly a slight turbidity due to the presence of mucus. Various abnormal constituents may affect clarity and those which can be detected by naked-eye examination include:
   - blood may give the urine a smoky appearance
   - mucus appears white and flocculent
   - pus is thick yellow, greenish-yellow or white and makes the urine cloudy

Odour

Freshly voided urine has a faint aromatic odour, but if left to stand the bacterial conversion of urea produces the odour of ammonia. Other odours include:

- 'fishy' odour in the presence of infection
- certain foods, e.g. asparagus, produce a characteristic odour
- the presence of abnormal substances in the urine can affect odour

1. high levels of glucose can produce a sweet-smelling urine in diabetes mellitus. **2.** the presence of ketones, such as in diabetic ketoacidosis, can produce a characteristic odour variously described as being like nail polish remover or newly cut hay. **3.** in maple syrup disease the urine smells of maple syrup due to presence of amino acids.

Specific Gravity (SG)

Specific gravity of urine is normally within the range 1.005–1.030 (distilled water has a SG of 1.000) and depends upon the amount of soluble solid material, e.g. salts, urea and any abnormal constituents. Specific gravity is measured using a urinometer or with a suitable reagent strip.

Generally the specific gravity becomes lower as the volume of urine increases, except in uncontrolled diabetes mellitus where a large volume of high-specific-gravity urine is produced due to the presence of glucose. Pale dilute urine has a low specific gravity and dark concentrated urine has a high specific gravity.

pH

Normally the pH of urine is around 6.0 (slightly acidic), but the kidneys are able to vary the pH within the range 4.5–8.0 depending upon homeostatic needs.

Acid urine may be produced:
- where the diet contains large quantities of protein and whole wheat foods (acid-ash diet)

Alkaline urine may be produced:
- where a vegetarian diet is consumed (alkaline-ash diet)
- with excessive or prolonged vomiting
- with bacterial infection of the urinary tract
- with intake of alkalis

Testing Urine

To obtain accurate results try to test a fresh specimen collected in a clean container.

1. Note the:
   - volume
   - colour
   - clarity and presence of any deposits
   - odour
2. Measure specific gravity if using a urinometer.
3. Measure pH if using separate pH papers. Litmus paper can be used if it is sufficient to have an indication of acidity or alkalinity without a precise pH.
4. Most testing for constituents (normal and abnormal) is now performed using commercially prepared reagent strips/sticks or tablets. It is vital that any instructions regarding use, including health and safety aspects, storage and shelf-life, provided by the manufacturers are followed where these products are in use. Various products are available to measure specific gravity and pH, and detect the presence of substances which include:
   - bilirubin
   - blood
   - sugar (glucose)
   - ketones
   - leucocytes
   - nitrites
   - phenylketone (phenylpyruvic acid)
   - protein (albumin)
   - urobilinogen

Possible significance of some abnormal constituents in urine

Protein
   - infection
   - renal disease
   - febrile illness
   - cardiac failure
   - contamination from vaginal discharges may give inaccurate results

Blood
   - cystitis
   - renal disease
   - trauma
   - renal calculi

- urinary tumours
- certain drugs, e.g. anticoagulants
- coagulation disorders
- contamination from menstrual flow may give inaccurate results

Sugar
- diabetes mellitus
- low renal threshold (renal glycosuria)
- associated with increased glomerular filtration rate (GFR) during pregnancy
- alimentary glycosuria (lag storage)

Ketones
- diabetes mellitus
- starvation
- excessive or prolonged vomiting
- high fat/low carbohydrate diet

Bilirubin
- biliary obstruction
- hepatocellular disease

Urobilinogen (normally present)
- absent in biliary obstruction
- excessive amounts present in:
  haemolytic diseases
  hepatic disease

Nitrites
- infection

Appendix 7
Blood glucose monitoring
(self-monitoring of diabetes mellitus)

Regular blood glucose monitoring (BGM) is part of the day-to-day management of diabetes. It is useful in helping patients to meet targets for glycosylated haemoglobin (HbA₁); (Burden, 2001). Major trials have shown that keeping HbA₁ below 7.5% for type 1 diabetes and below 7% for type 2 diabetes reduces the risk of long-term vascular complications: microvascular, affecting the eye, nerves and kidneys, and macrovascular problems that lead to strokes, myocardial infarction and peripheral vascular disease (Diabetes Control and Complications Trial Research Group, 1993; United Kingdom Prospective Diabetes Study Group, 1998).

BGM is undertaken both by the individual and his or her family and by healthcare professionals. There are also many other situations where rapid blood glucose estimation may be required, e.g. in primary care, accident and emergency departments, intensive care units and special care baby units.

The amount of glucose in capillary blood can be measured using test strips (a variety of simple-to-use test strips are available) which are either read by eye or, more usually, by use of a colorimetric meter. Current meters of increasing sophistication are able to store previous results, alert the user to abnormal levels and record events that are significant to the management of diabetes, e.g. insulin doses. Future trends include the development of non-invasive devices capable of measuring capillary blood glucose through the skin, without the need to prick the skin to obtain a drop of blood.

The following points are important if optimal results are to be obtained:

– users need adequate training and regular updates;
– storage of test strips must be according to manufacturer's advice;
– test strips and meters are used according to manufacturer's advice;

- meters are maintained and checked at recommended time intervals;
- quality control procedures are undertaken, where patients buy the quality control solutions to check their devices; however, the Medical Devices Agency advises that all such devices are subject to independent quality control by the pathology laboratory.

References

Burden M (2001) Diabetes: blood glucose monitoring. *Nursing Times* 97 (8): 37–39.

Diabetes Control and Complications Trial Research Group (1993) The effect of intensive treatment of diabetes on the development and progression of long-term complication in insulin dependent diabetes. *New England Journal of Medicine* 329: 977–985.

United Kingdom Prospective Diabetes Study Group (1998) Intensive blood glucose control with sulphonylureas or insulin compared with conventional treatment and risk of complications in patients with type 2 diabetes. *Lancet* 352: 837–853.

Appendix 8
Nutrition

For information regarding specific dietary regimens and further nutritional data it is necessary to consult professionals in the field of nutrition such as dietitians and specialist publications (*see* Further Reading).

The basic nutrients and other substances necessary for the production of energy, for growth, the replacement of tissues and the maintenance of health are:

Carbohydrates (starches and sugars)
Proteins
Fats
Vitamins
Minerals/electrolytes
Non-starch polysaccharide (NSP) or dietary fibre
Water

The first three nutrients are energy-yielding. The energy value of food is measured in the SI unit kilojoules (kJ).

N.B. 4.186 kJ (4.2 approx) = 1 kcal or Calorie. Energy requirements vary greatly according to gender, size, activity and health status, e.g. a raised body temperature increases the energy requirement.

Carbohydrates (1 g carbohydrate yields 17 kJ or 4 kcal)
They contain carbon, hydrogen and oxygen. They may be monosaccharides (glucose, fructose and galactose); disaccharides (maltose, lactose and sucrose) which are sugars; or polysaccharides such as starch or glycogen. During digestion available carbohydrates are broken down to simple monosaccharide molecules which are used in the body for energy. Some are stored as glycogen in the liver and skeletal muscles, but any excess is converted to fat.

Carbohydrates are obtained from sugar, pulses, potatoes and other vegetables, fruit, cereals such as wheat, rice and maize etc. plus products made from flour, e.g. bread, pasta and chapatis.

NSP or dietary fibre is that part of the polysaccharide molecule which is not digested in the human gut.

Proteins (1 g protein yields 17 kJ or 4 kcal)

Proteins contain carbon, hydrogen, oxygen, nitrogen and sometimes sulphur and phosphorus. They are broken down during digestion to provide the amino acids required by the body for protein synthesis, growth and repair and under certain conditions for energy. In adults eight amino acids are indispensable or essential; during childhood, histidine is essential and arginine is also considered to be essential because it is only synthesized in small amounts; the remainder can be synthesized by the body.

Currently the reference nutrient intake for protein in adults is between 45.0 and 55.5 g/day depending upon gender and age. This requirement increases during growth, pregnancy, lactation and illness.

Protein may be obtained from both animal and vegetable sources, e.g. meat, milk, cheese, fish, eggs, nuts, legumes and cereals. It is however vital that those who rely on vegetable sources obtain a balanced intake as some cereals are deficient in lysine and legumes in methionine.

Fats (1 g fat yields 37 kJ or 9 kcal)

Fats are a mixture of glycerol and fatty acids which are long hydrocarbon chains (containing carbon, hydrogen and oxygen).

Fatty acids may be:
- Saturated: when all the chemical bonds are single.
- Monounsaturated: when there is one double bond.
- Polyunsaturated: when there are two or more double bonds.

Saturated fatty acids are usually solid at room temperature whereas polyunsaturated fatty acids (PUFAs) are liquid. There are two essential fatty acids (EFAs): linoleic and alpha-linolenic. Arachidonic acid, which is synthesized from linoleic acid, becomes essential when linoleic acid is in short supply.

Fats are emulsified by bile salts in the small bowel and broken down by lipases (enzymes) into glycerol and fatty acids. These fatty acids are used in the body: as a stored energy source in the form of triglycerides (triacylglycerols), to form substances such as prostaglandins and phospholipids and as a source of the fat-soluble vitamins A, D and E and cholesterol. When fat is oxidized it yields twice as much energy produced by the same weight of protein or carbohydrate; this makes it valuable when energy requirements are high, but in the sedentary individual an excessive intake leads to obesity.

Fat is obtained from: dairy products such as milk, cream, butter and cheese; in and around meat; in nuts, pulses and seeds which produce oils, e.g. sunflower; and in oily fish such as herring and salmon.

Alcohol (1 g alcohol yields 29 kJ or 7 kcal)

Alcohol is not a nutrient but its consumption can substantially increase the total energy taken in by the body, e.g. 100 ml of bitter has 30 kcal and 100 ml red wine contains 68 kcal.

Non-starch polysaccharide (NSP) or dietary fibre

NSP is the indigestible plant material which consists of cellulose and certain other polysaccharides which are vital components of the diet. It adds bulk to the faeces, reduces bowel transit times, ensures slow constant absorption of nutrients such as glucose and gives a feeling of fullness without excessive energy intake. The recommendations suggest a daily intake of 12–24 g/day in adults with an average of 18 g/day. Good sources of NSP include: wholegrain cereals, legumes, vegetables and fruit. A diet consisting of meat, eggs, cheese, fats and refined carbohydrates provides little or no NSP. Certain substances present in a diet which is high in NSP, e.g. phytic acid, can inhibit the absorption of minerals such as calcium and zinc.

Vitamins

Fat-soluble

Vitamin A

Retinol (the precursor carotene can be converted to retinol)

Physiological action/function: Acts as an antioxidant. Needed for retinal function (as a component of rhodopsin). Healthy epithelial cells.

Sources: Retinol from animal sources and carotene from orange, yellow and dark green vegetables. Milk, eggs, cheese, butter, liver, fish oil, margarine (added in manufacture), dark green vegetables, carrots etc.

Deficiency: Night blindness. Blindness due to keratomalacia. Hyperkeratosis of the skin.

Excess: May occur if excessive supplements are taken. Accumulates in the liver. Retinol has been linked to birth defects and women are advised not to take extra vitamin A or eat liver if they are pregnant or planning to become pregnant.

Vitamin D

D_3 cholecalciferol* D_2 ergocalciferol

*Made in the skin by the action of ultraviolet light on 7-dehydrocholesterol.

Physiological action/function: Control of calcium homeostasis by increasing absorption.

Sources: Made in the skin. Fatty fish and fish oil, margarine (added in manufacture), butter and eggs.

Deficiency: Rickets, osteomalacia and poor muscle tone.

Excess: Causes: hypercalcaemia; calcium deposits in blood vessels and kidney, renal failure if intake is excessive.

Vitamin E

Tocopherols, tocotrienes

Physiological action/function: Acts as an antioxidant, which prevents oxidation in cell membranes, by disarming free radicals.

Sources: Wholegrain cereals, dark green vegetables, nuts and vegetable oils.

Deficiency: Haemolytic anaemia in infants and where malabsorption exists.

Excess: No consistent ill effects seen with high doses.

Vitamin K

Phylloquinone and menaquinone

Physiological action/function: Blood clotting. Required for the formation of coagulation factors and proteins in the liver.

Sources: Made in the bowel by the action of bacteria (gut flora). Present in many vegetables and cereals.

N.B. Requires bile in the bowel for absorption.

Deficiency: Tendency to bleed. May cause intestinal haemorrhage, epistaxis, bruising, haematuria and menorrhagia.

Excess: Naturally occurring forms are generally non-toxic, but synthetic supplements may cause problems in neonates, e.g. liver damage.

Water-soluble

Vitamin C

Ascorbic acid

Physiological action/function: Acts as an antioxidant. Required for healthy connective tissue. Also needed for iron absorption.

Sources: Fruit such as blackcurrants and citrus fruits, vegetables, e.g. potatoes, green vegetables and tomatoes.

N.B. Amounts in fruits and vegetables depends on the time of year. Destroyed by heat and alkalis in cooking.

Deficiency: Scurvy, poor wound healing and hair growth.

Excess: Kidney stones, diarrhoea.

Vitamin B Group

(i) B$_1$ Thiamin

Physiological action/function: Coenzyme required in the formation of acetyl coenzyme A (CoA), energy release from carbohydrates. Metabolism of fats and alcohol.

Sources: Cereals, green vegetables, nuts, milk, liver, lean meat, legumes, eggs.

Deficiency: Beriberi, Wernicke's encephalopathy, Korsakoff's psychosis.

Excess: Headache, tachycardia, weakness and irritability.

(ii) Riboflavin

Physiological action/function: Constituent of flavoproteins needed for the utilization of energy.

Sources: Liver, kidney, meat, eggs, yeast extracts, fortified, cereals, milk*.

Deficiency: Angular stomatitis, glossitis, skin lesions and eye problems.

Excess: None known

* losses occur if exposed to sunlight such as milk left on the doorstep.

(iii) Niacin (nicotinic acid and nicotinamide)

Physiological action/function: A constituent of the important coenzymes, NAD and NADP.

Sources: Wholegrain cereals, meat, fish, pulses, vegetables. Nicotinic acid can be synthesized from the amino acid tryptophan.

Deficiency: Pellagra (diarrhoea, dermatitis and dementia).

Excess: Liver damage, hyperglycaemia, flushing.

(iv) B$_6$ (Pyridoxine, pyridoxal, pyridoxamine)

Physiological action/function: A coenzyme required for amino acid metabolism. Also needed for glycogenolysis.

Sources: Widely distributed in foods, e.g. meat, eggs, fish, wholegrain cereals and some vegetables.

Deficiency: Not fully understood but pregnancy and the oral contraceptive do affect requirements. Causes weakness, depression and tiredness. Convulsions in infants.

Excess: Peripheral sensory neuropathy.

(v) Biotin

Physiological action/function: Needed for gluconeogenesis, lipogenesis and amino acid metabolism.

Sources: Egg yolk, legumes, offal. Can be synthesized by bowel (gut) flora.

Deficiency: Rare. Dermatitis, anorexia, nausea and fatigue. Deficiency may occur in long-term parenteral nutrition, and where large amounts of raw egg white are consumed.

Excess: None known.

(vi) Folate (folic acid)

Physiological action/function: Synthesis of purines and pyrimidines. Coenzyme required for red cell production.

Sources: Offal, green vegetables, pulses, bread and some fruit. Synthesized by bowel flora.

Deficiency: Megaloblastic anaemia, damage to intestinal mucosa and poor growth in children. Neural tube defects, e.g. spina bifida.

Excess: Possible reduction in zinc absorption.

(vii) B_{12} Cobalamins

Physiological action/function: Coenzyme required for red cell production and nerve myelination.

Sources: Liver, cheese, eggs, milk, meat and fish. Not found in plants.

N.B. Requires the gastric intrinsic factor for absorption.

Deficiency: Megaloblastic anaemia. Subacute combined degeneration of the spinal cord.

Excess: None known.

N.B. The metabolism of folate and B_{12} is linked.

(viii) Pantothenic acid

Physiological action/function: Coenzyme required for energy release from fats and carbohydrates.

Sources: Very widespread in cereals, legumes and animals products.

Deficiency: Unlikely, given very widespread sources. Vague fatigue, headache, muscle weakness and anorexia.

Excess: Possibly gastrointestinal disturbances such as diarrhoea.

Minerals/Electrolytes

Calcium (Ca)

Vitamin D controls absorption.

Physiological action/function: A constituent of bones and teeth, required for blood clotting, nerve and muscle activity. Various enzymes also require calcium.

Sources: Drinking water, milk, cheese, green vegetables.

N.B. Absorption may be inhibited by phytic acid present in cereal grains.

Deficiency/depletion: Rickets, osteomalacia (see vitamin D). A factor in the development of osteoporosis. Tetany.

Excess: Formation of renal calculi is linked with high intake.

Fluoride (F)

Physiological action/function: Small amounts present in bones and teeth. Increases resistance to dental caries.

Sources: Added to drinking water in some areas, sea fish and tea.

Deficiency/depletion: In areas where levels in drinking water are low there is an increased incidence of dental caries.

Excess: Mottling of the teeth. Poisoning may cause bone sclerosis.

Iodine (I)

Physiological action/function: Required by the thyroid gland for the production of the hormones T_3 and T_4.

Sources: Seafood, iodized table salt.

N.B. Amount present in vegetables depends upon the soil content.

Deficiency/depletion: Goitre. Hypothyroidism in infants born to iodine-deficient mothers.

Excess: Toxic goitre and hyperthyroidism.

Iron (Fe)

Physiological action/function: A constituent of haemoglobin and the muscle pigment myoglobin. Needed for many enzymes.

Sources: Meat, eggs, offal, wholegrain cereals, pulses, dried fruit.

N.B. Absorption increased by gastric acidity and adequate levels of vitamin C being present. Animal sources are absorbed more effectively.

Deficiency/depletion: Anaemia (normocytic or microcytic).

Excess: Siderosis: iron accumulates in the liver.

Magnesium (Mg)

Physiological action/function: Required for coenzymes necessary for energy utilization. Present in bone.

Sources: Green plants (constituent of chlorophyll), milk.

Deficiency/depletion: Neurological problems such as tremor, confusion, fits and agitation. Cardiac arrhythmias.

Excess: Seen with uraemia. Causes diarrhoea and toxicity.

N.B. Linked with the metabolism of calcium.

Phosphorus (P)

(as phosphates)

Physiological action/function: A constituent of bones and teeth. Present in all cells, it is vital for the utilization of energy from foods. Required for nucleic acids.

Sources: Cheese, eggs, peanuts, yeast extract, present in protein foods.

Deficiency/depletion: Rare, but may occur in premature infants fed on human milk. Also with renal loss of phosphates. Leads to muscle weakness.

Excess: May alter calcium:phosphorous ratio.

Potassium (K)

Physiological action/function: Mainly an intracellular electrolyte, it contributes to osmotic pressure. Muscle and nerve activity. Acid–base balance.

Sources: Vegetables, milk, meat, dried fruit, instant coffee.

Deficiency/depletion: Muscle weakness. Cardiac arrhythmias and cardiac arrest. Reduction in bowel peristalsis. Apathy and confusion.

Excess: Usually occurs with renal failure. Muscle weakness. Cardiac arrhythmias and cardiac arrest.

Sodium and chloride (Na and Cl)

Physiological action/function: Found mainly in the extracellular fluids where they contribute to osmotic pressure. Muscle and nerve activity depends upon sodium. Acid–base balance.

Sources: Salt added to food in preparation, storage, cooking and at the table. Bacon, butter, vegetables, cheese, kippers, some breakfast cereals and many processed foods.

Deficiency/depletion: Cramp.

N.B. Usually associated with water depletion which has other effects.

Excess: May contribute to hypertension. Oedema.

Zinc (Zn)

Physiological action/function: Involved in many enzyme-controlled reactions. Needed for insulin.

Sources: Wholegrain cereals, pulses, meat.

N.B. Absorption may be inhibited by phytic acid present in cereal grains.

Deficiency/depletion: Poor wound healing. Stunted growth. Acute deficiency causes diarrhoea, dermatitis, mental problems, immune system problems and hair loss.

Excess: Nausea, vomiting, anaemia.

In addition the following minerals are also required by the body:
Sulphur (S) – usually obtained from protein
Selenium (Se)
Copper (Cu)
Manganese (Mn)
Cobalt (Co) – utilized only as vitamin B_{12}
Chromium (Cr)
Molybdenum (Mo)

Assessment of nutritional status
Several methods exist for the assessment of nutritional status, including:

1. Biochemical, e.g. serum proteins, excretion of muscle breakdown products, etc. *N.B.* Findings may be of limited value and need very

careful interpretation as factors other than nutrition can influence results.
2. Anthropometric, e.g. body weight, body mass index (BMI), skin fold thickness, etc.
3. Dietary history, food intake analysis, etc.

Some guidelines for healthier eating

- reduction in the amount of energy obtained from fat: total fat intake to be decreased.
- reduction in the amount of saturated fats consumed.
- replacement of saturated fat such as lard with polyunsaturated and monounsaturated varieties, e.g. sunflower and olive oils.
- reduction in sugar (refined carbohydrates) intake.
- increase intake of NSP (unrefined carbohydrates).
- increase intake of fruit and vegetables to at least five portions each day.
- reduce salt intake.
- alcohol intake should be within the safe limits and should provide no more than 4% of the total energy.
- maintenance of a desirable body weight (BMI 20–25).

Further Reading

Bender, D. (1999) *Introduction to Nutrition and Metabolism*, 2nd edn. London: Taylor and Francis.

Department of Health (1991) *Dietary Reference Values for Food Energy and Nutrients for the United Kingdom. Report of the Panel on Dietary Reference Values of the Committee on Medical Aspects of Food Policy. Report on Health and Social Subjects, no. 41.* London: HMSO.

Department of Health (1994) *Nutritional Aspects of Cardiovascular Disease. Report of the Cardiovascular Review Group Committee on Medical Aspects of Food Policy. Report on Health and Social Subjects, no. 46.* London: HMSO.

Holland, B. Welch, A.A. Unwin, I.D. Buss, D.H. Paul, A.A. Southgate, D.A.T. (1991) *McCance and Widdowson's The Composition of Foods*, 5th edn. Cambridge: Royal Society of Chemistry and MAFF.

MAFF (1995) *Manual of Nutrition*, 10th edn. London: HMSO.

Morgan, S.L., Weinsier, R.H. (1998) *Fundamentals of Clinical Nutrition*, 2nd edn. London: Mosby.

National Heart Forum (1997) *At Least Five a Day: Strategies to Increase Vegetable and Fruit Consumption.* London: Stationery Office.

Appendix 9
Useful addresses

Action for Sick Children
300 Kingston Road, London
SW20 8LX.
www.actionforsickchildren.org

**Action on Smoking and Health
(ASH)**
109 Gloucester Place, London
W1H 4EJ.

Age Concern England
1268 London Road, London
SW16 4ER.
www.ace.org.uk

Age Concern Northern Ireland
3 Lower Crescent, Belfast,
BT7 1NR.

Age Concern Scotland
113 Rose Street, Edinburgh
EH2 3DT.

Age Concern Cymru
4th Floor, 1 Cathedral Road,
Cardiff CF1 9SD.

Al-Anon Family Groups
61 Great Dover Street, London
SE1 4YF.

Alateen
61 Great Dover Street, London
SE1 4YF.

Alcohol Concern
Waterbridge House, Loman
Street, London SE1 0EE.

Alcoholics Anonymous
PO Box 1, Stonebow House,
Stonebow, York YO1 2NJ.
www.alcoholics-
anonymous.org.uk

**Alcoholics Anonymous
(Scotland)**
50 Wellington Street, Glasgow
G2 6HJ.

Alzheimer's Disease Society
Gordon House, 10 Greencoat
Place, London SW1P 1PH.
www.alzheimers.org.uk

Arthritis Care
18 Stephenson Way, London
NW1 2HD
www.arthritiscare.org.uk

**Association of Radical
Midwives (ARM)**
62 Greetby Hill, Ormskirk,
Lancashire L39 2DT.

**Association to Aid the Sexual
and Personal Relationships of
People with a Disability (SPOD)**
286 Camden Road, London
N7 0BJ.

BACUP (British Association of Cancer United Patients and their Families and Friends)
3 Bath Place, Rivington Street, London EC2A 3JR.
www.cancerbacup.org.uk

Breast Cancer Care
Kiln House, 210 New King's Road, London SW6 4NZ
www.breastcancercare.org.uk

British Association for Counselling
1 Regent Place, Rugby, Warwickshire CV21 2PJ.

British Epilepsy Association
New Anstey House,
Gate Way Drive,
Leeds LS3 1BE.
www.epilepsy.org.uk

British Heart Foundation
14 Fitzhardinge Street, London W1H 4DH.
www.bhf.org.uk

British Medical Association (BMA)
BMA House, Tavistock Square, London WC1H 9JP.

British Pregnancy Advisory Service (BPAS)
Austy Manor, Wootton Wawen, Solihull, West Midlands B95 6BX.
www.bpas.org

British Red Cross Society (BRCS)
Grosvenor Crescent, London W1X 7EJ.
www.redcross.org.uk

Brook Advisory Centres
Central Office, 165 Grays Inn Road, London WC1X 8UD.

Carers UK
20–25 Glasshouse Yard, London EC1A 4JS.

Childline
Royal Mail Building, Studd Street, London N1 0QW.

Cruse Bereavement Care
126 Sheen Road, Richmond, Surrey TW9 1UR.
www.crusebereavementcare.org.uk

Department of Health
General Enquiries, Richmond House, 79 Whitehall, London SE1 6LW.
www.doh.gov.uk

NHS Management Executive
Quarry House, Quarry Hill, Leeds LS2 7EU.

Diabetes UK
10 Queen Anne Street, London W1M 0BD.
www.diabetes.org.uk

Disabled Living Foundation
380–384 Harrow Road, London W9 2HU.
www.dlf.org.uk

Down's Syndrome Association
155 Mitcham Road, London SW17 9PG.

Eating Disorders Association
Sackville Place, 44 Magdalen Street, Norwich NR3 1JE.

Family Planning Association (FPA)
Margaret Pyke House, 27–35 Mortimer Street, London W1N 7RJ.

Foundation for the Study of Infants Deaths (Cot Death Research and Support)
14 Halkin Street, London SW1X 7DP.

General Medical Council (GMC)
44 Hallam Street, London W1N 6AE.

Gingerbread (Association for One Parent Families)
49 Wellington Street, London WC2E 7BN.

Haemophilia Society
Chesterfield House, 385 Euston Road, London NW1 3AU.
www.haemophilia.org.uk

Headway National Head Injuries Association
7 King Edward Court, King Edward Street, Nottingham NG1 1EW.

Health and Safety Executive
Rose Court, 2 Southwark Bridge, London SE1 9HS
www.hse.gov.uk

Health Development Agency
Trevelyan House, 30 Great Peter Street, London SW1P 2HW.
www.hea.org.uk

Health Visitors' Association
50 Southwark Street, London SE1 1UN.

Help the Aged
16–18 St James's Walk, London EC1R 0BE.

Hospice Information Service
St Christopher's Hospice, 51 Lawrie Park Road, London SE26 6DZ.

Ileostomy and Internal Pouch Support Group
PO Box 23, Mansfield, Notts NG18 4TT.

International Council of Nurses (ICN)
3 Place Jean Marteau, 1201 Geneva, Switzerland.

King's Fund Centre
11–13 Cavendish Square, London, W1M 0AN

Leukaemia Care Society
14 Kingfisher Court, Venny Bridge, Pinhoe, Exeter EX4 8JN.

Macmillan Cancer Relief
89 Albert Embankment, London SE1 7UQ
www.macmillan.org.uk

Marie Curie Cancer Care
28 Belgrave Square, London SW1X 8QG.

MENCAP (Royal Society for Mentally Handicapped Children and Adults)
123 Golden Lane, London
EC1Y 0RT.

MIND (National Association for Mental Illness)
Granta House, 15–19 Broadway, London E15 4BQ.
www.mind.org.uk

Multiple Sclerosis Society
National Centre, 372 Edgeware Road, London NW2 6ND.
www.mssociety.org.uk

National Association for the Welfare of Children in Hospital (NAWCH)
Argyle House, 29–31 Euston Road, London NW1 2SD.

National Asthma Campaign
Providence House, Providence Place, London N1 0NT.
www.asthma.org.uk

National Autistic Society
276 Willesden Lane, London NW2 5RB.

National Childbirth Trust (NCT)
Alexandra House, Oldham Terrace, London W3 6NH.

National Eczema Society
163 Eversholt Street, London NW1 1BU.

National Meningitis Trust
Fern House, Bath Road, Stroud, Gloucestershire GL5 3TJ.

National Mobility Centre
Unit 2A, Atcham Estate, Shrewsbury SY4 4UG.

National Osteoporosis Society
PO Box 10, Radstock, Bath BA3 3YB.

National Society for the Prevention of Cruelty to Children (NSPCC)
42 Curtain Road, London EC2A 3NH.
www.nspcc.org.uk

Nursing and Midwifery Council
(replacing the UK Central Council for Nursing Midwifery and Health Visiting)
23 Portland Place, London W1B 1PZ.
www.ukcc.org.uk

Pregnancy Advisory Service
11–13 Charlotte Street, London W1P 1HD.

Relate (National Marriage Guidance Council)
Herbert Gray College, Little Church Street, Rugby, Warwickshire CV21 3AP.

Royal Association for Disability and Rehabilitation (RADAR)
Unit 12, City Forum, 250 City Road, London EC1V 8AF.

Royal College of Midwives (RCM)
15 Mansfield Street, London W1M 0BE.

Royal College of Nursing and Council of Nurses of the United Kingdom (RCN)
20 Cavendish Square, London W1M 0AB.
www.rcn.org.uk

Royal National Institute for the Blind (RNIB)
224 Great Portland Street, London W1N 6AA.
www.rnib.org.uk

Royal National Institute for the Deaf (RNID)
19–23 Featherstone Street, London EC1Y 8SL
www.rnid.org.uk

Royal Society for the Prevention of Accidents (RoSPA)
Cannon House, Priory Queensway, Birmingham B4 6BS.

Royal Society of Health
RSH House, 38a St George's Drive, London SW1Y 4BH.
www.rfph.org

Royal Society of Medicine
1 Wimpole Street, London W1M 8AE.

St John Ambulance Association and Brigade
1 Grosvenor Crescent, London SW1X 7EF.
www.sja.org.uk

Salvation Army
101 Queen Victoria Street, London EC4P 4EP.

Samaritans
10 The Grove, Slough, Berkshire SL1 1QP.

Spinal Injuries Association
Newpoint House, 76 St James's Lane, London N10 3DF.

Stillbirth and Neonatal Death Society (SANDS)
28 Portland Place, London W1N 4DE.

Stroke Association
123–127 Whitecross Street, London EC1Y 8JJ.
www.stroke.org.uk

Terrence Higgins Trust
52–54 Grays Inn Road, London WC1X 8JU.
www.tht.org.uk

World Health Organization
Avenue Appia, 1211 Geneva 27, Switzerland.
www.who.org